MEDICAL
SECRETS

MEDICAL SECRETS

Third Edition

ANTHONY J. ZOLLO, JR., MD

Assistant Professor
Department of Internal Medicine
Baylor College of Medicine
Houston, Texas
Chief Medical Officer
Lufkin VA Outpatient Clinic
Lufkin, Texas

HANLEY & BELFUS, INC./Philadelphia

Publisher: HANLEY & BELFUS, INC.
                 Medical Publishers
                 210 South 13th Street
                 Philadelphia, PA 19107
                 (215) 546-7293; 800-962-1892
                 FAX (215) 790-9330
                 Web site: http://www.hanleyandbelfus.com

Note to the reader: Although the information in this book has been carefully reviewed for correctness of dosage and indications, neither the authors nor the editor nor the publisher can accept any legal responsibility for any errors or omissions that may be made. Neither the publisher nor the editor makes any warranty, expressed or implied, with respect to the material contained herein. Before prescribing any drug, the reader must review the manufacturer's current product information (package inserts) for accepted indications, absolute dosage recommendations, and other information pertinent to the safe and effective use of the product described.

Library of Congress Cataloging-in-Publication Data

Medical secrets / edited by Anthony J. Zollo, Jr.—3rd ed.
     p. ; cm—(The Secrets Series®)
   Includes bibliographical references and index.
   ISBN 1-56053-476-1 (alk. paper)
     1. Internal medicine—Examinations, questions, etc. I. Zollo, Anthony J., 1954- II.
Series.
   [DNLM: 1. Internal Medicine—Examination Questions. WB 18.2 M4885 2001]
RC58.M43 2001
616'.0076—dc 21

                                                          2001024686

MEDICAL SECRETS, 3rd edition   ISBN 1-56053-476-1

Last digit is the print number: 9   8   7   6   5   4   3   2   1

CONTENTS

DEDICATION

To my wife, Mary, without whose help and support
this book, and many other things, would not be possible.

CONTRIBUTORS

Hamid Afsharkharaghan, M.D.
Clinical Fellow, Department of Cardiology, Ochsner Clinic, New Orleans, Louisiana

Amelita Lourdes P. Basa, M.D.
Clinical Instructor, Department of Endocrinology, Baylor College of Medicine; Veterans Affairs Medical Center, Houston, Texas

Rhonda A. Cole, M.D.
Assistant Professor, Department of Medicine–Gastroenterology, Baylor College of Medicine; Chief, GI Endoscopy, Houston VAMC, Houston, Texas

Charlene M. Dewey, M.D., F.A.C.P.
Assistant Professor of Medicine, Department of Medicine, Baylor College of Medicine; Assistant Director, General Internal Medicine Clinic, Ben Taub General Hospital, Houston, Texas

Mary Anne Doherty, M.D.
Late Associate Clinical Professor, Section of Oncology, Department of Internal Medicine, Boston University School of Medicine, Boston; Associate Chief of Staff for Ambulatory Care, Edith Nourse Rogers Memorial Veterans Hospital, Bedford, Massachusetts

Jane M. Geraci, M.D., M.P.H.
Assistant Professor of Medicine, Department of General Internal Medicine, Ambulatory Treatment and Emergency Care, The University of Texas MD Anderson Cancer Center, Houston, Texas

Sheila Goodnight-White, M.D.
Associate Professor and Vice-Chair, Undergraduate Education, Department of Medicine, Baylor College of Medicine; Houston Veterans Affairs Medical Center, Houston, Texas

Gabriel B. Habib, M.D., M.S.
Associate Professor of Medicine, Section of Cardiology, Department of Medicine, Baylor College of Medicine; Director of Coronary Care Unit and Acting Chief of Section of Cardiology, VA Medical Center, Houston, Texas

Richard J. Hamill, M.D.
Associate Professor, Departments of Medicine and Molecular Virology and Microbiology, Baylor College of Medicine; Veterans Affairs Medical Center, Houston, Texas

Mary P. Harward, M.D.
Clinical Assistant Professor, Internal Medicine, University of California–Irvine, Irvine, California; Medical Staff, St. Joseph Hospital, Orange, California

Teresa G. Hayes, M.D., Ph.D.
Assistant Professor, Internal Medicine Department, Hematology-Oncology Section, Baylor College of Medicine; Houston Veterans Affairs Medical Center, Houston, Texas

Christopher J. Lahart, M.D.
Assistant Professor of Medicine, Department of Medicine/Infectious Diseases, Baylor College of Medicine; Medical Director, Thomas Street Clinic, Houston, Texas

Sharma S. Prabhakar, M.D.
Assistant Professor, Division of Nephrology, Department of Internal Medicine, Texas Tech University Health Sciences Center; Medical Director, Dialysis Center of Lubbock, Lubbock, Texas

Wayne J. Riley, M.D., M.P.H., F.A.C.P.
Assistant Professor of Medicine, Department of Medicine, Baylor College of Medicine; Assistant Chief, Medicine Service, Ben Taub General Hospital, Houston, Texas

Loren A. Rolak, M.D.
Director, Marshfield Multiple Sclerosis Center, The Marshfield Clinic, Marshfield, Wisconsin

Roger Downey Rossen, M.D.
Professor, Immunology and Medicine, Baylor College of Medicine; Chief, Allergy and Immunology, and Director, Research Center for AIDS and HIV Infections, Houston Veterans Affairs Medical Center, Houston, Texas

Richard A. Rubin, M.D.
Clinical Assistant Professor of Medicine and Rheumatology, Baylor College of Medicine; The Methodist Hospital, Houston, Texas

Sarah E. Selleck, M.D.
Assistant Professor of Medicine, Geriatric Section of Department of Internal Medicine, Baylor College of Medicine, Houston, Texas

Mark M. Udden, M.D.
Associate Professor of Medicine, Internal Medicine, Baylor College of Medicine; The Ben Taub General Hospital, Houston, Texas

Anthony J. Zollo, Jr., M.D.
Assistant Professor, Department of Internal Medicine, Baylor College of Medicine, Houston, Texas; Chief Medical Officer, Lufkin Department of Veterans Affairs Outpatient Clinic, Lufkin, Texas

PREFACE TO THE THIRD EDITION

Editing this book remains a labor of love. This edition contains a great deal of new material and updated question-and-answer sets. The Allergy and Immunology, Medical Consultation and Endocrinology chapters have new contributors who have brought a fresh perspective to their chapters. There have been tremendous advances in diagnosis and treatment in all areas of Internal Medicine, and we have tried to reflect those advances in the third edition. I think we have succeeded!

I want to again thank an excellent group of contributors. It is not easy to carve out time from busy clinical and academic careers to work on a new edition, but each of them rose to the occasion to produce yet another edition in which we can all take pride.

Anthony J. Zollo, Jr., M.D.

PREFACE TO THE SECOND EDITION

The editing of the first edition of this book was an act of love. The tasks of assembling a team of contributors, collecting suggestions for question and answer sets, developing the final list of Q&A sets for each chapter, writing my share of those sets, and editing the overall manuscript was thoroughly enjoyable, albeit very time-consuming. This has been true for the second edition as well. I would like to acknowledge again the hard work and dedication of all of the contributors to this book. Only by utilizing the talents of experts in various subspecialties, with up-to-date knowledge of current developments, was it possible to complete this revision. Although many questions are the same, the answers often required revision. We are all proud of the finished product.

I would like to thank Linda Belfus, President of Hanley & Belfus, Inc., and her entire staff for their assistance and support. I would like to thank the readers of the first edition for their positive response to our work. After the countless hours spent producing the manuscript, one loses the ability to view the final result objectively. The success of the first edition was a validation of our hard work. I am confident you will receive the second edition with equal enthusiasm.

PREFACE TO THE FIRST EDITION

The art of Internal Medicine involves questions. It involves questions asked when taking a medical history, when forming a differential diagnosis, or when planning a diagnostic and therapeutic plan. Students of Internal Medicine, regardless of their level of training, are constantly confronted with questions posed from patients, from mentors, and from within themselves. The time-honored, question-based, Socratic approach to teaching is alive and well in the academic and clinical world of Internal Medicine. This book is intended to provide the reader with many of the questions (and answers) commonly encountered in training.

The knowledge base of Internal Medicine is substantial, probably more than any other specialty. Its acquisition is the goal of medical students, house officers, and all others who endeavor to learn and practice the discipline. There are many formal textbooks of internal medicine that provide complete coverage of all topics within the field. This work is not meant to replace the use of those texts. Rather, it is intended to focus on the lead-in questions and topics commonly encountered on teaching rounds, in clinical situations, and in examinations.

In preparing this text, we have attempted to take a middle ground between over-simplification and over-complication. We have included questions on common subjects and on "zebras," which, owing to their academic interest, are frequently discussed. We are grateful to our patients, our teachers, and our students for these questions and answers. As editor, I am indebted to my contributors on the faculty of Baylor College of Medicine for their assistance in this enjoyable and educational undertaking.

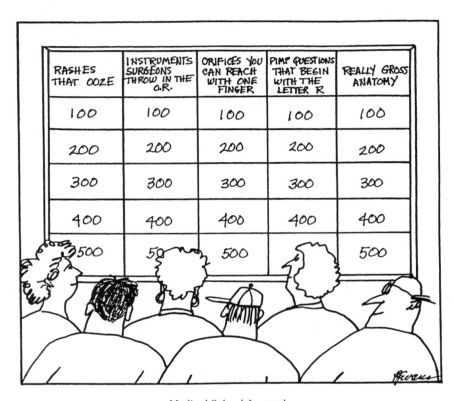

Medical School Jeopardy

1. GENERAL INTERNAL MEDICINE

Charlene M. Dewey, M.D., Wayne J. Riley, M.D., and Anthony J. Zollo, Jr., M.D.

> *The extraordinary development of modern science may be her undoing. Specialism, now a necessity, has fragmented the specialties themselves in a way that makes the outlook hazardous. The workers lose all sense of proportion in a maze of minutiae.*
> Sir William Osler (1849–1919)
> *Address, Classical Association, Oxford, May 16, 1910*

> *To my sons: Whatever specialty they follow, may they never forget to be doctors.*
> Harry E. Mock
> *Dedication to Skull Fractures and Brain Injuries*

1. What are Loeb's Laws of Medicine?
1. If what you're doing is working, keep doing it.
2. If what you're doing is not working, stop doing it.
3. If you don't know what to do, don't do anything.
4. Above all, never let a surgeon get your patient.

Matz R: Principles of medicine. NY State J Med 77:99–101, 1977.

2. What are the predominant organisms constituting the normal flora of the human body?

Oropharynx
Streptococcus viridans (α-hemolytic)
Staphylococci
Str. pyogenes
Str. pneumoniae
Moraxella catarrhalis
Neisseria sp.
Lactobacilli
Corynebacteria
Haemophilus sp.
Obligate anaerobes (not *Bacteroides fragilis*)
Candida albicans
Various protozoa

Upper intestine
Streptococci
Lactobacilli
Candida sp.

Lower genitourinary tract
Staphylococci
Streptococci (incl. enterococci)
Lactobacilli (vaginal)
Corynebacteria
Neisseria sp.
Obligate anaerobes
Aerobic gram-negative bacilli
C. albicans
Trichomonas vaginalis

Conjunctiva
Staphylococci
Corynebacteria
Haemophilus sp.

Nasopharynx
Staphylococci (incl. *S. aureus*)
Streptococci (incl. *S. pneumoniae*)
M. catarrhalis
Neisseria sp.
Haemophilus sp.

Skin
Staphylococci (incl. *S. aureus*)
Corynebacteria
Propionibacteria
Candida sp.
Malassezia furfur
Dermatophytic fungi

Large intestine and feces
Obligate anaerobes (incl. *B. fragilis*)
Aerobic gram-negative bacilli
Streptococci (incl. enterococci)
C. albicans
Various protozoa

Adapted from Rosebury T: Microorganisms Indigenous to Man. New York, McGraw-Hill, 1962, pp 310–384.

Mackowiak PA: The normal microbial flora. N Engl J Med 307:83–93, 1982.

1

3. What are the principles of "diagnostic roundsmanship"?

1. Common things occur commonly.
2. The race may not always be to the swift nor the battle to the strong, but it's a good idea to bet that way.
3. When you hear hoofbeats think of horses, not zebras.
4. Place your bets on uncommon manifestations of common conditions rather than common manifestations of uncommon conditions.

Matz R: Principles of medicine. NY State J Med 77:99–101, 1977.

4. What are the risk factors for thromboembolism?

Age greater than 40 years

Heart conditions: myocardial infarction (MI), atrial fibrillation, cardiomyopathy, and congestive heart failure (CHF)

Postoperative states: especially abdominal or pelvic operations; splenectomy, orthopedic procedures of the lower extremities: total hip or knee replacements

Neoplastic diseases, especially adenocarcinomas of lung, breast, viscera

Fractures, especially pelvic, hip, leg

High estrogen states: pregnancy and parturition

Prolonged immobilization or paralysis

Previous deep venous thrombosis (DVT)/pulmonary embolism (PE)

Nephrotic syndrome

Inflammatory bowel disease

Femoral vein catheters

Varicose veins

Drugs, especially oral contraceptives and estrogens

Hyperviscosity syndromes and abnormal flows

Myeloproliferative disorders with thrombocytosis, polycythemia vera

Antithrombin III deficiency

Protein C and protein S deficiencies

Activated protein C resistance (Factor V Leiden)

Abnormal fibrinolysis

Disorders of plasminogen and plasminogen activation

Antiphospholipid antibodies and lupus anticoagulant

Heparin-induced thrombocytopenia

Hyperhomocystinemia

Others: obesity, hemorrhage after strokes (CVA)

Clagett, GP et al: Prevention of venous thromboembolism. Chest 114(5)S:531S–560S, 1998.

5. How are prothrombin times (PT) standardized for monitoring patients on anticoagulant therapy with warfarin?

The International Normalization Ratio (INR) system standardizes the (PT) for different thromboplastin reagents, thus providing a universal standard by which to compare any given laboratory's results with that of the World Health Organization standard. The INR is calculated as follows:

$$INR = (\text{patient PT/normal PT})^{ISI}$$

where normal PT = mean PT of the target population (in sec) and ISI = International Sensitivity Index (provided with each batch of thromboplastin reagent).

Potential Problems with the INR

---

1. Lack of reliability of the INR system when used at the onset of warfarin therapy and for screening for a coagulopathy in a patient with liver disease
2. Relationship between precision of the INR determination and the reagent ISI

(*Table continued on next page.*)

3. Effect of instrumentation in ISI values
4. Lack of reliability of the ISI result provided by the manufacturer
5. Incorrect calculation of the INR resulting from the use of inappropriate control plasma
6. Problems with citrate concentrations and interference with lupus anticoagulants with thromboplastins with low ISI values

Hirsh J: Oral Anticoagulants: Mechanism of action, clinical effectiveness, and optimal therapeutic range. Chest 114(suppl 5):445S–469S, 1998, with permission.

6. What are the advantages of using the INR system?
1. Easier, smoother regulation of anticoagulation.
2. Traveling patients will have a standard regardless of the laboratory used.
3. Standardization for research and publication efforts.
4. Reduced risks of complications associated with higher doses of oral anticoagulants.

7. What is the appropriate response to an elevated INR?
a. **INR < 5 without bleeding:** No rapid reduction needed, decrease dose or skip next dose
b. **INR 5–9 without bleeding:** [A] Omit next 1–2 doses; monitor and restart at lower dose—no increased risk of bleed
[B] Next dose omitted and administer vitamin K_1 (1–2.5 mg) orally if at increased risk of bleeding
Urgency (i.e., dental surgery, urgent surgery): give vitamin K_1 orally at 2–4 mg, check INR at 24 hours; if still high, give another 1–2 mg vitamin K_1
c. **INR > 9 without bleeding:** Vitamin K_1 (3–5 mg) orally; monitor and repeat if needed in 24–48 hours
d. **Serious bleed or INR > 20:** Vitamin K_1, 10 mg slow IV and supplement with fresh plasma transfusion or prothrombin complex; concentrate depending on urgency; may need to be repeated at 12 hours
e. **Life threatening bleed or serious warfarin overdose** Replacement with prothrombin complex concentrate, supplemented with 10 mg vitamin K_1 by slow IV infusion; can be repeated based on INR

If warfarin is to be continued after a high dose of vitamin K_1, heparin can be used until the effects of vitamin K_1 are reversed and the patient becomes responsive to warfarin therapy.

Adapted from: Hirsh J: Oral anticoagulants: Mechanism of action, clinical effectiveness, and optimal therapeutic range. Chest 114(suppl 5):445S–469S, 1998, with permission.

8. What drugs are known to potentiate the effects of warfarin, usually requiring a lower dosing regimen? A higher dosing regimen?

Many commonly used drugs can interact to potentiate or inhibit warfarin and its effect on the prothrombin time (PT). Drugs can prevent the absorption of warfarin (such as cholestyramine) or alter its clearance from the body. Warfarin clearance is altered when drugs interact or inhibit the S-isomer or R-isomer form of warfarin. The S-isomer is most important due to its strong anti-vitamin K potential. Drugs that inhibit the S-isomer can seriously potentiate its effect and prolong the PT. Drugs that inhibit the S-isomer include amiodarone, metronidazole, trimethoprim-sulfamethoxazole, phenylbutazone, sulfinpyrazole and disulfuram. Drugs that inhibit the R-isomer resulting in less potentiation of the PT include cimetidine and omeprazole.

Drugs that can inhibit the effect of warfarin and may result in the need for higher doses include barbiturates, carbamazepine, cholestyramine, rifampin, sucralfate, griseofulvin, nafcillin, chlordiazepoxide and food with large amounts of vitamin K.

Other drugs such as acetaminophen, anabolic steroids, and erythromycin can potentiate the warfarin anticoagulant effect via unknown mechanisms.

Kelly WN: Textbook of Internal Medicine, 3rd ed. Philadelphia, Lippincott-Raven, 1997, p 574.

Hirsh J: Oral anticoagulants: Mechanism of action, clinical effectiveness, and optimal therapeutic range. Chest 114(suppl 5):445S–469S, 1998.

9. What are the benefits and limitations of the available screening tests for deep venous thrombosis and thromboembolism?

STUDY	PPV/NPV*	BENEFITS	LIMITATIONS
Contrast venography	Gold standard, 100% sensitive and specific	Highly specific, useful from IVC to calf	Invasive, painful and expensive; therefore not first line. Contra-indicated in renal failure and chronic renal insufficiency
Venous ultrasound	Sensitivity: 80–100% Specificity: 86–100% PPV: 92–100%	Highly accurate for proximal DVT, noninvasive; allows differentiation of fresh vs. old DVT; compression with venous imaging has best prediction, portable	Insensitive for DVT suspected in the calf; reader-dependent, less accurate for chronic DVT, massive obesity, severe edema, casts
Impedance plethysmography	Sensitivity: 93% Specificity: 94%	Reliable for proximal DVT; excellent screening test when used with I^{125}-labeled fibrinogen scan; less expensive and portable; non-invasive; no radiation exposure	Insensitive for calf; sensitivity/specificity dependent on ad-herence to study protocol; potential false positives; can-not be used to assist with other potential diagnoses
I^{125}-labeled fibrinogen scan (sympto-matic)	Sensitivity: 56% Specificity: 84%	Sensitive for calf and distal thigh DVT	Insensitive for proximal and iliac vein thrombosis; may not become positive until 72 hours; cannot be used with leg casts or bandages
D-dimer (ELISA, e.g., VIDAS DD)	Sensitivity: 94–100% NPV: 92–100%	Minimally invasive; suggests thrombus; acts as marker of activation of coagulation; newer tests are rapid, costly	Negative D-dimer (normal level) cannot rule out DVT; non-specific; currently not endorsed for widespread use in screening; restrict to low–moderate risk patients; can be timely
Latex (e.g., SimpleRed)	Sensitivity: 89–100% NPV: 95–100%	Minimally invasive; rapid, economical	Subjective; non-specific; cur-rently not endorsed for wide-spread use in screening; re-strict to low–moderate risk patients
Spiral (helical) CT	Sensitivity: 64–100% Specificity: 89–97%	Rapid; non-invasive; actually identifies thrombus; identi-fies other disease states; can be used in face of abnor-mal chest films; can provide alternative causes for symp-toms; possibly cost effective	Cannot detect emboli in sub-segmental pulmonary arteries where up to 36% of emboli are located; use as a "rule-in" study; cannot rule out secondary to unable to detect in the subsegmental areas; expensive, reader-dependent
MRI	Sensitivity: near 100% Specificity: 90–100%	Demonstrates an actual clot in leg or lung simultane-ously; non-invasive; no nephrotoxic iodine; excel-lent sensitivity/specificity for DVT; safe; can detect	Limited studies on use; less sensitive for calf and pul-monary emboli; not as sensi-tive as angiography for pul-monary emboli; insufficient evidence for replacement of

(Table continued on next page.)

STUDY	PPV/NPV*	BENEFITS	LIMITATIONS
MRI (cont.)		alternative diagnoses; no contrast or radiation needed	previous standards (V/Q and angiogram; restricted among patients who are claustrophobic, morbidly obese, have metallic implants

* PPV = Positive predictive value, NPV = Negative predictive value

Kelley WN (ed): Textbook of Internal Medicine, 3rd ed. Philadelphia, Lippincott-Raven, 1997.
Van der Graaf F et al: Exclusion of deep venous thrombosis with D-dimer testing. Thromb Haemost 83:191–198, 2000.
Gill P, Nahum A: Improving detection of venous thromboembolism. Post Grad Med 108(4):24–40, 2000.
Tapson V: The diagnostic approach to acute venous thromboembolism: Clinical practice guideline. Am J Respir Crit Care Med 160(3):1043–1066, 1999.

10. What is a Baker's cyst? What condition can its rupture simulate?

Baker's cysts result from the build-up of synovial fluid in the knee. Also called popliteal bursitis, it is most common in males 15–30 years of age. Symptoms consist of local pain, limitation of knee extension, and symptoms related to compression of adjacent structures (i.e., popliteal artery, deep veins, and tibial nerve). The cyst can be felt as a swelling in the popliteal space. When a non-ruptured cyst softens with knee flexion, it is known as Foucher's sign. Rupture of a Baker's cyst, usually due to trauma, can cause acute inflammation, pain, and swelling that can extend down into the posterior calf. This presentation can be confused with **venous thrombophlebitis**.

11. When is anticoagulation contraindicated?

Anticoagulation should be considered contraindicated whenever the risk of bleeding outweighs the benefit of the therapy. While the rules are not absolute, consider the following situations as probable contraindications to warfarin therapy:
- Pregnancy, or in women who may become pregnant, in which case, proper procedures to prevent pregnancy should be instituted
- Hemorrhagic tendencies or blood dyscrasias
- Surgery of non-compressible sites such as the central nervous system or eye
- Traumatic surgery resulting in large open surfaces
- Lumbar punctures
- Active bleeding of the gastrointestinal, genitourinary, or respiratory tracts
- Cerebrovascular hemorrhage, large embolic or ischemic strokes with uncontrolled hypertension, cerebral aneurysms
- Dissecting aortic aneurysms
- Pericarditis, pericardial effusions, and bacterial endocarditis

Anticoagulation with warfarin also should be reconsidered in patients at risk for chronic anticoagulation such as alcoholics who are frequently intoxicated, uncontrolled psychosis, demented patients in uncontrolled environments, or in situations where laboratory facilities or regular monitoring is not adequate.

Physician's Desk Reference, 54th ed. Montvale, NJ, Medical Economics Company, 2000.

12. How do you convert deciliters to milliliters? Grains to milligrams? Teaspoons to milliliters?

Useful Calculations and Conversions

• Swallow, avg (not a mouthful)		• Milligram (mg)	= 0.001 gm
Adult ≈ 10 ml		1 mg	= 1000 µg
Child ≈ 5 ml			= 0.015 grain
• 1 teaspoon (tsp) = 5 ml			
1 tablespoon (tbsp) = 15 ml		• Microgram (µg)	= 0.001 mg

(Table continued on next page.)

Useful Calculations and Conversions (cont.)

• Grain	= 64.8 mg		1 µg/ml	= 0.1 mg%
1/65 grain	= 0.015 grain	= 1 mg		= 0.1 mg/dl
1/150 grain	= 0.0067 grain	= 0.3 mg		= 1 mg/liter
1/400 grain	= 0.0025 grain	= 0.15 mg		
			• Nanogram (ng)	= 0.001 µg
• Percent solution	1% solution	= 1 gm/100 ml	1 ng/ml	= 0.001 µg/ml
	= 10 mg/1 ml			= 0.1 µg
	= 10 mg/liter			= 0.1 µg/dl
				= 1 µg/liter
• Milligram percent (mg%) 1 mg%	= mg/100 ml	= 0.001 mg%		
	= 10 µg/ml			
	= 1 mg/dl	• Milliequivalent (meq)		
	= 10 mg/liter	1 meq		$= \dfrac{MW\ gm}{valence \times 1000}$
• Deciliter (dl) = 100 ml				
1 mg/dl = 1 mg/100 ml		1 meq/L		$= \dfrac{mg/L \times valence}{MW}$
= 1 mg%				
= 10 µg/ml				
• Part per million (ppm) = 1 part in a million		mg/100 ml		$= \dfrac{meq/L\ 3\ MW}{10 \times valence}$
1 ppm = 1 mg/liter				
= 0.1 mg%				
= 1 µg/ml				

Flomenbaum NE, Roberts JR: Emergency Department Reference Guide, 2nd ed. New York, Cahners Publishing, 1989, p 20.

13. Who was Baron von Münchausen? Why is a syndrome named after him?

Baron von Münchausen, an 18th century German soldier/storyteller, is reputed to have been prone to wild exaggeration. Patients with a history of repeated factitious symptoms, illnesses, and accidents, usually of a dramatic or emergency nature, are said to have Münchausen's syndrome. The history often includes multiple invasive procedures with negative findings. Münchausen's syndrome is seen in women more frequently than men. It is considered a psychiatric condition and must be separated from malingering, which involves a conscious intent to deceive.

14. What criteria should be used to evaluate any preventive health care intervention?

Frame proposed the following six criteria:

1. The condition must have a significant effect on the quantity or quality of life.

2. Acceptable methods of treatment must be available.

3. The condition must have an asymptomatic period during which detection and treatment can significantly reduce the morbidity or mortality.

4. Treatment during the early asymptomatic period must yield a therapeutic result superior to that obtained if treatment is delayed until symptoms appear.

5. Tests to detect the condition in the asymptomatic period must be acceptable to patients and available at a reasonable cost.

6. The incidence of the condition must be sufficient to justify the cost of a screening program.

Frame PS: A critical review of adult health maintenance (pts 1-4). J Fam Pract 22:341, 417, 511, 1985; 23:29, 1986.

15. Define sensitivity, specificity, and predictive value of a test. How are they calculated?

These terms are frequently used in the assessment of a test and its ability to rule in or rule out a given condition (also called the **accuracy** of the test). To use these values, you must understand how they are derived. Since a test can be positive or negative (if we disregard inconclusive results), and a patient either has or does not have a condition, there are four possible outcomes in any test situation:

Disease:

	Present	Absent
+	a	b
−	c	d

Test result

a = True positive

b = False positive

c = False negative

d = True negative

Sensitivity	=	$\dfrac{a}{a+c}$	=	Percentage of patients who have the disease and test positive
Specificity	=	$\dfrac{d}{b+d}$	=	Percentage of persons who do not have the disease and test negative (True-Negative).
Positive predictive value	=	$\dfrac{a}{a+b}$	=	Percentage of patients who test positive and actually do have the disease.
Negative predictive value	=	$\dfrac{d}{c+d}$	=	Percentage of patients who test negative and really do not have the disease.

Last JM: A Dictionary of Epidemiology, 2nd ed. New York, Oxford University Press, 1988.

16. What is the pneumococcal polysaccharide vaccine (Pneumovax 23, Pneu-Imune 23)?

This vaccine is composed of 25 µg of purified capsular polysaccharide antigens from 23 types of *Streptococcus pneumoniae*. When introduced in 1983, this vaccine replaced the older 14-valent type (released in 1977). These 23-capsular types represent 85–90% of the causes of bacteremic pneumococcal disease in the U.S. Cross-reactivity with other capsular types may increase this coverage by another 8%. In healthy adults, antibody levels remain elevated for at least 5 years but then may fall to pre-vaccination levels within 10 years in some patients. Revaccination is recommended if more than 5 years have elapsed since the previous dose. The overall protective efficacy of the vaccine against pneumococcal bacteremia is approximately 60%.

17. Who should get this vaccine?

The Advisory Committee on Immunization Practices (ACIP) recommends that the vaccine be used more extensively and administered to all persons in the following groups:

1. Persons aged ≥ 65 years.
2. Immunocompetent persons aged ≥ 2 years who are at increased risk for illness and death associated with pneumococcal disease because of chronic illness.
3. Persons aged ≥ 2 years with functional or anatomic asplenia.
4. Persons aged ≥ 2 years living in environments in which the risk of disease is high.
5. Immunocompromised persons aged ≥ 2 years who are at high risk for infection.

Prevention of pneumococcal disease: Recommendations of the Advisory Committee on Immunization Practices (ACIP). MMWR 46(RR-08):1–24, 1997.

18. Are routine, periodic chest x-rays recommended as screening for lung cancer?

No. Most lung cancers are already systemic diseases at the time of earliest possible detection by chest x-rays, and the outcome as a result of screening by routine chest x-rays is not changed.

19. Outline the current recommendations by the various organizations for colorectal cancer screening in patients who are asymptomatic and not members of a high-risk group.

Recommendations for Colon Cancer Screening in Persons at Average Risk

American Cancer Society	Starting at age >50 with either (1) fecal occult blood test (FOBT) yearly plus flexible sigmoidoscopy every 5 years or (2) full colonoscopy every 10 years or double-contrast barium enema (DCBE) every 5–10 years
U.S. Preventive Services Task Force	Starting at age >50 with annual FOBT or sigmoidoscopy or both.
American College of Physicians	Between 50–70 years with flexible sigmoidoscopy, colonoscopy, or DCBE. FOBT for those who refuse.

American Cancer Society Colon and Rectum Resource Center. www3.cancer.org
Guide to Clinical Preventive Services, 2nd ed. Report of the US Preventive Services Task Force. Baltimore, Williams & Wilkins, 1996, pp 89–103.

20. What conditions can lead to false-positive or false-negative results with the HemOccult Slide Test?

The HemOccult Slide Test (Smith-Kline Diagnostics) detects the presence of hemoglobin in feces. **False-negative** results are obtained in patients with colonic neoplasms that are not bleeding (lesions < 1–2 cm, non-ulcerated lesions), that bleed intermittently, or that are not producing the 20 ml of blood per day required for a reliably positive result. Stool that is stored prior to testing and large doses of ascorbic acid may also lead to false-negative results.

False-positive results can be produced by the dietary intake of rare beef or fruits and vegetables that contain peroxidases. This effect is seen mainly in tests performed on rehydrated stool specimens. Oral iron preparations also have been implicated in some studies but not in others. **False-positive** results can occur due to blood from sources other than colorectal carcinoma, such as gastric blood loss caused by nonsteroidal anti-inflammatory drugs (NSAIDs).

Fleischer DE, et al: Detection and surveillance of colorectal cancer. JAMA 261:580–586, 1989.

21. What screening programs for colorectal cancer are recommended for patients in high-risk groups according to the American Cancer Society?

ACS Guidelines for Screening and Surveillance for Early Detection of Colorectal Polyps and Cancer

RISK CATEGORY	RECOMMENDATION[1]	AGE TO BEGIN	INTERVAL
Family history of familial adenomatous polyposis	Early surveillance with endoscopy, counseling to consider genetic testing and reference to a specialty center	Puberty	If genetic test (+) or polyposis confirmed, consider colectomy, once weekly endoscopy for 1–2 years
Family history of hereditary nonpolyposis colon cancer	Colonscopy and counseling to consider genetic testing	Age 12	If genetic test (+) or if patient has had genetic testing, colonoscopy every 2 years until age 40, then every 1 year
Inflammatory bowel disease	Colonoscopies with biopsies for dysplasia	Eight years after start of pancolitis. Twelve to 15 years after start of (L) side colitis	Every 1–2 years

[1] Digital rectal exam should be done at the time of each sigmoidoscopy, colonoscopy, or DCBE.
Copyright American Cancer Society (from their website at www.cancer.org, reproduced with permission).

22. What is the erythrocyte sedimentation rate (ESR)? What causes it to increase or decrease?
The ESR is a nonspecific index of inflammation. The normal values for patients under age 50 are 0–15 mm/hr in men and 0–20 mm/hr in women. The normal values increase with age and may be higher in individuals over age 60, even in the absence of disease.

Whether the ESR is normal, increased, or decreased depends on the sum of forces acting on the erythrocytes (RBCs). These include the downward force of gravity (dependent on the mass of the RBC), upward buoyant forces (dependent on the density [mass/volume] of the RBC), and bulk plasma flow (created by the downward-moving RBCs).

Conditions that Increase and Decrease the ESR

INCREASE	DECREASE
Inflammatory disorders	Increased serum viscosity
Hyperfibrinogenemia	Hypofibrinogenemia
Rouleaux formation	Sickle cell disease
Anemia (hypochromic, microcytic)	Leukemoid reaction
Pregnancy	Polycythemia
Hyperglobulinemia	Spherocytosis
Hypercholesterolemia	Anisocytosis
	High-dose corticosteroids
	Congestive heart failure
	Cachexia

23. Is the ESR useful in screening for any conditions?
The ESR is of little value in screening asymptomatic patients. It also is of little value in screening for malignancy, since it is often normal in patients with cancer. It is indicated in the diagnosis and monitoring of temporal arteritis and polymyalgia rheumatica. It may also be of value in monitoring the course and therapy of rheumatoid arthritis, Hodgkin's disease, other malignancies, and inflammatory disorders.

24. Which disease is associated with pagophagia (ice-eating)?
Iron-deficiency anemia (IDA). Patients with IDA may also crave other food and nonfood substances (**pica**). Although this behavior is rarely volunteered, it is found in approximately 50% of such patients. The pica of IDA responds to iron-repletion therapy.

Rector WG: Pica: Its frequency and significance in patients with iron-deficiency anemia due to chronic gastrointestinal blood loss. J Gen Intern Med 4:512–513, 1989.

25. Describe the four stages of alcohol withdrawal.
1. **Tremulousness** occurs 8–12 hours after cessation of drinking. The tremor is aggravated by intention or agitation and may be accompanied by nausea and vomiting, insomnia, headache, diaphoresis, tachycardia, and anxiety. The symptoms usually subside within 24 hours, unless the patient progresses to the next stage.

2. **Alcoholic hallucinosis** usually occurs 12–24 hours after the cessation of drinking but may take 6–8 days to develop. Auditory or visual hallucinations alternate with periods of lucidity. The symptoms of the first stage continue and worsen.

3. **Grand mal seizures** ("rum fits") occur in 90% of cases between 6–48 hours after cessation of drinking. The seizures are generalized and usually multiple. This stage occurs in 3–4% of untreated patients.

4. **Delirium tremens** usually occurs 3–4 days after the cessation of drinking but may not develop for up to 2 weeks. It manifests as confusion, hallucinations, tremors, and signs of autonomic hyperactivity (fever, tachycardia, dilated pupils, diaphoresis). It is a medical emergency and carries a mortality of 5–15% despite treatment. Death is usually due to cardiovascular collapse.

26. What is the LD_{50} for ethanol?

Five hundred mg/dl is the serum level that will be lethal in 50% of patients who ingest a sufficient quantity of ethanol to achieve such a serum level. The amount of orally ingested ethanol needed to produce this serum level (LD_{50}) varies with the size of the person, rates of ingestion, absorption, hepatic metabolism, and other factors.

27. Which organs are directly affected by chronic alcohol abuse?

Alcohol has pathologic effects in nearly every organ system:

CNS	Alcohol withdrawal "blackouts"	Hallucinations
	Dementia	Seizures
	Wernicke-Korsakoff syndrome	Peripheral neuropathy
Gastrointestinal	Esophageal varices	Neoplasm
	Esophagitis, gastritis	Cirrhosis
	Vitamin deficiencies (niacin, B_{12}, thiamine)	Chronic pancreatitis
Cardiovascular	Arrhythmias	Cardiomyopathy
	Congestive heart failure	Hypertension
Pulmonary	Pneumonia (aspiration)	Tuberculosis
Genitourinary	Impaired spermatogenesis	Testicular atrophy
	Impotence/infertility	Amenorrhea
Musculoskeletal	Myopathy	Rhabdomyolysis
	Higher incidence of gout	Osteonecrosis
Endocrine	Increased cortisol	Hyperglycemia
	Decreased T4 and T3	
Hematopoietic	Impaired granulocyte function	Anemia (iron, B_{12}, and folate deficiency, sideroblastic)
	Thrombocytopenia	

28. How quickly can a healthy person clear ethanol from his or her body?

A normal person can metabolize 150 mg of ethanol/kg body weight/hr. In a normal 70-kg person, this leads to a decrease in blood ethanol level of approximately 20 mg/dl/hr.

29. What laboratory data support a diagnosis of liver disease due to chronic alcohol abuse?

- Elevated gamma-glutamyl transpeptidase (GGT)
- Aspartate aminotransferase alanine aminotransferase ratio > 2:1
- Hypoalbuminemia
- Prolonged prothrombin time (PT)
- Low blood urea nitrogen (BUN)
- Low glucose
- Thrombocytopenia
- Macrocytosis of RBCs

30. What constellation of symptoms comprise the Wernicke-Korsakoff syndrome?

This syndrome most commonly occurs in the malnourished, alcoholic patient and includes the following symptoms:

Symptoms of the Wernicke-Korsakoff Syndrome

Ocular	**Altered mental status**
Horizontal/vertical nystagmus	Alcohol withdrawal
Paralysis of conjugate gaze	Global confusion (apathetic, inattentive, lethargic, slurred
External rectus muscle paralysis	speech, irrational)
Ataxia	Korsakoff's amnesic psychosis
Stance and gait affected	Anterograde amnesia (impairment of learning new ideas)
Cannot walk without assistance	Past memory disturbances (confabulation)

31. Which laboratory tests should be done when evaluating a person with altered mental status?

Complete blood count (CBC)
Full chemistry panel
Vitamin B_{12}
Serum folate
Urinalysis
Urine toxicology screen
Electrocardiogram
CT scan (in selected patients)
Electroencephalogram (in selected patients)
Erythrocyte sedimentation rate (ESR)
Serologic test for syphilis (VDRL)
Thyroid function tests (thyroid-stimulating hormone, free thyroxine)
Arterial blood gas
HIV test
Lumbar puncture (in selected patients)
Chest x-ray
MRI scan (in selected patients)

32. What are the causes of dementia?

Causes of Dementia

METABOLIC-TOXIC	STRUCTURAL	INFECTIOUS
Anoxia	Alzheimer's disease	Neurosyphilis (general paresis)
Pernicious anemia	Vascular disease	Tuberculous and fungal meningitis
Pellagra	Multi-infarct dementia	Viral encephalitis
Folic acid deficiency	Binswanger's dementia	HIV-related disorders
Hypothyroidism	Huntington's chorea	Gerstmann-Sträussler syndrome
Bromide intoxication	Multiple sclerosis	
Hypoglycemia	Pick's disease	
Hypercalcemia associated	Cerebellar degeneration	
with hyperparathyroidism	Wilson's disease	
Organ system failure	Amyotrophic lateral sclerosis	
Hepatic encephalopathy	Progressive multifocal	
Uremic encephalopathy	leukoencephalopathy	
Respiratory encephalopathy	Progressive supranuclear palsy	
Chronic drug-alcohol-nutritional	Brain tumor	
abuse	Irradiation to frontal lobes	
	Surgery	
	Normal-pressure hydrocephalus	
	Brain trauma	
	Chronic subdural hematoma	
	Dementia pugilistica	

33. Which etiologies of dementia can be treated?

Treatable Causes of Dementia

Medications	**Chemical intoxication**	**Infections**
Psychoactive agents	Alcohol	Neurosyphilis
Tricyclic antidepressants	Carbon monoxide	Meningitis
Tranquilizers	Lead	Abscess
Lithium carbonate	Arsenic	
Sedatives	Mercury	**Miscellaneous**
Methyldopa	Organophosphates	Depression
Clonidine	Trichloroethylene	Pellagra
Propranolol		Wernicke-Korsakoff syndrome
Phenytoin	**Endocrinopathies**	Schizophrenia

(Table continued on next page.)

Treatable Causes of Dementia (cont.)

Barbiturates	Hypo- or hyperthyroidism	Changes in environment
Corticosteroids	Addison's disease	Nursing home placement
Digitalis	Cushing's disease	Hospitalization
Quinidine	Hypoglycemia	
NSAIDs	Panhypopituitarism	
Cimetidine		
Diuretics	**Intracranial lesions**	
	Subdural hematomas	
Metabolic derangements	Cerebrovascular disease	
Hepatic encephalopathy	Brain tumor	
Hypercalcemia	Brain abscess	
Hyponatremia	Multiple sclerosis	
Uremia	Hydrocephalus	

34. What is the risk of recurrence after a first unprovoked seizure?

In a study of 224 patients with a first unprovoked seizure, the overall recurrence rate was 16% at 12 months, 21% at 24 months, and 27% at 36 months. Patients with a history of prior neurologic insult had a higher rate of recurrence (34%), all of which occurred within 20 months. Among those without a history of neurologic insult ("idiopathic"), patients free of recurrence at 36 months did not have a subsequent seizure. Among the idiopathic cases, recurrence risk was higher in those with generalized spikewave EEGs (50% at 18 months) and in those who had a sibling with seizures.

Hauser WA, et al: Seizure recurrence after a first unprovoked seizure. N Engl J Med 307:522–527, 1982.

35. What are the causes of delirium?

Differential Diagnosis of the Acute Confusional State (Delirium)

NEUROLOGIC

Trauma
  Concussion
  Intracranial hematoma
  Subdural hematoma
Vascular disorders
  Multiple infarctions
  Right hemisphere or posterior circulation infarcts
  Hypertensive encephalopathy
  Vasculitis (e.g., systemic lupus erythematosus (SLE) polyarteritis nodosa, giant-cell arteritis)
  Air and fat embolism
  Subarachnoid hemorrhage

Neoplasia
  Multiple parenchymal metastases
  Meningeal carcinomatosis
  Midline brain tumors
  Brain tumors causing brainstem compression, edema, or hydrocephalus
  Paraneoplastic syndromes (limbic encephalitis)
Infections
  Meningitis and encephalitis (viral, bacterial, fungal, protozoal)
  Multiple abscesses
  Progressive multifocal leukoencephalopathy
Inflammations
  Acute disseminated encephalomyelitis
  Postinfectious encephalitis
Epilepsy
  Postictal state
  Temporal lobe status (complex partial status)

SYSTEMIC

Substrate depletion
  Hypoglycemia

Endocrine, over- or underactivity
  Thyroid

(Table continued on next page.)

Differential Diagnosis of the Acute Confusional State (Delirium) (cont.)

SYSTEMIC (cont.)

Substrate depletion (cont.)
  Diffuse hypoxia (pulmonary, cardiac, CO
  poisoning)
Metabolic encephalopathy
  Diabetic ketoacidosis
  Renal failure
  Liver failure
  Electrolyte, fluid, and acid-base imbalance
  (esp. Na$^+$, Ca^{2+}, Mg^{2+})
  Hereditary metabolic disease (e.g., porphyria,
  metachromatic leukodystrophy, mitochon-
  drial cytopathy)
Vitamin deficiency
  Thiamine (Wernicke's encephalopathy)
  Nicotinic acid (pellagra)
  B$_{12}$

Endocrine, over- or underactivity (cont.)
  Parathyroid
  Adrenal
Infection
  Septicemia
  Malaria
  Subacute bacterial endocarditis
  Focal infection (e.g., pneumonia)
Thermal injuries
  Hypothermia
  Heat stroke
Hematologic disorders
  Hyperviscosity syndrome
  Severe anemia
Toxic causes
  Drug and alcohol intoxication (therapeutic,
  social, illegal)
  Drug withdrawal (e.g., alcohol, barbiturates,
  narcotics)
  Chemical toxins (e.g., heavy metals, organic
  toxins)

PSYCHIATRIC

Acute mania
Depression or extreme anxiety

Schizophrenia
Hysterical fugue states

From Brown MM, Hachinski VC: Acute confusional states, amnesia, and dementia. In Isselbacher KJ, et al:
Harrison's Principles of Internal Medicine, 13th ed. New York, McGraw-Hill, 1994, p 140; with permission.

36. What is St. Anthony's dance? St. Guy's dance? St. Vitus' dance?

They are all chorea. The following is a list of diseases and syndromes named after the saints:

Saint Syndromes

PATRONYMIC NAME	DISEASE OR SYNDROME
St. Agatha's	Mastopathic inflammatory disease
St. Aignan's or Agnan's	Favus ringworm, tinea
St. Arman's	Pellagra
St. Anthony's	
St. Anthony's dance	Chorea (see also St. Vitus)
St. Anthony's fire	Ergotism (epidemic gangrene and psychotic alterations)
St. Anthony's fire	Erysipelas
St. Apollonia's	Toothache
St. Avertin's	Epilepsy
St. Avidus'	Deafness
St. Blasius'	Quinsy (peritonsillar abscess)
St. Dymphna's	Mental derangements
St. Erasmus'	Colic pain
St. Fiacre's or Flacre's	Hemorrhoids
St. Francis'	Erysipelas

(Table continued on next page.)

Saint Syndromes (cont.)

PATRONYMIC NAME	DISEASE OR SYNDROME
St. Gervasius'	Juvenile or adult rheumatic pains
St. Gete's	Carcinoma
St. Giles'	Leprosy
St. Gothard's	Ancylostomiasis (hookworm)
St. Guy's dance	Chorea
St. Hubert's	Rabies
St. Ignatius'	Pellagra
St. Kilda's	Colds, infections
St. Louis'	Encephalitis
St. Main's	Scabies
St. Martin's	Alcoholism
St. Mathurin's	Idiocy
St. Modestus'	Chorea
St. Roch's or Roche's	Plague
St. Sebastian's	Plague
St. Valentine's	Epilepsy
St. Vitus' dance	Chorea
St. Zachary's	Mutism

Magalini SI, Magalini SC: Dictionary of Medical Syndromes, 4th ed. Philadelphia, Lippincott-Raven, 1997, pp 13–714, with permission.

37. What is Bell's palsy?

Bell's palsy is a demyelinating viral inflammatory disease that is the most common ailment of the facial nerve (cranial nerve [CN] VII). It is characterized by the following:

Bell's Palsy

Onset	Usually preceded by viral prodrome
	Onset is acute
Duration	Approximately 5 days
	Peak symptoms at 48 hrs
Findings	Unilateral
	Loss of facial expression
	Widened palpebral fissure
	Diminished taste
	Difficulty in chewing (food collects between lips and teeth)
	Hyperesthesia in ≥ 1 branch of CN V
	Hyperacusis
Treatment	Protect the affected eye
	Prednisone (if patient presents within first 2 days)
	Symptoms are self-limited

Adam KK: Current concepts in neurology: Diagnosis and management of facial paralysis. N Engl J Med 307:348–351, 1982.

38. Which organisms are implicated in meningitis of the adult?

Streptococcus pneumoniae is the most common cause of bacterial meningitis in the adult, followed by *Neisseria meningitis*. *Haemophilus influenzae* has decreased in frequency by 82%

due to the vaccination available against this organism. A newer epidemic is being seen with antibiotic resistant strains of *Streptococcus pneumoniae*.

Organisms Implicated in Adult Meningitis

Bacterial	**Viral**
S. pneumoniae	Enterovirus (polio, coxsackie, echo)
N. meningitis	Herpes simplex types 1 and 2
H. influenzae	Varicella-zoster virus
S. aureus	Adenoviruses
Treponema pallidum	Epstein-Barr virus
Enterobacteriaceae	Lymphocytic choriomeningitis virus
Klebsiella sp.	Human immunodeficiency virus
Pseudomonas sp.	Influenza virus types A and B
L. monocytogenes	
Borrelia burgdorferi	**Fungal**
N. gonorrhoeae	*Cryptococcus neoformans*
Clostridium sp.	*Histoplasma capsulatum*
Mycobacterium tuberculosis	*Coccidioides immitis*
Proteus sp.	*Blastomyces dermatitidis*
Ehrlichia bruella	
Parasites	
Toxoplasma gondii	
T. soleum (cysticercosis)	

Pruitt AA: Infections of the nervous system. Neurol Clin North Am 16(2):419–447, 1998.

39. Do the cerebrospinal fluid (CSF) findings differ among bacterial, tuberculous, fungal, and viral meningitis?

CSF Findings in Bacterial and Nonbacterial Meningitis

	BACTERIAL	VIRAL	MYCOBACTERIAL OR FUNGAL
Total cells (per ml)	Usually > 500	Usually < 500	Usually < 500
WBCs	Predominantly PMN	Predominantly mononuclear	Predominantly mononuclear
Glucose (% of blood)	≤ 40%	> 40%	≤ 40%
Protein (mg/dl)	> 50	> 50	> 50
Gram stain	Positive (65–95%)	Negative	Negative

Differential Diagnosis of CSF Pleocytosis

PREDOMINANTLY POLYMORPHONUCLEAR (> 90%)	PREDOMINANTLY MONONUCLEAR (< 90% PMNS)
Bacterial meningitis	Viral meningitis or encephalitis
Early viral meningitis	Tuberculous or fungal meningitis
Early tuberculous or fungal meningitis	Partially treated bacterial meningitis
Brain abscess or subdural empyema with rupture into subarachnoid space	Brain abscess or subdural empyema
Chemical arachnoiditis	Listeriosis (variable)
	Neurosyphilis
	Neuroborreliosis (Lyme disease)
	Neurocysticercosis
	Neurosarcoidosis

(Table continued on next page.)

Differential Diagnosis of CSF Pleocytosis (cont.)

PREDOMINANTLY POLYMORPHONUCLEAR (> 90%)	PREDOMINANTLY MONONUCLEAR (< 90% PMNS)
	Primary amoebic meningoencephalitis
	Guillain-Barré syndrome
	CNS vasculitis, tumor, hemorrhage
	Multiple sclerosis
	Others

From Kelly WN (ed): Textbook of Internal Medicine, 3rd ed. Philadelphia, Lippincott-Raven, 1997, p 2373, with permission.

40. Name the five leading etiologies of cerebrovascular disease (stroke).
- Embolism
- Atherosclerotic disease
- Lacunar infarcts
- Hypertensive hemorrhage
- Ruptured aneurysms/AV malformation

Cerebrovascular disease is the third leading cause of adult deaths. The major risk factors include hypertension, hypercholesterolemia, smoking, and cardiovascular disease (particularly atrial fibrillation and recent MI). Other causes include advanced age, diabetes mellitus, migraine headaches, and the use of oral contraceptive agents.

41. What are the types and causes of peripheral neuropathies in the adult?

MOTOR	SENSORY	SENSORIMOTOR	
Guillain-Barré syndrome	Alcohol	Diabetes mellitus	Alcohol
	Diabetes mellitus	Uremia	Inherited neuropathies
Porphyria	Vascular disease	Chronic inflammatory	Metronidazole
Lead poisoning	Neoplasm	polyradiculopathy	Colchicine
Sulfonamides	Uremia	Clofibrate	Chlorambucil
Amphotericin B	Arsenic	Chlorpropamide	Tolbutamide
Dapsone		Phenytoin	Ergotamine
Imipramine		Nitrofurantoin	Streptomycin
Amitriptyline		Ethambutol	Ethionamide
Gold		Penicillamine	Gold
		Indomethacin	Phenylbutazone

Farrante JA: Focusing on peripheral neuropathies. Emerg Med 22:57–62, 1990, with permission.

42. Which cranial nerves (CN) are commonly affected in tuberculous meningitis?

These CN palsies may be either unilateral or bilateral and most commonly occur in CN VI (abducens, usually bilateral). Palsies may also develop in CN III (oculomotor) > CN IV (trochlear) > CN II (optic).

Johnson JL, Ellner JJ: Tuberculous meningitis. In Evans RW, Baskins DS, Yatsu FM: Prognosis of Neurological Disorders. Oxford, Oxford University Press, 1992.

43. Which common viral illnesses are frequently seen in adults?

Influenza A > influenza B	Respiratory viruses
Epstein-Barr virus	Rhinoviruses
Herpes simplex virus I and II	Coronaviruses
Varicella-zoster virus	Respiratory syncytial virus
Cytomegalovirus	Parainfluenza virus
	Adenoviruses

44. Which groups are most susceptible to infection by the herpes zoster virus?

Elderly (age > 60)
Patients with Hodgkin's and non-Hodgkin's lymphoma
Immunocompromised patients
    Cancer
    Organ transplant
    AIDS and HIV infection
Patients on high-dose steroid therapy

45. Which organism is responsible for the cellulitis of marine workers and fishermen?

Vibrio vulnificus is a ubiquitous, invasive, gram-negative rod found in warm, salty, coastal waters. It is found in zooplankton and shellfish and has been associated with two disease syndromes: (1) sepsis in alcoholics and persons with liver disease, and (2) wound infections from minor abrasions and/or lacerations. Advanced cases can result in necrotizing vasculitis and gangrene.

46. What organism is the usual pathogen involved in pneumonia in the following scenarios?

Adult viral pneumonia	Influenza, parainfluenza, RSV, adenovirus, hanta virus

Community-Acquired Pneumonia

Smoker	*S. pneumoniae, H. influenzae, Moraxella catarrhalis*
Post-viral bronchitis	*S. pneumoniae*, rarely *Staphylococcus aureus*
Alcoholic	*S. pneumoniae*, anaerobes, coliforms
IV drug abuser	*S. aureus*
Epidemics	Legionnaire's
Bird handlers	Psittacosis
Rabbit handlers	Tularemia
COPD patients	Anaerobes
No co-morbid diseases/risks	Mycoplasma, chlamydia, viral

Hospital-Acquired Pneumonia

Mechanical ventilator	Coliforms, *P. aeruginosa, S. aureus*
Steroid use	Yeast, PCP
Airway obstruction	Anaerobes
Post-stroke (CVA)	*S. pneumoniae*, anaerobes

Eilbert DN, Moellening RC Jr, Sande MA: Sanford Guide to Antimicrobial Therapy, 30th ed. Hyde Park, NY, Antimicrobial Therapy Inc., 2000, p 28, with permission.

47. What factors predispose to acquiring the toxic shock syndrome (TSS)?

TSS is secondary to infection caused by *Staphylococcus aureus*. It should be considered in any patient presenting with fever, rash, and hypotension. Risk factors include:

- Use of high-absorbency tampons
- Diaphragm placement for contraception
- Postoperative wounds (breast augmentation, cesarean section, indwelling catheters)
- Cutaneous infections (especially in the axillary or perianal areas)

Cellulitis	Insect bites
Burns	Abscess

Cunha BA: Case studies in infectious diseases: Toxic shock syndrome. Emerg Med 21:119–126, 1989.

48. Which organisms are commonly implicated in infective endocarditis?

Incidence of Microbial Pathogens in Infective Endocarditis

ORGANISMS	NATIVE VALVE (%)		PROSTHETIC VALVE (%)	
	NONADDICTS	ADDICTS	EARLY (< 2 MOS)	LATE (> 2 MOS)
Streptococci	50–70	20	5–10	25–30
Enterococci	10	8	< 1	5–10

(*Table continued on next page.*)

Incidence of Microbial Pathogens in Infective Endocarditis (cont.)

ORGANISMS	NATIVE VALVE (%)		PROSTHETIC VALVE (%)	
	NONADDICTS	ADDICTS	EARLY (< 2 MOS)	LATE (> 2 MOS)
Staphylococci	25	60	45–50	30–40
(*S. aureus*)	(90)	(99)	(15–20)	(10–12)
(*S. epidermidis*)	(10)	(1)	(25–30)	(23–28)
Gram-negative bacilli	< 1	10	20	10–12
Fungi	< 1	5	10–12	5–8
Diphtheroids	<1	2	5–10	4–5
Miscellaneous organisms	5–10	1–5	1–5	1–5
Multiple	< 1	5	8	8
Culture negative	5–10	10–20	5–10	5–10

From Gorbach, et al (eds): Infectious Diseases. Philadelphia, W.B. Saunders, 1992, 549, with permission.

49. What is the differential diagnosis of generalized lymphadenopathy?

Causes of Generalized Lymphadenopathy*

INFECTIONS		NEOPLASMS	MISCELLANEOUS
Bacterial		Lymphoma	Sarcoidosis
Scarlet fever	Tuberculosis	Acute lymphocytic	Other chronic
Syphilis	Atypical mycobacteria	leukemia	granulomatous
Brucellosis	(Melioidosis)	Chronic lymphocytic	disorders
Leptospirosis	(Glanders)	leukemia	Systemic lupus erythe-
Viral		Other lymphopro-	matosus
HIV/AIDS	Rubella	liferative disorders	Rheumatoid arthritis
Epstein-Barr virus	(Dengue fever)	Immunoblastic	Hyperthyroidism
Cytomegalovirus	(West Nile fever)	lymphadenopathy	Lipid storage diseases
Hepatitis B	(Epidemic hemorrhagic fever)	Reticuloendothelioses	Generalized dermatitis
Measles	(Lassa fever)		Serum sickness
Parasitic			Phenytoin
Toxoplasmosis	(African trypanosomiasis)		
(Kala azar)	(Filariasis)		
(Chagas' disease)			
Rickettsial	**Fungal**		
(Scrub typhus)	Histoplasmosis		

* Parentheses indicate infections that are uncommon or not reported in the United States. Other infections that characteristically may produce regional lymphadenopathy (e.g., tularemia, Lyme disease, lymphogranuloma venereum) rarely cause generalized lymphadenopathy.
Adapted from Libman H: Generalized lymphadenopathy. J Gen Intern Med 2:48–58, 1987.

50. Describe the clinical features of cat scratch fever.

Who: Children represent 75% of the cases
When: Following a cat scratch, bite, or close contact with a cat (in 93% of cases). Usually occurs in fall or winter.
What: Pleomorphic, gram negative, bacillary organism (*Bartonella henselae*)
Symptoms: Primary lesion is raised, slightly tender papule or pustule that:
    May be single or multiple
    Appears 3–10 days after contact with cat
Regional lymphadenopathy including axillary (most common), cervical, preauricular, submandibular, inguinal, femoral, and epitrochlear nodes
Other symptoms and signs: Fever, headache, malaise, rash, anorexia, emesis, splenomegaly, sore throat

Atypical presentations < 5%: lung nodules, liver and spleen lesions; Parinaud's oculoglandular syndrome, CNS manifestations. Ten percent of lesions/nodes suppurate

Diagnosis: Exclude other possibilities
History of contact with a cat
Primary lesion on skin
Regional lymphadenopathy
(+) IFA serology
Skin biopsy or node biopsy—rarely needed
Positive intradermal skin test

Therapy: Azithromycin: Adults (> 45.5kg): 500mg PO × 1 then 250mg/d for 4 days; Children (< 45.5kg): liquid azithromycin 10mg/kg then 5mg/kg/day for 4 days
Treatment is controversial
Will spontaneously resolve without treatment in 2–6 mo
Needle aspiration relieves pain in suppurative nodes; avoid I & D

Gilbert DN, Moellering RC Jr, Sande MA: Sanford Guide to Antimicrobial Therapy, 13th ed. Hyde Park, Antimicrobial Therapy, Inc., 2000, p 31.

51. What are the most frequent presenting clinical features in Lyme disease?

Lyme disease, named after a town on the Connecticut shoreline where the disease was first identified in 1975, is a tick-borne spirochetal infection caused by the fastidious, microphilic bacterium *Borrelia burgdorferi*. Occurrences are more common in the summer and fall. The incidence of Lyme disease corresponds to the habitat of the *Ixodes* tick.

Clinical Features of Lyme Disease

SYMPTOMS		PHYSICAL FINDINGS	
Fatigue	54%	Erythema migrans	75%
Arthralgias	44%	At least one finding	42%
Myalgia	44%	Local lymphadenopathy	23%
Headache	42%	Fever	16%
Fever/chills	39%	Tender neck flexion	9%
Stiff neck	35%		

Nadelman RB: The clinical spectrum of early Lyme Borreliosis in patients with culture-confirmed Erythema Migrans. Am J Med May 100:502–508, 1996.

52. How many clinical stages are observed in Lyme disease?

Clinical Stages of Lyme Disease

STAGE	TIMING	SYMPTOMS
Stage 1 (Localized infection)	Days after tick bite	Erythema migrans (EM), headache, lethargy, malaise, fever, chills
Stage 2 (Disseminated infection)	Days–weeks after tick bite	Cardiac symptoms: prolonged PR interval, fluctuating degrees of AV block, palpitations, syncope. These symptoms can last 6 months or more Neurologic symptoms: usually occur while EM is still present. Include headache, stiff neck, photophobia, CN palsies (Bell's palsy), radiculoneuritis, encephalitis. Skin: multiple annular secondary lesions Joints: arthralgias, joint swelling, muscle pain Eyes: conjunctivitis

(*Table continued on next page.*)

Clinical Stages of Lyme Disease (cont.)

STAGE	TIMING	SYMPTOMS
Stage 3 (Persistent infection)	Months–years after tick bite	Arthritis: asymmetric mono- or oligoarticular pattern with swelling and pain; primarily affects the large joints, (e.g., knees) CNS: memory loss, mood and sleep disturbances Skin: acrodermatitis chronica atrophicans

Steere AC: *Borrelia burgdorferi* (Lyme Disease, Lyme Borreliosis).In Mandell GL, Douglas GD (eds): Bennett's Principles and Practice of Infectious Disease, 5th ed. New York, Churchill Livingstone, 2000, pp 2504–2518.

53. How is spontaneous bacterial peritonitis (SBP) diagnosed?

SBP is an infection of preexisting ascites without an obvious cause for peritoneal contamination (such as trauma or perforation) and has an incidence of 10–25% among patients with liver disease and ascites. It occurs most frequently in patients with Laennec's cirrhosis but also has been described in patients with other types of liver disease, such as chronic active hepatitis, acute viral hepatitis, and metastatic disease. Children with ascites due to nephrosis are also at risk.

SBP usually presents as fever, chills, and abdominal pain or tenderness, but it may be asymptomatic and should be looked for in any patient with ascites who presents with a sudden onset of hypotension or hepatic encephalopathy. It can be diagnosed by demonstrating an ascitic fluid leukocyte count of > 1000/µl or an absolute PMN cell concentration of > 250 µl.

54. Which organisms are most likely to cause SBP? How is this different in selective intestinal decontamination (SID)?

Greater than 60% of SBP cases are due to gram-negative enteric bacteria with *E. coli* and *K. pneumoniae* being the most likely organisms isolated. About 25% of cases are due to gram-positive cocci with streptococcal species topping the list. Anaerobic isolates are infrequently found.

SID, generally accomplished with fluorinated quinolones, suppresses gram-negative bacteria but not gram-positive bacteria. Therefore, patients on SID may have an increased frequency of gram-positive organisms as the etiology for their SBP episodes.

Such J, Rungon BA: Spontaneous bacterial peritonitis. Clin Infect Dis 27:669–676, 1998.

55. Which areas of the GI tract can be involved in Crohn's disease?

Crohn's disease had been reported to affect all areas from the mouth to the anus. The major site of involvement is the **colon**.

56. What is the most common cause of infectious diarrhea?

Enterotoxigenic *Escherichia coli* is the most frequently documented pathogen and the most likely cause of "traveler's diarrhea." There are also a host of viral, bacterial, protozoal, and parasitic causes.

57. What is the significance of projectile emesis?

Projectile emesis is characterized by the forceful expulsion of material from the mouth. It is most commonly observed in gastric outlet obstruction but also may occur in persons with increased intracranial pressure.

58. Name the common etiologies of GI hemorrhage.

UPPER GI HEMORRHAGE	LOWER GI HEMORRHAGE
Peptic ulcer disease	Hemorrhoids
Varices	Angiodysplasia
Esophagitis	Diverticulosis
Mallory-Weiss tear	Carcinoma
Erosive gastritis	Inflammatory bowel disease (Crohn's and ulcerative colitis)
Carcinoma	Polyps
AV malformation	Ischemic colitis

The first four conditions listed in each column are the most common causes, in order of frequency.

59. What symptoms are suggestive of peptic ulcer disease?

Epigastric pain that is described as deep, aching, or gnawing; is relieved with food or antacids; and awakens the patient at night.

60. What conditions precipitate hepatic encephalopathy?

Hepatic encephalopathy is a syndrome comprised of altered mentation (lethargy, obtundation), fetor hepaticus (peculiar odor of the breath in patients with liver disease), and asterixis ("wrist-flapping" tremor) occurring in the patient with underlying hepatic insufficiency. The causes are multifactorial and include:

Factors causing increased blood ammonia:

GI hemorrhage
Constipation
Onset of renal insufficiency (dehydration, diuretics, or acute tubular necrosis)

Increased dietary protein
Metabolic alkalosis
Insufficient treatment with laxatives and lactulose

Factors leading to worsened hepatic insufficiency:

Sedatives and tranquilizers
Analgesics
Viral hepatitis

Hepatorenal syndrome
Progressive hepatocellular dysfunction
Ethanol use

Systemic factors:

Infections
Electrolyte abnormalities
Hypoxemia

Hypercarbia
Hypokalemia

Fraser CL: Hepatic encephalopathy. N Engl J Med 313:865–873, 1985.

61. What are the characteristics of liver diseases associated with pregnancy?

Characteristics of Liver Diseases in Pregnancy

DISEASE	SYMPTOMS	JAUNDICE	TRIMESTER INCIDENCE IN PREGNANCY		LABORATORY VALUES	ADVERSE EFFECTS
Hyperemesis gravidarum	Nausea, vomiting	Mild	1 or 2	0.3–1.0%	Bilirubin < 4 mg/dl, ALT < 200 U/L	Low birth weight
Intrahepatic cholestasis of pregnancy	Pruritus	In 20–60%, 1–4 wk after pruritus starts	2 or 4 in US	0.1–0.2%	Bilirubin < 6 mg/dl, ALT < 3000U/L Increased bile acids	Stillbirth, prematurity, bleeding; fetal mortality 3.5%
Biliary tract disease	Right upper quadrant pain, nausea, vomiting, fever	With common bile duct obstruction	Any	Unknown	If CBD stone, increased bilirubin and GGT	Unknown
Drug-induced	None or nausea, vomiting, pruritus	Early (in cholestatic hepatitis)	Any	Unknown	Variable	Unknown

(Table continued on next page.)

Characteristics of Liver Diseases in Pregnancy (cont.)

DISEASE	SYMPTOMS	JAUNDICE	TRIMESTER INCIDENCE IN PREGNANCY		LABORATORY VALUES	ADVERSE EFFECTS
Acute fatty liver of pregnancy	Upper abdominal pain, nausea, vomiting, confusion late in disease	Common	3	0.008%	ALT < 500 U/I, low glucose; DIC in > 75%, increased bilirubin and ammonia late in disease	Increased maternal mortality (≤ 20%) and fetal mortality (13–18%)
Preeclampsia and eclampsia	Upper abdominal pain, edema, hypertension, mental status changes	Late, 5–14%	2 or 3	5–10%	ALT < 500 U/L (unless infarction), proteinuria, DIC in 7%	Increased maternal mortality (~1%)
HELLP syndrome	Upper abdominal pain, nausea, vomiting, malaise	Late, 5–14%	3	0.1% (4–12% of women with pre-eclampsia)	ALT < 500 U/L, platelets < 100,000/mm^3, hemolysis; increased LDH; DIC in 20–40%	Increased maternal mortality (1–3%) and fetal mortality (35%)
Viral hepatitis	Nausea, vomiting, fever	Common	Any	Same as general population	ALT greatly increased (> 500 U/L), increased bilirubin; DIC rare	Maternal mortality increased with hepatitis E

Knox TA, Olans LB: Liver diseases in pregnancy. N Engl J Med 335:569–576, 1996, with permission.

62. What are the common etiologies of acute pancreatitis?

Alcoholism and gallstones are the most common causes, accounting for 60–80% of cases, and idiopathic acute pancreatitis is the third leading etiology, representing up to 15% of cases.

Causes of Acute Pancreatitis

Alcohol ingestion (acute and chronic alcoholism)

Biliary tract disease (gallstones)

Postoperative state (after abdominal or non-abdominal operation)

Endoscopic retrograde cholangiopancreatography (ERCP), especially manometric studies of sphincter of Oddi trauma (especially blunt abdominal type)

Metabolic causes: hypertriglyceridemia, apolipoprotein CH deficiency syndrome, hypercalcemia (e.g., hyperparathyroidism), drug-induced, renal failure, after renal transplantation, acute fatty liver of pregnancy[**]

Hereditary pancreatitis

Infections: mumps, viral hepatitis, other viral infections (coxsackievirus, echovirus, cytomegalovirus), ascariasis, infections with *Mycoplasma*, *Campylobacter*, *Mycobacterium avium* complex, other bacteria

(Table continued on next page.)

Causes of Acute Pancreatitis (cont.)

Drugs

  Drugs for which association is definite: azathioprine, 6-mercaptopurine, sulfonamides, thiazide diuretics, furosemide, estrogens (oral contraceptives), tetracycline, valproic acid, pentamidine, dideoxyinosine (ddl)

  Drugs for which association is probable: acetaminophen, nitrofurantoin, methyldopa, erythromycin, salicylates, metronidazole , nonsteroidal anti-inflammatory drugs, angiotensin-converting enzyme (ACE) inhibitors

Vascular causes and vasculitis:

  Vascular: ischemic-hypoperfusion state (after cardiac surgery), atherosclerotic emboli

  Connective tissue disorders with vasculitis: systemic lupus erythematosus, necrotizing angiitis, thrombotic thrombocytopenic purpura

Penetrating peptic ulcer

Obstruction of the ampulla of Vater: regional enteritis, duodenal diverticulum

Pancreas divisum

Causes to be considered in patients having recurrent bouts of acute pancreatitis without an obvious cause: occult disease of the biliary tree or pancreatic ducts, especially occult gallstones (microlithiasis, sludge), drugs, hypertriglyceridemia, pancreas divisum, pancreatic cancer, sphincter of Oddi dysfunction, cystic fibrosis, truly idiopathic

---

* Pancreatitis occurs in 3 percent of renal transplant patients and is due to many factors, including surgery, hypercalcemia, drugs (glucocorticoids, azathioprine, L-asparaginase, diuretics), and viral infections.
** Pancreatitis also occurs in otherwise uncomplicated pregnancy and is most often associated with cholelithiasis.
Fauci AS, et al: Harrison's Principles of Internal Medicine, 14th ed. New York, McGraw-Hill, 1998, p 1742, with permission.

63. What are common causes of jaundice in adults?

Biliary tract obstruction	Hepatocellular dysfunction
Gallstones	Hepatitis
Tumor	Viral
Pancreatic neoplasm	Alcohol-induced
Congestive heart failure	Drug-induced
Hepatocellular carcinoma	Cirrhosis

64. What is the carcinoid syndrome?

The carcinoid syndrome is a symptom complex caused by carcinoid tumors, which are the most common endocrine tumors of the digestive tract. These tumors arise from enterochromaffin cells and have the ability to produce a wide variety of biologically active amines and peptides, including serotonin, bradykinin, histamine, ACTH, prostaglandins, and others. Because the liver, via the portal circulation, receives blood from the digestive tract and clears these products from the blood prior to their entry into the systemic circulation, most patients do not manifest symptoms until hepatic metastases occur.

Patients usually present with "cutaneous flushing" episodes, which typically are red in the beginning and then become purple, start on the face and then spread to the trunk, and last several minutes. These episodes are often accompanied by tachycardia and hypotension. Symptoms are paroxysmal in character and provoked by alcohol, stress, or palpation of the liver and may be triggered by the administration of catecholamines, pentagastrin, or reserpine. The tumors can also cause diarrhea, crampy abdominal pain, obstruction, GI bleeding, and malabsorption.

65. Discuss the two theories of site-specific tumor metastases.

Certain tumors exhibit site-specific metastases, indicating a tendency of these tumors to spread preferentially to specific sites. The two theories proposed to explain this phenomenon, both of which are valid in selected cases, are:

1. The **seed and soil hypothesis** was proposed by Stephen Paget in 1889 and hypothesizes that certain tumors tend to spread to tissues that have the ability to support the tumor's growth.

2. The **mechanical hypothesis**, proposed by James Ewing in 1928, theorizes that certain tumors spread to specific tissues because these tissues lie in the path of blood flow that carries tumor cells away from the primary site.

Zetter BR: The cellular basis of site-specific tumor metastases. N Engl J Med 322:605–612, 1990.

66. Which drugs can cause gingival hyperplasia?

Phenytoin, cyclosporine, and nifedipine.

Butler RT, et al: Drug-induced gingival hyperplasia: Phenytoin, cyclosporine and nifedipine. J Am Dent Assoc 114:56–60, 1987.

67. Which drugs are frequently abused in the U.S.? What are some of their common street names?

DRUG	COMMON STREET NAMES/TERMS
Alcohol	Booze, spirits
Marijuana (#1 illegal drug used)	Weed, joints, grass, pot, reefers, Acapulco gold, Mary Jane, blunts
Cocaine	Crack, rock
PCP (phencyclidine)	Angel dust, hog, dust, bromide fluid, elephant tranquilizer, animal tranquilizer, or monkey dust, killer weed, rocket fuel, supergrass
Amphetamines	
Amphetamine	White crosses, black beauties
Dextroamphetamine	Dexies
Methamphetamine	Speed, Ice, crystal, meth, Hawaiian ice, crank
Designer drugs	
Gamma-hydroxybutyrate (GHB)	Easy lady, liquid x, Georgia home boy, gamma-oh, everclear, water, wolfies, vita G, poor man's heroin, goop
Flunitrazepam (rohypnol)	Rophies, circles, forget pill, Mexican valium, "drop drug," roaches
Amphetamine analogues	
3,4 methylenedioxyamphetamine (MDA)	Love drug, love pulls
3,4-methylenedioxymethamphetamine (MDMA)	Ecstasy, XTC, Adam, California sunrise, E, hug drug, love drug, M&M, ice
3,4-methylenedioxymethamphetamine (MDEA)	Eve
Alphamethyl fentanyl	White china
Hallucinogens (psychedelics)	
LSD (lysergic acid diethylamide)	Acid, dots, microdots, cubes, window panes or blotters, acid, doses, trips
Psilocybin (psychedelic mushrooms)	Shrooms
Volatile substances	Glue, cement, gasoline, airplane glue (toluene), amyl nitrate; fluorinated hydrocarbons (freon), typewriter fluid (trichloroethylene) Sniffing, huffing, bagging are terms identifying how they are inhaled
Prescription drugs	Benzodiazepines: diazepam (Valium) and alprazolam (Xanax), narcotic analgesics: codeine, morphine, fentanyl, meperidine, hydrocodone, etc.

Schulz JE: Illicit drugs of abuse. Substance abuse. Prim Care 20(1):221–230, 1993.
Drug Enforcement Administration, US Department of Justice www.usdoj.gov/dea/index.htm
Ropero-Miller JD, Goldberger BA: Recreational drugs: Current trends in the 90's. Toxicol Clin Lab Med 18(4):727–746, 1998.
Finen J: Prescription drug abuse. Substance abuse. Prim Care 20(1):231–239, 1993.

68. What are the stages of cocaine use and cessation?

The high: Euphoria, increased self-confidence, increased energy, increased ability to do work

Levels drop: Feel depressed, irritable, restless and generally uncomfortable

Abstinence syndrome: Crash, cravings, withdrawal, and extinction

1. The "crash": depression, anxiety, and agitation
2. Prolonged sleeping followed by intense food cravings
3. Withdrawal: decreased energy, anhedonia, dysphoria, and reduced normal activities lasts 6–18 weeks after last use (a common time for relapse)
4. Extinction phase: return to usual state of activities, energy, and interests

A major side effect with continued abuse is paranoia, aka "armed paranoia." Combined with their increased energy levels, abusers often exhibit erratic and aggressive or violent behaviors.

69. How do overdoses of tricyclic antidepressant (TCA) medications cause death?

TCAs are the third most frequent cause of drug-related deaths. More than two-thirds of deaths occur in women. The agents most commonly implicated are amitriptyline, desipramine, and nortriptyline. The pathogenetic mechanisms of death include:

Cardiovascular arrhythmias	Respiratory arrest
Ventricular fibrillation	Intractable seizures
Prolonged QRS	CNS depression/coma
Asystole	

70. What antidotes are available for common drug and chemical overdoses?

DRUG	ANTIDOTE AND DOSAGE
Acetaminophen	N-acetylcysteine (Mucomyst, Mucosil-10): 140 mg/kg initially, followed by 70 mg/kg every 8 hrs for 17 doses
Narcotics	Naloxone (Narcan): 0.4–2.0 mg IV. Can be repeated at 2–3-min intervals
Benzodiazepines	Flumazenil (Romazicon): 0.3 mg IV. Additional doses of 0.5 mg over 30 sec at 1-min intervals to a cumulative dose of 3 mg
Anticholinergic agents	Physostigmine: 2 mg by slow IV. Repeat in 20 min; if no improvement, followed by 1–2 mg IV for recurrent symptoms
Methanol, ethylene glycol	Ethanol (absolute): 1 ml/kg in D_5W IV over 15 min. Maintenance dose: 125 mg/kg/hr IV in D_5W
Digoxin	Digoxin immune FAB (ovine): (Digibind). Can vary by serum concentration of digoxin, but on average, ten (10) vials can be given to start. For large unknown amounts of digoxin, give 20 vials (760 mg) IV reconstituted with sterile water for injection, preferably through a micron membrane
Phenothiazines, haloperidol, Loxitane	Diphenhydramine: 25-50 mg; or benztropine: 1–2 mg (may be given IV or IM)
Cyanide	Sodium nitrite: 300 mg IV; or sodium thiosulfate: 12.5 gm
Organophosphates (insecticides)	Atropine sulfate: 2–5 mg IV. Repeat every 10–30 min to maintain a decrease in bronchial secretions. After atropine, pralidoxime: 1 mg IV for 2 doses. Repeat every 8–12 hrs for 3 doses if muscle weakness is not relieved

Guzzardi LJ: Role of the emergency physician in poisoning. Med Clin North Am 2:10–11, 1982.
Physician's Desk Reference, 54th ed. Montvale, NJ, Medical Economics Company, Inc., 2000.

71. A 19-year-old girl is admitted with salicylate poisoning. What acid-base disturbances are seen in this condition on serial blood gas monitoring?

Acute salicylate intoxication is characterized by profound effects on acid-base balance. Early in the course of intoxication, there is a primary **respiratory alkalosis** resulting from direct stimulation of the respiratory center in the medulla by salicylates. This causes an increase in pH and fall in $PaCO_2$. A compensatory **metabolic acidosis** due to renal excretion of bicarbonate may be seen, which tends to bring the pH back toward normal. In young adults and children (especially with toxic doses), a primary metabolic acidosis ensues due to:

1. Impaired hepatic carbohydrate metabolism leading to accumulation of ketones and lactate in plasma.
2. Accumulated salicylic acid itself, which displaces several meq of bicarbonate.
3. Dehydration and hypotension impair renal excretion of inorganic acids and cause further metabolic acidosis.

The resulting primary metabolic acidosis is normochloremic and associated with a high anion gap. The continuation of primary respiratory alkalosis and metabolic acidosis should give a clue to the diagnosis of acute salicylate intoxication. In more severe cases, primary respiratory acidosis occurs due to the depression of the respiratory center at very high salicylate levels.

72. What are the initial steps in the assessment and treatment of a patient with a suspected drug overdose?

- Control airway
- Check vital signs (blood pressure, respiration, pulse, temperature)
- Stabilize any abnormalities in vital signs
- Check mental status/level of consciousness
- Obtain blood for laboratory studies (chemistries, arterial blood gases, toxicology screen)
- IV fluid: D5W with thiaminenaloxone
- Quick physical exam (heart, lungs, abdomen, neurologic)

Goldfrank LJR, et al: Management of overdose with psychoactive medications. Med Clin North Am 2:65, 1982.

73. Which organs are frequently damaged by intravenous drug abuse (IVDA)?

In descending order of frequency: the lung, heart, and kidneys.

74. Which infectious diseases are commonly observed among IVDAs?

Persons who are IVDAs run a high risk of acquiring serious infections from all classes of pathogens, and any organ system may be affected.

Common Infections in IV Drug Abusers

CNS	Lungs	Heart
Meningitis	Septic pulmonary emboli	Endocarditis
Mycotic aneurysm	Pneumonia	*S. aureus* (> 50% of cases)
Focal neurologic infections:	*S. pneumoniae*	Strep. groups A, B & G (2nd
1. Abscess	*S. aureus*	most common)
2. Subdural empyema	Aspiration (anaerobes)	Polymicrobial
Eye	*P. aeruginosa*	Noncandidal sp. (5%)
Endophthalmitis	Abscess	Enterococcus ($\downarrow$ frequency)
Fungal (candida)	Empyema	Gram-negative bacilli
Bacterial (*S. aureus*)	Tuberculosis	(infrequent)
Abdomen	**Muscle**	**Noncardiac Vascular Infections**
Hepatitis A, B, C, D, G	Necrotizing fascitis ± myositis	Septic thrombophlebitis
Splenic abscess	Pyomyositis	Mycotic aneurysms
		Both due to *S. aureus*
		(Table continued on next page.)

Common Infections in IV Drug Abusers (cont.)

Skin	Joints	HIV Infection
Cellulitis	Osteomyelitis (esp. LS spine)	(most common infection in IVDAs)
S. aureus	Septic arthritis (mostly knee)	AIDS
Streptococci	**Genitourinary**	AIDS-related
Gram negative bacilli	Sexually transmitted diseases	*Pneumocystis carinii*
Suppurative phlebitis	(GC & syphilis)	pneumonia
Skin ulcers	Renal abscesses	Cytomegalovirus
		Toxoplasmosis
		Cryptococcal meningitis
		Mycobacterium avium complex
		H. influenzae pneumonia

Levine DP, Brown PD: Infections in injection drug users. In Mandell GL, Bennett JE, Dolin R (eds): Principles and Practice of Infectious Disease, 5th ed. New York, Churchill Livingstone, 2000, pp 3112–3126.

75. What factors indicate a poor prognosis in hypertension?

1. Black race
2. Youth
3. Male sex
4. Persistent diastolic pressure > 115 mmHg
5. Smoking
6. Diabetes mellitus
7. Hypercholesterolemia
8. Obesity
9. Excessive alcohol intake
10. Evidence of end-organ damage
   a. Cardiac (cardiac enlargement, ECG changes of ischemia or left ventricular strain, MI, CHF)
   b. Eyes (retinal exudates, hemorrhages, and papilledema)
   c. Renal (impaired renal function)
   d. Nervous system (cerebrovascular accident)

Williams GH: Hypertensive vascular disease. In Fauci AS, et al (eds): Harrison's Principles of Internal Medicine, 14th ed. New York, McGraw-Hill, 1998, p 1383, with permission.

76. Which valves are most frequently affected in rheumatic heart disease?

In order of frequency: the mitral valve is the most commonly involved. The aortic valve is often involved, and the tricuspid, although rare, is more frequently involved than the pulmonic valve.

77. What are the etiologies of the common cardiac arrhythmias seen in adults?

ARRHYTHMIA	RATE (BPM)	ETIOLOGIES
Sinus tachycardia	100–200	Fever, pain, drugs, hyperthyroidism, hypotension
Paroxysmal supraventricular tachycardia (PSVT)	130–220 (usually 160)	Pre-excitation syndrome (Wolff-Parkinson-White syndrome), AV nodal re-entry, congenital abnormalities, atrial septal defect, concealed accessory bypass tracts
Atrial flutter	Atrial, 250–350 Ventricular, 150–220	Mitral valve disease, COPD, pulmonary embolus, alcohol abuse, organic heart disease, MI, cardiac surgery
Atrial fibrillation	Atrial, 350–500 Ventricular, 100–160	Myocardial ischemia, MI, organic heart disease, rheumatic heart disease, alcohol abuse, CHF, elderly patients, febrile illness, hyperthyroidism, chest surgery

(Table continued on next page.)

ARRHYTHMIA	RATE (BPM)	ETIOLOGIES
Ventricular tachycardia	100–230	Ischemic heart disease, MI, mitral valve prolapse, cardiomyopathy, hypercalcemia, hypokalemia, hypomagnesemia, hypoxemia

78. How do you differentiate the common tachyarrhythmias?

	SINUS TACHYCARDIA	PAROXYSMAL ATRIAL TACHYCARDIA	ATRIAL FIBRILLATION	ATRIAL FLUTTER	VENTRICULAR TACHYCARDIA
Rate	100–200	169–190	160–190	140–160	100–230
Rhythm	Regular	Regular	Irregular	Regular	Slightly irregular
QRS shape	Normal[*]	Normal[*]	Normal[*]	Normal[*]	Abnormal
Atrial activity	Sinus P wave[†]	Absent or nonsinus P wave[†]	Absent	Flutter waves	Sinus P waves[†]
P-QRS relation	Yes	May be masked by rapid ventricular rate	No	May be masked by rapid ventricular rate	No
Carotid massage	Slows	No response, or converts to sinus rhythm	No response	Increased block	No response

[*] Unless intraventricular conduction disturbance.
[†] Sinus P waves are upright in lead II and occur at least 0.12 sec before the QRS complex begins.
From Gottlieb AJ, et al: The Whole Internist Catalog. Philadelphia, W.B. Saunders, 1980, p 158, with permission.

79. Discuss the mechanism of Cheyne-Stokes breathing in patients with severe CHF.

In the patient with left ventricular failure, the circulation time between the lungs and respiratory center of the brain is slowed. This delay causes the system to respond sluggishly, leading to the oscillations in breathing patterns observed in Cheyne-Stokes respiration. Cheyne-Stokes breathing, also known as periodic or cyclic breathing, is characterized by periods of apnea alternating with hyperpnea. During apnea, the PCO_2 rises and PO_2 falls, causing stimulation of the brain center. The end result is hyperventilation. This results in a fall in the PCO_2, which results in suppression of the respiratory drive, and another period of apnea ensues.

80. Which classes of medications should be given cautiously to persons with a prolonged QT interval?

Antiarrhythmic drugs from class IA, IC and III can prolong QT intervals and should be avoided or withdrawn if prolongation of the QT interval develops. Example of class IA include: quinidine, procainamide, disopyramide; class IC: flecainide, propafenone; class III: amiodarone, sotalol, bretylium tosylate. Others include phenothiazines, certain antibiotics, pentamidine, terfenadine, antidepressants, and cocaine.

81. What are the causes of prolonged QT intervals?

The QT interval can be prolonged due to congenital (Romano-Ward syndrome and Jervell-Lange-Nielson syndrome) or acquired (usually secondary to medications) causes. Hypomagnesemia, hypokalemia, and bradycardia can contribute to the risk.

82. What are the manifestations of digitalis toxicity?

1. **Arrhythmias:** the most dangerous and, unfortunately, often the first manifestation. Many different brady- and tachyarrhythmias have been described. The more common include supraventricular tachycardia with AV block, ventricular ectopy, all degrees of AV block, and sinoatrial or AV nodal exit block.

2. **Neurologic:** headache, fatigue, lethargy, confusion, delirium, seizures, and malaise

3. **Gastrointestinal:** nausea, vomiting, diarrhea, anorexia

4. **Visual:** disturbed color vision (greenish or yellow tinting, halos around objects), blurred vision, photophobia

5. **Endocrine:** gynecomastia in males

83. What special management does a non-Q-wave MI require?

A non-Q-wave MI (NQWMI) has a better short-term prognosis, but these patients are at higher risk of reinfarction or extension of the infarct area, early onset of postinfarction pain, and an overall higher late mortality rate.

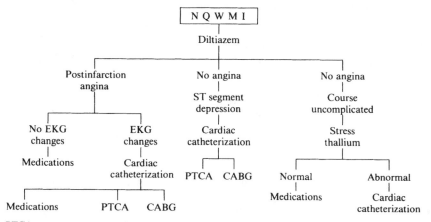

PTCA = percutaneous transluminal coronary angioplasty; CABG = coronary artery bypass grafting.

84. When is corrective surgery indicated in patients with aortic stenosis?

Once symptoms of aortic stenosis (AS) develop, patients should be considered for valve replacement. The typical symptoms include heart failure, angina, and syncope. Any of these symptoms depict severe AS (estimated valve area < 0.8 cm^2) and has an estimated 3-year mortality of 50%.

85. When do ventricular premature depolarizations (VPDs) warrant medical therapy?

VPDs, or premature ventricular contractions (PVCs), occur in asymptomatic individuals without cardiac problems, in acute situations such as post-myocardial infarctions, and in patients with cardiac diseases. Each is treated differently. When they occur in asymptomatic individuals, therapy is usually not warranted, and patients should be counseled to avoid aggravating factors (caffeinated products, tobacco, stimulants, etc.) and given reinforcement. PVCs after a myocardial infarction are usually accepted as a "warning arrhythmia" and treated with IV lidocaine as the drug of choice. In cardiac conditions, patients face a higher risk of sudden death, and PVCs are usually suppressed with beta-blockers. Newest data conclude that asymptomatic middle-aged men with PVCs during exertion may have an increased risk of death from cardiovascular diseases long-term.

Myerburg RJ, Kessler KM, Castellanos A: Recognition, clinical assessment, and management of arrhythmias and conduction disturbances. In Alexander RW, et al (eds): Hurst's The Heart, 9th ed. New York, McGraw-Hill, 1998, pp 905–909.

Jouven X, et al: Long-term outcome in asymptomatic men with exercise-induced premature ventricular depolarizations. N Engl J Med 343(12):826–833, 2000.

86. What is torsade de pointes?

Torsade de pointes (pronounced *tōr-sahd' dĕ pwahnt*), or "twisting of the points," is a polymorphic ventricular tachycardia characterized by QRS complexes that change in amplitude and electrical polarity, appearing to "twist" around the isoelectric line. A prolonged QT interval must be present. There may also be U waves.

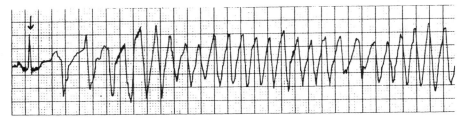

Torsade de pointes. A single sinus beat (arrow) is followed by ventricular tachycardia with an oscillating or swinging pattern of QRS complexes. (From Seelig CB: Simplified EKG Analysis. Philadelphia, Hanley & Belfus, 1992, p 75, with permission.)

87. What are the etiologies of torsade de pointes?

Quinidine	Hypokalemia	Amiodarone	Hypomagnesemia
Psychotropic drugs	Myocardial ischemia	Procainamide	Myocarditis
Phenothiazines	Tumors	Subarachnoid hemorrhage	Trauma
Lithium	Severe bradycardia	Third-degree heart block	CNS lesions
Tricyclic antidepressants	Disopyramide		

Saffer J, et al: Polymorphous ventricular tachycardia associated with normal and long Q-T intervals. Am J Cardiol 49:2021–2029, 1982.

88. Name the risk factors for the development of coronary artery disease (CAD).

Positive Risk Factors (increase risk)

Age

Male: 45 years

Female: 55 years or premature menopause without estrogen replacement therapy

Family history of premature CAD (definite MI or sudden death before age 55 in father or other male first-degree relative, or before age 65 in mother or other female first degree relative)

Current cigarette smoking

Hypertension (BP 140/90 mmHg confirmed by several measurements or taking anti-hypertensive medication)

Elevated LDL cholesterol

Low HDL cholesterol (< 35 mg/dl or 0.9 mmol/L confirmed by several measurements)

Diabetes mellitus

Negative Risk Factor (decrease risk)

High HDL cholesterol (> 60 mg/dl or 1.6 mmol/L)

Summary of the second report of the National Cholesterol Education Program (NCEP) expert panel on detection, evaluation, and treatment of high blood cholesterol in adults (Adult Treatment Panel II). JAMA 269:3015–3023, 1993, with permission.

89. What hormonal change in women increases their risk of coronary artery disease (CAD)?

Menopause. The risk of CAD, while lower in premenopausal females than in age-matched males, rapidly increases in postmenopausal females.

90. A 35-year-old black man with a past history of nephrotic syndrome is admitted for elective knee surgery. He has been taking ibuprofen for 3 weeks. His admission serum creatinine is 3 mg/dl. What points help you to differentiate acute renal failure (ARF) from chronic renal failure (CRF)?

This patient with a previous history of nephrotic illness has been taking an NSAID and has a moderate degree of renal insufficiency. This could be ARF induced by the NSAID or could be an unrecognized progressive CRF. Urinary sediment can be useful in this situation. Acute interstitial nephritis is associated with red and white blood cell casts, whereas CRF is associated with broad casts (usually two to three times the diameter of a WBC). The presence of significant anemia, hyperphosphatemia, hypocalcemia, and changes of renal osteodystrophy are suggestive of advanced CRF. The most important confirmation of chronicity is demonstration of shrunken or small kidneys by ultrasound or CT scanning.

91. How do nonsteroidal anti-inflammatory drugs (NSAIDs) cause acute renal failure?

The NSAIDs inhibit cyclooxygenase, an enzyme responsible for synthesizing prostaglandins from arachidonic acid. The intrarenal production of prostaglandins, especially PGE_2, contributes significantly to the maintenance of renal blood flow (RBF) and glomerular filtration rate (GFR) in states of diminished effective arterial blood volume. In any of the prerenal states, angiotensin II and norepinephrine production is increased, which in turn increases renal vasodilator prostaglandin synthesis and thus leads to improvement of renal ischemia. The NSAIDs have the potential to significantly lower RBF and GFR in certain disease states (such as hypovolemia, CHF, nephrotic syndrome, and lupus nephritis) and to produce ARF. An acute interstitial nephritis associated with nephrotic syndrome may also occur, particularly after the use of fenoprofen.

92. Who is at highest risk for NSAID-induced renal failure?

Elderly patients
Patients on angiotensin-converting enzyme (ACE) inhibitors and/or beta-blockers
Patients receiving > 1 NSAID (i.e., aspirin and indomethacin)
Diabetics
Patients on diuretics or who are dehydrated
Patients with underlying CHF

93. Which conditions related to pregnancy predispose to acute renal failure (ARF)?

Although its incidence has declined markedly with control of septic abortions and antenatal care, ARF is not uncommon in pregnancy. Toxemia of pregnancy, antepartum hemorrhage, and postpartum hemorrhage are associated with an increased risk of ARF. Other predisposing factors include postpartum sepsis, abortion, postpartum hemolytic uremia syndrome, and amniotic fluid embolism. In addition, acute fatty liver and urinary tract obstruction are occasionally associated with ARF during pregnancy.

94. Describe the physiologic changes in the kidney during pregnancy.

Pregnancy is associated with an increase in GFR of about 50% and a mild decrease in plasma creatinine and BUN. There is a slight increase in kidney size (about 1 cm) and dilation and tortuosity of the ureters. These changes were believed secondary to pressure by the gravid uterus, but it is now known that these changes can be related to increased progesterone levels. Other physiologic changes include increased uric acid clearance, resulting in slight hypouricemia.

95. How does aging affect the kidney?

1. Diminished glomerular filtration rate (GFR)
2. Decreased creatinine production (due to decreased muscle mass)
3. Obstructive uropathy (due to benign prostatic hypertrophy)
4. Urinary incontinence

96. List the most common etiologies of ARF in hospitalized patients.

- Hypoperfusion (approximately 50%)
  - Dehydration
  - CHF
- Postoperative renal failure
- Obstruction

- Drugs (especially aminoglycosides)
- Sepsis
- Arrhythmia
- IV contrast dye
- Hepatorenal syndrome

97. Which class of antihypertensive agents is contraindicated in patients with bilateral renal artery stenosis?

Angiotensin-converting enzyme (ACE) inhibitors. In bilateral renal artery stenosis or stenosis to a solitary kidney, the renal perfusion pressure (and thus GFR) depends on the local renin-angiotensin system. When the system is blocked by an ACE inhibitor, a marked decrease in the efferent arterial pressure with subsequent decrease in renal perfusion pressure results, causing a diminished GFR.

98. What does the presence of eosinophils in urine denote?

Normal urine does not contain eosinophils, so their presence in a urine sample points to renal disease. The contribution of eosinophils to the immune response is not clearly known, but they are activated by antigens and antigen-induced hypersensitivity reactions. Eosinophils in the urine are characteristic of tubulo-interstitial disease (i.e., interstitial nephritis), especially if they comprise > 5% of the total number of WBCs in the sample. Eosinophils in the urine are seen in:

Interstitial nephritis   Acute tubular necrosis
Urinary tract infections   Hepatorenal syndrome
Kidney transplant rejection
Carwin HL, et al: Clinical correlates of eosinophiluria. Arch Intern Med 145:1097–1099, 1985.

99. What three findings comprise the hyporeninemic-hypoaldosteronism syndrome?

1. Low serum aldosterone levels (due to impaired secretion)
2. Low serum renin levels
3. Hyperkalemia (which is more severe than expected by the degree of renal insufficiency)

Clinical Characteristics in Patients with Hyporeninemic Hypoaldosteronism

Mean age	65 yrs
Asymptomatic hyperkalemia	75%
Chronic renal insufficiency	70%
Diabetes mellitus	50%
Cardiac arrhythmias	25%
Normal aldosterone response to ACTH	25%

100. In CRF patients, what is the importance of the $Ca^{++} \times PO_4^-$ product (calcium-phosphate product)?

When the product of the serum concentrations of calcium and phosphate exceeds 70, metastatic calcifications are more likely to occur. Calcium phosphate ($CaPO_4$) may precipitate out of the plasma and deposit in arteries, soft tissues, periarticular areas, and viscera.

101. Which organisms typically colonize the bronchioles of smokers?

Haemophilus influenzae
Streptococcus pneumoniae
Moraxella catarrhalis
A variety of respiratory viruses

102. What are the common etiologies of diffuse bilateral interstitial lung infiltrates?

Pulmonary edema

Miliary tuberculosis

Pneumocystis carinii pneumonia

Lymphangitic spread of carcinoma
(breast, gastric)

Sarcoidosis

Lymphoma

Idiopathic

Drugs/toxins

Nitrofurantoin

Amiodarone

Sulfonamides

Zidovudine

Bleomycin

Methotrexate

Cyclophosphamide

Chlorambucil

Crystal RG, et at: Interstitial lung disease of unknown cause. N Engl J Med 310:154–166, 235–244, 1984.

103. Where do you find Hampton's hump?

Hampton's hump, named after Aubrey Otis Hampton (1900–1955), a U.S. radiologist, is a radiographic finding that is highly suggestive of a pulmonary infarction. It is a dense, homogeneous, wedge-shaped consolidation occurring in the middle and lower lobes. The base is contiguous with the pleura, but the apex points, in a convex fashion, toward the hilum. This gives the appearance of a hump.

104. How are lung cancers classified? What are the most common types?

Lung cancers are classified into small cell lung cancer (SCLC) and non-small cell lung cancer (NSCLC). NSCLC accounts for over 80% of all lung cancers. There are several types of non-small cell cancers; adenocarcinoma makes up the majority of the NSCLC (32%). Others include squamous cell, large cell, epidermoid, bronchioloalveolar carcinoma and mixed versions of all of these.

105. Which skin cancer is most common in adults?

Non-melanoma skin cancers are the most common and include basal cell carcinoma (the most common skin neoplasm worldwide), and squamous cell carcinoma. Basal cell carcinoma occurs 4–10 times as frequently as squamous cell carcinoma. The primary risk factor is excessive sun exposure, especially in fair-skinned individuals, and 90% of tumors occur in sun-exposed areas of the skin. Basal cell carcinomas are divided into six types: nodular, pigmented, cystic, sclerosing, superficial, and nevoid. Metastasis is very rare, and the prognosis is usually excellent, although deaths from local extension do occur. Therapy is based on location and extent of the tumor. Removal of the tumor, by a variety of means, is curative in 90% of the cases.

Jerant AF, et al: Early detection and treatment of skin cancer. Am Fam Physician 62(2):357–368, 2000.

106. Which skin cancer is associated with the highest mortality? What are its risk factors?

Melanoma causes the largest number of deaths related to skin cancer.

Risk Factors for Cutaneous Melanoma

High risk (> 50-fold increased risk)

Persistently changing mole

Atypical moles in patients with 2 family members with melanoma

Adulthood (vs. childhood)

> 50 nevi ≥ 2 mm

Intermediate risk (approximately 10-fold increased risk)

Family history of melanoma

Sporadic atypical moles

Congenital nevi (?)

Whites (vs. black or East Asian ethnicity)

Prior history of melanoma

(Table continued on next page.)

Risk Factors for Cutaneous Melanoma (cont.)

Low risk (2–4-fold increase in risk)
Immunosuppression
Sun sensitivity or excess exposure

Sober AJ, et al: Melanoma and other skin cancers. In Fauci AS, et al (eds): Harrison's Principles of Internal Medicine, 14th ed. New York, McGraw-Hill, 1998, p 544, with permission.

107. What criteria should be remembered when evaluating a lesion suspicious for a melanoma?

The **ABCD** rule lists the key criteria for evaluating these lesions:

A = Asymmetry
B = Border irregularity
C = Color variation (usually purple/black)
D = Diameter > 6 mm

Jerant AF, et al: Early detection and treatment of skin cancer. Am Fam Physician 62(2):357–368, 2000.

108. What are actinic keratoses? In whom do they occur?

What:	Benign dysplasia of the epidermis. Multiple erythematous or tan plaques with an adherent scaly surface
Whom:	Most common in elderly patients
Where:	Sun-exposed areas: face, dorsal surface of hands, forearms, balding scalp
Risk:	< 1% risk of developing squamous cell carcinoma in early lesions and up to 20% in late lesions
Treatment:	Primary prevention: use of sunscreens and protective clothing and prophylaxis (topical vitamin C) Medical: 2–% topical 5-fluorouracil twice daily for 2–5 weeks Surgical: excision

109. Are tinea versicolor and vitiligo manifestations of the same disease?

No. The differences are shown in the following table.

	VITILIGO	TINEA
Etiology	? Autoimmune	Fungal infection
Pathology	Destruction of melanocytes	Decreased melanosomes in the stratum corneum
Incidence	1%	Common
Age of onset	Young adults	Young adults
Description	Macular depigmented areas Absence of melanin	Small hypopigmented-to-tan macules with a bran-like scale
Associated conditions	Graves' disease, pernicious anemia, diabetes mellitus, Addison's disease	Seborrhea
Diagnosis	Chalk-white under Wood's lamp Absence of melanocytes on skin biopsy	Gold fluorescence on Wood's lamp Spores/hyphae on skin biopsy KOH = positive, "spaghetti and meatballs" appearance
Therapy	Trioxsalen with sun exposure at least two times a week	Selenium sulfide, sulfur ointments, ketoconazole, salicylic acid

110. How do a chancre and a chancroid ulcer differ?

	CHANCRE	CHANCROID ULCER
Disease	Syphilis	Chancroid (a disease in itself)
Organism	*Treponema pallidum*	*Haemophilus ducreyi*
Description	Painless papule that rapidly erodes. Edge feels cartilaginous. Indurated.	Painful, superficial ulcer with ragged edges. Base is covered by necrotic exudate. More often multiple.
Location	Penis, cervix/labia, and anus/rectum/ mouth in homosexuals	Males: Preputial orifice, prepuce, frenulum Females: labia, clitoris, vestibule
Treatment	Penicillin G, tetracycline	Trimethoprim/sulfamethoxazole, erythromycin

111. What are petechiae?
Small, 1–3 mm, round, reddish or brown lesions that do not blanch. They are caused by hemorrhage into the skin. They are commonly seen in platelet disorders and vasculitic processes.

112. When should a mole be removed?

Indications for Removal of a Mole

Change in size or diameter	Onset of bleeding, itching, or pain
Color becomes darker or lighter	Increase in height
Development of irregular borders	Congenital moles after one reaches adulthood
Elevation of the surface	(> 50 yrs)

Rhodes AR, et al: Risk factors for cutaneous melanoma. JAMA 258:3146–3154, 1987.

113. What are cutaneous manifestations of hyperthyroidism?

Warm, moist, "velvety" texture of skin	Vitiligo
Increased palmar/dorsal sweating	Altered hair texture
Facial flushing	Alopecia
Palmar erythema	Pretibial myxedema

114. Which cardiac abnormality is a common cause of CHF in the elderly hypertensive patient?
Hypertensive hypertrophic cardiomyopathy. The disease is characterized by:
1. Severe concentric cardiac hypertrophy
2. Small left ventricular cavity
3. Elevated left ventricular ejection fraction

Tapale J, et al: Hypertensive hypertrophic cardiomyopathy of the elderly. N Engl J Med 312:277–283, 1985.

115. What is the frequency of asymptomatic bacteriuria in patients over age 65? Is treatment necessary?
Asymptomatic bacteriuria is present in at least 20% of women and 10% of men over age 65. Treatment is not necessary unless it is associated with an obstructive uropathy.

Boscia JA, et al: Asymptomatic bacteriuria in the elderly. Infect Dis Clin North Am 1:893–905, 1987.

116. Headaches in an elderly patient should always alert one to the possibility of which illness?
Temporal (giant cell) arteritis should be considered in any patient over age 50 with a headache. Untreated temporal arteritis can result in irreversible monocular blindness. Symptoms include:

- Continuous, throbbing, unilateral "temporal" headache
- Claudication of jaw when chewing and/or talking
- Transient loss of vision (amaurosis fugax), visual-field deficits, diplopia, sudden visual loss
- Symptoms of polymyalgia rheumatica (girdle-hip pain) seen in 50% of patients
- Tender, swollen, red, nodular temporal artery with decreased pulsation on palpation seen in two-thirds of patients
- Fever
- Weight loss

117. What are the leading causes of blindness in the elderly?
- Cataracts
- Glaucoma
- Retinopathies
- Temporal arteritis
- Diabetes mellitus (DM)

118. What are the common presentations of type 1 DM versus type 2 DM?

	TYPE 1	TYPE 2
Age	< 40 years	> 40 years, elderly
Onset	Short period	Insidious, found incidentally on lab tests
Complications	Diabetic ketoacidosis	Hyperosmolar coma
Body habitus	Normal, thin	Obese (generally)
Pathology	Islet cells destroyed	Insulin resistance, low insulin secretion, islet cells intact
Ketosis prone	Yes	Yes, but much less common than type 1
Therapy	Insulin	Weight loss, balanced diet, oral hypo-glycemic agents, perhaps insulin

119. List the contraindications to sulfonylurea (hypoglycemic) drugs.
1. Type 1 DM or pancreatic diabetes
2. Pregnancy
3. Major surgery
4. Severe infections, stress, or trauma
5. History of severe adverse reaction to sulfonylurea or similar compound (sulfa drug)
6. Predisposition to severe hypoglycemia (e.g., patients with significant liver or kidney disease)

Lebovitz HE, et al: Therapy for Diabetes Mellitus and Related Disorders, 3rd ed. Alexandria, VA, American Diabetes Association, 1998, p 165.

120. What are the proposed mechanisms of action and the advantages of metformin in diabetes therapy?

Proposed Mechanisms for Antidiabetic Action of Metformin

Increase insulin receptors on cell surface or insulin-sensitive tissues
Increase glucose-transport units in insulin-sensitive cells
Increase glucose uptake of muscle and adipose tissue
Decrease hepatic glucose production
Potentiate insulin action
Decrease GI absorption of glucose
Cause anorexia

Advantages of Metformin Therapy in Type 2 Diabetes

Usually modest weight loss
No hypoglycemia
Decreased plasma VLDL cholesterol and increased HDL cholesterol
Unchanged or slightly decreased plasma insulin levels

Lebovitz HE, et al: Therapy for Diabetes Mellitus and Related Disorders, 3rd ed. Alexandria, VA, American Diabetes Association, 1998, p 171–175.

121. Why are oral agents useful in the treatment of type 2 diabetes mellitus?

Patients with Type 2 DM still have functioning beta cells in the islets of Langerhans of the pancreas. Therefore, some endogenous insulin production remains. The oral hypoglycemic agents' primary mechanism of action is thought to include:
- Stimulation of insulin release from islet cells
- Increased insulin receptors in target tissues
- Improved action of insulin
- Decrease in the previously increased rates of hepatic glucose production

122. What are the end-organ effects/complications of chronically elevated blood glucose?

Skin
Dermopathy
Diabetic foot/leg ulcers
Lower susceptibility to skin infections
Necrobiosis lipoidica diabeticorum

Eyes
Cataracts
Retinopathy

Peripheral nerves
Peripheral neuropathy
Mononeuropathy (median nerve)

Genitourinary
Impotence
Retrograde ejaculation
Neurogenic Bladder
Diabetic amyotropy
Neuropathic cachexia

GI
Gastroparesis
Diabetic diarrhea
Constipation
Esophageal dysfunction
Gastroesophageal reflux disease (GERD)

Kidneys
Renal insufficiency
End-stage renal disease
Nephrotic syndrome
Repeated urinary tract infections

CNS
Coma (due to diabetic ketoacidosis or
  hyperosmolar coma)
Personality changes
Autonomic insufficiency

Cardiovascular
Increased risk of CAD, CVA, DVT
Silent MI
Cardiomyopathy
Hypertriglyceridemia
Elevated total cholesterol
Lowered HDL cholesterol
Hypertension
Peripheral vascular disease
Impaired cardiovascular reflexes

123. What recommendations on foot care should the diabetic receive?

1. Check feet daily.
2. Wear cushioned shoes that fit properly. (Jogging shoes are great!)
3. Always turn shoes over and shake them out before putting them on.
4. Never go barefoot.
5. Use cotton socks and cornstarch powder to reduce moisture in shoes.
6. Report redness, skin breakdown, or trauma to a physician immediately.
7. Soak feet in warm water 15–20 minutes daily, followed by lubrication with lotion for dry skin, but not between toes.
8. Test bath water temperature with hands, not feet.

9. Calluses should be treated by a physician, nurse, or podiatrist (no bathroom surgery!).
10. Trim nails squarely (do not round edges).

124. What are the clinical stages of hypoglycemia? How are they characterized?

Characterization of Mild, Moderate, and Severe Hypoglycemia

Mild	Symptoms related to stimulation of the adrenergic or cholinergic system or CNS in response to a low blood sugar.
Moderate	Symptoms related to CNS effects of hypoglycemia are more pronounced, but patient is still capable of assisting him- or herself. Symptoms include impaired motor function, confusion, and inappropriate behaviors.
Severe	Symptoms of hypoglycemia result in coma, seizure, or altered mental status, impairing the patient's ability to seek help or get a sugar source.

Hypoglycemia unawareness: an iatrogenic syndrome usually occurring in type 1 DM where patients become resistant/unaware of early defense signs like tachycardia and sweats. Patients may progress to coma and/or seizures without warning signs.

Lebovitz HE, et al: Therapy for Diabetes Mellitus and Related Disorders, 3rd ed. Alexandria, VA, American Diabetes Association, 1998, p 241–251.

125. What are consistent laboratory findings in adrenal insufficiency?
Hyponatremia (rarely < 120 mEq/L)
Hyperkalemia (rarely > 7 mEq/L)
Hypocarbia (HCO_3 ~15–20 mEq/L)
Hypoglycemia
Elevated BUN
Elevated eosinophils
Elevated lymphocytes

126. Which hormonal imbalance can cause obstructive sleep apnea?
Severe hypothyroidism associated with myxedema. The upper airway constriction is caused by myxedematous swelling of the face, tongue, and pharyngeal structures.
Brown LK: Sleep apnea syndromes: Overview and diagnostic approach. Mt Sinai Med 61(2):99–112, 1994.

127. What complaints in elderly hypothyroid patients most commonly bring them to medical attention?
Constipation   Lethargy, easy fatigability
Difficulty in thinking   Cold intolerance
Bartuska DG: Thyroid disease in the news. Contemp Intern Med (Jun):23–32, 1989.

128. What protection is afforded to patients with the heterozygous sickle cell gene?
The high frequency of the sickle cell gene in areas endemic for malaria is an example of balanced polymorphism. The sickle cell gene protects the host from lethal *Plasmadium falciparum* malaria. The actual mechanism is not fully understood, but it is postulated that the entry of the parasite into the host cell lowers RBC oxygen saturation. This desaturation leads to sickling and arrests the maturation of the parasite. The sickled cells are cleared by the phagocytic system.
Luzzatto L: Genetics of red cells susceptibility to malaria. Blood 54:961–976, 1979.

129. Name the five types of crises in sickle cell disease.
1. Vaso-occlusive (painful): The typical "sickle crisis" whose symptoms depend on the location of occlusion.
2. Aplastic: Bone marrow suppression due to infection.
3. Sequestration: Seen in younger patients (aged 1–5 yr) while the spleen is still intact.

4. Hemolytic: Look for G6PD deficiency or malaria.
5. Megaloblastic: Seen in conditions of increased folate requirements (as in pregnancy).

130. How quickly does a megaloblastic bone marrow recover after the deficient vitamins are added to the patient's diet?
Within 6–8 hours after ingestion of even small amounts of vitamin B_{12} or folate, the bone marrow begins to normalize.

131. Which drugs are most commonly implicated in drug-induced immune thrombocytopenia?

Antibacterials	**Anticonvulsants**	**Cinchona alkaloids**
Sulfonamides	Carbamazepine	Quinine
Rifampin	Phenytoin	Quinidine
Trimethoprim	Sodium valproate	
Ampicillin	Diphenylhydantoin	**Miscellaneous**
Cephalosporins	Phthalazinol	Heroin
p-Aminosalicylate		Chlorpropamide
Nitrofurantoin	**Antihypertensives**	Bleomycin
Isoniazid	Methyldopa	Desipramine
	Chlorothiazide	Gold
NSAIDs	Hydrochlorothiazide	Heparin
Aspirin	Diazoxide	Cimetidine
Indomethacin	Furosemide	Digitoxin
Phenylbutazone		Acetaminophen
Sulindac		

132. What are the differential diagnoses of macrocytic and microcytic anemias?

Macrocytic Anemia	Microcytic Anemia
Liver disease	Iron deficiency (most common type of
Vitamin B_{12} deficiency	anemia worldwide)
Folate deficiency	Hemoglobinopathies
Myelodysplastic syndrome	Thalassemia
Drugs that impair DNA synthesis	Sickle cell
6-Mercaptopurine	SC disease
Zidovudine	Sideroblastic anemias
5-Fluorouracil	Anemia of chronic disease
Hydroxyurea	

133. What are the characteristics of anemia of chronic disease?

Hemoglobin 7–10%	Reticulocyte count < 2%
RBC normochromic/normocytic	Saturated Fe-binding capacity < 20%
Total Fe-binding capacity ↓	Tissue storage Fe: ↑ bone marrow Fe
In hospital, without renal failure	Mild hypochromia and microcytosis
Serum Fe < 60 mg/100 ml	
Ferritin > 100 ng/ml	

134. What criteria must be met to make the diagnosis of systemic lupus erythematosus (SLE)?
SLE is a chronic, inflammatory disease that results from an immunoregulatory disturbance and is characterized by an exaggerated production of autoantibodies. There is a marked female predominance of the disease, with a female:male ratio of 9:1. For a definitive diagnosis, 4 of the following 11 criteria must be met:

1982 Revised Criteria for Classification of SLE

CRITERION	DEFINITION
1. Malar rash	Fixed erythema, flat or raised, over the malar eminences, tending to spare the nasolabial folds
2. Discoid rash	Erythematous raised patches with adherent keratotic scaling and follicular plugging; atrophic scarring may occur in older lesions
3. Photosensitivity	Skin rash as a result of unusual reaction to sunlight, by patient history or physician observation
4. Oral ulcers	Oral or nasopharyngeal ulceration, usually painless, observed by a physician
5. Arthritis	Nonerosive arthritis involving 2 or more peripheral joints, characterized by tenderness, swelling, or effusion
6. Serositis	Pleuritis—convincing history of pleuritic pain or rub heard by a physician or evidence of pleural effusion, or Pericarditis—documented by ECG or rub or evidence of pericardial effusion
7. Renal disorder	Persistent proteinuria > 0.5 gm/day or > 3+ if quantitation not performed, or Cellular casts—may be red cell, hemoglobin, granular, tubular, or mixed
8. Neurologic disorder	Seizures—in the absence of offending drugs or known metabolic derangements (e.g., uremia, ketoacidosis, or electrolyte imbalance), or Psychosis—in the absence of offending drugs or known metabolic derangements (e.g., uremia, ketoacidosis, or electrolyte imbalance)
9. Hematologic disorder	Hemolytic anemia—with reticulocytosis, or Leukopenia—< 4,000/mm^3 total on two or more occasions, or Lymphopenia—< 1,500/mm^3 on two or more occasions, or Thrombocytopenia—< 100,000/mm^3 in the absence of offending drugs
10. Immunologic disorder	Positive LE cell preparation, or Anti-DNA: antibody to native DNA in abnormal titer, or Anti-Sm: presence of antibody to Sm nuclear antigen, or False-positive serologic test for syphilis known to be positive for at least 6 months and confirmed by *Treponema pallidum* immobilization or FTA-ABS test
11. Antinuclear antibody (ANA)	Abnormal titer of ANA by immunofluorescence or equivalent assay at any time and in the absence of drugs known to be associated with "drug-in duced lupus"

Tan EM, Cohen AS, Fries JF, et al: The 1982 revised criteria for the classification of systemic lupus erythematosus (SLE). Arthritis Rheum 25:1271–1277, 1982, with permission.

135. Which enzyme is usually elevated in lymphoma?

Lactate dehydrogenase (LDH) is elevated in many lymphomas and other lymphoproliferative disorders. The source is believed to be tumor cells, and LDH is used as a measurement of disease activity.

136. Neutropenia is most commonly observed in which peoples?

Africans, West Indian blacks, and African-Americans. This is not a genetic trait but rather an acquired one. The neutropenia probably results from an abnormal release of neutrophils by the bone marrow. The WBC count ranges from 3,000–4,000 in African-Americans. There is a normal response to infections, steroids, and pregnancy.

137. What causes the hyperpigmentation of chronic venous stasis?

The breakdown of RBCs as they pass through small blood vessels in the dermis, over a long period of time, leads to the hyperpigmentation.

138. What is the classic tetrad in Henoch-Schönlein purpura?
Palpable purpura, arthralgia or arthritis, abdominal pain, and hematuria.

139. Name the three phases of discoloration in Raynaud's phenomenon.
Pallor (white)—Vasospasm
Cyanosis (blue)—Digital ischemia
Rubor (red)—Reperfusion

140. What criteria must be met to diagnose rheumatoid arthritis (RA)?
RA affects 0.3–1.5% of the U.S. population, most commonly women in the fourth to sixth decades. For a definitive diagnosis, at least 4 of the following 7 criteria must be met:

American Rheumatism Association 1987 Revised Criteria for the
Classification of Rheumatoid Arthritis

CRITERION	DEFINITION
1. Morning stiffness	Morning stiffness in and around the joints, lasting at least 1 hr before maximal improvement
2. Arthritis of ≥ 3 joint areas	At least 3 joint areas simultaneously have had soft tissue swelling or fluid (not bony overgrowth alone) observed by a physician. The 14 possible areas are right or left PIP, MCP, wrist, elbow, knee, ankle, and MTP joints
3. Arthritis of hand joints	At least 1 area swollen (as defined above) in a wrist, MCP, or PIP joint
4. Symmetric arthritis	Simultaneous involvement of the same joint areas (as defined in 2) on both sides of the body (bilateral involvement of PIPs, MCPs, or MTPs is acceptable without absolute symmetry)
5. Rheumatoid nodules	Subcutaneous nodules, over bony prominences, extensor surfaces, or in juxta-articular regions, observed by a physician
6. Serum rheumatoid factor (RF)	Demonstration of abnormal amounts of serum RF by any method for which the result has been positive in < 5% of normal control subjects
7. Radiographic changes	Radiographic changes typical of RA on posteroanterior hand and wrist radiographs, which must include erosions or unequivocal bony decalcification localized in or most marked adjacent to the involved joints (osteoarthritis changes alone do not qualify)

Criteria 1–4 must have been present for at least 6 weeks.
Klippel JH (ed): Primer on the Rheumatic diseases, 11th ed. Atlanta, GA, The Arthritis Foundation, 1997, p 328, with permission.

BIBLIOGRAPHY

1. Alexander RW, et al (eds): Hurst's The Heart, 9th ed. New York, McGraw-Hill, 1998.
2. Beers MH, Berkow R: The Merck Manual of Diagnosis and Therapy, 17th ed. Whitehouse Station, NJ, Merck Research Laboratories, 1999.
3. Fauci AS, et al (eds): Harrison's Principles of Internal Medicine, 14th ed. New York, McGraw-Hill, 1998.
4. Guide to Clinical Preventive Services, 2nd ed. Report of the US Preventive Services Task Force. Baltimore, Williams & Wilkins, 1996.
5. Kelley WN (ed): Textbook of Internal Medicine, 3rd ed. Philadelphia, Lippincott-Raven, 1997.
6. Klippel JH (ed): Primer on the Rheumatic diseases, 11th ed. Atlanta, GA, The Arthritis Foundation, 1997.
7. Lebovitz HE, et al: Therapy for Diabetes Mellitus and Related Disorders, 3rd ed. Alexandria, VA, American Diabetes Association, 1998.
8. Mandell GL, Douglas GD, Bennett JE (eds): Principles and Practice of Infectious Disease, 5th ed. New York, Churchill Livingstone, 2000.

 9. Physician's Desk Reference, 54th ed. Montvale, NJ, Medical Economics Company, Inc., 2000.
10. Sanford Guide to Antimicrobial Therapy, 13th ed. Hyde Park, NY Antimicrobial Therapy, Inc., 2000.
11. Tapson VP (Committee chair): The Diagnostic Approach to Acute Venous Thromboembolism: Clinical Practice Guidelines. Am J Respir Crit Care Med 160(3):1043–1066, 1999.
12. Tierney LM, McPhee SJ, Papdakis MA: Current Medical Diagnosis and Treatment, 38th ed. Norwalk, CT, Appleton & Lange, 1999.

2. ENDOCRINOLOGY

Amelita Lourdes P. Basa, M.D., and Hamid Afsharkharaghan, M.D.

> *"It would indeed be rash for a mere pathologist to venture forth on the uncharted sea of the endocrines, strewn as it is with the wrecks of shattered hypotheses, where even the most wary mariner may easily lose his way as he seeks to steer his bark amid the glandular temptations whose siren voices have proved the downfall of many who have gone before."*
> William Boyd (1885–1972)
> *Pathology for the Surgeon, 7th edition, Ch. 32*

> *"One of the essential qualities of the clinician is interest in humanity, for the secret of the care of the patient is in caring for the patient."*
> Frances Weld Peabody (1881–1927)

1. Who was William of Ockham (or Occam)? What was his razor? How did he die?

William of Ockham, known as Doctor Invincibilis, was a 14th century philosopher. His "razor," a philosophical means of choosing doctrinal postulates, was *"Essentia non sunt multiplicanda praetor necessitatum,"* or "Entities [or postulates] are not to be multiplied without necessity." We use Occam's razor to choose the fewest etiologies to explain multiple problems. Ironically, William of Ockham died of multiple causes.

2. What is the most important thing in approaching a patient (according to Zen master Ikkyu)?

Attention. Before one takes the history or does the physical, one should attend fully to the patient and thereby maximize the appreciation of the sensory data that are incoming. Failure to do so leads to the prejudicial selection of data and may bring about an erroneous or incomplete diagnosis.

DIABETES MELLITUS, METABOLISM AND HYPOGLYCEMIA

3. How does one calculate caloric needs in prescribing a diet?

Make an initial estimate of caloric needs by multiplying the patient's weight by the energy use per kilogram based on activity level. Bedrest is estimated to use 20–25 cal/kg/day; desk work uses 30; work including walking uses up to 35; very active physical labor uses 40–50. These estimates may be used as a first approximation but should be adjusted as the patient demonstrates his or her own caloric needs.

4. How many calories must one lack each day to lose 1 lb a week?

One pound of fat stores approximately 3,500 cal. Thus, one must establish a deficit of 500 cal each day to lose 1 lb of fat each week. Of course, overall weight loss entails a day-to-day balance of salt, water, and muscle, as well as fat, so that this calculation may not match changes in the actual measured body weight.

5. What are the current recommendations for the distribution of dietary nutrients?

Protein	10–20%
Fat**	30%
Carbohydrate*	45–50%

* The carbohydrate portion is preferably made up of complex carbohydrates. ** The fat component should mostly be monounsaturated fat (e.g., olive, canola and peanut oils) with less than 10% saturated fat and up to 10% polyunsaturated fat.

43

6. What is C-peptide?

C-peptide is the fragment that is clipped out of the center of the original insulin polypeptide after sulfhydryl bonding has connected what will become the α and β chains. It is secreted from the pancreatic β-cells with insulin on an equimolar basis and may be used in assessing endogenous insulin secretion.

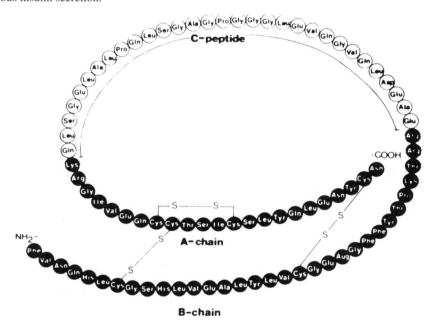

Amino acid sequence and covalent structure of human proinsulin. (From Skyler JS: Insulin dependent diabetes mellitus. In Kohler PO (ed): Clinical Endocrinology. New York, Churchill Livingstone, 1986, p 505; with permission.)

7. What factors influence glucose control? Which factors may be modulated?

Glucose control is an overall result of the balance between glucose production and disposal. Glucose production is controlled by gluconeogenic substrate supply and the hormonal environment, including insulin, growth hormone, cortisol, glucagon, and catecholamines.

Glucose disposal may be divided into two processes. The first is cellular uptake, governed by actual caloric needs created by exercise and by circulating insulin. Second, disposal is controlled in part by renal losses when the circulating glucose concentration exceeds the maximum renal threshold (T_{max}).

In the diabetic patient, production may be modulated by diet, exercise, insulin, or hypoglycemic agent selection and by the avoidance of stressors.

8. What is the average hepatic glucose production per day? What does this suggest about hyperglycemia attributed to routine intravenous fluids?

Within the first 24 hours of fasting, the liver generates roughly 180 gm of glucose for metabolic support. The usual regimen of 125 ml/hr of 5% dextrose would provide 150 gm of glucose per day. Obviously this amount should be easily tolerated, so hyperglycemia cannot be attributed to the IV fluids used.

9. Where does the major clearance of insulin occur?

Insulin has approximately 50% clearance on first pass through the liver. Once in the periphery, roughly 30% of the remainder is cleared by the kidney.

10. What is the new classification of diabetes mellitus? How is it differentiated from the others?

In July 1997, the American Diabetes Association (ADA) classified diabetes mellitus into one of four types based on etiology: **Type 1** diabetes (previously called insulin-dependent, IDDM or juvenile-onset DM) is associated with either an autoimmune destruction of the pancreatic β-cells or an idiopathic variety. Patients usually are diagnosed before age 30 and are more prone to ketoacidosis/ketosis because of insulinopenia at its onset. **Type 2** diabetes (previously called non-insulin dependent, NIDDM or adult-onset DM) is associated with defects in insulin secretion (patients still have pancreatic β-cell insulin secreting capacity) and insulin action (insulin resistance). Patients usually are diagnosed after age 30, are obese, and are not prone to develop ketoacidosis except during periods of severe stress, such as caused by infection, trauma or surgery. Other specific types of diabetes (secondary diabetes) are usually caused by another underlying disease process affecting the pancreas, or insulin secretion and action. **Gestational diabetes** is diabetes diagnosed during pregnancy.

11. What are some causes of secondary diabetes?

Causes of Secondary Diabetes

Processes causing reduced insulin secretion:

Pancreatitis or pancreatectomy	Somatostatinoma
Cystic fibrosis	Aldosteronoma
Hemochromatosis	Hypokalemia
Pheochromocytoma	

Processes producing impairment of insulin action:

Insulin receptor defects	Diseases producing excess anti-insulin hormones
With acanthosis nigricans	Pheochromocytoma
Insulin receptor antibodies	Cushing's syndrome
Anti-insulin antibodies	Acromegaly
	Glucagonoma
	Thyrotoxicosis

Diseases producing secondary diabetes by unknown mechanism:

Muscular dystrophy	Friedreich's ataxia	Chromosomal abnormalities
Myotonic dystrophy	Lawrence-Moon-Biedl syndrome	Klinefelter's syndrome
Acute intermittent porphyria	Progeria	Turner's syndrome
Glycogen storage disease, type I	Prader-Willi syndrome	Down's syndrome
Hyperlipidemia		Sexual ateliotic dwarfism

From Garber AJ: Diabetes mellitus. In Stein JH (ed): Internal Medicine, 3rd ed. Boston, Little, Brown, 1990, p 2244, with permission.

12. How is Type 2 diabetes diagnosed?

The diagnosis can be made one of three ways:

1. Symptoms of diabetes plus casual plasma glucose (PG) concentration ≥ 200 mg/dl (11.1 mmol/l). Casual is defined as any time of day without regard to time since last meal. The classic symptoms of diabetes include polyuria, polydipsia, and unexplained weight loss.

OR

2. Fasting PG ≥ 126 mg/dl (7.0 mmol/l). Fasting is defined as no caloric intake for at least 8 hours.

OR

3. 2-hour PG ≥ 200 mg/dl (11.1 mmol/l) during an OGTT. The test should be performed as described by the World Health Organization using a glucose load containing the equivalent of 75 g anhydrous glucose dissolved in water.

* In the absence of unequivocal hyperglycemia with acute metabolic decompensation, these criteria should be confirmed by repeat testing on a different day. The third measure (OGTT) is not recommended for routine clinical use.

13. In diabetic ketoacidosis, what are the usual deficits of sodium, potassium, and water?

	TOTAL	PER KG BODY WEIGHT
Water	5–11 liters	100 ml
Sodium	300–700 meq	7 meq
Chloride	350–500 meq	5 meq
Potassium	200–700 meq	5 meq
Phosphate	70–100 mmole	1 mmole

14. Continuous IV insulin is the usual treatment during DKA. What dose should be used, and what should be monitored during insulin infusion?

After an IV bolus of 0.1 U/kg, infusion should begin at 0.1 U/kg/hr. After this rate is initiated, blood glucose should be carefully followed and insulin administration tailored to the individual patient. Insulin can drive potassium into the cell, so frequently checking electrolytes in addition to glucose is mandatory in managing a patient on an insulin drip.

15. How does one convert to intermittent insulin after IV therapy?

Begin a regimen of intermediate and short-acting insulins, starting with 75% of the IV dose administered over the previous 24 hours. On discontinuing IV insulin, be sure to give the subcutaneous (SC) insulin for a long enough period before stopping the IV insulin to allow the SC insulin to act.

16. Why is there a high frequency of recurrent DKA in the alcoholic or malnourished patient? How can this complication be avoided?

Such patients are often depleted of potential glucogenic substrates, with low liver glycogen stores and even frank muscle wasting. If adequate glucose is not administered during the first 24–48 hours of therapy, there will be a tendency for recrudescence of the ketosis, burning adipose tissue because of the lack of gluconeogenic substrate. This may be prevented by glucose loading during this period, using insulin to ensure repletion of glycogen. Avoid cutting back on glucose therapy in an attempt to modulate circulating glucose levels. This should be accomplished by using insulin.

17. What are the features of hyperosmolar hyperglycemic nonketotic syndrome?

- Severe hyperglycemia with blood glucose > 600 mg/dl and generally between 1,000–2,000 mg/dl
- Absence of or only slight ketosis
- Plasma hyperosmolarity > 340 mOsm/l
- Profound dehydration

Treatment includes determination of the precipitating event, combined with correction of the dehydration, electrolyte imbalance and hyperglycemia with IV fluids, potassium, phosphate, and insulin, respectively.

18. When does one start insulin therapy in type 2 diabetes? When would one choose human insulin over another source?

The main indication for insulin use is poor glucose control with lifestyle modifications and oral agents. Insulin can be used by itself or in combination with oral agents during periods of acute injury, stress, infection, surgery, and glucocorticoid treatment, in pregnancy, and in patients with renal or hepatic disease or allergies that preclude use of oral therapies. Patients started on insulin should be started on human insulin. Patients experiencing lipodystrophy or in whom insulin resistance becomes problematic may benefit from switching to human insulin. Otherwise, there is no pressing reason to change insulin species in a well-controlled diabetic.

19. What are the kinetics of action of the different types of insulin?

TYPE	ONSET	PEAK	DURATION
Short acting			
Lispro	5 min	0.5–1 h	3 h
Regular	30 min	2–5 h	5–8 h
Intermediate acting			
NPH	1–2 h	6–10 h	16–20 h
Lente	1–2 h	8–12 h	18–24 h
Long-acting			
Ultralente	4-6 h	10–18 h	24–28 h
Mixtures			
70/30, 50/50	30 min	7–12 h	16–24 h

NPH = neutral protamine Hagedorn.
These values are highly variable among individuals. Even in a given person, these values vary depending on the site and depth of injection, skin temperature and exercise. (From Medical Management of Type 2 Diabetes, 4th edition. American Diabetes Association Clincal Education Series 1998, with permission.)

20. How is the management of hypertension different in the diabetic? Why?

Hypertension is implicated in accelerating the microvascular complications of diabetes (mainly retinopathy, nephropathy and neuropathy). Blood pressure should be maintained at < 130/85 mmHg. In isolated systolic hypertension (systolic BP > 180 mmHg) the goal is a blood pressure of < 160 mmHg or a reduction of 20 mmHg for SBP between 160–179 mmHg. Once achieved, further blood pressure lowering is pursued. It may take 3 or more different classes of antihypertensive agents to control the blood pressure of a typical type 2 diabetic.

21. What are the antihypertensives of choice for diabetics? Which ones should be avoided and why?

In the diabetic, the antihypertensives chosen should not worsen glucose or lipid control, they should not block normal "alerting" or counter-regulatory mechanisms if hypoglycemia should occur, and they should not antagonize common neurologic defects in diabetes, such as autonomic insufficiency and impotency.

Among the most-used agents in hypertensive diabetics, angiotensin-converting enzyme (ACE) inhibitors have been shown to slow the progression of diabetic nephropathy. Calcium-channel blocking agents provide pressure reduction without adverse effects on lipids, glucose control, or autonomic interference. Alpha-blocking agents may also provide smoother control and an improved lipid profile. Beta-blocking agents should be used with extreme care because of their blockade of hypoglycemic responses, degraded lipid profile, and incidence of impotence. Thiazide diuretics may also worsen glucose and lipid profiles. The United Kingdom Diabetic Prospective Study (UKDPS) proved that microvascular complications are prevented in type 2 diabetes irrespective of the anti-hypertensive agent used as long as the blood pressure was well-controlled.

22. How is diabetic nephropathy screened? When is screening indicated?

Routine urinalysis should be performed at diagnosis for every type 2 diabetic or for type 1 diabetes that has been present for more than 5 years and after puberty. If positive for proteins, quantitative measurement is helpful to develop a treatment plan. If negative for proteins, a test for the presence of microalbuminuria is necessary. Microalbuminuria can be detected by three methods: measuring albumin to creatinine ratio in a random spot collection, measuring a 24-hour urine for albumin and creatinine, or measuring albumin during a timed urine collection.

CATEGORY	24-H COLLECTION (mg/24 h)	TIMED COLLECTION (µg/min)	SPOT COLLECTION (µg/mg CREATININE)
Normal	< 30	< 20	< 30
Microalbuminuria	30–300	20–200	30–300
Clinical albuminuria	> 300	> 200	> 300

Definition of abnormalities in albumin excretion (Diabetes Care 23 (Suppl 1):January 2000, p S70).

Albumin excretion varies from day to day and can be transiently elevated during acute hyperglycemia, urinary tract infections, heart failure, marked hypertension, exercise, and febrile illness. It is therefore necessary to have two of three collections within a 3–6 month period showing elevated levels before designating a patient as having microalbuminuria.

23. What steps can be taken to avoid or slow the progression of diabetic nephropathy?
Excellent glucose control
Excellent blood pressure control
ACE inhibitors
Protein restriction

24. How often should diabetics see an ophthalmologist?
Type 1 diabetics—after 5 years of disease and at least yearly thereafter.
Type 2 diabetics—start yearly check-ups at diagnosis.

25. To which type of ear infection is the diabetic predisposed? How is it treated?
Malignant otitis externa, an infection of the external auditory canal due to *Pseudomonas aeruginosa*, is mainly seen in elderly diabetic patients. It is an invasive and necrotizing infection with a high mortality, mainly due to meningitis. The typical clinical presentation consists of pain in the ear with or without a purulent drainage, swelling of the parotid gland, trismus, and paralysis of the 6th through 12th cranial nerves. Treatment consists of antipseudomonal antibiotics with or without surgical debridement.

26. Why might a diabetic's insulin requirement drop?
Success in weight control
Improved exercise program
Change in type or brand of insulin
Decrease in renal function (lessened insulin clearance)

27. What is a reliable sign that the house officer has done a good job in seeing a diabetic patient in clinic?
The patient has his or her shoes off. A careful examination of the feet of a diabetic is a necessary part of comprehensive care. The patient must be taught to self-examine the feet and to administer proper foot care.

28. When are multiple injection regimens indicated for diabetes?
Inability to maintain pre- and postprandial glucose levels to near normal levels on single-dose regimens.

29. When is an insulin pump indicated?
Patient and physician preference may lead a patient to use a pump instead of an intensive regimen (preprandial regular insulin plus intermediate or long-acting insulin). Failure of a well-monitored and executed intensive SC regimen is a reasonable indication for a pump. Pregnant patients often do well with insulin pumps.

30. What is MODY?

MODY or maturity onset diabetes of the young is a specific type of diabetes caused by several distinct genetic defects of β-cell function leading to impaired release of insulin. This is transmitted in an autosomal dominant fashion. Patients may present with mild to moderate hyperglycemia and are usually ketosis-resistant. To date, abnormalities in three different genes on three different chromosomes have been described.

31. What is the Somogyi phenomenon? What are its signs and symptoms? How is it differentiated from the Dawn phenomenon?

Somogyi phenomenon is hyperglycemia following hypoglycemia, known parochially as "the bounce." The overuse of insulin with attendant hypoglycemia causes counter-regulatory stress hormone secretion, most notably glucagon, growth hormone, cortisol, and catecholamines. These agents lead to a rebound hyperglycemia, which may be confused with under-insulinization and result in mistaken therapy with larger doses of insulin at night. This hypoglycemia and rebound hyperglycemia phenomenon often occurs at night or early morning, with high glucose on awakening. The symptoms include poor sleep, nightmares, nighttime diaphoresis, and morning headache. The signs include hyperglycemia with positive urine ketones, the latter related to the hypoglycemia and fatty acid released.

The dawn phenomenon is hyperglycemia caused by the early morning surge of counter-regulatory stress hormones (growth hormone, cortisol, and catecholamines) resulting from inadequate amount of insulin at night to counteract this effect. This can be differentiated from the Somogyi phenomenon by checking an early morning (3 a.m.) blood glucose.

32. How may type 2 diabetes be treated?

Diet, exercise, oral agents, and insulin can be used.

33. What are the common oral diabetic agents used for type 2 diabetes?

CLASS	GENERIC NAME (BRAND NAMES)	SIDE EFFECTS
Augments insulin release		
Sulfonylureas (SUR)	Glipizide (Glucotrol, Glucotrol XL)	Hypoglycemia
	Glyburide (Micronase, Diabeta, Glynase)	
	Glimepiride (Amaryl)	
Meglitinides	Repaglinide (Prandin)	Hypoglycemia
Enhances insulin effect (insulin sensitizers)		
Thiazolidinediones	Rosiglitazone (Avandia)	Weight gain, hypoglycemia
	Pioglitazone (Actos)	when used in conjuction with insulin or sulfonylureas; possible idiosyncratic hepatocellular damage
Biguanides	Metformin (Glucophage)	Anorexia, diarrhea, GI upset; rarely lactic acidosis
α-Glucosidase inhibitor	Acarbose (Precose)	
	Miglitol (Glyset)	Flatulence, abdominal distress or distention, diarrhea

34. How often does lactic acidosis develop in metformin-treated patients? How can lactic acidosis be prevented?

Lactic acidosis associated with metfomin treatment is extremely rare. Since metformin is primarily excreted by the kidneys, it should not be given in patients with impaired renal function (serum creatinine > 1.4 mg/dl for women and > 1.5 mg/dl for men) or to those with serious hepatic or cardiovascular and pulmonary decompensation. Patients undergoing cardiac catheterization (or any procedures involving the use of radiocontrast agents), with its attendant risk of going into renal failure, should stop metformin during the procedure and resume the drug only after adequate renal function is assured post-procedure.

35. How is the diagnosis of hypoglycemia established?

Hypoglycemia is established when it is based on the Whipple's triad: presence of symptoms consistent with hypoglycemia (such as sweating, hunger, palpitations, weakness), a documented low plasma glucose at the time of symptoms, and relief of symptoms when the plasma glucose concentration is raised to normal levels.

36. What are the clinical classifications of hypoglycemia? What are some of the causes of each?

Hypoglycemia can be classified as either **postabsorptive** (fasting) or **postprandial**. Postabsorptive hypoglycemia develops in the absence of substrate intake and is aggravated by prolonged fast and is usually caused by a more serious underlying problem. Some of its causes include drugs (sulfonylurea, insulin, alcohol, sulfonamides, or salicylates), critical illnesses including hepatic or renal failure, sepsis, hormone deficiency states (cortisol, growth hormone), non-beta cell tumors (mesenchymal tumors such as fibrosarcoma, mesothelioma, leiomyosarcoma that produce insulin-like growth factor-II or IGF-II), insulinoma, or metabolic disorders of infancy and childhood.

Postprandial or reactive hypoglycemia occurs exclusively after meals, typically within 4 hours after eating. This may be attributed to alimentary dysfunction (e.g., gastrectomy, pyloroplasty, gastroenterostomy) where rapid movement of ingested food into the small intestine causes a sudden surge of insulin or other insulinotropic gut hormones, rare congenital enzyme deficiency states (galactosemia or hereditary fructose intolerance), and the idiopathic or functional form, which remains a diagnosis of exclusion. Postabsorptive hypoglycemia can also manifest as postprandial hypoglycemia and should always be considered.

37. What is a possible cause of low plasma glucose in a patient with leukemia without hypoglycemic symptoms?

Artifactually low measured glucose levels can result from enhanced glycolysis in vitro (pseudohypoglycemia) in the presence of leukocytosis or polycythemia. It is therefore important to separate the plasma from the formed elements of the blood as soon as possible in these states.

38. How is C-peptide useful in assessing the etiology of fasting hypoglycemia?

C-peptide is absent in commercial insulin preparations. High endogenous insulin levels (as in insulinoma, sulfonylurea ingestion) are accompanied by high C-peptide levels. High insulin levels with low C-peptide levels are strongly suggestive of exogenous insulin use. Serum or urine sulfonylurea levels can be measured to rule out surreptitious ingestion.

39. Describe the biochemical mechanism for alcohol-induced hypoglycemia.

The oxidation of alcohol to acetaldehyde increases the NADH:NAD ratio, which in turn pushes the lactate:pyruvate redox pair toward lactate. Low pyruvate levels slow gluconeogenesis; this can lead to hypoglycemia.

40. What is hemoglobin A1c? What does it reflect?

Hemoglobin A1c (glycohemoglobin) is hemoglobin glycosylated by nonenzymatic means. The percentage of glycohemoglobin in the circulation is indicative of the average ambient glucose concentration over the prior 6–12 weeks. The measurement of hemoglobin A1c can be used as an indicator of the degree of glucose control over that time period.

PITUITARY

41. What is pituitary apoplexy? How is it managed?

This condition is an acute, life-threatening hemorrhagic infarction of the pituitary gland usually in the setting of a pituitary tumor, irradiated pituitary adenoma, pregnancy, anticoagulation, increased intracranial pressure, vascular disease (e.g., diabetes mellitus) or vasculitis. Patient presentation may range from asymptomatic to symptoms of severe retro-orbital headache, visual defects, meningeal signs, altered sensorium, seizure, or coma depending on the extent of the lesion. Clinical symptoms and signs plus CT scan or MRI of the pituitary aid in the diagnosis. Treatment consists of stress doses of steroids (to decompress the cerebral edema and to treat presumed adrenal insufficiency) and/or neurosurgical decompression.

42. How is prolactin secretion regulated, and how is it different from the other anterior pituitary hormones? Name the other anterior pituitary hormones.

Prolactin is primarily controlled by tonic inhibition from the hypothalamus via the portal system. Prolactin inhibitory factor (PIF) has been identified as dopamine, so that dopamine and dopamine agonists suppress the secretion of prolactin. Thyrotropin-releasing hormone (TRH) is a mild positive modulator of prolactin secretion.

The other anterior pituitary hormones are positively stimulated by hypothalamic-releasing hormones: luteinizing (LH) and follicle-stimulating hormones (FSH) by gonadotropin-releasing hormone (GnRH), thyroid stimulating hormone (TSH or thyrotropin) by thyrotropin-releasing hormone (TRH), growth hormone (GH) by growth-hormone-releasing hormone (GH-RH) (and negatively by somatostatin), and ACTH by corticotropin-releasing hormone (CRH).

43. How does hyperprolactinemia present?

The clinical picture of hyperprolactinemia is highly variable depending on age, sex, duration of hyperprolactenemia, and tumor size. Hypogonadism is a very common manifestation in both men and women. Women of reproductive age usually present with interference of the menstrual cycle and galactorrhea (amenorrhea-galactorrhea syndrome). Men and postmenopausal women usually present with mass effect such as headache and visual deficits.

44. Why should we check thyroid function in a patient with elevated prolactin level?

Primary hypothyroidism causes lack of feedback inhibition at the hypothalamic-pituitary level. This causes a rise in TRH from the hypothalamus which is a positive modulator of prolactin release. Primary hypothyroidism may also cause an enlargement of the pituitary (from thyrotrope hyperplasia) which, together with an elevated prolactin level, may be mistaken as a prolactinoma.

45. What is the "stalk effect"?

Large non-prolactin secreting tumors compress the pituitary stalk thus interrupting the tonic inhibitory effect of dopamine (or prolactin-inhibiting factor) on the pituitary causing elevation of prolactin levels up to 200 ng/mL.

46. What are the therapeutic options for prolactinomas?

Bromocriptine, a dopamine agonist, is very effective in shrinking prolactinomas, even those of very large size. Other dopamine agonist include lisuride, pergolide, metergoline, quinagoline, and cabergoline. **Surgery** is usually an option for tumors resistant to dopamine agonist therapy and in enlarging and compressing tumors during pregnancy. Surgery is associated with a high rate of recurrence in cases of macroadenoma.

47. What are the therapies used in acromegaly?

Acromegaly usually requires more than one approach. **Transsphenoidal surgery** is the primary therapeutic modality in acromegaly. **Radiation therapy** is reserved for patients with persistent disease following surgery. **Medical therapies** are used in conjunction with surgery and/or radiotherapy and include bromocriptine (a dopamine agonist), and somatostatin analogues, such as octreotide and lanreotide.

48. How is IGF-1 (somatomedin C) used in the management of acromegaly?

Monitoring IGF-1 (insulin-like growth factor-1) levels allows assessment of the efficacy of initial therapy and follow-up in the posttherapeutic period.

49. Why is colonoscopy warranted in patients with acromegaly?

Acromegaly has been associated with increased incidence of colonic polyps and colon cancer.

50. Which circulating protein may help in diagnosing a glycoprotein-secreting pituitary tumor?

The α-subunit, which is common to the glycoprotein hormones LH, FSH, and TSH, is elevated in many of these cases.

51. What causes panhypopituitarism?

Etiologies of Hypopituitarism

Tumors	**Infarction (cont.)**	**Infiltrative disease (cont.)**
Pituitary adenomas	Diabetes necrosis	Lymphoma
Craniopharyngioma	Trauma with stalk section	Lymphocytic hypophysitis
Metastatic carcinoma	Epidemic hemorrhagic fever	Hemochromatosis
Primary pituitary carcinoma	Malaria	
Meningioma	Arteritis	**Miscellaneous causes**
	Sickle cell anemia (crisis)	Pituitary abscess
Infarction		Aneurysm
Pituitary adenomas (pituitary	**Infiltrative disease**	Radiation therapy
apoplexy)	Sarcoidosis	Congenital absence of pituitary
Postpartum pituitary necrosis	Eosinophilic granuloma	Therapeutic ablation
(Sheehan's syndrome)	Leukemia	Hypothalamic disease

Boyd, et al: Disorders of the hypothalamus and anterior pituitary. In Kohler PO (ed): Clinical Endocrinology. New York, John Wiley, 1986, p 44.

52. How closely is vasopressin (AVP, antidiuretic hormone or ADH) release related to osmolarity? How much volume must one lose to trigger AVP release?

An osmolarity change of 1–2% will produce changes in AVP secretion. A loss of 10–15% of circulating volume will trigger AVP secretion. Volume stimuli can override the effects of osmolality stimuli.

53. Why is cortisol deficiency associated with hyponatremia?

It appears that cortisol negatively modulates the release of AVP, and that its deficiency is associated with a syndrome of inappropriate antidiuretic hormone-like (SIADH-like) effect. This is distinguished from the hyponatremia and hyperkalemia seen in primary adrenal deficiency with both cortisol and aldosterone deficiency. In that setting, aldosterone deficiency leads to potassium retention and sodium loss. The loss of sodium and volume contributes to an appropriate increase in ADH.

54. What is DDAVP? How is it used?

DDAVP, or desmopressin, is 1-desamino-8-D-arginine vasopressin, a long-acting ADH analogue, which may be administered intranasally, IV, SC, or PO. Its long action allows it to be used intranasally once- or twice-daily for diabetes insipidus.

55. What is diabetes insipidus (DI)? What are the clinical manifestations of DI?

It is a condition characterized by inability to conserve water secondary to absence or lack of AVP secretion (central DI) or unresponsiveness of the kidney to AVP action (nephrogenic DI). These conditions are manifested by polyuria and polydipsia. Hypernatremia and hyperosmolarity with circulatory collapse and hypertonic encephalopathy develop without free water replacement. This is differentiated from psychogenic polydipsia which is functional suppression of AVP secondary excessive water intake.

56. What is an interesting observation of the pituitary MRI of patients with central DI?

Normally, there is a hyperintense signal of the posterior pituitary on T1-weighted images by MRI caused by AVP storage granules. In central DI, this hyperintense signal is absent.

ADRENAL

57. How much cortisol can the normal adrenal axis make during stress in one day? How, then, should "stress steroids" be administered for patients adrenally insufficient for surgery or in sepsis?

Estimates of maximal adrenal output range from 125–300 mg cortisol/24 hrs. The usual approach for treatment of a high-stress period in a patient deemed adrenally insufficient is to administer 100 mg of hydrocortisone IV every 6–8 hrs.

58. What is the distinction between Cushing's syndrome and Cushing's disease?

Cushing's syndrome is the symptom complex produced by an excess of adrenal corticosteroids. **Cushing's disease** is the most common cause of Cushing's syndrome, accounting for about two-thirds of all cases. It is caused by pituitary overproduction of ACTH, leading to bilateral adrenal hyperplasia. Other causes of Cushing's syndrome include excess cortisol production originating in the adrenal gland (adrenal adenoma or carcinoma), excess production of ACTH from a nonpituitary source (ectopic ACTH syndrome), and iatrogenic or factitious ingestion of excess exogenous corticosteroids.

59. Is there an indication for a random cortisol or ACTH measurement in the diagnosis of Cushing's disease?

No. These tests are not reliable in screening for Cushing's disease.

60. What are the signs and symptoms of Cushing's disease?

Skin	Endocrine	Adipose tissue
Atrophic, thin skin	Amenorrhea	Weight gain
Easy bruising	Diabetes	Truncal obesity
Broad, purple striae on hips, abdomen, axillae	Hypertension	Fat deposition in supraclavicular area and dorsum of
Hair loss	**Immune system**	back (buffalo hump)
Tinea versicolor	Susceptible to infections	Moon facies
	Poor wound healing	

Muscles	Skeleton	Psychiatric	Sexual characteristics
Muscle wasting	Osteoporosis	Psychosis	(women)
Decreased strength	Chronic backache	Paranoia	Hirsutism
	Bone pain	Mood swings	Deepened voice
			Clitoral enlargement

61. What are the most reliable physical findings in Cushing's syndrome?

Purple striae (usually > 1 cm in width) and thinning of the skin. Proximal muscle weakness also may be striking and unexpected until tested. The presence of supraclavicular fullness may be more specific for Cushing's than the dorsal cervical fat pad ("buffalo hump").

62. How should one screen for Cushing's syndrome?

1. Low-dose dexamethasone suppression test: 1 mg of dexamethasone at 11 p.m. the night before should suppress 8 a.m. cortisol to < 5 µg/dl, *or*

2. Collection of a 24-hr urine for urinary free cortisol should be < 100 µg/24 hr.

The dexamethasone suppression test may yield false-positive results (unsuppressed cortisol) in conditions that increase dexamethasone's metabolic clearance such as concomitant alcohol, rifampin, phenytoin or phenobarbital use (induce the cytochrome P450-related enzymes) while renal and hepatic failure that retard dexamethasone clearance may give a false-negative result.

63. What is Carney's complex?

It is a rare autosomal dominant syndrome causing Cushing's syndrome secondary to adrenal overproduction of cortisol. Other features of the complex include myxomas of the skin, breast, and heart; spotty pigmentations (such as lentigines and blue nevi); and other endocrine overactivity (such as acromegaly and testicular tumors).

64. What condition should you consider in a patient who has had bilateral surgical adrenalectomy as part of the treatment for Cushing's disease?

Nelson's syndrome. This is manifested by hyperpigmentation caused by an enlarging, locally invasive pituitary corticotrope tumor which produces high levels of ACTH (which also has melanocyte-stimulating activity, hence the hyperpigmentation) because of the lack of inhibition from adrenal cortisol. This condition is prevented by pituitary irradiation prior to adrenalectomy.

65. What is Addison's disease? What causes it?

Addison's disease is primary adrenal insufficiency. It is due to a failure of the adrenals to produce sufficient amounts of adrenal corticosteroids. Autoimmune destruction is responsible in approximately 80% of cases, and adrenal destruction by tuberculosis (TB) in approximately 20% of cases. Other rare causes include adrenal destruction by bilateral hemorrhage or infarction, tumor, infections (other than TB), surgery, radiation, drugs, amyloidosis, sarcoidosis, hyporesponsiveness to ACTH, and congenital abnormalities. Symptoms of adrenal insufficiency require loss of 90% of both adrenal cortices.

66. What are the major symptoms and signs of Addison's disease?

Symptoms	Signs
Hyperpigmentation	Hyperpigmentation (most prominent on
Weakness	skinfolds, extensor surfaces, pressure points,
Fatigue	buccal mucosa and gums, nipples, areolae,
Anorexia	perivaginal and perianal mucosa, and newly
Weight loss	formed scars)
Salt craving	Hyperkalemia (usually mild)
Nausea	Weight loss
Diarrhea	Orthostatic hypotension
Postural dizziness	Adrenal calcifications
	Vitiligo

67. How do primary and secondary adrenal insufficiency differ in their presentation? Why?

Primary adrenal insufficiency (Addison's disease) is caused by failure or destruction of the adrenal glands, leading to underproduction of glucocorticoids and mineralocorticoids. This results in an increase in ACTH production by the pituitary. Its signs and symptoms are described in question 66. **Secondary** adrenal insufficiency (SAI) is caused by deficient production of ACTH, leading to underproduction of glucocorticoids. The manifestations are the same as those of Addison's disease, except for the following:

1. Hyperpigmentation is not seen. This is a product of the hypersecretion of ACTH and its related peptides (including melanocyte-stimulating hormone), which is not present in SAI.

2. Hyperkalemia due to mineralocorticoid deficiency is not usually seen. Since mineralocorticoid activity is largely regulated by the renin-angiotensin system and not ACTH, this is not present in SAI.

3. Other manifestations of hypopituitarism may be seen with SAI.

4. Hypoglycemia is more commonly seen with SAI due to the presence of combined ACTH and growth hormone deficiency.

68. How is the pituitary-adrenal axis reserve tested?

The insulin tolerance test (ITT) is the gold standard to test adequacy of the axis. The principle of the test is to induce hypoglycemia (plasma glucose ≤ 40 mg/dl) by IV insulin which acts as a major stress to stimulate increase production of ACTH, cortisol, and growth hormone. It is contraindicated in patients with seizure disorders or cardiovascular/cerebrovascular disease.

69. What does metyrapone do? How is it used?

Metyrapone inhibits the 11-hydroxylase step of cortisol synthesis, causing accumulation of 11-deoxycortisol, which does not provide feedback inhibition at the hypothalamus. The administration of metyrapone therefore causes an intact axis to hyperfunction, with accumulation of 11-deoxycortisol, which may then be measured.

It is also important to measure cortisol, which should be low. If cortisol is not low, there has been inadequate enzyme inhibition, and the test is not adequate.

70. How do you wean a patient off corticosteroids?

First, place the patient on a short-acting corticosteroid, such as prednisone or hydrocortisone, on a twice daily basis. Next, the evening dose should be weaned down, leaving a solitary morning dose. By this time, hydrocortisone should be substituted for prednisone. As the morning dose is weaned toward a physiologic level (20 mg), the next morning's cortisol may be measured. When a normal a.m. cortisol is attained, daily supplementation may be stopped. However, the patient should still use supplements for stress until an insulin tolerance test or a metyrapone test or, recently, a low dose (1 µg) ACTH stimulation test documents adequate hypothalamic-pituitary-adrenal axis response to stress.

71. How should an incidentally found adrenal mass be evaluated? What parameters are of importance?

Because roughly 0.1–1% of patients demonstrate an incidental adrenal tumor by CT done for other reasons, the work-up of this finding must be individualized. A careful history and physical exam are required to assess the possible functional status of the tumor. The most common functioning adrenal tumor secretes corticosteroids which produce overt or subclinical Cushing's syndrome. Therefore, low-dose dexamethasone suppression test or 24-hour urine free cortisol screening may be appropriate. In the absence of family history, hypertension, or symptoms, pheochromocytoma is unlikely. Otherwise, urinary metanephrines and catecholamines may be obtained. In the presence of isolated hypertension with or without attendant hypokalemia, a single plasma aldosterone concentration (PAC) and plasma renin activity (PRA) may be used to test for an aldosterone-secreting tumor, looking for an PAC:PRA ratio > 25.

Tumors > 4–5 cm are almost always an indication for surgery after the functional status of the tumor is evaluated. FNA of the tumor is helpful to rule-out metastasis from an extra-adrenal tumor. Otherwise, FNA should not be routinely performed because of the possibility of seeding the peritoneum with adrenocortical cancer cells or for an unsuspected pheochromocytoma, provoking a hypertensive crisis.

72. What are the differences among the high dose 250 µg ACTH stimulation test, insulin tolerance test (ITT), and metyrapone test? What are the appropriate settings for their use?

ITT and metyrapone tests evaluate the response of the entire adrenal axis. The high dose 250 µg ACTH stimulation test stimulates only the adrenal glands. This test will suggest adrenal insufficiency when there has been prolonged defect anywhere in the adrenal axis or when there has been direct adrenal damage. Recently, a low dose 1 µg ACTH stimulation test has been developed which has shown comparative results to the ITT for testing pituitary corticotrope reserve.

73. What is the rapid ACTH stimulation test?

This test is used to assess adrenal function and is useful as an initial screening test. 250 µg of synthetic ACTH (Cosyntropin, Cortrosyn) is administered to the patient, and cortisol levels are measured at 0, 30, and 60 min. A normal cortisol response (> 20 µg/dl) to the ACTH rules out primary adrenal insufficiency. Lack of a normal response indicates decreased adrenal reserve but does not differentiate between primary and secondary adrenal insufficiency.

74. How do you differentiate primary and secondary adrenal insufficiency?

Plasma ACTH levels can be used in this differentiation. In the face of adrenal insufficiency, ACTH levels > 250 pg/ml are associated with primary adrenal insufficiency (usually 400–2000 pg/ml), and ACTH levels of 0–50 pg/ml are associated with pituitary or secondary ACTH deficiency (usually 20 pg/ml).

75. Describe the recovery of the hypothalamic-pituitary-adrenal (H-P-A) axis after glucocorticoid withdrawal.

Recovery of the H-P-A axis appears to recapitulate its suppression. The first to recover is the hypothalamic corticotropin-releasing hormone (CRH) synthesis and secretion. This is followed by restoration of normal ACTH secretion from the pituitary. After several weeks, adrenal steroidogenesis begins to recover. The whole process may take 6–9 months to complete.

76. How does late-onset congenital adrenal hyperplasia present? How is it diagnosed?

This presents as hirsutism and a mild form of virilization in the female. ACTH-stimulated 17-OH-progesterone levels will be elevated.

77. What gene do familial Hirschsprung's disease and multiple endocrine neoplasia (MEN) type 2B have in common?

The *RET* proto-oncogene is mutated in both conditions. Familial Hirschsprung's disease has a mutation that causes nonexpression with resultant disordered neuronal development of the colon. An activating mutation results in MEN 2B.

78. Categorize the MEN syndromes.

MEN 1	Variants of MEN 2A
Parathyroid neoplasia	Familial medullary thyroid carcinoma only
Pituitary neoplasia	MEN 2A with Hirschsprung's disease
Pancreatic islet-cell tumors	MEN 2A with cutaneous lichen amyloidosis
Other manifestations	**MEN 2B**
Carcinoid	Medullary thyroid carcinoma
Lipomas	Pheochromocytoma
MEN 2A	Mucosal and alimentary tract ganglioneuromatosis
Medullary thyroid carcinoma	Marfanoid features
Pheochromocytoma	Absence of parathyroid neoplasia
Parathyroid neoplasia	

Gagel RF: Multiple endocrine neoplasia. Endocrinol Metabol Clin North Am 23:1994.

79. Why is β-blockade of a pheochromocytoma a bad idea as initial therapy?

Pheochromocytomas may secrete epinephrine, norepinephrine, or both. Because β-adrenergic activity dilates peripheral blood vessels, β-adrenergic blockade in the presence of unopposed α-agonists may lead to net peripheral vasoconstriction and an exacerbation of the patient's hypertension. α-blockade comes before β-blockade (A comes before B). In addition, it is important to keep the patient adequately hydrated since pheochromocytoma patients often have reduced plasma volume.

80. What are the diseases associated with pheochromocytoma?

MEN 2A (Sipple's syndrome)
MEN 2B (mucosal neuroma syndrome)
Von Hippel-Lindau disease (retinal cerebellar hemangioblastomatosis)
Neurofibromatosis type 1

81. What are the organs of Zuckerkandl?

These are rests of chromaffin tissue located in the para-aortic sympathetic chain in which extra-adrenal pheochromocytomas may arise.

82. What is the best screening test for primary hyperaldosteronism? How should a positive test be followed up?

An upright plasma aldosterone concentration and plasma renin activity (PRA) taken in the absence of drugs that alter the renin-aldosterone axis (such as most antihypertensives, e.g., spironolactone and ACE inhibitors and diuretics). A ratio of plasma aldosterone concentration (ng/dl) to plasma renin activity (ng/ml/hr) of 25 is nearly 100% sensitive but has inadequate specificity (75–80%) for a definitive diagnosis. Confirmation requires a high 24-hour urine aldosterone level in the presence of normokalemia and adequate volume status.

83. How do you decide whether to treat hyperaldosteronism medically or surgically? What is the drug of choice?

Patients with unilateral aldosteronomas (Conn syndrome) are best treated surgically. Patients who are poor operative risks or who have bilateral adrenal hyperplasia are best treated with a specific aldosterone receptor antagonist, spironolactone. Keep in mind, however, that these patients may have concomitant essential hypertension and may need more than one treatment regimen.

84. What is the differential diagnosis of hypertension, hypokalemia, and a suppressed plasma renin activity (PRA)?

- Primary aldosteronism
- Deoxycorticosterone (DOC)-secreting tumors
- Some forms of congenital adrenal hyperplasia (11β-hydroxylase and 17α-hydroxylase deficiencies)
- Syndrome of apparent mineralocorticoid excess including licorice ingestion
- Cushing's syndrome
- Liddle's syndrome

85. What is glucocorticoid-remediable aldosteronism (GRA)?

This is a rare form of hyperaldosteronism transmitted in an autosomal dominant fashion by a chimeric gene that synthesizes aldosterone in response to ACTH stimulation. Its treatment is by ACTH suppression with dexamethasone.

86. What are the most common settings for hyporeninemic hypoaldosteronism?

Type 2 diabetes
Interstitial nephritis
AIDS

THYROID

87. How much does the normal adult thyroid gland weigh?

15–20 grams

88. What are the goals and limitations of the various tests of the thyroid gland?

Comparison of Thyroid Tests

TEST	GOAL	COMMENTS
Total T_4	T_4 level	Detects 90% of hyperthyroid cases; affected by alterations of TBG and can be misleadingly high or low; FT_4 is only a fraction of the total T_4.

(Table continued on next page.)

Comparison of Thyroid Tests (cont.)

TEST	GOAL	COMMENTS
Free T_4 (FT_4)	Assessment of FT_4	Directly measures FT_4; independent of TBG levels.
Serum T_3	T_3 level	Used to detect hyperthyroidism; misleadingly low in patients with non-thyroidal illness (i.e., low value does not usually indicate hypothyroidism). Do not confuse with RT_3U.
RT_3U	Assessment of FT_4	Clarifies whether alterations in T_4 are due to thyroid disease or alteration in T_4 binding proteins. Does not measure T_3.
Radioactive iodine uptake (RAIU)	Extent of thyroid function	Normal range must be determined for each population district. Difficult to distinguish low from low-normal values when dietary iodine is high. Hyperthyroidism does not always cause high iodine uptake.
TSH level	Index of thyroid status	Most sensitive test for primary hypothyroidism (TSH high before other tests show low T_4).
Thyroid scan	Functional status of nodular goiter	Often not needed in other types of thyroid disease.
Ultrasound	Status of single nodule	Reliably discriminates between cystic and solid nodules in 90% of cases.

TBG = Thyroxine-binding globulin; RT_3U = resin T_3 uptake test; TSH = thyroid-stimulating hormone.
Rubenstein E, et al (eds): Scientific American Medicine. New York, Scientific American, 1989.

89. What causes hyperthyroidism?

Hyperthyroidism is a syndrome resulting from the response to excess thyroid hormone levels. The excess thyroid hormone can come from hyperfunction of the thyroid gland, inflammation, destruction of all or part of the gland with resultant release of stored hormone, or from a source outside the thyroid. Separation of the causes by a low or high RAIU can help narrow the differential diagnosis:

Normal or High RAIU
Graves' disease
Toxic multinodular goiter
Solitary toxic nodule
Hypothalamic-pituitary disease
Choriocarcinoma or hydatidiform mole
Tumor metastases to the thyroid

Low RAIU
Subacute thyroiditis
Hyperthyroiditis
Factitious thyrotoxicosis
Jod-Basedow phenomenon (iodine-induced thyrotoxicosis)
Metastatic thyroid carcinoma
Struma ovarii (teratoma)

Kohler PO (ed): Clinical Endocrinology. New York, John Wiley, 1986, p 90.

90. Name the major signs and symptoms of hyperthyroidism.

Signs and Symptoms of Hyperthyroidism

SYSTEM	SYMPTOMS	SIGNS
↑ metabolic rate	Heat intolerance, increased appetite, weight loss	Sweating, ↓ muscle mass and fat; rarely fever
Cardiovascular	Palpitation; may have symptoms of heart failure	Tachycardia; hypertension (esp. systolic); arrhythmia (esp. atrial fibrillation); heart murmur or rub

(Table continues on next page.)

Signs and Symptoms of Hyperthyroidism (cont.)

SYSTEM	SYMPTOMS	SIGNS
Neuromuscular	Fatigue, muscular weakness	Tremor; ↑ deep tendon reflexes; proximal muscle weakness; rarely paralysis
Neuropsychiatric	Nervousness, irritability, depression, difficulty sleeping	Emotional lability, frank psychosis
Ophthalmologic	Eye irritation and stare,* photophobia,* diplopia,* brittle nails	Stare, lid retraction, lid lag, Graves' ophthalmopathy (proptosis, extra-ocular muscle dysfunction, optic neuropathy, chemosis)*
Skin, hair, nails	Alopecia, rash of pretibial myxedema,* ankle swelling	Smooth, soft, warm skin; hair of fine texture and easily removable; edema; pretibial myxedema in Graves' disease*; onycholysis
Respiratory	Dyspnea	↑ respiratory rate
Gastrointestinal	↑ frequency and softening of stools	Usually normal; may be splenomegaly*
Reproductive	Oligomenorrhea, impotence	Gynecomastia
Other	Anorexia, constipation	Lymphadenopathy*

* These findings are not manifestations of increased circulating thyroid hormone levels but are related to the disturbance in the immune system that occurs in Graves' disease.
From Kohler PO (ed): Clinical Endocrinology. New York, John Wiley, 1986, p 93, with permission.

91. What is a thyroid storm?

Thyroid storm is a dramatic, life-threatening exacerbation of **thyrotoxicosis**. It is characterized by fever, altered mental status, and signs of one or more organ decompensation such as cardiovascular (e.g., atrial fibrillation, congestive heart failure) and/or gastrointestinal (hepatitis, jaundice) dysfunction.

Thyroid storm is usually not associated with T_4 and T_3 levels markedly higher than the "pre-storm" values, so its diagnosis must be made on clinical grounds. Thyroid storm is often precipitated by another acute illness, such as infection, surgery, trauma to the thyroid, or withdrawal of partially effective antithyroid therapy.

92. How do you treat thyroid storm?

Treatment involves the use of propranolol to control the hyperadrenergic state, propylthiouracil (PTU) to block thyroid hormone synthesis and/or saturated solution of potassium iodide (SSKI) or other iodine-rich compounds (gastrograffin, ipodate) to block the release of preformed thyroid hormones. The peripheral conversion of T_4 to T_3 is partially blocked by PTU, propranolol, and hydrocortisone. Steroids may also be part of the initial management since thyroid hormones increase metabolism of endogenous cortisol in addition to its T_4 to T_3 blocking effect. Supportive therapy, IV fluids, antipyretics, cooling blankets, and sedatives also play a role. In extreme cases, plasmapheresis or peritoneal dialysis have been used to remove the thyroid hormone. In all cases, a search for and treatment of the initiating condition should be undertaken.

93. Why is aspirin not the antipyretic of choice in thyroid storm?

It can displace thyroid hormones from their protein binding and further increase free thyroid hormone levels.

94. Name the four basic mechanisms that lead to hypothyroidism.

Hypothyroidism is a clinical syndrome caused by the cellular responses to a deficiency of thyroid hormone. It can be produced by the following four mechanisms:

1. **Primary:** due to a pathologic process intrinsic to the thyroid gland, leading to defective production of thyroid hormone or destruction of the gland

2. **Secondary:** due to a deficiency of thyroid stimulating hormone from the pituitary (central hypothyroidism)

3. **Tertiary:** due to a deficiency of thyrotropin-releasing hormone (TRH) from the hypothalamus (central hypothyroidism)

4. **Peripheral resistance to the action of thyroid hormone:** a rare cause of hypothyroidism (Refetoff syndrome)

95. What are the causes of hypothyroidism?

Causes of Hypothyroidism

CLASSIFICATION	SPECIAL FEATURES
Primary	
Autoimmune (chronic thyroiditis, idiopathic, "burnt out" Graves' disease)	Thyroid antibodies positive in most cases; pernicious anemia and other primary endocrine deficiencies may coexist
Postablative	After radioactive iodine or surgery
Subacute thyroiditis	Transient phase, usually preceded by sore neck and thyrotoxicosis with low ^{131}I uptake
Drugs (iodines, lithium, thionamides)	Coexistent thyroiditis (autoimmune) prior to ablative therapy; recent history of drug administration
Thyroid agenesis	Most common cause in neonates
Thyroid dysgenesis	May cause juvenile hypothyroidism
Dyshormonogenesis	Goiter, family history
Head and neck irradiation	History of treatment with radiation
Neoplasia	Primary or metastatic tumor (rare)
Secondary	Associated with low TSH; impaired TSH response to TRH, when present, is helpful in diagnosis. Requires thorough evaluation for underlying cause of pituitary failure
Tertiary	Same as secondary, except TSH response to TRH is usually preserved
Peripheral resistance	Raised levels of thyroid hormone and TSH

From Kohler PO (ed): Clinical Endocrinology. New York, John Wiley, 1986, p 105, with permission.

96. What are the major signs and symptoms of hypothyroidism?

Signs and Symptoms of Hypothyroidism

SYSTEM	SYMPTOMS	SIGNS
↓ Metabolic rate	Cold intolerance, ↓ appetite, weight gain	Obesity, hypothermia
Neuromuscular	Muscle cramps, joint stiffness, paresthesias, weakness	Delayed deep tendon reflexes, ↑ muscle mass and rigidity, myotonia, joint effusions, carpal tunnel syndrome
		In infants: mental retardation, short stature

(*Table continued on next page.*)

Signs and Symptoms of Hypothyroidism (cont.)

SYSTEM	SYMPTOMS	SIGNS
Neuropsychiatric	Lethargy, ↓ energy, ↑ sleeping	Delirium, dementia, frank psychosis
Skin, hair, and nails	Dry skin, hair loss, straightened hair, brittle nails, edema	Cool, thin, scaling skin; alopecia; coarse hair; myxedema (esp. face and periorbital tissues)
Cardiovascular	Angina	Bradycardia, hypertension, cardio-megaly with effusion ("myxedema heart")
Ear, nose and throat	Hoarseness, hearing loss, altered taste/smell, vertigo	Deep voice, slow speech, conductive hearing loss, enlarged tongue
Respiratory	Dyspnea	Reduced inspiratory effort, pleural effusion
Gastrointestinal	Epigastric pain, constipation	Abdominal distention rarely toxic megacolon
Reproductive	Infertility, impotence In children: precocious puberty, delayed puberty	Galactorrhea

From Kohler PO (ed): Clinical Endocrinology. New York, John Wiley, 1986, p 109, with permission.

97. What is Pendred's syndrome?

Hypothyroidism (from organification defect) plus sensorineural deafness.

98. Describe the pathogenesis of Graves' disease. Give the characteristic triad of Graves'.

Graves' disease is an autoimmune disease in which T lymphocytes produce antibodies to certain thyroid antigens. Thyroid-stimulating immunoglobulin (TSI) is an antibody to the TSH receptor on the thyroid cells, which results in stimulation of growth and function. The cause of the autoimmune process is not known. The characeristic triad includes hyperthyroidism, diffuse goiter, and mesenchymal extrathyroid effects, namely ophthalmopathy, acropachy or dermopathy.

99. What is the NO-SPECS classification for Graves' ophthalmopathy?

	CHANGE	CLASS
N	No signs or symptoms	0
O	Only signs	1
S	Soft tissue involvement	2
P	Proptosis	3
E	Extraocular muscle involvement	4
C	Corneal involvement	5
S	Sight loss in visual acuity	6

Graves' ophthalmopathy does not necessarily progress in order of the NO-SPECS classes.

100. Which antithyroid drugs are used for hyperthyroidism? Which is unsafe in pregnancy?

Methimazole (Tapazole) and propylthiouracil (PTU). Methimazole has been associated with aplasia cutis in the newborn and is therefore not used in pregnancy in the U.S.

101. Which characteristics are predictive of spontaneous remission in Graves' disease?

Small thyroid gland	Female sex	Low antithyroid antibody titers
Young age	Acute onset of disease	

102. What therapies are available for Graves' ophthalmopathy? What are their indications?

Medical therapy may include the use of corticosteroids and/or cyclosporine. High dose steroids may be useful in moderate-to-severe disease. Cyclosporine may be useful as an adjunct in therapeutic failure.

Nonmedical therapy includes radiotherapy to the orbit and surgical decompression. These methods are usually reserved for more severe complications, such as corneal involvement or visual compromise.

103. How do the antibody profiles differ in Graves' disease, Hashimoto's thyroiditis, and subacute thyroiditis?

Hashimoto's thyroiditis has an increased prevalence of high titers of antimicrosomal and antithyroid antibodies. Graves' patients often have high titers of antithyroid antibodies and thyroid-stimulating immunoglobulin. Subacute thyroiditis is rarely associated with short-lived elevations of antithyroid antibodies, usually in low titers.

104. What is hashitoxicosis?

This term is used when Hashimoto's thyroiditis is associated with hyperthyroidism secondary to uncontrolled release of thyroid hormone.

105. What is Jod-Basedow phenomenon? What is its mechanism of occurrence?

Jod-Basedow phenomenon is hyperthyroidism resulting from an iodine load. It is usually seen in the setting of endemic goiter, multinodular goiter, or Graves' disease previously treated with antithyroid drugs. Any source of iodine, including contrast media, iodine-containing expectorants, or kelp, may induce this process.

106. Discuss the natural history and treatment of subacute thyroiditis.

Subacute thyroiditis, also called de Quervain's thyroiditis, usually begins as a prodromal viral-like syndrome followed 2–3 weeks later by thyroid or ear pain, sometimes with dysphagia. The thyroid gland is slightly enlarged, firm, and tender. The patient may range from euthyroid to thyrotoxic. The active phase lasts from days to months and may recur before final resolution.

Nonsteroidal anti-inflammatory drugs are usually sufficient to relieve the pain. Hyperthyroidism is usually treated with β-blockers. Antithyroid medications are poorly effective. More severe pain or active thyroiditis may be treated with a tapering dose of corticosteroids.

107. What historical and physical findings are suggestive of malignancy in a thyroid nodule?

Risk factors include positive family history of thyroid cancer, extremes of age (< 20 yrs or > 70 yrs), male sex, rapid growth of a preexisting nodule, invasive and compressive symptoms, and history of head and neck irradiation.

108. What should be your clinical approach to a patient who presents with a thyroid nodule?

After a thorough history and physical exam (focusing on signs and symptoms of hyperthyroidism) and normal thyroid function test, the single best way to assess a thyroid nodule is to do a fine needle aspiration biopsy of that nodule.

109. How is thyroid cancer staged?

STAGE	PAPILLARY (AGE ≤ 45 Y)	OR	FOLLICULAR (AGE ≥ 45 Y)	MEDULLARY (ANY AGE)	ANAPLASTIC (ANY AGE)
I	M0		T1	T1	—
II	M1		T2-T3	T2-T4	—
III	—		T4 or N1	N1	—
IV	—		M1	M1	Any

AJCC Stage Groupings for Thyroid Carcinoma: T, size of primary thyroid tumor (T1 ≤ 1 cm; T2 > 1 ≤ 4 cm; T3 > 4 cm; T4, extrathyroid invasion); N, regional nodal metastasis (0, absent; 1, present); M, distant metastases (0, absent; 1, present). (From Wilson JD, et.al (eds): Williams Textbook of Endocrinology, 9th ed. Philadelphia, W.B. Saunders, 1998, p 486, with permission.)

110. How should you follow-up thyroid carcinoma?

Physical examination, thyroid function tests to keep the TSH suppressed, thyroglobulin levels, and whole-body radioiodine scanning at 6–9 months, 1 year, 3 years, and then at 5-year intervals.

111. What is struma ovarii?

Ectopic thyroid tissue in an ovarian teratoma producing a hyperthyroid state. It is one of the rare causes of low radioactive iodine uptake hyperthyroidism. Other causes of low-uptake hyperthyroidism are thyroiditis, Jod-Basedow phenomenon, and exogenous thyroxine.

112. What is Reidel's thyroiditis?

A rare thyroiditis in which the gland has extensive fibrosis with adherence to adjacent structures, producing a characteristic "woody" consistency.

113. How is the TRH stimulation test useful in hyperthyroidism and hypothyroidism?

The pituitary gland is less responsive to TRH in the presence of high circulating levels of T_4. A "flat" TRH stimulation test suggests that the patient's axis is suppressed. On the other hand, the pituitary will be hyperresponsive to TRH with low circulating T_4, allowing the assessment of subtle hypothyroidism or an interpretation of an axis with altered binding proteins or T_4 metabolism, such as in phenytoin or amiodarone use. It is rarely used now with the advent of the ultrasensitive TSH assays.

114. What does "euthyroid sick" mean? What are the usual findings?

Euthyroid sick designates the changes in thyroid hormone levels in patients with severe systemic illness. T_4 and T_3 will decrease, with increased reverse T_3. Despite maintenance of a functional euthyroid state, T_4 to T_3 conversion is decreased, with shunting to reverse T_3. TSH is low, normal, or mildly elevated depending on what phase of the illness the thyroid function was checked. Recovery may be associated with a self-limited rise in TSH. No treatment is necessary other than repeating thyroid function check once the patient has recovered from the illness.

115. What is the earliest means of detecting medullary carcinoma of the thyroid (MCT)? What is the best therapy?

Pentagastrin stimulation testing. This test provokes an exaggerated rise in calcitonin, even in very early MCT. Surgery is the best therapy when seeking a cure.

116. What is McCune-Albright syndrome?

It is the constellation of bone tumors (polyostotic fibrous dysplasia), café-au-lait spots, and signs of endocrine hyperactivity (such as hyperthyroidism, precocious puberty or adrenocortical hyperplasia) caused by an activating mutation in the α-subunit of the G_S protein.

MALE AND FEMALE REPRODUCTIVE ENDOCRINOLOGY

117. Discuss the differential diagnosis for erectile dysfunction (ED).

ED may have vascular, neurogenic, hormonal, pharmacologic, local, and psychiatric components. A drug history, particularly noting antihypertensives (e.g., β-blocker, Ca-channel blockers, diuretics) and alcohol, may be key in evaluating the source. Studies on REM-associated erections may help differentiate between psychogenic causes and other reasons. Barring patients with drug-induced ED or those with normal nocturnal erections, further evaluation of hormone status, local factors, and neurocirculatory problems need to be investigated.

118. What is nocturnal penile tumescence?

This describes erections associated with REM sleep. This phenomenon is detected using penile strain gauges and EEG in a sleep laboratory.

119. What does the Lyon hypothesis have to do with a buccal mucosal scraping in a man with long arms and infertility?

The Lyon hypothesis predicts random inactivation of an X chromosome in XX women, producing the distinctive Barr body in somatic cells. Men should not have Barr bodies, but men with Klinefelter's syndrome, XXY, will have them on a smear of buccal cells.

120. What does obesity have to do with a hypogonadal male who cannot smell well?

These findings suggest Kallmann's syndrome, a defect in midline hypothalamic development that produces obesity, hypogonadotropic hypogonadism, and disordered smell.

121. What is the difference between hirsutism and virilization?

Hirsutism is excess hair only. Virilization includes increased androgen response, including increased muscle mass, lowered voice, clitoral enlargement, and behavioral changes.

122. What is the differential diagnosis for hirsutism in a woman?

Racial or familial predilection	Polycystic ovarian syndrome
Ovarian or adrenal neoplasm	Late onset congenital adrenal hyperplasia

123. What are the causes of gynecomastia?

1. Idiopathic
2. Physiologic
   Puberty
   Aging
   Newborn
3. Drugs
   Drugs with estrogen activity: conjugated or synthetic estrogens, oral contraceptives, digitalis (digitoxin only, not digoxin)
   Drugs that stimulate estrogen synthesis or effect: clomiphene citrate, HCG, LHRH
   Drugs that decrease testosterone synthesis or effect: cimetidine, spironolactone, ketoconazole, cancer chemotherapeutic agents
   Unknown mechanisms: methyldopa, marijuana, testosterone, isoniazid, diazepam, ethionamide, tricyclic antidepressants, D-penicillamine, ?heroin, ?phenothiazines, ?amphetamines
4. Tumors with increased HCG or estrogen formation
   Choriocarcinoma (testicular or teratoma)
   Other testicular tumors
   Bronchogenic carcinoma
   Adrenal carcinoma
5. Increased estrogen synthesis
   Liver disease (may be combined with decreased androgens)
   Thyrotoxicosis
   Obesity (presumed)
   True hermaphroditism
   Familial
6. Decreased androgen synthesis or androgen resistance
   Testicular failure: orchitis, trauma or castration, granulomatous disease, myotonic dystrophy, neurologic disorders
   Klinefelter's syndrome
   Defects in testosterone synthesis
   Congenital anorchism
   Androgen resistance syndromes
   Renal failure
7. Altered testosterone and estrogen binding
   Thyrotoxicosis

8. Unknown mechanism
   Starvation-refeeding
   HCG = human chorionic gonadotropin; LHRH = luteinizing hormone-releasing hormone.
   From: Kohler PO (ed): Clinical Endocrinology. New York, John Wiley, 1986, p 373, with permission.

124. What are the causes of amenorrhea?

It is important to differentiate whether amenorrhea is primary (never had menses before) versus secondary (cessation of menses after they have started). It is always important to rule out pregnancy as a cause of amenorrhea. After pregnancy is ruled out, the following causes are taken into consideration:

1. Outflow tract defects
   Imperforate hymen   Asherman's syndrome
   Cervical agenesis/stenosis   Transverse vaginal septum
   Mullerian agenesis
2. Ovarian failure or hypergonadotropic hypogonadism
   Congenital   *Acquired*
     Turner's syndrome   Irradiation
     Enzyme deficiencies   Chemotherapy
                                                Mumps orchitis
3. Chronic anovulation with estrogen present
   Polycystic ovary syndrome   Hypothyroidism or hyperthyroidism
   Cushing's disease   Functional ovarian tumors
   Congenital adrenal hyperplasia
4. Chronic anovulation with estrogen absent or hypogonadotropic hypogonadism
   Hypothalamic   *Pituitary*
     Tumors (e.g., craniopharyngioma,   Tumors (prolactinoma, nonfunctional macro-
       metastasis)   adenoma, metastasis)
     Infection (TB, syphilis, meningitis)   Necrosis/autoimmune (Sheehan's, lymphocytic
     Sarcoidosis   hypophysitis)
     Functional (e.g., anorexia nervosa,   Inflammatory/infiltrative (sarcoidosis, hemo-
       malnutrition)   chromatosis

125. Describe the polycystic ovary syndrome (PCOS).

Hyperandrogenism and chronic anovulation characterize this syndrome. Other conditions such as adult-onset congenital adrenal hyperplasia, hyperprolactinemia, and androgen-secreting neoplasms must be ruled-out first before this diagnosis is given. Insulin resistance has also been associated with PCOS, and insulin sensitizers such as metformin or thiazolidinediones (drugs used in diabetes) now play a role in the management of this syndrome.

PARATHYROID HORMONE, CALCIUM, AND BONE DISORDERS

126. List the mediators of hypercalcemia of malignancy.

Interleukin 1   Tumor necrosis factor
Lymphotoxin   Parathyroid hormone-related protein (PTH-rp)
Prostaglandins   1,25-dihydroxy Vitamin D

127. What are bisphosphonates?

Bisphosphonates are a class of compounds whose backbone is modeled on pyrophosphate in which the bridge oxygen is replaced by carbon. These compounds generally inhibit bone resorption through multiple mechanisms and differ in potency and side-effect profiles. They are generally useful in conditions of high bone turnover, such as humoral hypercalcemia and Paget's disease, and are now being used in osteoporosis.

128. When is medical therapy indicated for Paget's disease of bone? What medicines are available?

Pain, deformity, nerve entrapment, and cranial involvement indicate the need for medical therapy. Calcitonin and bisphosphonates are indicated for suppression of disease activity.

129. How may bone density be measured and why? Isn't there anything easier?

Bone density is now most commonly measured by dual-energy x-ray absorptiometry (DEXA) scanning, although quantitative CT may also be used. Bone mass has been shown prospectively to correlate with skeletal fragility and fracture risk. Typically, bone mass is compared to the "peak" bone mass achieved in a person's second and third decade, with deviations from peak described in standard deviations (SD). Responses to therapy may also be followed by bone densitometry.

Bone ultrasound is now being evaluated as another means of assessing bone quality. Prospective studies have shown a correlation between bone ultrasound attenuation and subsequent fracture risk. This technology will likely become more useful in the future.

130. What are the indications for bone biopsy?

Bone biopsy is best used for evaluation of bone disorders of unknown etiology. Direct sampling of bone allows assessment of bone architecture and qualitative disorders of formation. The use of timed fluorescent labels allows kinetic parameters to be assessed, including turnover rate and bone formation rate. Special stains can detect aluminum and other heavy metals.

Indications for Bone Biopsy in the Clinical Setting

- Suspected osteomalacia
- Diagnostic classification of renal osteodystrophy
- Osteopenia in young individuals (< 50 yrs)
- Osteopenia in individuals with abnormal calcium metabolism
- Hereditary childhood bone diseases that are classification problems
- Evaluation of treatment in certain diseases (e.g., osteomalacia, hypophosphatasia)

Eriksen EF, Axelrod DW, Melsen F: Bone Histomorphometry. New York, Raven Press, 1994, p 35.

131. How do osteopenia and osteoporosis differ?

Osteopenia only denotes loss of bone mass. This may or may not be accompanied by an increase in fragility. For example, hyperparathyroidism is accompanied by some degree of osteopenia but is not associated with increased fragility, probably because of maintained microarchitecture.

In osteoporosis, bone mass and architecture are progressively lost with a resultant increase in susceptibility to fracture. According to the WHO nomenclature, osteoporosis denotes a loss of bone mass > 2.5 SD from the peak achieved earlier in life, and established or severe osteoporosis denotes the additional presence of osteoporotic (fragility) fracture.

Assessment of Fracture Risk and Its Application to Screening for Postmenopausal Osteoporosis: Report of a WHO Study Group. Geneva, World Health Organization, 1994.

132. What is the differential diagnosis of osteoporosis?

	Primary Osteoporosis	
Juvenile	Idiopathic (young adults)	Involutional
	Secondary Osteoporosis	
Endocrine diseases		
Hypogonadism	Hyperadrenocorticism	Hyperthyroidism
Hyperparathyroidism	Diabetes mellitus	
Gastrointestinal diseases		
Subtotal gastrectomy	Malabsorption syndromes	Chronic obstructive jaundice
Primary biliary cirrhosis	Severe malnutrition	Anorexia nervosa

Bone marrow disorders

Multiple myeloma	Mastocytosis	Metastatic carcinoma

Connective tissue diseases

Osteogenesis imperfecta	Homocystinuria	Ehlers-Danlos syndrome
Marfan's syndrome		

Miscellaneous causes

Immobilization	Rheumatoid arthritis	Chronic alcoholism
Chronic heparinization	Chronic obstructive pulmonary disease	

Riggs BL: Osteoporosis. In DeGroot LJ (ed): Endocrinology, 2nd ed. Philadelphia, W.B. Saunders, 1989, p 1196.

133. Why are women more prone to osteoporosis than men?

They are not. Men are equally prone to osteoporosis, just later in life. Men develop the classical fractures of osteoporosis (Colles', vertebral, and hip) later in life than do women.

In women, the loss of sex steroids at menopause or through medical or surgical causes leads to an increase in bone turnover through activation of bone remodeling. This itself causes an overall loss of bone and loss of cancellous (trabecular) bone. Further, with loss of estrogen, the amount of bone resorbed is greater than that replaced, leading to a continuing decline in overall bone mass and worsening microarchitecture.

134. What is the principle of the intact parathyroid hormone (PTH) assay? Why is it particularly useful in renal failure?

Antibodies to one end of the PTH molecule are attached to a solid phase, such as beads or the inside of the test tube. The patient's serum is then added, incubated, and washed out, leaving PTH attached to the solid phase. A radiolabeled antibody to the other end of the PTH molecule is then added. This antibody only binds to intact PTH, the other end of which is attached to the solid phase. Any fragments bound to the solid phase will not be recognized by the second antibody. In this manner, only "intact" PTH produces a signal. Renal failure causes poor clearance of PTH fragments, which produce large signals on one-site PTH assays, but which do not interfere with the two-site assay.

135. How does magnesium deficiency cause hypocalcemia?

Magnesium deficiency inhibits PTH release from the parathyroid glands; it also interferes with its action at bone and kidney.

136. How should surgery for sporadic primary hyperparathyroidism differ from surgery for MEN syndrome?

Sporadic hyperparathyroidism is almost always secondary to an isolated parathyroid adenoma, which leads to cure on its resection. MEN is associated with diffuse parathyroid hyperplasia and hyperfunction. The therapy of choice is resection of $3\frac{1}{2}$ glands, usually with implantation of the remaining $\frac{1}{2}$ gland in the sternomastoid muscle or forearm.

137. What are the indications for surgical intervention in primary hyperparathyroidism?

Surgery remains the mainstay of treatment for hyperparathyroidism, although, because of the slow progression of the disease, some clinicians and patients opt for medical management. The following schema shows the need for surgery:

Serum calcium > 12 mg/dl	Marked hypercalciuria > 400 mg/24-hours
Overt manifestation of hyperparathyroidism (kidney stones, osteitis fibrosa cystica, classic neuromuscular disease)	Reduced creatinine clearance in the absence of other causes
	Age < 50 years old
Markedly reduced cortical bone density	

138. What do you monitor after parathyroidectomy from hyperparathyroidism?

Calcium and phosphate. Postoperatively, patients are at increased risk of hypocalcemia because of several factors. These factors include suppression of the remaining parathyroid function after single parathyroid adenoma excision causing a state of temporary hypoparathyroidism; inadvertent or intentional removal of all parathyroid glands causing permanent hypoparathyroidism; and "hungry bone syndrome," which can develop in those patients severely hyperparathyroid before surgery. This is due to bone depletion of mineral content (Ca^{++} and $Phos^{++}$) by the excessive parathyroid hormone. Hence, with the removal of the excess parathyroid source, the bones avidly take up all the minerals that have been "robbed" from them.

139. What is familial hypocalciuric hypercalcemia (FHH)? How can it be differentiated from hyperparathyroidism?

FHH is a familial-dominant disorder in which the calcium level is set higher than normal in the face of high-normal PTH levels. Urine calcium levels are remarkably low, in contrast to those seen in hyperparathyroidism. Patients give a long history, usually from birth, of mildly elevated calcium levels without any symptoms. No long-term morbidity is associated with FHH. All patients with suspected hyperparathyroidism should be checked for FHH by urine calcium determination to avoid misdiagnosis of hyperparathyroidism and inadvertent surgery.

140. How does sarcoidosis cause hypercalcemia?

Sarcoid tissue is able to hydroxylate 25-hydroxyvitamin D to the active 1,25-dihydroxy form and produce an endogenous hypervitaminosis D.

141. What are the most common causes of hypercalcemia?

Hyperparathyroidism and malignancy.

142. How is acute symptomatic hypercalcemia managed?

Remember that patients who present with symptomatic hypercalcemia are volume-depleted; hence, first line therapy is IV fluid hydration with normal saline (up to 2–4 L/day). Once adequately hydrated, furosemide, a loop diuretic, may be added to increase calcium loss from the kidneys. Other agents may be used in conjunction with hydration to inhibit osteoclastic bone resorption and thus decrease serum Ca^{++}, including bisphosphonates, calcitonin, and, rarely, gallium nitrate and plicamycin. In severe cases, hemodialysis may be required. Steroids may be useful if the hypercalcemia is secondary to vitamin D intoxication or noninfectious granulomatous disease such as sarcoidosis.

LIPIDS

143. What are the major lipoproteins and their compositions?

Lipoproteins are composed of nonpolar (and therefore water-insoluble) cholesterol esters and triglycerides (TG) surrounded by a layer of polar (and therefore water-soluble) proteins and lipids (unesterified cholesterol and phospholipids). This structure allows the entire particle to remain miscible in serum. The major lipoproteins are:

COMPOSITION (%)

TYPE	DIAMETER Å	ELECTRO-PHORETIC MOBILITY	PROTEIN	TG	CHOLESTEROL FREE	ESTER	PHOSPHO-LIPID
Chylomicrons	5000	Origin	1–2	85–95	1–3	2–4	3–6
VLDL	2000	Pre-b	6–10	50–65	4–8	16–22	15–20
LDL	250	b	18–22	4–8	6–8	45–50	18–24
HDL	80	a	45–55	2–7	3–5	15–20	26–32

144. Compare familial hypercholesterolemia (FHC) and primary moderate (polygenic) hypercholesterolemia (PHC). How does the latter contrast with primary (familial) combined hyperlipidemia (PCHL)?

FHC stems from a LDL receptor defect leading to diminished LDL-cholesterol uptake at the liver and increased cholesterol synthesis. Homozygotes have extremely elevated cholesterol levels and accelerated atherosclerosis in childhood. Heterozygotes show LDL-cholesterol levels of about twice normal.

PHC is much more common, presenting with LDL-cholesterol levels of 160–220 mg/dl. This syndrome probably represents several defects in LDL receptors, receptor binding, or intracellular cholesterol metabolism. It may be differentiated from PCHL syndrome in that the latter also incorporates elevated triglycerides through elevated LDL and/or VLDL levels.

145. Which apolipoprotein directs LDL binding to its receptor?

Apolipoprotein B-100 directs LDL binding to its cellular receptor and its subsequent uptake into the cell.

146. What is the chylomicronemia syndrome and its differential diagnosis?

The syndrome is characterized by markedly elevated triglyceride levels (often > 1,000 mg/dl), eruptive xanthomas, and pancreatitis. It may be a primary disease caused by deficiency of lipoprotein lipase or apoprotein C-II but is more commonly seen in the setting of excessive alcohol intake, uncontrolled diabetes, or use of oral contraceptives.

147. What are the noncholesterol risk factors used in assessing treatment modalities for hypercholesterolemia?

Atherosclerotic disease in the patient
    Definitive coronary artery disease (CAD)
    Peripheral vascular disease
Positive risk factors (increase risk of morbidity/mortality)
    Men > 45 yrs old
    Women > 55 yrs old or premature menopause without estrogen replacement
    Premature CAD in first-degree relatives (male relatives < 55 y/o, female relatives < 65 yrs)
    Current cigarette smoking
    Type 2 diabetes
Hypertension
    Low HDL-cholesterol (35 mg/dl or less)
Negative risk factors (decrease risk of morbidity/mortality)
    High HDL-cholesterol (60 mg/dl or more)

Summary of the second report of the National Cholesterol Education Program (NCEP) expert panel on detection, evaluation, and treatment of high blood cholesterol in adults (Adult Treatment Panel II). JAMA 269:3015–3023, 1993.

148. At what LDL levels should dietary and pharmacologic treatments for hyperlipidemia be initiated? What are the treatment goals?

Risk Factors and Treatment of Hyperlipidemia

	INITIATION LEVEL	LDL-C GOAL
Diet and Exercise		
No CAD and < 2 CAD risk factors	> 160 mg/dl	< 160 mg/dl
No CAD and 2 or more CAD risk factors	> 130 mg/dl	< 130 mg/dl
CAD present	> 100 mg/dl	< 100 mg/dl
Pharmacologic		
No CAD and <2 CAD risk factors	> 190 mg/dl	< 160 mg/dl
No CAD and 2 or more CAD risk factors	>160 mg/dl	<130 mg/dl
CAD present	>130 mg/dl	<100 mg/dl

149. How can you estimate a patient's LDL from measurements of total cholesterol, HDL, and triglyceride?

LDL = Total cholesterol − HDL − Triglycerides/5

150. Who should have their cholesterol measured? How often?

All adults aged 20 and older should have their total and LDL cholesterol tested at least once every 5 years. These may be tested in a nonfasting state.

The Expert Panel: Report of the National Cholesterol Education Program (NCED) Expert Panel on detection, evaluation and treatment of high blood cholesterol in adults. JAMA 269:3015–3023, 1993.

151. List the currently available lipid-lowering agents, their mechanism of action, and their side effects.

Summary of Lipid-Lowering Agents

CLASS	AGENT(S)	MECHANISM	ACTIONS	SIDE-EFFECTS & CONSIDERATIONS
Bile-acid resins	Cholestyramine Colestipol	Bind bile acids in gut, with resultant ↑ cholesterol utilization, ↑ LDL receptor activity, and ↑ LDL clearance from circulation	LDL ↓ VLDL, TG ↑ HDL ↔	Constipation Bloating Impaired absorption of some medications
Nicotinic acid (Niacin)	Nicotinic acid (slow-release forms available)	Inhibits hepatic secretion of VLDL and FFA release from fat	LDL ↓ TG ↓ HDL ↑	Flushing (suppressed with low-dose aspirin) Worsening of glucose tolerance Elevated LFTs
HMG-CoA reductase inhibitors	Lovastatin Pravastatin Simvastatin Fluvastatin	Inhibit cholesterol formation through inhibition of HMG-CoA reductase, with ↑ LDL receptor activity.	LDL ↓ TG ↓ (small) HDL ↑	Myositis Elevated LFTs
Gemfibrozil	Gemfibrozil	↑ activity of lipoprotein lipase, may inhibit hepatic secretion of VLDL	TG ↓↓ HDL ↓ (variable) LDL ↓	Myositis, diarrhea Nausea, skin rash (rare)

LFT, liver function tests; FFA, free fatty acids.

152. What effect does alcohol use have on lipids?

Alcohol causes an increase in triglyceride levels but does not affect LDL levels. It does cause an increase in HDL levels through an unknown mechanism. This may lead to a reduction of the risk of CAD, although use of alcohol is not specifically recommended for this purpose.

The Expert Panel: Report of the National Cholesterol Education Program Expert Panel on detection, evaluation and treatment of high blood cholesterol in adults. Arch Intern Med 148:36–69, 1988.

153. Can other factors increase HDL levels?

The following have been found to elevate HDL levels:
• Weight loss
• Aerobic exercise (however, mild to moderate exercise may have little effect)
• Discontinuation of cigarette smoking
• Drugs (nicotinic acid, gemfibrozil)

154. What are prostaglandins (PGs)?

PGs are oxygenation products of 20-carbon (eicosanoic) fatty acids that produce a wide variety of biologic effects. They are part of a group of compounds derived from eicosanoic fatty acids (called eicosanoids) that also includes thromboxanes and leukotrienes. PGs are produced by many different tissues and have regulatory actions throughout the body. They are produced and exert their effects locally rather than systemically.

155. What are some of the medical conditions that present primarily with increasd LDL, increased triglycerides, and decreased HDL?

Increased LDL	Increased triglycerides	Decreased HDL
Hypothyroidism	Type 2 diabetes	Hypertriglyceridemia
Nephrotic syndrome	Obesity	Cigarette smoking
Obstructive liver disease	Hypothyroidism	Sedentary life style
Anabolic steroids	Estrogens	Type 2 diabetes
Glucocorticoid therapy	Alcohol	
	β-blockers	
	Thiazides	
	SLE	

156. What are the some of the physical findings associated with the different lipid disorders?

Type IIa (predominantly LDL) or FH	Tendon xanthomas of the Achilles tendons and extensor tendons of the hands
Type III (IDL excess) or dysbetalipo-proteinemia	Palmar xanthomas
Type I (hyperchylomicronemia)	Eruptive xanthomas
Tangier disease (low HDL)	Orange tonsils

BIBLIOGRAPHY

1. DeGroot LJ (ed): Endocrinology, 3rd ed. Philadelphia, W.B. Saunders, 1995.
2. Eriksen EF, Axelrod DW, Melsen F: Bone Histomorphometry. New York, Raven Press, 1994.
3. Kohler PO (ed): Clinical Endocrinology. New York, John Wiley, 1986.
4. Stein JH (ed): Internal Medicine, 4th ed. St. Louis, Mosby, 1994.
5. Wilson ID, et al: Williams Textbook of Endocrinology, 9th ed. Philadelphia, W.B. Saunders, 1998.

3. CARDIOLOGY

Gabriel B. Habib, M.D., and Anthony J. Zollo, Jr., M.D.

Of all the ailments which may blow out life's little candle, heart disease is the chief.

William Boyd
Pathology for the Surgeon

Art is long and Time is fleeting
And our hearts, though stout and brave,
Still, like muffled drums are beating
Funeral marches to the grave.

Henry Wadsworth Longfellow
A Psalm of Life

PHYSICAL EXAM

1. What are the cardiac physical examination findings in cardiac tamponade?
When the clinical triad of cardiac tamponade was first described by Beck in 1935, it consisted of hypotension, elevated systemic venous pressure, and a small quiet heart and was commonly due to penetrating cardiac injuries, aortic dissection, or intrapericardial rupture of an aortic or cardiac aneurysm. Today, the most common causes are neoplastic disease, idiopathic pericarditis, acute myocardial infarction (MI), and uremia. The physical findings are:

1. **Jugular venous distension**. It is almost universally present except in patients with severe hypovolemia.

2. **Pulsus paradoxus**, defined as a decrease in systolic BP in excess of 10 mmHg during quiet inspiration. Pulsus paradoxus is difficult to elicit in volume-depleted patients.

3. **Tachycardia**, with a thready peripheral pulse. Sometimes, severe cardiac tamponade may restrict LV and RV filling enough to cause hypotension, but a thready and rapid pulse is almost invariably present.

Kussmaul's sign, an inspiratory increase in systemic venous pressure, is commonly present in chronic constrictive pericarditis but is rarely detected in acute cardiac tamponade.

2. What is the third heart sound (S_3)? What is a physiologic S_3?
An S_3 (or ventricular gallop) is a low-frequency sound that is heard just after the second heart sound (S_2). It is found in normal young patients (called a **physiologic S_3**) and also in a variety of pathologic conditions (**pathologic S_3**), including congestive heart failure (CHF), mitral valve prolapse, thyrotoxicosis, coronary artery disease (CAD), cardiomyopathies, pericardial constriction, mitral or aortic insufficiency, and left-to-right shunts.

The mechanism behind an S_3 is controversial. It may be due to an increase in the velocity of blood entering the ventricles (rapid ventricular filling). It usually represents myocardial decompensation when associated with heart disease.

3. What is an S_4?
An S_4, or atrial gallop, occurs just before S_1 and reflects decreased ventricular compliance (a stiff ventricle). It is associated with CAD, pulmonic or aortic valvular stenosis, hypertension, and ventricular hypertrophy from any cause.

4. How are heart murmurs graded?

Grading System for Heart Murmurs

GRADE	PHYSICAL EXAMINATION FINDINGS
1	Barely audible intensity (only a cardiologist can hear it!)
2	Low-intensity murmur (the upper-level resident can hear it)
3	Loud murmur (everyone can hear it)
4	Loud murmur with palpable thrill
5	Loudest murmur audible (still requires a stethoscope placed on the chest)
6	Murmur loud enough to be heard with the stethoscope off the chest

5. What is paradoxical splitting of S_2? What are its causes?

S_2 is normally split into aortic (A_2) and pulmonic components (P_2) caused by the closing of the two respective valves. The degree of splitting varies with the respiratory cycle (physiologic splitting). With inspiration, the negative intrathoracic pressure leads to increased venous return to the right side of the heart and a decrease to the left side; this causes P_2 to occur slightly later and A_2 to occur slightly earlier, which leads to a widening of the splitting of S_2. With expiration, the negative intrathoracic pressure is eliminated and A_2 and P_2 occur almost simultaneously. **Paradoxical splitting** of S_2 refers to the situation in which the split of A_2 and P_2 seems to widen with expiration and shorten with inspiration (the opposite of normal). This is caused by P_2 preceding A_2 during expiration and is usually due to conditions that delay A_2 by delaying ejection of blood from the left ventricle (LV) and therefore closure of the aortic valve. Causes include aortic insufficiency, aortic stenosis, hypertrophic obstructive cardiomyopathy, myocardial ischemia, left bundle branch block, or a right ventricular (RV) pacemaker.

6. What causes fixed splitting of S_2?

In fixed splitting of S_2, the interval between A_2 and P_2 does not change with the respiratory cycle. It is typically associated with atrial septal defects or RV dysfunction.

7. How do you measure the jugular venous pulse at the bedside?

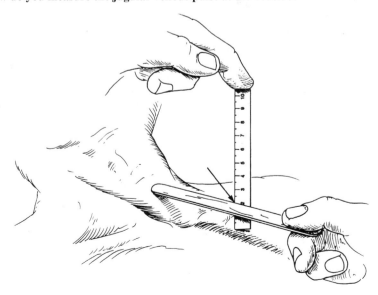

The patient's chest should be elevated to the point where the pulsations are maximally visualized (usually 30–45° of elevation). The height of this oscillating venous column above the sternal angle (angle of Louis) can then be measured. Since the sternal angle is about 5 cm from the right atrium (regardless of elevation angle), central venous pressure can be estimated by adding 5 cm to the measurement. Normal central venous pressure is 5–9 cm H_2O.

From Adair OV, Havranek EP: Cardiology Secrets. Philadelphia, Hanley & Belfus, 1995, p 6; with permission.

8. Name the three waves comprising the jugular venous pulse.

1. **a-wave**, produced by right atrial contraction, occurs just before S_1.

2. **c-wave** is caused by bulging upward of the closed tricuspid valve during RV contraction (often difficult to see).

3. **v-wave** is caused by right atrial filling just before opening of the tricuspid valve.

9. What are "cannon" a-waves?

These very large and prominent a-waves occur when the atria contract against a closed tricuspid valve. Irregular "cannon" a-waves are seen in AV dissociation or ectopic atrial beats. Regular "cannon" a-waves are seen in a junctional or ventricular rhythm in which the atria are depolarized by retrograde conduction.

10. What is the likely cause of a systolic ejection murmur, best heard at the second right intercostal space, in an 82-year-old symptomatic man?

By far, the most common cause in this situation is aortic sclerosis. This valvular abnormality is characterized by thickening and/or calcification of the aortic valve, and unlike valvular aortic stenosis, it is typically *not* associated with any significant transvalvular systolic pressure gradient. On physical examination, aortic sclerosis can be differentiated from aortic stenosis as follows:

	AORTIC STENOSIS	AORTIC SCLEROSIS
Diminished carotid upstroke	Yes	No
Diminished peripheral pulses	Yes	No
Late peaking of systolic murmur	Yes	No
Loud S_4	Yes	No
Syncope, angina, or heart failure	Yes	No
Loud systolic murmur and thrill	Yes	No

11. How do standing, squatting, and leg-raising affect the intensity and duration of the systolic murmur heard on dynamic auscultation in a patient with idiopathic hypertrophic subaortic stenosis (IHSS)?

In IHSS, a decrease in the size of the LV increases the dynamic LV outflow obstruction, leading to an increased intensity of the murmur. A decrease in LV volume occurs on standing. In contrast, leg-raising and squatting increase venous return and thereby increase LV volume, decreasing the dynamic LV obstruction and the murmur intensity.

12. What is the mechanism of pulsus paradoxus? What medical diseases can present with pulsus paradoxus?

Pulsus paradoxus was first described by Kussmaul in 1873 as the apparent disappearance of the pulse during inspiration despite persistence of the heartbeat. In fact, pulsus paradoxus is an exaggeration of the normal decline in systolic BP and LV stroke volume on inspiration. The fall in intrathoracic pressure is rapidly transmitted through the pericardial effusion and results in an exaggerated increase in venous return to the right side of the heart. This, in turn, causes bulging of the interventricular septum toward the LV, thereby resulting in a smaller LV volume and LV stroke volume during inspiration.

Pulsus paradoxus is **not** a *sine qua non* of cardiac tamponade. It may also occur in patients with severe chronic obstructive pulmonary disease complicated by the need for large negative intrathoracic pressures on inspiration. Interestingly, pulsus paradoxus is usually absent in chronic constrictive pericarditis.

ELECTROCARDIOGRAPHY

13. Describe the sequence of ECG changes in an acute transmural MI. What is their timing in relation to the onset of symptoms?

The evolution of an acute MI consists of three phases on ECG:

1. **Abnormal T wave**, which is tall, prolonged, inverted, or upright. Hyperacute tall T waves are typically seen in the first hour or two of MI evolution. The T wave usually becomes inverted after ST-segment elevation has occurred and may remain inverted for days, weeks, or years.

2. **ST-segment elevations** in leads facing the infarcted myocardial wall and reciprocal ST depressions in opposite leads. ST-segment changes are the most common ECG signs of acute MI. ST-segment elevations rarely persist > 2 weeks except in patients with a ventricular aneurysm.

3. **Appearance of new Q waves**, often several hours or days after the onset of MI symptoms. Alternatively, the amplitude of the QRS complex is decreased. Q waves may develop earlier when thrombolytic therapy is administered.

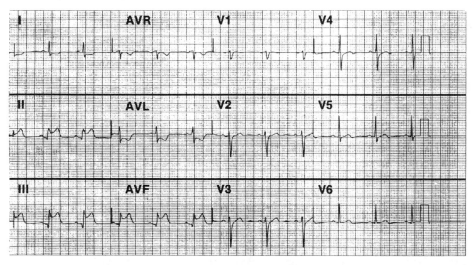

Acute MI localized to inferior leads (II, III, and aVF). The ECG shows ST elevation with hyperacute peaked T waves and the early development of significant Q waves. Reciprocal ST depression is also seen (leads I and aVL). (From Seelig CB: Simplified EKG Analysis. Philadelphia, Hanley & Belfus, 1992, p 13; with permission.)

14. What are the ECG manifestations of atrial infarction?

1. Depressed or elevated PR segment
2. Atrial arrhythmias:
   a. Atrial flutter
   b. Atrial fibrillation
   c. AV nodal rhythms

15. Where does an S_3 occur in relation to the QRS complex? Where does the venous a-wave appear in the cardiac cycle?

During the course of one cardiac cycle, note that the electrical events (ECG) initiate and therefore precede the mechanical (pressure) events and that the latter precede the auscultatory events (heart sounds) they produce. Shortly after the P wave, the atria contract to produce the a-wave; S_4 may succeed the latter. The QRS complex initiates ventricular systole, followed shortly by LV contraction and the rapid build-up of LV pressure. Almost immediately, LV pressure exceeds left atrial (LA) pressure to close the mitral valve and produces S_1. When LV pressure exceeds aortic pressure, the aortic valve opens (AVO), and when aortic pressure is once again greater than LV pressure, the aortic valve closes to produce S_2 and terminate ventricular ejection. The decreasing LV pressure drops below LA pressure to open the mitral valve (MVO), and a period of rapid ventricular filling commences. During this time, an S_3 may be heard. (For simplification, right-sided heart pressures have been omitted.)

From Andreoli TE, et al (eds): Cecil Essentials of Medicine, 2nd ed. Philadelphia, W.B. Saunders, 1990, p 8; with permission.

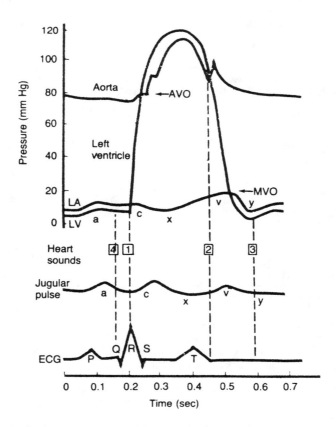

16. Which arrhythmias can be detected in young patients without apparent heart disease?

In a study of 24-hour continuous ECG monitoring performed on 50 male medical students, severe sinus bradycardia (40 bpm or fewer), sinus pauses of up to 2 sec, and nocturnal AV nodal block were frequently found. Frequent premature atrial or ventricular beats were not commonly found.

Brodsky M, et al: Arrhythmias documented by 24-hour continuous electrocardiographic monitoring in 50 male medical students without apparent heart disease. Am J Cardiol 39:390–395, 1977.

17. How do you differentiate among the various types of supraventricular tachycardias (SVTs)?

   Atrial fibrillation (AF) differs from all other SVTs by having totally disorganized atrial depolarizations without effective atrial contraction. An ECG may occasionally show small, irregular waves of variable amplitude and morphology, occurring at a rate of 350–600/min, but these are often difficult to recognize on a routine 12-lead ECG.

   Atrial tachycardia (or paroxysmal atrial tachycardia) and **atrial flutter**, unlike AF, demonstrate a regular ventricular rhythm and are characterized by regular and slower atrial rhythms. The flutter rate (i.e., the atrial rate) in atrial flutter ranges between 250–350 bpm. The most common flutter rate is 300 bpm, and the most common ventricular rates are 150 and 75 bpm, respectively. Atrial tachycardias have slower atrial rates, ranging from 150–250 bpm. The most common cause of atrial tachycardia with block is digitalis toxicity.

Comparison of Supraventricular Tachycardias

	ATRIAL FIBRILLATION	ATRIAL FLUTTER	ATRIAL TACHYCARDIA
Atrial rate	> 400	240–350	100–240
Atrial rhythm	Irregular	Regular	Regular
AV block	Variable	2:1, 4:1, 3:1, or variable	2:1, 4:1, 3:1, or variable
Ventricular rate	Variable	150, 75, 100, or variable	Variable

18. What is the significance of capture and fusion beats on ECG in differentiating between ventricular tachycardia (VT) and SVT with aberrancy?

Distinguishing Features of Wide-Complex VT and SVT

	VT	SVT
History of MI	Yes	No
Ventricular aneurysm	Yes	No
Fusion beats	Yes	No
Capture beats	Yes	No
Complete AV dissociation	Yes	No
Similar QRS when in sinus rhythm	No	Yes
RBBB + QRS > 0.14 sec	Yes	No
LBBB + QRS > 0.16 sec	Yes	No
Positive concordance in V_1–V_6	Yes	No
LBBB + right QRS axis	Yes	No
Intermittent cannon waves	Yes	No

LBBB = left bundle branch block; RBBB = right bundle branch block.

   Three ECG findings are virtually pathognomonic of VT: AV dissociation, capture beats, and fusion beats. A capture beat is a normally conducted sinus beat interrupting a wide-complex tachycardia. A fusion beat has a QRS morphology intermediate between a normally conducted narrow beat and a wide-complex ventricular beat. The clinical hallmark of AV dissociation is the presence of intermittent cannon waves in the jugular neck veins.

19. What are the medical contraindications to exercise ECG testing?

   Exercise stress testing is widely used to detect and assess the functional significance of CAD. It also has been shown to predict survival in patients recovering from an acute MI. Because exercise stress testing is commonly requested, its contraindications should be widely known and clearly understood so that use of this test is appropriate and safe. Contraindications include:

   1. Myocardial infarction acute or pending
   2. Unstable angina
   3. Acute myocarditis or pericarditis
   4. Left main coronary artery disease
   5. Severe aortic stenosis
   6. Uncontrolled hypertension
   7. Uncontrolled cardiac arrhythmias
   8. Second- or third-degree AV block
   9. Acute non-cardiac illness

20. What are the types of AV block?

1. **First-degree AV block:** Prolongation of the PR interval due to a conduction delay at the AV node.

2. **Second-degree AV block:** Manifested by dropped beats in which a P wave is not followed by a QRS complex (no ventricular depolarization and therefore no ventricular contraction). It is divided into two types:

    a. **Type I:** (Wenckebach phenomenon): The PR interval lengthens with each successive beat until a beat is dropped and the cycle repeats itself.

    b. **Type II:** The PR intervals are prolonged but do not gradually lengthen until a beat is suddenly dropped. The dropped beat may occur regularly, with a fixed number (X) of beats for each dropped beat (called an X:1 block). Type II is much less common than Type I and is commonly associated with bundle branch blocks.

3. **Third-degree AV block** (complete heart block): The atria and ventricles are controlled by separate pacemakers. It is associated with widening of the QRS complex and a ventricular rate of 35–50 bpm.

21. What ECG changes are seen in hyperkalemia?

A tall, peaked, symmetrical T wave with a narrow base (so-called tented T wave) is the earliest ECG abnormality and is usually present in leads II, III, V_2, V_3, and V_4. Shortening of the QT

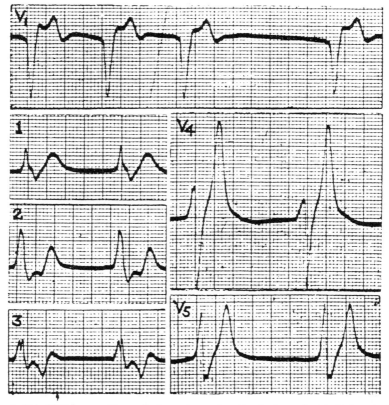

Hyperkalemia. This ECG shows evidence of advanced potassium intoxication: tall peaked T waves, absent P waves, widened QRS complexes, and irregular rhythm. The patient's serum K+ level was 8.1 mEq/L. (From Marriott HJL: Practical Electrocardiography, 9th ed. Baltimore, Williams & Wilkins, 1994, p 183; with permission.)

interval, widening of the QRS interval, ST-segment depression, flattening of the P wave, and PR-interval prolongation follows this. Eventually, the P waves disappear and the QRS complexes assume a configuration similar to a sine wave, eventually degenerating into ventricular fibrillation (VF). Widening of the QRS complex can assume a configuration consistent with atypical RBBB or LBBB, making the recognition of hyperkalemia more difficult. Unlike typical RBBB, hyperkalemia often causes prolongation of the entire QRS complex.

Sequence of ECG Changes in Experimental Hyperkalemia

Tall, symmetrical T waves	$K^+ > 5.7$ mEq/L
Reduced P wave amplitude	$K^+ > 7.0$ mEq/L
Prolongation of PR interval	$K^+ > 7.0$ mEq/L
Disappearance of P waves	$K^+ > 8.4$ mEq/L
Widening of QRS interval	$K^+ = 9–11$ mEq/L
Ventricular fibrillation (VF)	$K^+ > 12$ mEq/L

22. What ECG signs suggest hypercalcemia? Are similar changes seen in other conditions?

Hypercalcemia shortens the QT interval, particularly the interval between the beginning of the QRS complex and the peak of the T wave. The abrupt slope to the peak of the T wave is most characteristic of hypercalcemia. Another cause of shortened QT interval is digitalis toxicity.

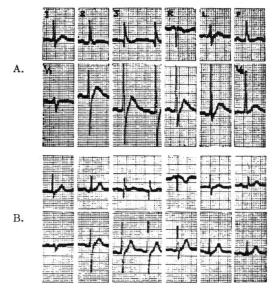

Hypercalcemia in a patient with hyperparathyroidism. *A*, Before parathyroidectomy (serum calcium, 15 mg/dl). Note virtual absence of ST segment, early peak of T wave, and relatively gradual downslope of descending limb of T wave. *B*, After parathyroidectomy (serum calcium, 10.7 mg/dl). Note normal contour of ST-T pattern. (From Marriott HJL: Practical Electrocardiography, 9th ed. Baltimore, Williams & Wilkins, 1994, p 185; with permission.)

23. What is the normal range for PR and QT intervals on a 12-lead ECG? Do these intervals vary with heart rate, sex, or age?

The normal range for the **PR interval** is 0.12–0.20 sec. It is not significantly related to age, sex, or heart rate.

The normal range for the **QT interval** also is unrelated to age, but it does vary with heart rate. As the heart rate increases, the QT interval shortens. To help evaluate a QT interval independent of heart rate, the corrected QT interval (QTc) can be calculated:

QTc (in msec) = measured QT (in msec)/square root of the R-R interval (in sec)

The normal range for the **QTc** is 0.36–0.44 sec. A prolonged QTc is defined as QTc > 0.39 sec in men or > 0.44 sec in women.

24. In the frontal plane, is a QRS axis of +120° compatible with a diagnosis of left anterior hemiblock?

This diagnosis requires the presence of a QRS of –60° to –90° in the frontal plane. A frontal plane QRS axis of +120° is consistent with right axis deviation and is therefore not compatible with a diagnosis of left anterior hemiblock (left anterior fascicular block).

Diagnostic criteria for left anterior fascicular block include:
1. QRS axis –60° to –90°
2. Small q-wave in lead I
3. Small r-wave in lead III

25. Describe the ECG manifestations of RV hypertrophy.
1. R wave > S wave in V_1 or V_2
2. R wave > 5 mm in V_1 or V_2
3. Right axis deviation
4. Persistent rS pattern (V_1–V_6)
5. Normal QRS duration

26. What are the causes of a prolonged QT interval?
Congenital causes
1. With deafness: Jervell syndrome
2. Without deafness: Romano-Ward syndrome

Acquired causes
1. Drugs: Class IA/IC antiarrhythmics, tricyclic antidepressants and phenothiazines
2. Electrolyte abnormalities: low K^+, Ca^{2+}, Mg^{2+}
3. Hypothermia
4. CNS injury (least common cause)
5. Liquid diets
6. CAD
7. Cardiomyopathy
8. Mitral valve prolapse

Prolongation of the QT interval is associated in certain patients with a definite increase in risk of VF and death.

DIAGNOSIS

27. How are cardiac and non-cardiac causes of chest pain differentiated?

Cardiac Causes of Chest Pain

CONDITION	LOCATION	QUALITY	DURATION	AGGRAVATING/ RELIEVING FACTORS	ASSOCIATED SIGNS AND SYMPTOMS
Angina	Retrosternal, radiates to neck, left	Pressure, burning, squeezing	< 10 min	Aggravated by exercise, cold, emotional stress, after meals Relieved by rest, nitroglycerin	S_4, paradoxically split S_2, murmur of papillary muscle
Rest or crescendo angina	Same as angina	Same as angina	> 10 min	Same as angina with gradually decreasing tolerance for exertion	Same as angina

(*Table continued on next page.*)

Cardiac Causes of Chest Pain (cont.)

CONDITION	LOCATION	QUALITY	DURATION	AGGRAVATING/ RELIEVING FACTORS	ASSOCIATED SIGNS AND SYMPTOMS
Myocardial infarction	Substernal; may radiate like angina	Heaviness, pressure, burning, constriction	30 min or longer, variable	Unrelieved	Shortness of breath, diaphoresis, nausea, vomiting, weakness, anxiety
Pericarditis	Substernal or cardiac apex; may radiate to left arm	Sharp, stabbing, knifelike	Hours to days	Aggravated by deep breathing, rotating chest, or supine position. Relieved by sitting up and leaning forward.	Pericardial friction rub, cardiac tamponade, pulsus paradoxsus
Dissecting aortic aneurysm	Anterior chest, back, abdominal	Excruciating, tearing, knifelike	Sudden onset, lasts for hours	Unrelated to anything	Lower BP in one arm, absent pulses, murmur of aortic insufficiency, paralysis, pulsus paradoxsus

Noncardiac Causes of Chest Pain

CONDITION	LOCATION	QUALITY	DURATION	AGGRAVATING/ RELIEVING FACTORS	ASSOCIATED SIGNS AND SYMPTOMS
Pulmonary embolism	Substernal or over area of pulmonary infarction	Pleuritic or like angina	Sudden onset, min to > 1 hr	May be aggravated by breathing	Dyspnea, tachypnea, tachycardia, hypotension, signs of right-sided (CHF), rales, pleural rub, hemoptysis (with infarction)
Pulmonary hypertension	Substernal	Pressure	—	Aggravated by effort	Dyspnea, signs of pulmonary hypertension
Pneumonia with pleuritis	Over area of consolidation	Pleuritic, well-localized	—	Aggravated by breathing	Dyspnea, cough, fever, dull to percussion, bronchial breath sounds, pleural rub
Spontaneous pneumothorax	Unilateral	Sharp, well-localized	Sudden onset, hours	Painful breathing	Dyspnea, hyperresonance, and decreased breath and voice sounds
Musculoskeletal	Variable	Aching	Short or long	Aggravated by movement, history of muscle exertion	Tender to pressure or movement
Herpes zoster	Dermatomal distribution	—	Prolonged	None	Rash appears in area of discomfort
GI disorders (esophageal reflux, ulcer)	Lower substernal, epigastric	Burning, colicky, aching	—	Precipitated by recumbency or meals, partial relief with antacids	Nausea, vomiting, food intolerance, melena, hematemesis, jaundice
Anxiety	Often localized to a point, moves	Sharp, burning, variable	Variable	Situational anger, usually brief	Sighing respirations, often chest wall tenderness

From Andreoli TE, et al (eds): Cecil Essentials of Medicine, 2nd ed. Philadelphia, W.B. Saunders, 1990, pp 12–13; with permission.

28. A 31-year-old man complains of a sudden onset of sharp left chest pain, increased by deep inspiration and coughing. Physical findings, chest x-ray, and the ECG are all normal. What is your differential diagnosis?

Differential Diagnosis of Pleuritic Chest Pain

1. Acute pleuritis (coxsackievirus A, B)	4. Pulmonary embolus or infarction
2. Acute pericarditis (coxsackievirus B)	5. Pneumothorax
3. Pneumonia (viral, bacterial)	

In this patient, the most likely clinical diagnosis causing pleuritic chest pain in the presence of a normal physical, chest x-ray, and ECG findings is acute viral pleuritis or pericarditis.

29. A 56-year-old man presents to the emergency center with acute onset of squeezing, diffuse, anterior chest pain associated with diaphoresis and dyspnea. What is your differential diagnosis? Which tests will help confirm your clinical suspicions?

The differential diagnosis consists of the following:

1. Acute MI	4. Acute pericarditis
2. Angina pectoris	5. Acute pulmonary embolus
3. Acute aortic dissection	6. Acute pneumothorax

Among these diagnoses, the first three are most common and should be carefully considered in the diagnostic work-up of this patient. A **12-lead ECG** is performed to look for ST-segment elevations (evidence of acute myocardial injury due to infarction or pericarditis), ST-segment depressions (evidence of subendocardial ischemia), or T-wave changes. Determination of **serial cardiac enzymes** (creatine kinase and MB isoenzyme) over the first 24–48 hours of hospitalization will help to confirm a diagnosis of acute MI. The absence of any ECG changes of acute MI or ischemia in a patient with severe anterior chest pain radiating to the back should suggest the clinical diagnosis of acute aortic dissection. Finally, a **chest x-ray** is helpful in the work-up of patients with acute chest pain to look for evidence of pneumothorax, cardiac enlargement suggestive of cardiac failure, or wedge-shaped pulmonary consolidation suggestive of acute pulmonary embolus.

30. Identify the types of shock and their causes.

Classification of Shock States

TYPE	PRIMARY MECHANISM	CLINICAL CAUSES
Hypovolemic	Volume loss	Exogenous Blood loss due to hemorrhage Plasma loss due to burn, inflammation Fluid/electrolyte loss due to vomiting, diarrhea, dehydration, osmotic diuresis (diabetes) Endogenous Extravasation due to inflammation, trauma, tourniquet, anaphylaxis, snake venom, and adrenergic stimulation (pheochromocytoma)
Cardiogenic	Pump failure	MI, CHF, cardiac arrhythmias, intracardiac obstruction (incl. valvular stenosis)
Distributive (vasomotor dysfunction)		
1. High or normal resistance	Expanded venous capacitance	Hypodynamic septic shock due to gram-negative enteric bacillemia; autonomic blockade; spinal shock; tranquilizer, sedative, or narcotic overdose

(Table continued on next page.)

Classification of Shock States (cont.)

TYPE	PRIMARY MECHANISM	CLINICAL CAUSES
2. Low resistance	AV shunting	Pneumonia, peritonitis, abscess, reactive hyperemia
Obstructive	Extracardiac obstruction of main blood flow channels	Vena caval obstruction (supine hypotensive syndrome), pericarditis (tamponade), pulmonary embolism, dissecting aortic aneurysm, aortic compression.

From: Weil MH, et al: Acute circulatory failure (shock). In Braunwald E (ed): Heart Disease: A Textbook of Cardiovascular Medicine, 3rd ed. Philadelphia, W.B. Saunders, 1988, p 569; with permission.

31. What is a pseudoinfarction? What is its differential diagnosis?

Some patients exhibit ECG changes similar to those of MI but do not have any other definitive evidence of an MI. These patients are said to have ECG evidence of "pseudoinfarction." Causes include:

1. LV or RV hypertrophy
2. Left bundle branch block
3. Wolff-Parkinson-White syndrome
4. Hypertrophic cardiomyopathy
5. Hyperkalemia
6. Early repolarization
7. Cardiac sarcoid or amyloid
8. Intracranial hemorrhage

32. A patient presents to the cardiac care unit with clinical signs and symptoms suggestive of acute right ventricular MI. How would an ECG help to confirm this clinical diagnosis?

About one-third of patients with acute inferior wall MI develop a RV infarction. The clinical syndrome of RV MI should be suspected when the following clinical triad is present in a patient suffering from an inferior wall MI:

1. Hypotension
2. Elevated jugular veins
3. Clear lungs

The clinical recognition of RV infarction is important. The clinical suspicion can be confirmed by performing a right-sided ECG. The presence of at least 1 mm of ST-segment elevation in lead V_3R or V_4R is characteristically present in RV MI. Further confirmation can be derived from noninvasive assessment of RV systolic function using radionuclide techniques or two-dimensional echocardiography.

33. Name the three types of cardiomyopathies. How are they distinguished?

Classification of Cardiomyopathy

TYPE	CHARACTERISTICS	SYMPTOMS AND SIGNS	LABORATORY DIAGNOSIS
Dilated (congestive)	Cardiac dilation, generalized hypocontractility	LV and RV failure	X-ray: cardiomegaly with pulmonary congestion ECG: sinus tachycardia, nonspecific ST-T changes, arrhythmias, conduction disturbances, Q waves Echo: dilated LV, generalized decreased wall motion, mitral valve motion consistent with low flow Catheterization: dilated hypocontractile ventricle, mitral regurgitation

(Table continued on next page.)

Classification of Cardiomyopathy (cont.)

TYPE	CHARACTERISTICS	SYMPTOMS AND SIGNS	LABORATORY DIAGNOSIS
Hypertrophic	Ventricular hypertrophy, esp. of the septum, with or without outflow tract obstruction Typically good systolic but poor diastolic (compliance) ventricular function	Dyspnea, angina, presyncope, syncope, palpitations Large jugular a-wave, bifid carotid pulse, palpable S4 gallop, prominent apical impulse, "dynamic" systolic murmur and thrill, mitral regurgitation murmur	X-ray: LV predominance, dilated left atrium ECG: LV hypertrophy, Q waves, nonspecific ST-T waves; ventricular arrhythmias Echo: hypertrophy, usually asymmetric (septum > free wall); systolic anterior motion of mitral valve; midsystolic closure of aortic valve Catheterization: provokable outflow tract gradient; hypertrophy with vigorous systolic function and cavity obliteration; mitral regurgitation
Restrictive	Reduced diastolic compliance impeding ventricular filling; normal systolic function	Dyspnea, exercise intolerance, weakness Elevated jugular venous pressure, edema, hepatomegaly, ascites, S_4 and S_3 gallops, Kussmaul's sign	X-ray: mild cardiomegaly, pulmonary congestion ECG: low voltage, conduction disturbances, Q waves Echo: characteristic myocardial texture in amyloidosis with thickening of all cardiac structures Catheterization: square root sign, M-shaped atrial waveform, elevated left and right filling pressures

From Andreoli TE, et al (eds): Cecil Essentials of Medicine, 2nd ed. Philadelphia, W.B. Saunders, 1990, p 106; with permission.

34. An 89-year-old woman was found unconscious in her backyard. She "woke up" a few minutes after arrival to the ED. Physical, neurologic, ECG, and chest x-ray findings are all normal. She feels fine and demands to be released. Would you admit her to the hospital?

Syncope, defined as a transient loss or impairment of consciousness, can be due to a wide variety of etiologies, both cardiovascular and noncardiovascular. Patients most likely to have cardiovascular syncope are older and may or may not have a prior history of documented cardiac disease (manifested by angina pectoris, MI, or sudden cardiac death). Common cardiovascular causes of syncope include:

1. **Tachyarrhythmias**, such as VT or SVT (AF, atrial flutter, or paroxysmal SVT).

2. **Bradyarrhythmias**, such as second- or third-degree AV block, AF with a slow ventricular response rate, or sinus bradycardia due to sick sinus syndrome.

3. **LV outflow obstruction** due to fixed lesions (valvular, subvalvular, or supravalvular aortic stenosis) or dynamic obstruction such as hypertrophic cardiomyopathy. Characteristically, these patients present with syncope during or immediately after exercise.

4. **LV inflow obstruction** due to severe mitral stenosis or a large left atrial myxoma.

5. **Primary pulmonary hypertension**

It is desirable to hospitalize patients who are at high risk for cardiovascular syncope, since they have a much worse prognosis and may have potentially life-threatening complications of their underlying cardiovascular disease. This elderly woman should be hospitalized since she is at high risk for cardiovascular syncope.

35. Should a thorough work-up be done on all patients with syncope?

No. The routine use of expensive or invasive studies into the cause of syncope is not warranted. The etiology of syncope will be undetermined in 30–50% of cases even after a thorough (and expensive) work-up. In up to 85% of cases in which an etiology is identifiable, it will be identified or at least suggested by the initial history, physical exam, and ECG. Further studies should be ordered on the basis of the results of this initial evaluation.

36. A 68-year-old man with hypertension presents with a 2-week history of progressive exertional dyspnea, orthopnea, and paroxysmal nocturnal dyspnea. What is the differential diagnosis?

Differential Diagnosis of CHF in Hypertensive Patients

1. Coronary artery disease
2. Diastolic dysfunction associated with hypertension
3. Dilated cardiomyopathy (idiopathic or alcoholic)
4. Valvular heart disease (mitral regurgitation, aortic stenosis, aortic insufficiency)
5. Restrictive heart disease (amyloidosis)
6. Hypertrophic cardiomyopathy (idiopathic hypertrophic subaortic stenosis)

37. What is a hyperdynamic precordial impulse?
It is a thrust of exaggerated height that falls away immediately from the palpating fingers. It is typically found in patients with a large stroke volume. The clinical conditions include thyrotoxicosis, anemia, beriberi, AV shunts or grafts, exercise, or mitral regurgitation. A hyperdynamic precordial impulse should be differentiated from the sustained apical impulse, a graphic equivalent of a heave, detected in the presence of LV hypertrophy due to hypertension or aortic stenosis.

38. What is the differential diagnosis of an abnormal early diastolic sound heard at the apex and lower left sternal border?
1. Loud P_2
2. S_3 gallop
3. Opening snap
4. Pericardial knock
5. Tumor plop (atrial myxoma)

An early diastolic sound may be due to wide splitting of S_2, with or without a loud pulmonic closure sound. An atrial septal defect (ASD) causes wide and fixed splitting of S_2.

A **loud P_2** usually indicates the presence of pulmonary hypertension, whether primary or secondary to chronic pulmonary disease.

Unlike other causes of an early diastolic sound, a **third heart sound** (S_3) can best be heard using the bell of the stethoscope. Unlike a physiologically split A_2–P_2, the A_2–S_3 interval does not change during respiration. Associated physical findings of CHF, such as pulmonary rales, distended neck veins, or edema are usually present along with an S_3.

An **opening snap** may be the only finding in a patient with a mild non-calcified and pliable mitral valve. In such a patient, a loud S_1 is also commonly present. A diastolic rumble at the apex confirms the physical diagnosis of mitral stenosis.

In patients with chronic constrictive pericarditis, the sudden slowing of LV filling in early diastole associated with the restriction of a rigid pericardium acting as "a rigid shell" causes the **pericardial knock**.

In some patients with large atrial myxomas protruding through the mitral valve during diastole, the sudden cessation of LV filling, caused by the tumor's obstruction to the flow of blood, creates an audible tumor plop. Cardiac auscultation in various positions helps to detect a tumor plop. Likewise, cardiac symptoms in these patients are often related to body position.

39. In patients with mitral stenosis, what are the pathophysiology and significance of an opening snap? Does its presence imply a more severe degree of stenosis?
An opening snap is typically present only when the mitral valve leaflets are pliable, and it is therefore usually accompanied by an accentuated S_1. Diffuse calcification of the mitral valve can

be expected when an opening snap is absent. If calcification is confined to the tip of the mitral valve, an opening snap is still commonly present.

The interval between the aortic closure sound and opening snap (A_2–OS) is inversely related to the mean left atrial pressure. A short A_2–OS interval is a reliable indicator of severe mitral stenosis; however, the converse is not necessarily true.

40. What is the "figure 3" sign? What congenital cardiac disease does it most likely suggest?
A routine chest x-ray may reveal a characteristic "3" sign. This is the result of post-stenotic dilatation of the descending aorta and the dilated left subclavian artery. A barium swallow may reveal a reverse "3" sign. Along with rib notching, the presence of the "3" sign is almost pathognomonic for **aortic coarctation**.

41. What are the major and minor Jones criteria for diagnosing acute rheumatic fever?

Major Jones Criteria	Minor Jones Criteria
Carditis	Fever
Polyarthritis	Arthralgia
Chorea	Prolonged PR internal
Erythema marginatum	Elevated ESR or positive C-reactive protein
Subcutaneous nodules	Previous rheumatic fever or rheumatic heart disease

The clinical diagnosis of acute rheumatic fever is made if two major criteria or one major and two minor criteria are present in a patient with a preceding streptococcal infection (as evidenced by recent scarlet fever, positive throat culture for group A Streptococcus, or increased ASO or other streptococcal antibody titer).

CORONARY ARTERY DISEASE

42. Is aspirin effective in the treatment of unstable angina pectoris?
There is unequivocal evidence from two clinical trials, the VA and Canadian cooperative trials, that aspirin reduces subsequent MI and mortality in unstable angina patients. Both mortality and MI are reduced by about 50% in aspirin-treated patients. On the other hand, there is less evidence to suggest a beneficial effect of aspirin in chronic stable angina pectoris.

Lewis HD, et al: Protective effects of aspirin against acute myocardial infarction and death in men with unstable angina: Results of a Veterans Administration Cooperative Study. N Engl J Med 309:396–403, 1983.

Cairns JA, et al: Aspirin, sulfinpyrazone, or both in unstable angina: Results of a Canadian multicenter trial. N Engl J Med 313:1369–1375, 1985.

43. What is the pathophysiological mechanism of acute coronary syndromes? Compare and contrast acute coronary syndromes to acute ST-elevation myocardial infarction.
Acute coronary syndrome is a clinical syndrome characterized by ischemic cardiac chest pains associated with ST or T wave changes, but, unlike classic acute myocardial infarction, there is no acute ST segment elevation. Thus, it is called the non-ST elevation acute coronary syndrome. This includes two diseases: unstable angina and non-Q-wave myocardial infarction, which are differentiated based on the presence or absence of an elevation of the creatinine kinase MB fraction (MB CK).

The pathophysiologic mechanism of acute non-ST elevation coronary syndrome is intermittent and/or incomplete coronary occlusion by platelet-rich "white" recent thrombus resulting from platelet aggregation at the site of a damaged inner surface of a coronary artery. The trigger for this platelet aggregation is usually rupture of an atherosclerotic plaque. This type of thrombus is in sharp contrast to the mature red blood cell and fibrin-rich "red" or "mature" thrombus, which is the hallmark pathologic finding in patients with acute ST elevation myocardial infarction. Unlike the platelet-rich "white" thrombus, a mature "red" thrombus results in a complete and/or persistent coronary artery occlusion resulting in severe transmural ischemia characterized by acute ST segment elevation. An intermittent or incomplete occlusion of a coronary artery usually causes acute subendocardial ischemia, which presents with ST segment depression or T wave changes that are transient or dynamic in nature.

Interestingly, the clinical presentations of these pathophysiologically distinct clinical syndromes are quite different. Patients with acute ST elevation myocardial infarction present with a persistent relentless chest pain lasting for over 30 min (and up to several hours). In contrast, patients with non-ST segment elevation acute coronary syndromes usually present with a waxing and waning of intermittent and recurrent episodes of ischemic cardiac chest pains.

44. Does the addition of an inhibitor of platelet glycoprotein 2b/3a receptor to a thrombolytic (or fibrinolytic) drug improve the angiographic outcome of thrombolysis?

First why should one even want to add an inhibitor of platelet aggregation to a thrombolytic drug regimen?

The answer is now widely accepted in the cardiovascular community: thrombolysis as the sole reperfusion strategy has some important limitations. First, even the most potent available thrombolytics such as the third generation thrombolytics (r-PA, TNK-t-PA, see question 117 below) achieve a complete reperfusion (defined as normal flow in the infarct-related artery and referred to as TIMI Flow Grade 3) in only 55–63% of all patients treated. This falls short of mechanical reperfusion strategies such as primary angioplasty or primary stenting of the infarct related artery. Several trials have shown that the latter, balloon angioplasty, or stenting can achieve complete reperfusion in 80–90% of all patients treated. Moreover, 5–12% of successfully reperfused patients reinfarct within a few days after thrombolysis. We have learned that the major drawback of thrombolysis alone is that it increases platelet activation and aggregation because of an increase in free thrombin, a potent agonist of the platelet glycoprotein 2b/3a receptors. It is this induced platelet aggregation that limits the clot lytic effect of thrombolytics and predisposes to reinfarction due to rethrombosis. Thus, the addition of a potent inhibitor of platelet aggregation such as a platelet 2b/3a inhibitor is an effective means of further improving the limited efficacy of thrombolysis as the sole reperfusion strategy in acute myocardial infarction.

45. Has the combination of thrombolysis and 2b/3a inhibitors been tested in clinical trials? How successful is it?

Three clinical trials have evaluated the angiographic results of thrombolytics in combination with an inhibitor of the platelet glycoprotein 2b/3a receptor: the **TIMI 14**, **SPEED GUSTO**, and **INTRO-AMI** trials. All three specifically evaluated angiographic outcome at 60 and 90 min after thrombolytics, when combined with a platelet glycoprotein 2b/3a receptor. The TIMI 14 and GUSTO SPEED trials (reference below) revealed that the proportion of patients who completely reperfuse (as evidenced by a TIMI Flow Grade 3) is significantly higher with the combination of half-dose t-PA or r-PA with the platelet glycoprotein 2b/3a receptor inhibitor **abciximab** (Reopro). For example, 76% of patients treated with 50 mg t-PA combined with a 12-hour infusion of abciximab had a TIMI 3 flow at 90 minutes compared with only 57% of those who received full-dose t-PA alone. Similarly, in the SPEED GUSTO trial, half-dose r-PA combined with abciximab resulted in a TIMI 3 flow in 61% compared with 47% in those who received full dose r-PA alone. The INTRO-AMI trial confirmed these results using a different platelet glycoprotein 2b/3a receptor inhibitor eptifibatide (Integrelin) and showed a similar increase in rate and extent of thrombolysis at 90 min after thrombolysis is initiated.

Antman EM, Giugliano RP, Gibson CM, et al for the TIMI 14 Investigators: Abciximab facilitates the rate and extent of thrombolysis: Results of the Thrombolysis in Myocardial Infarction (TIMI) 14 trial. Circulation 99:2720–2732, 1999.

Trial of Abciximab with and without low-dose reteplase for Acute Myocardial Infarction: Strategies for Patency Enhancement in the Emergency Department (SPEED) Group. Circulation 101:2788–2794, 2000.

46. Thrombolytic therapy is the most life-saving pharmacologic therapy in acute ST elevation myocardial infarction. Is primary angioplasty (a mechanical reperfusion therapy) using a balloon tipped angioplasty catheter as effective as pharmacologic reperfusion therapy with a thrombolytic drug?

The **PAMI** trial is the first published clinical trial designed specifically to compare balloon angioplasty to t-PA as the primary reperfusion therapy in patients with acute ST elevation myocardial infarction. In this trial, 395 patients in 12 clinical sites who presented within 12 hr of the onset of myocardial infarction were randomized to undergo primary angioplasty (195 patients) or to receive tissue-type plasminogen activator (t-PA) (200 patients). The results of this trial were interesting both at the initial 30 day and after two years of follow-up. At 30 days and at two years, there was no difference in survival. At two years, patients undergoing primary angioplasty had less recurrent ischemia (36.4% vs. 48% for t-PA, p = 0.026), lower reintervention rates (27.2% vs. 46.5% for t-PA, p < 0.0001) and reduced hospital readmission rates (58.5% vs. 69.0% for t-PA, p = 0.035). The combined end point of death or reinfarction was 14.9% for angioplasty vs. 23% for t-PA (p = 0.034). Multivariate analysis revealed angioplasty to be independently predictive of a reduction in death, reinfarction, or target vessel revascularization (p = 0.0001). Thus, the initial benefit of primary angioplasty in acute myocardial infarction is maintained over a two-year follow-up period with improved infarct-free survival and reduced rate of reintervention.

Another important advantage of balloon angioplasty over thrombolytic drug therapy is freedom from intracranial hemorrhage, a dreadful complication of thrombolysis, particularly in elderly patients.

In conclusion, survival (at 30 days and at 2 years) after primary angioplasty is similar to that of t-PA in acute myocardial infarction, and angioplasty confers greater freedom from recurrent ischemia, reinfarction, need for readmission to the hospital, and greater freedom from intracranial hemorrhage.

Nunn CM, O'Neill WW, Rothbaum D, et al: Long-term outcome after primary angioplasty: Report from the primary angioplasty in myocardial infarction (PAMI-I) trial. J Am Coll Cardiol 33(3):640–646, 1999.

47. Do the various classes of antianginal drugs differ in their efficacy and safety when used in the management of vasospastic angina as compared with classic effort angina?

Patients with both forms of angina respond promptly to nitrates.

Although the response of patients with effort angina to beta-blockers is uniformly good, the response of patients with Prinzmetal's angina is variable. In some patients, the duration of episodes of angina pectoris may be prolonged during therapy with propranolol, a non-cardioselective beta-blocker. In others, especially those with associated fixed atherosclerotic lesions, beta-blockers may reduce the frequency of anginal episodes. Non-cardioselective beta-blockers may, in some patients with variant angina, leave a receptor mediated coronary arterial vasoconstriction unopposed and thereby worsen anginal symptoms.

In contrast to beta-blockers, calcium blockers are quite effective in reducing the frequency and duration of episodes of variant angina. Along with nitrates, calcium blockers are the mainstay of treatment of Prinzmetal's angina because of their proven efficacy and safety.

48. Is treadmill exercise ECG testing helpful in confirming the diagnosis of variant angina?

Exercise testing is the most common provocative test used by clinicians to confirm the clinical diagnosis of exertional angina pectoris. An exercise ECG test is considered positive for CAD if it shows at least a 1-mm ST-segment depression during exercise. Myocardial ischemia is induced in these patients by an increase in myocardial O_2 demand, primarily due to the increase in heart rate with exercise.

In patients with variant angina, myocardial ischemia is primarily due to a decrease in O_2 supply rather than to an increase in O_2 demand. Exercise testing is thus of limited diagnostic value in these patients. It may show ST-segment elevation, ST-segment depression, or no change in ST segments during exercise.

49. A 78-year-old asthmatic man has stable exertional angina of 3 years' duration. His past medical history reveals intermittent claudication after walking 50 yards. What is your approach to managing this patient's anginal symptoms?

This elderly man has three medical problems: asthma, intermittent claudication, and chronic stable angina.

Of the available antianginal drugs, beta-blockers are contraindicated because of the presence of asthma. Cardioselective beta-blockers, such as metoprolol (Lopressor) or atenolol (Tenormin), may be used cautiously in low doses in asthma, but non-cardioselective beta-blockers are not safe in this patient. However, the presence of peripheral vascular disease manifested by intermittent claudication also is a contraindication for the use of any beta-blocker. Calcium antagonists or nitrates are thus the antianginal drugs of choice in this patient.

50. Based on clinical history, physical examination, and initial admission ECG, which patients with unstable angina are at highest risk for death or acute MI?

Unstable angina is a common potentially life-threatening medical condition. In 1991, it accounted for 570,000 hospital admissions in the U.S. The risk of death or nonfatal MI is highest in patients with unstable angina complicated by any of the following features:
1. Ongoing prolonged chest pain > 20 min in duration
2. Acute pulmonary edema (by physical exam or chest x-ray)
3. New or worsening mitral regurgitation murmurs
4. Rest angina with dynamic ST-segment changes ≥ 1 mm
5. S_3 gallop or lung rales
6. Hypotension

Patients with one or more of these high-risk indicators should generally be admitted to the coronary care unit for ECG monitoring and intensive medical therapy with IV nitrates, heparin, aspirin, and calcium and/or beta-blockers.

Braunwald E, et al: Diagnosing and managing unstable angina. Circulation 90:613–622, 1994.

51. Which patients with unstable angina should undergo cardiac catheterization?

Cardiac catheterization should be entertained in patients with unstable angina refractory to medical management or with any of the following features:
1. Prior revascularization
2. Depressed LV function (LV ejection fraction < 50%)
3. Life-threatening "malignant" ventricular arrhythmias
4. Persistent or recurrent angina/ischemia
5. Inducible myocardial ischemia (provoked by exercise, dobutamine, adenosine, or dipyridamole)

Braunwald E, et al: Diagnosing and managing unstable angina. Circulation 90:613–622, 1994.

52. A 48-year-old man presents with acute severe epigastric pain, anorexia, nausea, vomiting, and diaphoresis. Which myocardial wall is likely affected? Explain the rationale for such an unusual clinical presentation.

Patients with an **acute inferior wall MI** sometimes present with epigastric pain associated with gastrointestinal symptoms, as in this patient. Less commonly, they present with hiccupping, which may at times be intractable. These unique clinical manifestations are thought to be related to increased vagal tone and irritation of the diaphragm by the adjacent infarcted inferior wall.

53. Does early administration of thrombolytic therapy after MI decrease mortality?

The effect of IV thrombolytic therapy on MI mortality is well established. In the GISSI trial published in 1986, 11,806 patients with acute MI presenting within 12 hours of symptom onset were randomly assigned to receive IV streptokinase or placebo. The hospital mortality was significantly reduced in patients treated with streptokinase within the first 6 hours. Most importantly, there was a remarkable 50% reduction in hospital mortality in patients treated within 1 hour of symptom onset. Subsequent clinical trials of various thrombolytic drugs including streptokinase, tissue plasminogen activator (t-PA, Activase), recombinant plasminogen activator (r-PA, Retavase) and the most recent FDA approved thrombolytic TNK-t-PA (Tenecteplase) conducted in the subsequent 15 years confirmed the consistent improvement in survival with thrombolytic therapy. In fact, thrombolysis is the most effective life-saving pharmacologic therapy in acute myocardial infarction. It saves about 40 lives for every 1,000 treated patients and reduces 30-day and one-year mortality by about 25%. Patients presenting up to 12 hours after symptom onset may benefit from thrombolysis.

The current standard of care for patients with acute ST elevation (or transmural) MI includes administration of IV thrombolytic therapy in all patients admitted within 12 hours of symptom onset (in the absence of contraindications). Contraindications include bleeding disorders, severe uncontrolled hypertension (blood pressure > 180/120 mmHg despite treatment), recent history of thromboembolic cerebrovascular accident (within 2 months), any prior history of a hemorrhagic cerebrovascular accident, prolonged cardiopulmonary resuscitation (over 10 min), or active bleeding from a peptic ulcer or other noncompressible source.

GISSI Trial: Effect of time to treatment on reduction in hospital mortality observed in streptokinase-treated patients. Lancet 1:397–401, 1986.

AHA/ACC Task Force: Guidelines for management of acute myocardial infarction. Circulation September 1999.

54. Which drug is more effective in achieving successful reperfusion of a thrombosed coronary artery: Streptokinase (SK), tissue plasminogen activator (t-PA, Activase), recombinant plasminogen activator (r-PA, retavase) or TNK-t-PA (tenectaplase)?

In the multicenter phase I TIMI trial, t-PA was shown to result in about twice as many successful reperfusions (due to clot lysis) as streptokinase. In the recent GUSTO trial, consisting of about 41,000 patients with acute MI, t-PA was more effective than streptokinase in opening coronary arteries and in preventing death in the first 30 days after acute MI. An open coronary artery (with a normal coronary flow: so-called TIMI Flow Grade 3) is an excellent predictor of short-term (hospital) and long-term (1 year post-discharge) survival, regardless of which thrombolytic drug is used.

Two angiographic clinical trials, the RAPID I and RAPID II trials, compared r-PA to t-PA in about 990 patients with acute myocardial infarction. In these trials, about 60% of r-PA treated patients experienced complete reperfusion (as evidenced by a TIMI Flow Grade 3) at 90 min compared with about 50–55% with t-PA.

However, despite the higher TIMI Flow Grade 3 in patients treated with r-PA, survival was similar in patients who received t-PA or r-PA in the large-scale GUSTO III trial of about 15,000 patients.

Angiographic trials of TNK-t-PA showed similar coronary angiographic success compared with t-PA, and the ASSENT-2 trial confirmed the equivalent efficacy of both TNK-t-PA and t-PA in improving survival.

In summary, t-PA is clearly angiographically superior to SK in opening arteries and saving lives, whereas the newer r-PA and TNK-t-PA thrombolytics are not clearly superior to t-PA in overall efficacy.

GUSTO Angiographic Investigators: The effects of tissue plasminogen activator, streptokinase, or both on coronary-artery patency, ventricular function and survival after acute myocardial infarction. N Engl J Med 329:1615–1622, 1993.

55. Should oral nitrates be administered routinely to all patients with uncomplicated MI?

IV, transdermal, and/or oral nitrates have traditionally been used routinely in all patients admitted with suspected acute MI. However, despite the encouraging results of early small clinical studies, two recent large clinical trials, ISIS-4 and GISSI-3, consisting of about 78,000 patients, showed no significant benefit of early oral nitrates on survival, infarct size, or ventricular function. Their routine administration should thus be limited to patients with well-established indications for nitrates, such as postinfarction angina pectoris or CHF.

Gruppo Italiano per lo Studio della Sopravivenza nell' Infarto Miocardio (GISSI-3): Effects of lisinopril and transdermal glyceryltrinitrate singly and together on 6-week mortality and ventricular function after acute myocardial infarction. Lancet 343:1115–1122, 1994.

ISIS-4: A randomized factorial trial assessing early oral captopril, oral mononitrate, and intravenous magnesium sulphate in 58,050 patients with suspected acute myocardial infarction. Lancet 345:669–685, 1995.

Morris JL, et al: Nitrates in myocardial infarction: Influence on infarct size, reperfusion, and ventricular remodeling. Br Heart J 73:319, 1995.

56. What is the most common cause of death in the first 48 hours after an acute MI?

Ventricular fibrillation (VF). Other causes of death include cardiac rupture, pump failure due to massive infarction, acute mechanical complication such as ventricular septal rupture or acute mitral regurgitation, and cardiogenic shock.

57. Which calcium antagonist, if any, reduces the risk of reinfarction during hospitalization for a non-Q-wave MI?

Non-Q-wave MI is more likely than Q-wave MI to be complicated by early recurrent infarction. The Diltiazem Reinfarction Study revealed a 50% reduction in recurrent infarction during hospitalization of patients with non-Q-wave MI treated with the calcium antagonist **diltiazem** compared with placebo. Based on the results of this study, administration of diltiazem, in doses of 60–90 mg orally every 6 hours, is generally used for the first year in patients who evolve a non-Q-wave myocardial infarction.

Gibson RS, Boden WE, Theroux P, et al and the Diltiazem Reinfarction Study Group: Diltiazem and re-infarction in patients with non-Q-wave myocardial infarction. N Engl J Med 315:423–429, 1986.

58. Cardiac rupture is almost always a fatal complication of acute MI. What are three risk factors for its development? What are its clinical features?

Risk Factors	Clinical Features
1. Female sex	1. LV to RV infarction ratio is 7:1
2. Hypertension	2. Seen in anterior or lateral wall MI
3. First MI	3. Usually with large MI (> 20%)
	4. Usually 3–6 days post-MI
	5. Rare with LV hypertrophy or good collateral vessels

59. What complication of acute inferior wall MI typically presents with hypotension, elevated neck veins, clear lungs, and a normal cardiac silhouette on chest x-ray?

This is the classic triad of right ventricular MI. The diagnosis can be confirmed by demonstrating at least 1-mm ST elevation in right-sided chest leads V_3R or V_4R. Clinical management consists of volume expansion in combination with IV dopamine. In these patients, we should avoid diuretics or preload reducing drugs such as nitrates, as they further worsen the low cardiac output state.

60. Which lipid-lowering drug, if any, has been proved in a prospective placebo-controlled clinical trial to reduce cardiovascular mortality in acute myocardial infarction survivors with "average" blood cholesterol levels?

Pravastatin, a potent HmG Co-A reductase inhibitor, has been evaluated in myocardial infarction patients in the CARE (Cholesterol and Recurrent Events) Trial. In this double-blind trial, 4,159 patients (3,583 men and 576 women) received pravastatin (40 mg/day) or placebo for five years. These patients survived a recent myocardial infarction and had plasma total cholesterol levels below 240 mg% (mean of 209 mg%) and low-density lipoprotein (LDL) cholesterol levels of 115 to 174 mg% (mean of 139 mg%). The primary end point was a fatal coronary event or a nonfatal myocardial infarction. The frequency of the primary end point was 10.2% in the pravastatin group and 13.2% in the placebo group, an absolute difference of 3 percentage points and a 24% reduction in risk (95% confidence interval, 9–36%; P = 0.003). Subgroup analysis revealed that most of the benefit occurred in patients with baseline serum LDL cholesterol levels > 125 mg%.

In practical terms, the implications of this clinical trial are that patients with LDL cholesterol > 125 mg% and prior myocardial infarction should receive an HmG CoA reductase inhibitor ("statin") for at least 5 years.

Sacks FM, Pfeffer MA, Moye LA, et al and the Cholesterol and Recurrent Events Trial investigators: The effect of pravastatin on coronary events after myocardial infarction in patients with average cholesterol levels. N Engl J Med 335:1001–1009, 1996.

61. Do angiotensin-converting enzyme (ACE) inhibitors improve survival in patients recovering from acute MI?

Long-term oral ACE inhibitors started 3–16 days after acute MI and maintained for about 3 years reduce mortality by about 19% in patients with asymptomatic LV systolic dysfunction (LVEF < 40%). This was demonstrated in the Survival and Ventricular Enlargement (SAVE) Trial. Subsequent trials, namely the ISIS-4 and GISSI-3 trials, specifically showed that even a short 6 week course of an ACE inhibitor started within 24 hours of infarct onset decreases 6-week mortality by 7–12%, corresponding to 5 deaths prevented for every 1,000 treated patients.

However, IV ACE inhibitors should be avoided in the first 24 hours of acute MI evolution since they may cause a potentially harmful acute decrease in BP with a resultant reduction in coronary blood flow, as was demonstrated in the CONSENSUS-II trial.

The current guidelines for the management of patients with acute myocardial infarction specifically recommend the routine use of an ACE inhibitor in the first 6 weeks after onset of a myocardial infarction. This is followed in those with an impaired left ventricular systolic function (as defined by an LVEF < 40%) by life-long use of an ACE inhibitor.

Pfeffer MA, Braunwald E, Moye LA, et al on behalf of the SAVE Investigators: Effect of captopril on mortality and morbidity in patients with left ventricular dysfunction after myocardial infarction. Results of the Survival and Ventricular Enlargement Trial. N Engl J Med 327:669–677, 1992.

ISIS-4: A randomized factorial trial assessing early oral captopril, oral mononitrate, and intravenous magnesium sulphate in 58,050 patients with suspected acute myocardial infarction. Lancet 345:669–685, 1995.

Gruppo Italiano per lo Studio della Sopravvivenza nell' Infarto Miocardio (GISSI-3): Effects of lisinopril and transdermal glyceryltrinitrate singly and together on 6-week mortality and ventricular function after acute myocardial infarction. Lancet 343:1115–1122, 1994.

Swedberg K, et al: Effects of the early administration of enalapril on mortality in patients with acute myocardial infarction: Results of the cooperative New Scandinavian Enalapril Survival Study II (CONSENSUS-II). N Engl J Med 327:678–684, 1992.

62. What is the differential diagnosis of a new systolic murmur and acute pulmonary edema appearing 3 days after an acute anterior wall MI?

(1) Acute mitral regurgitation due to papillary muscle rupture, and (2) interventricular septal rupture. Both are potentially fatal complications and are most common 3–6 days post-infarction.

Rupture of the posteromedial papillary muscle, associated with inferior wall MI, is more common than that of the anterolateral papillary muscle. Unlike rupture of the interventricular septum, which occurs with large infarcts, papillary muscle rupture occurs with a small infarction in about 50% of cases.

Differentiation between acute mitral regurgitation and ventricular septal rupture is difficult at the bedside. Two-dimensional and Doppler echocardiography at the bedside can demonstrate the presence and severity of mitral regurgitation and localize the site of a ventricular septal defect (VSD). Further confirmation of the presence of a left-to-right shunt across a VSD can be obtained by a step-up in blood oxygen saturation from the right atrium to the pulmonary artery, documented by blood sampling using a Swan-Ganz catheter.

63. What is the most likely cause of a persistent ST-segment elevation several weeks after recovery from a large transmural anterolateral wall MI?

Persistent ST-segment elevation is not an uncommon complication of a large anterolateral transmural MI. It may be a manifestation of dyskinesis of the thinned-out infarcted myocardium. However, persistent ST-segment elevations should suggest the presence of an **LV aneurysm**, and noninvasive confirmation of this diagnosis by two-dimensional echocardiography or radionuclide ventriculography should be sought.

64. Which myocardial infarctions are most commonly complicated by left ventricular (LV) aneurysms?

A ventricular aneurysm develops in 12–15% of survivors of an **acute transmural MI**. Aneurysms range from 1–8 cm in diameter. They are four times more common at the apex and anterior wall than in the inferoposterior wall, and they are more common in patients with larger infarcts. The mortality is about six times higher in patients with an LV aneurysm than in those with comparable global LV function. Death is often sudden, suggesting an increased risk of sustained VT and VF in these patients.

65. How do beta-blockers reduce cardiovascular mortality in survivors of acute MI?

There is a reduction in sudden cardiac deaths due to VF. Thus, the protective effect of oral beta-blockers in post-MI patients is primarily due to their "anti-fibrillatory" effects.

66. Beta-blockers are effective in the treatment of stable exertional angina pectoris. Would you recommend routine administration of oral beta-blockers in MI survivors who are angina-free?

Several large-scale, multicenter clinical trials conducted in the U.S. and abroad have shown a consistent reduction in total and cardiovascular mortality in survivors of acute transmural MI treated with oral beta-blockers for 1–3 years. The largest published U.S. trial is the Beta-Blocker Heart Attack Trial, which randomized 3,837 MI survivors to either propranolol (180 or 240 mg/day) or placebo. At 3 years of follow-up, a 26% reduction in mortality was found in those patients treated with propranolol compared to placebo-treated patients. Thus, regardless of the presence or absence of angina, the routine administration of oral beta-blockers—propranolol (180-240 mg), timolol (10 mg bid), or metoprolol (100 mg bid), to be started 5–21 days post-MI and continued for at least 7 years—is recommended in survivors of transmural MI.

Beta-Blocker Heart Attack Trial Research Group: A randomized trial of propranolol in patients with acute myocardial Infarction: 1. Mortality results. JAMA 247:1707–1714, 1982.

67. A 67-year-old man has stayed in bed for the last 3 days with flu-like symptoms. A 12-lead ECG reveals new Q waves in leads V_1 to V_6 and ST-segment elevation of 3 mm in leads V_2–V_5, I, and aVL. What do you suspect in this patient? Is plasma creatinine kinase (CK) likely to be high in this patient?

This patient has ECG changes indicative of the recent evolution of an extensive anterolateral MI, as evidenced by:

1. 3-mm ST-segment elevations in anterolateral leads V_2–V_5, I, and aVL
2. New Q waves in all anterolateral chest leads

The most likely clinical diagnosis is an acute, extensive anterolateral MI that occurred 3–4 days ago, when he first complained of flu-like symptoms.

The laboratory confirmation of this clinical diagnosis is routinely done by measuring serum CK levels at 6-hour intervals for 24–48 hours. Serum CK levels are elevated starting at 4–8 hours after symptom onset, reach a peak at 18–24 hours, and normalize within 3–4 days. Thus, serum CK levels in this patient are likely to be normal.

In these latecomers, a measurement of lactate dehydrogenase-1 (LDH-1) iso-enzyme or LDH-1/LDH-2 ratio is recommended. An LDH-1/LDH-2 ratio > 1.0 supports the clinical diagnosis of acute MI. Unlike serum CK, LDH is elevated at 1–2 days, reaches a peak at 3–6 days, and returns to normal 8–14 days after an acute MI. Newer, more specific enzymatic cardiac markers, such as cardiac troponins I or T are now the most commonly used enzymatic markers of acute MI in late cases presenting more than 12 hours after symptom onset.

68. What is Dressler's syndrome?

Dressler's syndrome, first described in 1854, is post-MI chest pain *not* due to coronary insufficiency. Its exact etiology is unclear, but it is characterized by inflammation of the pericardium and surrounding tissues. It occurs 2–10 weeks post-MI in 3–4% of cases and can be treated with corticosteroids and nonsteroidal antiinflammatory agents.

69. How does Bayes' theorem help determine the value of exercise ECG testing in the detection of CAD?

Bayes' theorem allows prediction of the presence or absence of CAD in a patient, given the prevalence of CAD in the population and the sensitivity and specificity of the diagnostic test used in that patient. In general, the ability of noninvasive stress tests (treadmill exercise ECG test, treadmill thallium myocardial scintigraphy, treadmill or dobutamine echocardiography, or bicycle exercise radionuclide ventriculography) to predict the presence or absence of CAD in patients with a very low or very high pretest probability of CAD is poor. Thus, at both ends of the spectrum of pretest probability, noninvasive testing does not help the clinician decide whether to perform or not perform a definitive diagnostic test, such as coronary arteriography. On the other hand, patients with a reasonable pretest probability of CAD (30–70%) are good candidates for noninvasive stress testing.

Probability of Coronary Artery Disease

PRETEST PROBABILITY	AFTER TREADMILL ECG		AFTER TREADMILL THALLIUM
80%	Positive test: 95%	→	Positive test: 99%
		→	Negative test: 85%
	Negative test: 60%	→	Positive test: 90%
		→	Negative test: 30%

In the patient with typical exertional angina pectoris (associated with an 80% pretest probability of CAD), a negative treadmill ECG and thallium myocardial scintigram predict only a 30% probability of CAD. However, a positive treadmill thallium test in the same patient predicts a 90% probability of CAD. In such patients, coronary angiography is recommended in the latter case (positive treadmill thallium test) but not in the former.

HYPERTENSION

70. A 45-year-old hypertensive woman has been treated with nifedipine, 30 mg po qid, for chronic stable angina pectoris. She complains of ankle edema that worsened after her dose of nifedipine was recently increased. Are diuretics indicated in this patient?
Edema is a common side effect of chronic nifedipine treatment, occurring in 10–30% of patients treated with oral nifedipine in daily doses of 30–120 mg. Unlike other side effects of nifedipine, edema is dose-dependent and commonly responds to decreasing the nifedipine dose. Characteristically, edema secondary to nifedipine is not associated with volume expansion and does not respond to diuretics.

71. Are there different types of hypertension (HTN)?
1. **Idiopathic or essential HTN** is the most common, affecting approximately 40 million American adults. Men are more frequently affected than women (until the postmenopausal age); Black and Hispanic men and women are more commonly affected than whites.

2. **Labile or intermittent HTN** occurs only in certain circumstances, such as visits to the physician, stress, or exercise. These patients are at increased risk for the development of chronic HTN.

3. In **isolated systolic HTN**, systolic BP is elevated but diastolic BP is < 90 mmHg. This type of HTN typically occurs in the elderly, in whom large-vessel compliance is decreased secondary to atherosclerosis and age. Systolic BP is usually > 160 mmHg.

4. **High-normal blood pressure** is defined as 130–139/85–89 mmHg. Usually, these patients are in transition from the normotensive to the hypertensive state and are at increased risk for the development of chronic HTN. Typically, they have a family history of essential HTN. Diabetics with high-normal blood pressure should receive antihypertensive drugs with a blood pressure goal of < 130/85 mmHg.

5. **Malignant HTN** is a medical emergency requiring immediate therapy. It is characterized by marked elevation in BP, usually > 180/120 mmHg, and is associated with evidence of acute end-organ damage, profound intravascular volume loss, and activation of the renin-angiotensin-aldosterone axis.

6. **Hypertensive urgency** is a milder form of malignant HTN in which the patient is not symptomatic. These patients should be treated in the doctor's office and generally do not require hospitalization.

7. **Hypertensive emergency** is associated with acute end-organ damage such as acute pulmonary edema, acute myocardial infarction, aortic dissection, acute renal failure, acute thrombotic or hemorrhagic stroke, and hypertensive encephalopathy.

72. Describe your approach to the initial evaluation of a patient with possible secondary causes of hypertension (HTN). What is the value of findings such as postural HTN, paroxysmal HTN, and hypokalemia in the diagnostic work-up of these patients?

The initial evaluation of the hypertensive patient should be focused on historical or physical clues to the various causes of secondary HTN, including:

Alcohol consumption	Dietary salt intake
Muscle weakness	Paroxysmal episodes of palpitation
Headache	Sweating
Nervousness	Nausea or vomiting
History of renal parenchymal disease	Concomitant history of generalized
Documented postural hypotension	atherosclerotic vascular disease

A careful history (including age at onset of HTN, and family history of HTN), physical examination, and laboratory panel consisting of urinalysis, microscopy, CBC, blood electrolytes, serum creatinine, chest x-ray, and 12-lead ECG should be obtained in all patients evaluated for HTN.

Paroxysmal HTN and postural HTN suggest pheochromocytoma. The presence of generalized atherosclerosis and abdominal or flank bruits suggest renal artery stenosis. Muscle weakness and unexplained hypokalemia suggest aldosteronism. Prior history of renal parenchymal disease and the presence of abnormal urine sediment suggest secondary HTN due to parenchymal renal disease.

73. It is generally accepted that antihypertensive therapy lowers the risk of stroke, but does it have any effect on risk of CAD (MI and angina)?

The Systolic HTN in the Elderly Program (SHEP) demonstrated that a thiazide-based antihypertensive regimen (chlorthalidone, 12.5–25 mg/day, alone or combined with atenolol, 25–50 mg/day) reduces stroke risk by 36% and nonfatal MI plus coronary death by 27% in older (> 60 yr) patients with isolated systolic HTN (systolic BP > 160 mmHg/diastolic BP < 90 mmHg). Major cardiovascular events were reduced by 32%. As a result, overall all-cause mortality was 13% lower. Similar studies in younger hypertensive patients have shown a smaller beneficial effect or no effect of antihypertensive drug therapy on CAD events.

SHEP Cooperative Research Group: Prevention of stroke by anti-hypertensive drug treatment in older persons with isolated systolic hypertension. Final results of the Systolic Hypertension in the Elderly Program (SHEP). JAMA 265:3255–3264, 1991.

74. A 42-year-old woman has an office BP reading of 150/90 mmHg. Would you initiate antihypertensive therapy in this patient?

Initiation of chronic antihypertensive drug therapy in a patient with a single office BP measurement of 150/90 mmHg is not recommended. Unlike diastolic BP, systolic BP is subject to wider variations between office visits and even between examiners during a single office visit. Among the factors that may affect systolic BP measurement and thus result in the erroneous diagnosis of systemic hypertension are:

- Patient's anxiety level
- Ambient temperature at the doctor's office
- Examiner (physician or nurse)
- Time of day
- Physical activity preceding BP measurement
- Size of cuff used
- Patient's posture (supine, sitting, or standing)
- Presence or coexistent medical problems, such as fever, thyrotoxicosis, anemia, AV fistula, etc.

Drug therapy for hypertension is recommended for sustained elevations of sitting BP exceeding 140/90 mmHg during at least 2 clinic visits.

75. Which antihypertensive drug classes are currently recommended as "preferred" first-line drugs in the treatment of hypertension?

In the last 3 decades, several clinical trials have conclusively demonstrated that antihypertensive drugs improve survival and reduce the risk of stroke, heart failure, and renal failure in HTN. All of these studies used a treatment strategy consisting of a thiazide diuretic or beta-adrenergic blocker alone or in combination with other drugs, if necessary. There are no published clinical trials demonstrating a favorable effect of newer antihypertensive drugs, such as ACE inhibitors, calcium antagonists, or alpha-adrenergic blockers, on fatal or morbid complications of HTN. The only exception is the SYST-EUR trial of a long-acting dihydropyridine calcium channel blocker showing a reduction of cardiovascular mortality and stroke risk in older patients with isolated systolic hypertension. Thus, The Sixth Report of the Joint National Committee on Detection, Evaluation and Treatment of High Blood Pressure recommended diuretics and beta-adrenergic blockers as "preferred" first-line antihypertensive drugs. In older patients with isolated systolic hypertension, a thiazide diuretic or a long-acting dihydropyridine calcium channel blocker are recommended since these drugs have been demonstrated to reduce cardiovascular mortality and stroke risk in these patients. Pharmacologic therapy should be considered after life-style modifications have failed to achieve a reduction of BP to < 140/90 mmHg.

Joint National Committee on Detection, Evaluation and Treatment of High Blood Pressure: The Sixth Report of the Joint National Committee on Detection, Evaluation, Treatment and Prevention of High Blood Pressure (JNCVI). Arch Intern Med 153:154–183, 1997.

Staessen JA, Fagard R, Thijs L, et al for the Systolic Hypertension–Europe (Syst-Eur) Trial Investigators: Morbidity and mortality in the placebo-controlled European Trial on Isolated Systolic Hypertension in the Elderly. Lancet 350:757–764, 1997.

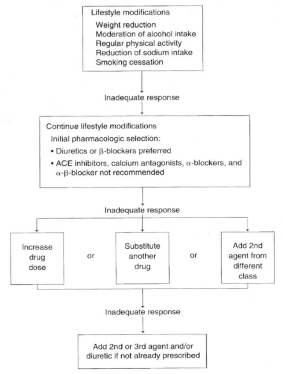

Treatment algorithm for HTN. (Adapted from Joint National Committee on Detection, Evaluation, and Treatment of High Blood Pressure: The fifth report of the Joint National Committee on Detection, Evaluation, and Treatment of High Blood Pressure (JNCV). Arch Intern Med 153:154–183, 1993.)

76. What classes of antihypertensive drugs are preferred for use in a patient with a known history of CHF? Which drugs should you avoid?

The following classes of antihypertensive drugs are desirable in patients with CHF:

Vasodilators

Direct vascular smooth-muscle-relaxing drugs (hydralazine and minoxidil)

Angiotensin-converting enzyme inhibitors (captopril, enalapril, lisinopril, or monopril)

Angiotensin receptor blockers (losartan, irbesartan, valsartan, candesartan)

Diuretics, such as thiazide diuretics (hydrochlorothiazide)

Drugs to *avoid* in these patients are those with negative inotropic effects:

Calcium channel blockers (verapamil or diltiazem)

Beta-blockers (propranolol, metoprolol, atenolol, etc.)

Not all calcium channel blockers are poorly tolerated and thus contraindicated in patients with heart failure. Amlodipine, a dihydropyridine calcium channel blocker with no clinically significant negative inotropic effects, has been extensively evaluated in two large prospective placebo-controlled clinical trials in heart failure patients. Unlike diltiazem and verapamil, non-dihydropyridine calcium channel blockers with significant negative inotropic effects, amlodipine can be used safely in patients with impaired systolic function who have an indication for the use of a calcium channel blocker, such as hypertension or angina pectoris.

Although beta blockers are generally considered to be contraindicated in patients with heart failure, an increasing number of clinical trials with beta blockers such as carvedilol and metoprolol—carefully and gradually titrated starting with very low doses—support a beneficial long-term effect of these beta blockers in patients with NYHA Functional Class II and III (mild to moderate symptomatic heart failure). The initiation of beta blockers even in low doses in patients with heart failure should be done very cautiously as a significant proportion of these patients (as high as 30–40%) may experience symptomatic hypotension or worsening heart failure symptoms in the first 4 weeks.

77. Discuss the effect of alcohol consumption on hypertension.

Alcohol intake is one of the most common causes of secondary HTN. A linear relationship between alcohol consumption and BP has been described, with even small quantities of alcohol sometimes raising BP. A threshold effect also has been described, with a lower BP observed in patients who consume 1–2 oz of alcohol a day, compared to those who do not drink any alcohol. It is likely that alcohol causes HTN by raising cardiac output and heart rate. The mechanism is probably a rapid rise in plasma epinephrine and cortisol levels.

Klatsky AL, et al: The relationship between alcoholic beverage use and other traits to blood pressure: A new Kaiser-Permanente study. Circulation 73:628, 1986.

78. Among the nonpharmacologic interventions for HTN, many popular beliefs, such as dietary garlic or onion intake and dietary magnesium or calcium in excess of RDA levels, have not withstood careful evaluation in controlled clinical trials. Which lifestyle modifications have proved beneficial to hypertensive patients?

Lifestyle Modifications for Hypertension Control and Overall Cardiovascular Health

- Lose weight if overweight
- Limit alcohol intake to 1 oz/day of ethanol (24 oz of beer, 8 oz of wine, or 2 oz of 100 proof whiskey)
- Exercise (aerobic) regularly
- Reduce sodium intake to < 100 mmol/day (< 2.3 gm of sodium or approximately 6 gm of NaCl)
- Maintain adequate dietary potassium, calcium, and magnesium intake
- Stop smoking and reduce dietary saturated fat and cholesterol intake for overall cardiovascular health (reducing fat intake also helps reduce caloric intake, which is important for control of weight and type II diabetes)

Joint National Committee on Detection, Evaluation and Treatment of High Blood Pressure: The Sixth Report of the Joint National Committee on Detection, Evaluation, Treatment and Prevention of High Blood Pressure (JNCVI). Arch Intern Med 153:154–183, 1997.

CONGESTIVE HEART FAILURE

79. What are some common signs and symptoms of CHF?
Listed in order of decreasing specificity:

Right Heart Failure	**Left Heart Failure**
Jugular vein distension	Chest x-ray with redistribution of perfusion
Hepatomegaly	or interstitial edema
Increased PT	Third heart sound (S_3)
Peripheral edema	Cardiomegaly
Increased AST/SGOT, bilirubin	Pulmonary rales
Pleural effusion	Paroxysmal nocturnal dyspnea, orthopnea
Decreased albumin	Dyspnea on exertion
Abdominal discomfort	
Anorexia	
Proteinuria	

80. What is the differential diagnosis of CHF?

Isolated Right Heart Failure	**Left or Biventricular Failure**
Pulmonary embolus	Aortic stenosis
Tricuspid stenosis	Aortic insufficiency
Tricuspid regurgitation	Mitral stenosis
Right atrial tumor	Mitral regurgitation
Cardiac tamponade	Most cardiomyopathies
Constrictive pericarditis	Acute MI
Pulmonic insufficiency	Myxoma
Right ventricular (RV) infarction	Hypertensive heart disease
Intrinsic lung disease	Myocarditis
Ebstein's anomaly	Supraventricular arrhythmias
High cardiac output states (anemia,	Left ventricular (LV) aneurysm
systemic fistulae, beriberi, Paget's	Cardiac shunts
disease, carcinoid, thyrotoxicosis, etc.)	High cardiac output states

81. What factors can precipitate an exacerbation of formerly well-controlled chronic CHF?
When patients with well-controlled chronic CHF experience sudden exacerbations, in addition to worsening of the underlying condition(s) that led to the CHF, a precipitating factor must be searched for and corrected. These factors include:

Increased consumption of salt	Paget's disease
Fluid overload	Poor compliance with medications
Pulmonary emboli	Arrhythmias
Fever, infection	Elevated BP
Anemia	High environmental temperature
Renal failure	Cardiac ischemia or MI
Pregnancy	Thyrotoxicosis

82. A 78-year-old man with a longstanding history of CHF presents with weakness, anorexia, nausea, and dizziness. He has been receiving digoxin, 0.5 mg po daily, and furosemide, 120 mg po twice a day. What specific tests would you request in your evaluation?
Any patient receiving digitalis who presents with GI symptoms, such as anorexia, nausea, or vomiting, should be suspected of having digitalis toxicity. The nausea and vomiting are thought to be mediated by stimulation of the area postrema in the medulla oblongata of the brainstem, rather than by any direct effects of digitalis on the GI mucosa. These GI manifestations may also occur in patients receiving excessive parenteral doses of digitalis.

Uncommonly, patients with chronic CHF complain of similar GI symptoms due to passive hepatic congestion or ascites. Differentiation of the various causes of nausea and vomiting in such patients, on clinical grounds alone, can be difficult. Other manifestations of digitalis toxicity include:

1. **Neurologic symptoms:** headache, neuralgia, confusion, delirium, and seizures
2. **Visual symptoms:** scotomata, halos, altered color perception
3. **Cardiac toxicity:**
   a. Ventricular or junctional tachyarrhythmias
   b. AV block
4. **Other manifestations:** gynecomastia, skin rash

The single most useful laboratory test to confirm the clinical suspicion of digitalis intoxication is a serum digoxin level. However, even serum digoxin levels in the "therapeutic range" may be toxic in elderly patients or in patients with hypokalemia, hypercalcemia, acid-base disorders, or thyroid disorders.

83. Describe the cardiac complications of digitalis intoxication.

Cardiac manifestations are by far the most life-threatening complications of digitalis intoxication. Almost any arrhythmia can be a manifestation of digitalis intoxication. Common ones include paroxysmal atrial tachycardia with AV block, junctional tachycardia with or without AV block, and first-degree or Mobitz I second-degree AV block. The coexistence of increased automaticity of ectopic pacemakers with impaired AV conduction is also very suggestive of digitalis intoxication.

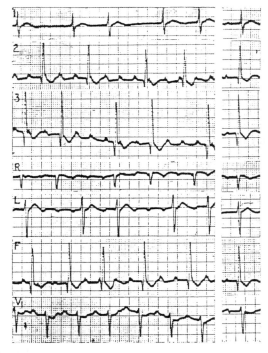

Digitalis intoxication presenting with paroxysmal atrial tachycardia with varying AV block. Note that the P waves are almost normally directed (axis +90°), the AV conduction ratio varies, and the atrial rhythm is not precisely regular. The single column of complexes on the right shows the form and direction of P waves (axis +60°) once sinus rhythm was restored. (From Marriott HJL: Practical Electrocardiography, 8th ed. Baltimore, Williams & Wilkins, 1988, p 488; with permission.)

84. A large variety of cardiac drugs are presently available for use in the treatment of CHF. Which one(s) has been proved to decrease mortality?

The drugs used to treat CHF include various classes of **vasodilators** (nitrates, hydralazine, prazosin, ACE inhibitors), digitalis, and diuretics. Unlike digitalis or diuretics, some vasodilators have been shown to reduce mortality in patients with CHF. **Enalapril**, an ACE inhibitor, reduces mortality in patients with moderate or severe CHF (NYHA Class II, III, or IV). A combination of **isosorbide dinitrate**, a predominant venous vasodilator, and **hydralazine**, an arteriolar vasodilator, reduces mortality in mildly to moderately severe CHF (NYHA Class II or III). Interestingly, not all vasodilators decrease mortality in patients with CHF. Prazosin, a postsynaptic alpha-1-receptor blocker, did not alter mortality when compared to placebo.

The Consensus Trial Study Group: Effects of enalapril on mortality in severe congestive heart failure: Results of the Cooperative North Scandinavian Enalapril Survival Study (CONSENSUS). N Engl J Med 316:1429–1435, 1987.

Cohn JN, et al: Effect of vasodilator therapy on mortality in chronic congestive heart failure: Results of a Veterans Administration Cooperative Study. N Engl J Med 314:1547–1552, 1986.

INFECTIONS

85. When is surgical intervention generally indicated in infectious endocarditis?

Most patients with infective endocarditis involving native heart valves can be successfully and effectively treated with a 4–6 week course of parenteral antibiotics. In contrast, patients with infective endocarditis involving prosthetic heart valves commonly are candidates for valve replacement. In both patient groups, however, the need for valve replacement depends most importantly on the evolution of major complications of endocarditis that are not generally appropriately managed with antiobitics. These complications consist of the following:

1. Heart failure refractory to adequate medical therapy
2. More than one major systemic embolic episode
3. Persistent bacteremia despite appropriate antibiotics
4. Severe valvular dysfunction by echocardiography
5. Ineffective antimicrobial therapy (e.g., fungal endocarditis)
6. Resection of mycotic aneurysm
7. Many cases of prosthetic valve endocarditis, especially with dehiscence or obstruction
8. Development of persistent heart block or bundle branch block, usually seen in aortic valve involvement and unrelated to drug therapy or ischemic heart disease
9. Extravalvular myocardial invasion, such as myocardial abscess or purulent pericarditis

86. What infectious pathogens may produce culture-negative endocarditis?

There are many potential reasons why blood cultures may be negative in the presence of infective endocarditis. They include prior administration of antibiotics, presence of uremia, and infection by fastidious organisms. Nutritionally deficient streptococci, *Brucella* sp., intracellular organisms (rickettsia and chlamydia), fungi, anaerobes, and the HACEK group of organisms (*Haemophilus* sp., *Actinobacillus actinomycetemcomitans*, *Cardiobacterium hominis*, *Eikenella corrodens*, and *Kingella kingae*) also must be considered when cultures are negative.

87. What does the new onset of conduction system abnormalities in the setting of endocarditis imply?

Perivalvular and/or myocardial abscesses. Surgical drainage and valve replacement are usually necessary.

88. What are the so-called immunologic manifestations of subacute bacterial endocarditis (SBE)?

Immunologic manifestations of infective endocarditis are believed to be mediated by the deposition of immune complexes within extracardiac structures, such as the retina, joints, fingertips, pericardium, skin, and kidney, rather than direct bacterial invasion. Interestingly, these immunologic manifestations of endocarditis are reported almost exclusively in patients with a prolonged course of SBE. They include:

1. **Roth spots:** cytoid bodies in the retina
2. **Osler nodes:** tender nodular lesions in the terminal phalanges
3. **Janeway lesions:** painless macular lesions on palms and soles
4. **Petechiae** and purpuric lesions
5. **Proliferative glomerulonephritis**

89. What are the most common causes of acute pericarditis?

In the outpatient setting, pericarditis is usually idiopathic. Many of these cases are probably due to viral infections. The coxsackie A and B viruses are highly cardiotropic and are two of the most common viruses to lead to pericarditis and myocarditis. Other responsible viruses include mumps, varicella-zoster, influenza, Epstein-Barr, and HIV.

In the inpatient setting, some of the more common etiologies can be recalled with the mnemonic TUMOR. "Tumor" also serves as a reminder that metastatic cancer is a frequent cause of pericarditis and pericardial effusion in hospitalized patients:

T = Trauma
U = Uremia
M = Myocardial infarction (acute and post), Medications (e.g., hydralazine and procainamide)
O = Other infections (bacterial, fungal, tuberculous)
R = Rheumatoid arthritis and other autoimmune disorders, Radiation

90. What is the major cardiac finding in Lyme disease?

Lyme disease is caused by the tick-borne spirochete, *Borrelia burgdorferi*. A rash, followed in weeks to months by involvement of other organ systems, including the heart, neurologic system, and joints, often marks the initial infection. About 1 in 10 patients manifest cardiac involvement, usually with severe AV block which is often associated with syncope, since there is concomitant depression of ventricular escape rhythms. Temporary pacing is indicated (the AV block usually resolves), as is antibiotic treatment with high-dose IV penicillin or oral tetracycline.

CONGENITAL HEART DISEASE

91. Which congenital cardiac lesions most often present in adulthood?

Bicuspid aortic valve and atrial septal defect (ASD) are the most common congenital heart diseases that present in adulthood. Congenital cyanotic cardiac lesions presenting in adulthood are distinctly uncommon. ASD alone accounts for about 30% of all congenital heart disease in adults.

The types and frequencies of ASDs are:

1. Ostium secundum   70%
2. Ostium primum   15%
3. Sinus venosus   15%

92. Coeur-en-sabot is a term coined in 1888 by a French scientist in his first report of a congenital cardiac disease. Which congenital heart disease is it?

"Coeur-en-sabot" was first coined by E.L. Fallot in a case report of Tetralogy of Fallot. It describes the typical configuration of the cardiac silhouette on chest x-ray in these patients. The four components of this malformation are:

1. Ventricular septal defect
2. Obstruction to RV outflow
3. Overriding of the aorta
4. RV hypertrophy

The most distinctive radiographic finding in Tetralogy of Fallot is RV hypertrophy. This results in a fairly classic boot-shaped (or wooden shoe-shaped) configuration of the cardiac silhouette, with prominence of the RV and a concavity in the region of the underdeveloped RV outflow tract and main pulmonary artery.

93. Which cardiac disease most commonly presents in adulthood with right bundle branch block (RBBB), first-degree AV block, and left axis deviation on ECG? Discuss the mechanism of these ECG findings.

The presence of complete or incomplete RBBB is an ECG hallmark of RV volume overload, often accompanied by rightward deviation of the QRS axis, except in patients with ostium primum ASD. Because of hypoplastic changes in the left anterior fascicle, patients with ostium primum ASD have left axis QRS deviation. Thus, the combination of RBBB and left axis QRS deviation is a fairly distinctive feature of ostium primum ASD, and it is often accompanied by first-degree AV block.

CARDIAC SYNDROMES AND OTHER ENTITIES

94. What are the cardiac manifestations of ankylosing spondylitis? What valvular dysfunction is commonly encountered in this syndrome?

The incidence of cardiovascular involvement in ankylosing spondylitis ranges from 3–10%, depending on the duration of the disease. The characteristic cardiac involvement consists of dilatation of the aortic valve ring and the sinuses of Valsalva, as well as inflammatory changes in the aortic valve ring. The resultant clinical hallmark is aortic root dilatation and aortic regurgitation, often rapidly progressive and ultimately requiring aortic valve replacement. Echocardiography is the diagnostic technique of choice in the evaluation and follow-up of these patients.

95. What is the ECG triad of Wolff-Parkinson-White (WPW) syndrome?
1. Short PR interval (< 0.12 sec)
2. Wide QRS complex (> 0.12 sec)
3. Delta wave or slurred upstroke of QRS complex

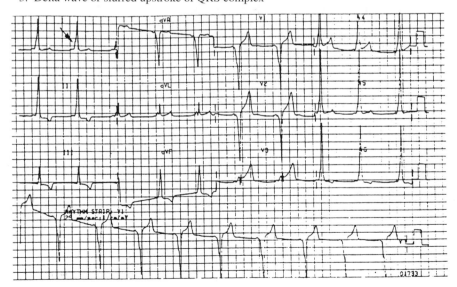

Right anteroseptal accessory pathway in WPW. The 12-lead ECG characteristically exhibits a normal to inferior axis. The delta wave is negative in V1 and V2; upright in lead I, II, AVL, and AVF; isoelectric in lead III; and negative in AVR. The arrow indicates delta wave (lead 1). (From Braunwald E (ed): Heart Disease: A Textbook of Cardiovascular Medicine, 3rd ed. Philadelphia, W.B. Saunders, 1988, p 686; with permission.)

96. Discuss the mechanism underlying sudden cardiac death in patients with WPW syndrome.

Patients with a pre-excitation syndrome such as WPW are at risk for developing AF with antegrade conduction along the accessory pathway. This tachycardia presents a serious risk because of its propensity to degenerate into VF due to very rapid conduction over the accessory pathway.

Patients with accessory pathways and short refractory periods (< 200 msec) are at highest risk for this antegrade conduction AF and therefore sudden cardiac death. Intermittent pre-excitation during sinus rhythm and loss of conduction along the accessory pathway during exercise or during administration of ajmaline or procainamide suggest that the refractory period of the accessory pathway is long (> 250 msec). These patients are not at risk of developing very rapid ventricular rates when AF or atrial flutter occurs and are therefore not at risk for sudden cardiac death.

97. How does Marfan's syndrome affect the heart?

Marfan's syndrome is a generalized disorder of connective tissue that is inherited as an autosomal dominant trait. Cardiac abnormalities occur in over 60% of these patients and are almost always responsible for early death when it occurs. The most common cardiac lesion is dilatation of the aortic ring, sinuses of Valsalva, and ascending aorta. This dilatation leads to progressive aortic regurgitation and may be complicated by acute aortic dissection. The risk of dissection is markedly increased during pregnancy.

Another common valvular dysfunction in Marfan's syndrome is mitral regurgitation due to a redundant myxomatous mitral valve (called "floppy" prolapsed mitral valve). In contrast to adults, children with Marfan's are much more likely to have severe isolated mitral regurgitation than aortic root or aortic valve disease.

98. To what does the term Marfan's syndrome-forme fruste refer?

Mitral valve prolapse (MVP) in the absence of other systemic manifestations of Marfan's syndrome has been referred to as Marfan's syndrome-forme fruste, in view of the similar pathologic appearance of the myxomatous mitral valve in both disorders. Isolated MVP is more common than Marfan's syndrome.

99. What are the three types of Takayasu's arteritis?

Type I involves primarily the aortic arch and brachiocephalic vessels. Type II affects the thoracoabdominal aorta and particularly the renal arteries. Type III combines features of both types I and II. Types I and III may be complicated by aortic regurgitation.

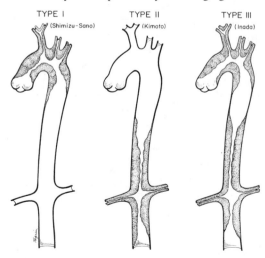

From Braunwald E (ed): Heart Disease: A Textbook of Cardiovascular Medicine, 3rd ed. Philadelphia, W.B. Saunders, 1988, p 1563; with permission.

100. Which age and gender groups most commonly present with Takayasu's arteritis? How does this differ from atherosclerosis and giant cell arteritis?

Takayasu's arteritis typically affects young women, with a female:male ratio of 8:1. In about three-fourths of all cases, onset is in the teenage years. This is in sharp contrast to atherosclerotic aortic disease, which usually affects older men, and giant cell arteritis, which usually affects women over age 50 years.

	TAKAYASU'S ARTERITIS	ATHEROSCLEROSIS	GIANT CELL ARTERITIS
Synonyms	Pulseless disease, reversed coarctation	—	Granulomatous arteritis
Age at onset	15–25 yrs	> 50 yrs	> 50 yrs
F:M ratio	8:1	1:4	2–3:1
Systemic prodrome	Fever, weight loss	None	Headache, fever
Site of involvement	Aortic arch, thoracoabdominal	Large arteries	Temporal arteries
Complications	Pulseless arms, aortic hypertension	Stroke, MI, claudication (leg)	Blindness, jaw or arm claudication, polymyalgia

101. What is the classic clinical prodrome associated with Takayasu's arteritis?

Patients with Takayasu's arteritis commonly present with a number of systemic manifestations. The classic clinical prodrome associated with Takayasu's arteritis consists of the following clinical features:

1. Fever and night sweats   4. Arthralgias
2. Anorexia and weight loss   5. Pleuritic pain
3. Malaise and fatigue

102. What is the holiday heart syndrome?

The holiday heart syndrome is characterized by the presence of supraventricular arrhythmias in alcoholic patients following an acute alcoholic binge, sometimes associated with holiday parties or long weekends. These arrhythmias are often transient and do not require long-term antiarrhythmic drug therapy. The most common arrhythmias are AF and atrial flutter. Digitalis and beta-blockers produce an effective and rapid therapeutic response. Supportive care is also essential to prevent alcohol withdrawal symptoms in these patients.

103. Which of the cardiac chambers is most frequently involved in an atrial myxoma?
Frequency of Location of Myxomas

1. Left atrium   86%
2. Right atrium   10%
3. Left ventricle   2%
4. Right ventricle   2%
5. Multiple locations   10%

The most common site of origin of atrial myxomas is the fossa ovalis. To prevent recurrence of myxoma, a wide resection of the fossa ovalis area of the interatrial septum is performed during surgical excision.

104. What is the most common cause of chronic mitral regurgitation in the U.S.?

Mitral valve prolapse. This has replaced rheumatic heart disease, which was the most common cause of chronic mitral regurgitation in the 1950s and 1960s.

105. What are the physical examination findings in mitral regurgitation?

Mitral regurgitation is associated with an apical holosystolic murmur. The intensity and radiation of the murmur vary with the cause and severity. Physical examination also may reveal an S_3, peripheral pulses with a quick upstroke and short duration, a widened pulse pressure, and a hyperdynamic precordium.

106. How is mitral regurgitation treated?

Medical management includes afterload reduction (to maximize "forward" cardiac output), salt restriction and diuretics (in the face of CHF), and digitalis (in the face of AF). Surgical mitral valve replacement should be performed in patients refractory to medical management before they enter the severely symptomatic stage, or in asymptomatic patients before they develop irreversible ventricular dysfunction as evidenced by left ventricular ejection fraction of less than 40% or progressive ventricular dilatation.

PACING

107. Describe the three-letter code used to indicate the essential functions of a cardiac pacemaker.

The Three-Letter Pacemaker Code

First letter	Chamber(s) paced	A–atrial V–ventricle D–dual chamber
Second letter	Chamber(s) sensed	A–atrial V–ventricle D–dual chamber
Third letter	Mode of response to sensed event	O–no response I–inhibition T–triggering D–dual response

The letters in the pacing code describe the different pacer functions. The first letter indicates the chamber paced, the second is the chamber in which electrical activity is sensed, and the third represents the response to a sensed event. Thus, for the two most commonly used pacemakers today, the code indicates:

VVI, a pacemaker that can pace and sense the right ventricle (VV) and has an inhibited mode of response (I).

DDD, the so-called dual-chamber AV sequential pacemaker, can pace and sense either right ventricle or right atrium (DD) and has both inhibited and triggered modes of response (D).

108. What do the different modes of response indicate?

I—Inhibited: Pacemakers with an inhibited mode of response do not pace when a spontaneous depolarization (atrial or ventricular) is sensed by the pacemaker. Following a fixed interval, if no spontaneous depolarization is sensed, pacing occurs. The inhibited mode of response is most commonly used.

T—Triggered: These pacemakers pace shortly after a spontaneous depolarization is sensed. After a fixed interval, pacing will occur if no spontaneous depolarization is sensed.

D—Dual-response: The pacemakers have both inhibited and triggered modes of response.

109. Who generally receives dual-chamber pacemakers?

Dual-chamber pacemakers (DDD) are more expensive, are more difficult to implant, and require greater expertise from the clinician in charge of the patient's follow-up as compared to ventricular-demand pacemakers (VVI). Insertion of a dual-chamber pacemaker is therefore reserved for patients who are not good candidates for ventricular-demand pacemakers. These include older patients, patients with CHF or LV hypertrophy, and physically active young adults who would not tolerate fixed-rate ventricular pacing. On the other hand, patients who have a history of recurrent SVT are not good candidates for any pacing modality that involves atrial sensing, such as dual-chamber pacemakers. The latter would be better served by a simpler ventricular-demand pacemaker (VVI).

110. What are the manifestations and pathophysiology of pacemaker syndrome?

Patients suffering from symptomatic bradyarrhythmias who receive ventricular demand pacemakers (VVI) sometimes report dizziness, palpitations, a pounding sensation in the chest or neck, and/or dyspnea associated with ventricular pacing. The underlying mechanism is the loss of the normal AV synchrony during ventricular pacing. An improvement in cardiac output has been documented in various studies when the pacing modality was changed from ventricular to dual-chamber or AV sequential pacing. It is likely that patients with LV hypertrophy or LV failure or older patients who have a large atrial contribution to LV filling are most prone to develop pacemaker syndrome. They may be better candidates for AV sequential pacing using a DDD pacemaker.

AORTA

111. What are the causes of acute, severe aortic regurgitation (AR)?

Infective endocarditis
Dissecting aneurysm
Rupture or prolapse of aortic leaflet(s)
Traumatic rupture
Spontaneous rupture of myxomatous valve
Spontaneous rupture of leaflet fenestrations
Sudden sagging of a "normal" leaflet
Postoperative—faulty incision of a stenotic aortic valve
Morganroth J, et al: Acute severe aortic regurgitation. Ann Intern Med 87:225, 1977.

112. Why is a wide pulse pressure, typically present in chronic severe AR, unlikely to be observed in patients with acute AR?

The absence of a wide pulse pressure, as well as the concurrent absence of the characteristic arterial auscultatory signs of chronic AR, in patients presenting with acute AR is thought to be due to the much higher LV end-diastolic pressure (LVEDP) in the acute form. The acute development of a severe aortic valvular leak causes a much higher LVEDP in the normal-sized LV of patients with acute AR. Patients with chronic AR commonly have a dilated LV with increased compliance capable of accommodating large blood volumes without a significant rise of LVEDP.

Salient Hemodynamic Features of Severe Aortic Regurgitation

	ACUTE	CHRONIC
LV compliance	Not ↑	↑
Regurgitant volume	↑	↑
LV end-diastolic pressure	Markedly ↑	May be normal
LV ejection velocity	Not significantly ↑	Markedly ↑
Aortic systolic pressure	Not ↑	↑
Aortic diastolic pressure	→ to ↑	Markedly ↓
Systemic arterial pulse pressure	Slightly to moderately ↑	Markedly ↑
Ejection fraction	Not ↑	↑
Effective stroke volume	↓	↔
Effective cardiac output	↓	↔
Heart rate	↑	↔
Peripheral vascular resistance	↑	Not ↑

↔ = unchanged, ↑ = increased, ↓ = decreased.
Morganroth J, et al: Acute severe aortic regurgitation. Ann Intern Med 87:225, 1977.

As a result of the rapid elevation of LVEDP in acute AR and its rapid equilibration with aortic pressure, the diastolic rumble of acute AR is much shorter and softer than that of chronic AR. Another auscultatory manifestation of the rapid rise of LVEDP is premature mitral valve closure. This is considered a reliable echocardiographic sign of acute AR.

113. What are the signs of chronic AR? What are their mechanisms?

Chronic AR is characterized by a dilated LV due to longstanding volume overload, with a large stroke volume and a wide pulse pressure. The peripheral arterial auscultatory signs of chronic regurgitation are primarily due to this wide pulse pressure of chronic AR.

Peripheral Arterial Signs of Chronic Aortic Regurgitation

1. **de Musset's sign:** bobbing of the head with each heartbeat
2. **Corrigan's pulse:** abrupt distension and quick collapse of femoral pulses (also called water-hammer pulse)
3. **Traube's sign:** booming, "pistol-shot" systolic and diastolic sounds heard over the femoral pulse
4. **Müller's sign:** systolic pulsations of the uvula
5. **Duroziez's sign:** systolic murmur over femoral artery when compressed proximally and diastolic murmur when compressed distally
6. **Quincke's sign:** capillary pulsations of fingertips
7. **Hill's sign:** popliteal cuff systolic pressure exceeding brachial cuff pressure by > 60 mmHg

114. What are the three types of aortic dissection according to the DeBakey classification? What are their clinical and therapeutic significance?

The DeBakey classification divides aortic dissections into three groups based on their location, with each type requiring a different therapeutic approach. In general, Types I and II are best managed surgically, whereas type III is best managed medically. These differences are based largely on the disparate natural history of proximal (types I and II) and distal (type III) dissections. Even minimal progression of a proximal dissection can cause potentially fatal complications, such as cardiac tamponade, acute aortic regurgitation, or neurologic compromise. On the other hand, patients with distal aortic dissections often have advanced cardiovascular and cardiopulmonary disease and are therefore poor surgical candidates.

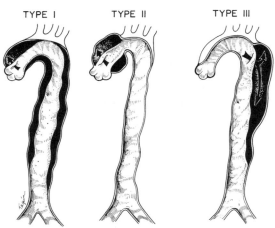

TYPE I   TYPE II   TYPE III

"PROXIMAL" or "ASCENDING"   "DISTAL" or "DESCENDING"

From Braunwald E (ed): Heart Disease: A Textbook of Cardiovascular Medicine, 3rd ed. Philadelphia, W.B. Saunders, 1988, p 1554; with permission.

115. What are the most common sites of aortic coarctation?

In descending order of frequency:

1. Postductal (adult-type coarctation)
2. Localized juxtaductal coarctation
3. Preductal (infantile-type coarctation)
4. Ascending thoracic aorta
5. Distal descending thoracic aorta
6. Abdominal aorta

116. Which congenital cardiac lesions are associated with coarctation of the aorta?

Aortic coarctation is frequently associated with other congenital cardiac lesions, including:

1. Bicuspid aortic valve
2. Patent ductus arteriosus
3. Ventricular septal defect
4. Berry aneurysms of circle of Willis

DRUG THERAPY

117. What are the advantages of third-generation thrombolytic drugs? Where do they come from?

Third-generation thrombolytics (better called fibrinolytics as they basically degrade fibrin) are mutants of wild-type tissue plasminogen activator. They are genetically engineered to confer two key properties: greater ability to dissolve the clot and longer half-life. There are three extensively evaluated third-generation thrombolytics:

1. Recombinant tissue plasminogen activator (r-PA, Retavase or Reteplase)
2. TNK tissue plasminogen activator (TNK-t-PA or Tenecteplase)
3. Novel plasminogen activator (n-PA or Lanoteplase)

r-PA and n-PA are deletion mutants of wild-type t-PA. They both lack the finger moiety of wild-type t-PA. Deletion of the finger moiety makes the drug less "sticky" to the fibrin on the surface of the clot. This ability of the drug to "stick" to the outer clot surface is called "fibrin affinity." Deletion of the finger moiety confers less fibrin affinity to the drug and is believed to potentiate the clot dissolving effect of r-PA and n-PA. Thus, r-PA achieves a statistically better angiographic outcome than t-PA in two large angiographic trials with 60–63% of patients achieving a complete reperfusion (referred to as TIMI Flow Grade 3) compared to 50–55% of those treated with t-PA. Similarly, n-PA results in a slightly but not statistically significantly better angiographic outcome compared to t-PA.

Only r-PA and TNK-t-PA are currently FDA approved and commercially available third-generation thrombolytic drugs; n-PA was found to cause an unacceptably high risk of intracranial hemorrhage and is not approved by the FDA for general use in the U.S.

The main advantages of third-generation thrombolytic drugs are:

1. Greater clot lytic effect.
2. Convenience: longer half-life makes these drugs "bolusable thrombolytics." Both r-PA and TNK-t-PA have longer half-lives than t-PA and can be given as "bolus" injections: r-PA is administered as a double-bolus (10 U IV every 30 minutes) and TNK-t-PA is administered as a single 5-second intravenous bolus.
3. Greater fibrin specificity: TNK-t-PA is 80-fold more fibrin specific than t-PA.
4. Greater resistance to PAI-1 (plasminogen activator inhibitor 1), making it more resistant to breakdown by naturally occurring inhibitors of plasminogen activator. This is the case for TNK-t-PA.

118. Give the mechanisms of action and usual doses of vasodilator drugs.

Effects and Dosages of Major Vasodilators

AGENT	MECHANISM OF ACTION	VENOUS DILATING EFFECT	ARTERIOLAR DILATING EFFECT	USUAL DOSAGE
Nitroglycerin	Direct	+++	+	25–500 µg/min IV
Isosorbide dinitrate	Direct	+++	+	5–20 mg q2h subling 10–60 mg q4h po
Hydralazine	Direct	—	+++	10–100 mg q6h po
Minoxidil	Direct	—	+++	10–40 mg/day po
Sodium nitroprusside	Direct	+++	+++	5–150 µg/min IV
Epoprostenol (prostacyclin)	Direct	+++	+++	5–15 ng/kg/min IV
Phenoxybenzamine	α-blockade	++	+	10–20 mg q8h po
Phentolamine	α-blockade	++	+	50 mg q4–6h po
Prazosin	α-blockade	+++	++	1–10 mg q8h po
Captopril	Inhibition of ACE	+++	++	6.25–50.0 mg q6–8h po
Enalapril	Inhibition of ACE	+++	+++	5–20 mg bid po
Lisinopril	Inhibition of ACE	+++	++	10–40 mg/day po
Quinapril	Inhibition of ACE	+++	++	10–40 mg/day po

From Rubenstein E, Federman D (eds): Scientific American Medicine. New York, Scientific American, 1988; with permission.

119. What is the mechanism of action of digitalis?

Digitalis and all the cardiac glycosides act by inhibiting Na^+-K^+ ATPase activity (the sodium pump). This blocks the transport of sodium and potassium across cell membranes, leading to an intracellular increase in sodium and decrease in potassium. The increase in intracellular sodium in turn leads to an exchange for calcium. The increased intracellular calcium, the contractile element of muscle, leads to increased contractility (positive inotropic effect).

The antiarrhythmic effects of the cardiac glycosides are probably not due to any direct effect of the drug. Rather, they are mediated by an increase in vagal tone in the atria and AV junction.

120. What factors contribute to digitalis toxicity?

Hypokalemia	Drugs
Hypercalcemia	Quinidine
Hypomagnesemia	Verapamil
Renal insufficiency (digoxin)	Amiodarone
Hepatic insufficiency (digitoxin)	Others

121. Name four classes of pharmacologic drugs that have proved effective in improving survival in acute myocardial infarction.

In 188 randomized controlled prospective trials conducted over three and a half decades in over 350,000 patients, 10 pharmacologic classes of drugs were evaluated in patients with acute myocardial infarction. Four classes of drugs proved effective in improving survival:

Thrombolytics
Beta-blockers
Anticoagulants (coumadin)
Antiplatelet drugs (aspirin)

Nitrates and early angiotensin-converting enzyme inhibitors improve survival but not drastically or consistently in various clinical trials.

Four other classes of drugs demonstrate no beneficial effect or may even cause an increase in mortality. They are:

Magnesium

Lidocaine (which is no longer routinely recommended in myocardial infarction)

Immediate and short-acting calcium channel blockers, especially nifedipine

Antiarrhythmic drugs

The latter four classes of drugs are no longer routinely recommended in acute myocardial infarction survivors in the most recently published guidelines for management of acute myocardial infarction.

Mortality is reduced about 15–25% with thrombolytics, beta-blockers, aspirin, or coumadin. This amounts to a saving of 20–40 lives per 1,000 treated patients. The single most life-saving pharmacologic therapy in acute myocardial infarction is thrombolytic drug therapy with a saving of 40 lives per 1,000 treated patients and a saving of 60–80 lives for every 1,000 patients treated within the first hour after symptom onset.

Guidelines for management of patients with acute myocardial infarction. Circulation August 31;100(9):1016–1030, 1999.

122. Patients maintained on digitalis commonly exhibit some changes on ECG referred to as "digitalis effect." What are these changes? How do they compare with those in myocardial ischemia?

Digitalis is to the ECG what syphilis once was to medicine, a great imitator. Digitalis can cause a variety of ECG abnormalities depending on the serum digoxin level. Administered in therapeutic doses, digoxin causes a characteristic sagging of the ST segment and flattening and inversion of the T waves. These changes typically occur in the inferolateral ECG leads.

These ST and T-wave changes are difficult to distinguish from those of subendocardial myocardial ischemia; however, some subtle differences exist. Typically, horizontal or down sloping ST-segment depression, sharp-angled ST-T junctions, and U-wave inversion are present in patients with subendocardial ischemia (coronary insufficiency). Less commonly, tall T waves may be a subtle ECG sign of myocardial ischemia.

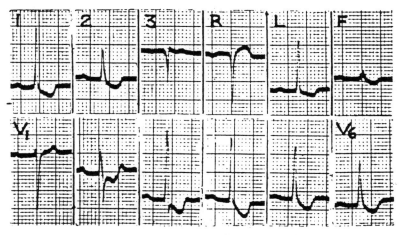

Digitalis effect. Note sagging ST segments in most leads with short QT interval. (From Marriott HJL: Practical Electrocardiology, 8th ed. Baltimore, Williams & Wilkins, 1988, p 478; with permission.)

123. In primary prevention trials aimed at reducing cardiovascular mortality with cholesterol-lowering drugs, which drugs have been shown to lower the risk of death from cardiac causes?

Coronary Primary Prevention Trials: LRC-CPPT vs. HHS

	LRC-CPPT	HHS
Cholesterol-lowering drug	Cholestyramine	Gemfibrozil
Average daily dose	24 gm	600 mg bid
Duration of follow-up	7.4 yrs	5 yrs
Reduction in cholesterol	8.5%	10%
Reduction in LDL cholesterol	13%	10%
Increase in HDL cholesterol	2%	10%
Reduction in CV mortality	19%	34%

Two primary prevention trials, the Lipid Research Clinic–Coronary Primary Prevention Trial (LRC–CPPT) and the Helsinki Heart Study (HHS), were designed to test the hypothesis that a reduction of serum cholesterol decreases cardiovascular mortality. Both clinical trials showed that cholesterol-lowering drugs, such as cholestyramine and gemfibrozil, effectively reduced serum cholesterol and decreased cardiovascular mortality.

A 1% reduction in serum cholesterol in the LRC–CPPT was associated with a 2% reduction in cardiovascular mortality. Overall, about a 10% reduction in serum cholesterol was accompanied by a 20% decrease in cardiovascular mortality. One of the most interesting findings in this trial was that the reduction in cardiovascular mortality was highest in those patients who had the lowest reduction in serum cholesterol levels, supporting the causal relationship between cholesterol and cardiovascular disease.

The LRC–CPPT and HHS were conducted in patients with markedly elevated LDL and cholesterol levels and used two drugs with a fairly modest LDL-lowering effect as reflected by the 10–13% reduction in LDL in these two trials. More recently, HmG Co-A reductase inhibitors (lovastatin, simvastatin, atorvastatin and pravastatin) have been shown to cause a greater reduction in LDL in the range of 20–65%, particularly when used in large doses. The largest recent primary prevention trial of a statin in "asymptomatic subjects" is the AFCAPS/TexCAPS Coronary Atherosclerosis Prevention Study. In this trial, lovastatin was evaluated in 5,608 men and 997 women with average TC and LDL-C and below-average HDL-cholesterol levels. Lovastatin reduced the risk for the first acute major coronary event in men and women with average TC and LDL-C levels and below-average HDL-C levels.

In summary, LDL reduction is effective in preventing the first coronary events in asymptomatic subjects with no previous known coronary artery disease. The use of a more effective LDL lowering HmG Co-A reductase inhibitor ("statin") is recommended in primary prevention in those asymptomatic subjects who are at greater risk of coronary disease as evidenced by a combination of an elevated LDL level and a below-average HDL level.

Lipid Research Clinics Program: The Lipid Research Clinics Coronary Primary Prevention Trial results: Reduction in incidence of coronary heart disease. JAMA 251:351, 1984.

Frick MH, et al: Helsinki Heart Study: Primary prevention trial with dyslipidemia. N Engl J Med 317:1237–1245, 1987.

Downs JR, Clearfield M, Weis S, et al: Primary prevention of acute coronary events with lovastatin in men and women with average cholesterol levels: Results of AFCAPS/TexCAPS. Air Force/Texas Coronary Atherosclerosis Prevention Study. JAMA 279:1615–1622, 1998.

124. Most lipid-lowering drugs lower serum cholesterol levels by reducing the LDL fraction, but some are capable of raising the serum HDL-cholesterol level as well. Which lipid-lowering drug is most effective in raising HDL cholesterol levels? Does this affect coronary mortality?

Among all available lipid-lowering drugs, **gemfibrozil** results in the most marked increase in HDL-cholesterol levels. A 600 mg-dose, taken twice a day, resulted in a 10% increase in HDL in the Helsinki Heart Study. In this trial, 4,081 asymptomatic men with hyperlipidemia were randomly assigned to receive gemfibrozil or placebo over 5 years. Unlike patients in the

LRC–CPPT, who received cholestyramine and experienced almost no change in the serum HDL level, gemfibrozil-treated patients experienced a 10% increase in HDL and a remarkable 34% reduction in coronary mortality. Cholestyramine-treated patients had only 19% reduction in mortality.

The 10% increase in HDL-cholesterol levels induced by gemfibrozil likely accounted for the additional 15% reduction in CHD mortality. This led to the so-called "HDL hypothesis,"— i.e., that an increase in HDL alone can decrease the risk of death from CAD.

The importance of raising HDL cholesterol with gemfibrozil was further evaluated in the more recent Veterans Affairs Cooperative Study called the HIT trial (High-Density Lipoprotein Cholesterol Intervention Trial). This was a double-blind trial comparing gemfibrozil (1200 mg per day) with placebo in 2,531 men with coronary heart disease, an HDL cholesterol level of 40 mg% or less, and an LDL cholesterol level of 140 mg% or less. The primary study outcome was nonfatal myocardial infarction or death from coronary causes. At the median follow-up of about 5 years, gemfibrozil resulted in a modest increase in HDL of 6% and no significant change in LDL. This was accompanied by a significant reduction in the risk of major cardiovascular events in patients with coronary disease whose primary lipid abnormality was a low HDL cholesterol level. There was a 24% reduction in the combined outcome of death from coronary heart disease, nonfatal myocardial infarction, and stroke (p < 0.001). The findings suggest that raising HDL cholesterol levels and lowering levels of triglycerides without lowering LDL cholesterol levels would reduce recurrent coronary events in patients with known coronary artery disease.

Lipid Research Clinics Program: The Lipid Research Clinics Coronary Primary Prevention Trial results: Reduction in incidence of coronary heart disease. JAMA 251:351, 1984.

Frick MH, et al: Helsinki Heart Study: Primary prevention trial with dyslipidemia. N Engl J Med 317:1237–1245, 1987.

Rubins HB, Robins SJ, Collins D, et al: Gemfibrozil for the secondary prevention of coronary heart disease in men with low levels of high-density lipoprotein cholesterol. Veterans Affairs High-Density Lipoprotein Cholesterol Intervention Trial Study Group. N Engl J Med 341:410–418, 1999.

125. Does lowering LDL cholesterol reduce the risk of further mortality in patients with preexisting CAD?

The first published randomized controlled clinical trial of the effect of lipid-lowering therapy on CAD and all-cause mortality is the 4S (Scandinavian Simvastatin Survival Study). In this clinical trial of 4,444 men and women, aged 35–70 years, with a history of angina pectoris or acute MI and serum cholesterol of 220–320 mg/dl, simvastatin lowered total cholesterol and LDL cholesterol by 25% and 35%, respectively, and increased HDL by 8%. This was accompanied by a 30% reduction in overall mortality (from 12% to 8%), a 42% reduction in CAD deaths (from 28% to 19%), and a 37% reduction in the need for myocardial revascularization procedures (coronary bypass or angioplasty).

Unlike the LRC–CPPT, the 4S study showed a 3-fold greater reduction in cardiovascular mortality over a shorter follow-up period (5 vs. 10 years). It is hypothesized that simvastatin lowered CAD events primarily by stabilizing atherosclerotic lesions, accounting for a lower incidence of CAD events as early as 2 years after starting lipid-lowering drug therapy.

Scandinavian Simvastatin Survival Study Group: Randomized trial of cholesterol lowering in 4444 patients with coronary heart disease: The Scandinavian Simvastatin Survival Study (4S). Lancet 344:1383–1389, 1994.

126. What does cardioselectivity of a beta-blocking drug mean? Which beta-blockers are cardioselective, and what are the clinical implications of this pharmacologic property?

CARDIO-SELECTIVE BETA-BLOCKERS	NON-CARDIOSELECTIVE BETA-BLOCKERS
Atenolol (Tenormin)	Propranolol (Inderal)
Metoprolol (Lopressor)	Timolol (Blocadren)
Acebutolol (Sectral)	Pindolol (Visken)
	Nadolol (Corgard)

Cardioselectivity refers to the predominant blockade of the β_1-adrenergic receptors, which are mostly present in the heart. Cardioselective beta-blockers, in low doses, have minimal blocking effects on β_2-receptors, the predominant β receptors in the lungs. However, cardioselectivity is only relative; when administered in large doses, cardioselectivity is markedly diminished. Despite these limitations, cardioselective beta-blockers are much safer than noncardioselective beta-blockers in patients with obstructive lung disease.

127. What is the importance of intrinsic sympathomimetic activity (ISA) as it applies to beta-blockers? Which beta-blockers possess ISA?

ISA refers to the partial beta-adrenergic agonist properties of some beta-blockers. When sympathetic activity is low (at rest), these beta-blockers produce low-grade beta-stimulation. However, under conditions of stress (exercise), beta-blockers with ISA behave essentially as conventional beta-blockers without ISA. The clinical significance of ISA is not clearly established.

Pindolol and acebutolol demonstrate ISA. All other beta-blockers currently available do not have any significant ISA.

128. Prior to elective cardioversion of a patient with atrial fibrillation (AF), a 4-week course of adequate anticoagulation decreases the risk of thromboembolic events during and shortly after cardioversion. Is anticoagulation similarly required in a patient with AF with a fast ventricular rate of 230 bpm and systolic BP of 70 mmHg?

The risks and benefits of cardioversion and anticoagulation must be weighed very carefully prior to elective cardioversion. A 4-week period of adequate anticoagulation is desirable before elective cardioversion of a patient with AF. However, in a patient with AF with a fast ventricular response rate, the most important question is how urgent is cardioversion? Whenever there is clinical evidence of hemodynamic compromise (such as CHF, hypotension or systemic hypoperfusion, acute anginal symptoms, or acute MI), urgent cardioversion should be administered immediately, regardless of left atrial or LV size, systolic LV function, or prior anticoagulation. In the patient in question with AF with a fast ventricular response rate of 230 bpm and severe hypotension, cardioversion absolutely should not be delayed.

129. How is acute pulmonary edema managed with digitalis, diuretics, and vasodilators?

The therapeutic approach to any patient with acute pulmonary edema must be individualized, but some general guidelines for therapy are helpful:

1. IV diuresis with a loop diuretic such as furosemide (20–60 mg IV push, to be repeated as necessary): IV furosemide lowers venous tone and thus lowers pulmonary wedge pressure even before inducing effective diuresis.

2. IV, cutaneous, or oral preload-reducing drug therapy: Nitrates are effective venodilators. In single oral doses of 40–60 mg (to be repeated 3 or 4 times daily), they are effective in lowering pulmonary capillary wedge pressure and thus improving congestive symptoms of dyspnea, orthopnea, paroxysmal nocturnal dyspnea, and nocturnal cough.

3. IV digitalization is recommended in patients with acute pulmonary edema with or without associated AF.

4. Oxygen therapy, depending on results of arterial blood gas measurements.

5. Bed rest and salt restriction.

6. Afterload-reducing drugs are effective in alleviating the signs and symptoms of CHF. ACE inhibitors such as captopril, enalapril, or lisinopril are effective afterload and preload-reducing drugs and can be administered orally in patients with overt CHF. Unlike other drugs that effectively improve the symptoms of heart failure (such as diuretics and digoxin), ACE inhibitors are the only class of vasodilators that have been demonstrated in a large number of randomized placebo-controlled clinical trials to reduce cardiovascular mortality in patients with heart failure and a depressed left ventricular systolic function.

BIBLIOGRAPHY

1. Braunwald E (ed): Heart Disease: A Textbook of Cardiovascular Medicine, 6th ed. Philadelphia, W.B. Saunders, 2001.
2. Hurst JW (ed): The Heart, 8th ed. New York, McGraw-Hill, 1994.
3. Marriott HJL: Practical Electrocardiography, 10th ed. Baltimore, Williams & Wilkins, 2000.
4. Johnson RA, et al: The Practice of Cardiology. Boston, Little, Brown, 1980.
5. Isselbacher KJ, et al (eds): Harrison's Principles of Internal Medicine, 14th ed. New York, McGraw-Hill, 1998.

4. INFECTIOUS DISEASES

Richard J. Hamill, M.D.

*Men take diseases, one of another. Therefore let me take heed of their
company.*

William Shakespeare
Henry IV

*Throughout nature, infection without disease is the rule rather than the
exception.*

Rene Dubos
Man Adapting

1. What is Luria's law?

Three antibiotics equals one fungal infection.

Matz RP: Principles of medicine. NY State J Med 77:99–101, 1977.

2. What role does the horseshoe crab, *Limulus polyphemus*, play in infectious diseases?

In 1956, Bang reported that gram-negative bacterial endotoxin caused gelation of a lysate
prepared from the blood cells (amebocytes) of the Limulus crab. This limulus amebocyte lysate
reaction is the basis of an assay now used to detect the presence of endotoxin in various body
fluids, pharmacologic products, and medical devices.

Bang FB: A bacterial disease of *Limulus polyphemus*. Bull Johns Hopkins Hosp 98:325–350, 1956.

3. What is Vincent's angina?

This is a necrotizing pharyngitis caused by a mixture of anaerobes and spirochetes. *Streptococcus pyogenes* and *Staphylococcus aureus* may also play a role. Symptoms include an extremely sore throat, fever, and foul breath. Physical examination reveals pharyngeal ulcerations
that are covered with a purulent exudate. Treatment with penicillin is curative.

4. Where and when was the last naturally occurring case of smallpox identified?

In Merka Town, Somalia, in October 1977.

5. What are the tick-borne infectious diseases seen in the U.S.?

Tick-borne Infectious Diseases in the U.S.

DISEASE	ORGANISM
Lyme disease	*Borrelia burgdorferi*
Q fever	*Coxiella burnetii*
Human ehrlichiosis	*Ehrlichia chaffeensis, Ehrlichia ewingii*
Rocky Mountain spotted fever	*Rickettsia rickettsi*
Tularemia	*Francisella tularensis*
Babesiosis	*Babesia microti*
Relapsing fever	*Borrelia hermsii*
Tick-borne encephalitis	A flavivirus
Colorado tick fever	An orbivirus

Taege AJ: Tick trouble: Overview of tick-borne diseases. Cleve Clin J Med 67:245–249, 2000.

6. What is tick paralysis?

Tick paralysis is a complication of prolonged attachment of certain species of ticks
(*Dermacentor andersoni* and *D. variabilis* in the U.S.). It is an ascending paralysis that begins in

117

the lower extremities and rapidly progresses to involve the upper extremities and head. It is thought to be caused by a neurotoxin in the tick's saliva, and it usually resolves quickly after the tick is removed.

Felz MW, et al: Brief report. A six-year-old girl with tick paralysis. N Engl J Med 342:90–94, 2000.

7. Post-splenectomy sepsis is caused by what organisms?

Splenectomy predisposes patients to sepsis by encapsulated organisms, including:

Streptococcus pneumoniae   *Neisseria meningitidis*
Haemophilus influenzae   *Escherichia coli*

Occasional cases due to *Staphylococcus aureus* and *Capnocytophaga canimorsus* (DF-2) have been described.

8. Infective endocarditis due to *Pseudomonas aeruginosa* occurs almost always in what risk group?

P. aeruginosa causes infective endocarditis on native heart valves in intravenous drug abusers. Rarely, it is a cause of prosthetic valve endocarditis. The occurrence of *P. aeruginosa* endocarditis varies regionally. The source of the organism is thought to be standing water that contaminates drug paraphernalia.

9. What are the causative organisms of prosthetic valve endocarditis and their time of appearance relative to valve replacement surgery?

Traditionally, prosthetic valve endocarditis has been classified according to the time of onset with respect to the replacement surgery, with 2 months being the division between early- and late-onset endocarditis:

Prosthetic Valve Endocarditis (PVE)

ORGANISM	EARLY PVE (%)	LATE PVE (%)	OVERALL (%)
Staphylococci			
S. epidermidis	35	26	29
S. aureus	17	12	14
Streptococci			
Group D and enterococci	3	9	7
S. pneumoniae	1	< 1	1
Other (incl. viridans streptococci)	4	25	17
Gram-negative bacilli	16	12	13
Diphtheroids	10	4	7
Other bacteria	1	2	2
Candida	8	4	5
Aspergillus	2	1	1
Other fungi	1	< 1	1
Culture negative	1	4	3

Mayer KH, et al: Evaluation and management of prosthetic valve endocarditis. Prog Cardiovasc Dis 25:43–62, 1982.

10. What are the causes of a biologic false-positive RPR?

The causes of biologic false-positive rapid plasma reagent (RPR) tests for syphilis can be divided into those of acute or chronic duration:

Acute (positive < 6 months)	**Chronic (> 6 months duration)**
Acute febrile illnesses	Chronic infections (lepromatous leprosy)
Recent immunizations	Autoimmune diseases (e.g., lupus)
Pregnancy	IV drug addiction

When false-positive tests occur, the titer is usually low (< 1:8).

11. Do the specific treponemal serologic tests for syphilis (i.e., MHA-TP, FTA-ABS) return to undetectable levels after appropriate antimicrobial therapy for syphilis?

No, the treponemal tests remain positive for life after initial infection. These tests should not be used to assess response to therapy.

12. What is the expected rate of fall of nontreponemal serologic tests after appropriate treatment of primary, secondary, and early latent syphilis?

Expect a four-fold decline in VDRL or RPR titers at three months and an eight-fold decline at six months.

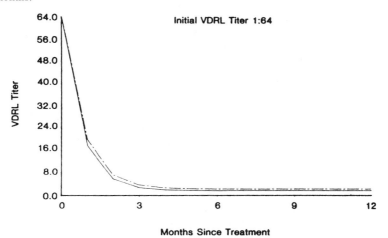

VDRL titer decline after treatment of primary or secondary syphilis with penicillin or tetracycline. (From Brown ST, et al: Serologic response to syphilis treatment. JAMA 253:1296–1299, 1985; with permission.)

13. What are the clinical settings and risk factors associated with *Candida* infections?

Clinical Settings and Risk Factors for Candida Infections

CLINICAL SETTING	RISK FACTORS
Chronic mucocutaneous infections	Defects in T-lymphocyte immunity, congenital (e.g., chronic mucocutaneous candidiasis) or acquired (e.g., AIDS)
Deeply invasive, disseminated infections	Peripheral neutrophil count <500/mm³ Mucosal barrier breakdown (burn, cytotoxic agents, GI surgery, IV catheter sites) Candidal overgrowth (broad-spectrum antibiotics)
Colonization of a catheter, with fever	Indwelling catheter

The difference between the first two categories may be difficult to distinguish clinically, and if there is doubt the patient should be treated for disseminated disease.

Crislip MA, et al: Candidiasis. Infect Dis Clin North Am 3:103–133, 1989.

14. Endophthalmitis is present in what percentage of patients with candidemia?

10–37%. Endophthalmitis is an important clue that the infection is disseminated.

15. Which species of *Candida* most commonly colonizes the skin?

C. parapsilosis. Its identification in blood cultures may suggest a contaminated intravascular line.

16. Which occupations are associated with *Erysipelothrix rhusiopathiae* infection?

Fishermen, fish handlers, butchers, meat-processing workers, poultry workers, farmers, veterinarians, and abattoir (slaughterhouse) workers. There are two major clinical syndromes: (1) localized cutaneous and (2) disseminated/endocarditis.

Brooke CJ, Riley TV: *Erysipelothrix rhusiopathiae:* Bacteriology, epidemiology and clinical manifestations of an occupational pathogen. J Med Microbiol 48:789–799, 1999.

17. What are the infusion-related syndromes associated with IV vancomycin administration?

1. Red-man syndrome is a histamine-mediated phenomenon that occurs with too rapid an infusion of vancomycin. It is characterized by the development of erythema, hives, and pruritus across the upper trunk and face.

2. The pain and spasm syndrome is characterized by throbbing chest pain that resolves when the antibiotic infusion is stopped. The pain is not secondary to myocardial ischemia.

3. Hypotension, a very rare infusion-related syndrome, can usually be treated with antihistamines, although pressor agents are occasionally needed.

18. How is the "bedside" cold agglutinin test performed? What does a positive result indicate?

Four to five drops of blood are added to a blood collection tube containing sodium citrate. The tube is immersed in an ice bath for 1–2 minutes. Floccular hemagglutination observed on the side of the tube is indicative of a positive reaction. Confirmation is provided if the agglutination disappears when the tube is warmed to 37°C. A positive test correlates with a cold agglutinin titer of ≥ 1:64, seen with *Mycoplasma pneumoniae* infections.

19. The commercial Monospot test for detection of heterophile antibodies is reactive in what percentage of patients with acute infectious mononucleosis?

Heterophile antibodies, as detected by the Monospot test, are present in approximately 90% of cases at some point in the illness.

20. What are the causes of a false-positive Monospot test?

Serum sickness, lymphoma, and acute hepatitis. One can distinguish false-positives from true-positives with differential adsorptions using guinea pig kidney and beef red cells as follows:

	UNADSORBED	ADSORPTION WITH GUINEA PIG KIDNEY	ADSORPTION WITH BEEF RBCS
Inf. mononucleosis	4+	3+	0
Lymphoma	3+	0	0
Serum sickness	3+	0	0
Hepatitis	3+	0	0
Normal	1+	0	1+

21. What is the differential diagnosis of exudative pharyngitis?

- Groups A, C, and G streptococci
- *Arcanobacterium hemolyticum*
- *Corynebacterium diphtheriae*
- Anaerobic bacteria
- *Yersinia enterocolitica*
- *Mycoplasma pneumoniae*
- Adenovirus, herpes simplex virus, Epstein-Barr virus

22. Patients with multiple myeloma are prone to develop infections due to what types of organisms?

Infections in patients with myeloma demonstrate a biphasic pattern. Infections with *Streptococcus pneumoniae* and *Haemophilus influenzae* occur at the time of initial presentation of myeloma, early in the disease, and during response to chemotherapy. Infections with *Staphylococcus aureus* and gram-negative bacilli (including *Escherichia coli, Pseudomonas aeruginosa, Klebsiella pneumoniae, Enterobacter* sp. and *Serratia marcescens*) cause approximately 80% of infections seen after diagnosis of myeloma and 92% of infectious deaths. These latter infections occur in patients with active and advancing disease and in those responding to chemotherapy in the period in which they are neutropenic.

Savage DG, et al: Biphasic pattern of bacterial infection in multiple myeloma. Ann Intern Med 96:47–50, 1982.

23. When examining a sputum specimen, how can you determine if a specimen originates from the lower respiratory tract and is adequate for culture?

Generally, a sputum is considered adequate when there are < 10 epithelial cells and > 25 polymorphonuclear leukocytes per low-power ($\times$ 100) field.

24. What is the differential diagnosis of trismus ("lockjaw")?

While tetanus is the best-known cause of trismus, other disorders must be considered in a patient with tonic spasm of the masticatory muscles:

- Tetanus
- Inflammatory lesions of the floor of the mouth, cheeks, pharynx, or external auditory canal (peritonsillar or dental abscess, Ludwig's angina, trichinosis)
- Malignancies (sarcoma of the jaw, squamous cell carcinoma of the oral cavity)
- Psychiatric disorders (hysteric tetanus)
- Mechanical problems (temporomaxillary ankylosis, dislocation of the jaw)
- Strychnine poisoning (a late manifestation)
- Phenothiazine drugs (part of a dystonic reaction)
- Encephalitis

25. Describe the different clinical presentations of tetanus in the adult.

Tetanus may present in three clinical forms:

1. **Generalized tetanus**, the most common form of the disease, is characterized by trismus, nuchal rigidity, dysphagia, irritability, and rigidity of the abdominal muscles.

2. **Localized tetanus** is manifested by persistent rigidity of a group of muscles close to the site of injury. It occasionally progresses to generalized tetanus.

3. **Cephalic tetanus** is a severe form of localized tetanus that occurs when the injury is on the head or neck. It usually presents with cranial motor nerve dysfunction (most commonly CN VII) and has a poor prognosis.

Bleck TP: Tetanus: Dealing with the continuing clinical challenge. J Crit Illness 2:41–52, 1987.

26. If a patient with no prior history of tetanus vaccination recovers from an episode of tetanus, is he or she at risk for a second episode?

Yes. The occurrence of tetanus does not prevent second episodes of clinical disease from occurring because the amount of toxin needed to produce the clinical syndrome is so small that it is usually not immunogenic. Hence, persons recovering from tetanus should be vaccinated with tetanus toxoid against future episodes of the disease.

27. What are the different types of clinically important antimicrobial resistance mechanisms displayed by *Staphylococcus aureus*?

1. Plasmid-mediated production of extracellular enzymes (β-lactamases) that act on the β-lactam ring.

2. Chromosomally mediated resistance (methicillin-resistance or intrinsic resistance) that results from production of penicillin-binding proteins with altered affinity for β-lactam antibiotics.

3. Tolerance, defined by a minimal bactericidal concentration to minimal inhibitory concentration (MBC/MIC) ratio > 32, which results from an inability of β-lactam antibiotics to activate autolytic enzymes.

4. Recently, several reports of *S. aureus* strains with intermediate resistance to vancomycin have appeared. These organisms have been called VISA (vancomycin-intermediate *S. aureus*) or

GISA (glycopeptide-intermediate *S. aureus*) strains. The minimal inhibitory concentrations (MICs) for vancomycin are typically in the range of 8–16 µg/ml; the mechanism of resistance has not been delineated, but may involve alterations in the cell wall and capture of antibiotic molecules distant from sites of cell wall synthesis.

28. *Staphylococcus saprophyticus* is most commonly associated with what infectious problem?

Urinary tract infections (UTI), usually in young women. There is a high correlation between genitourinary mucosal colonization with this organism and the subsequent development of UTI. Symptoms and urinalysis findings are indistinguishable from those of infections due to enteric organisms. This bacterium accounts for 20% of UTIs in women 16–35 years old.

29. Discuss the etiologic and epidemiologic associations in the toxic shock syndrome (TSS).

Approximately 70% of cases occur in women < 30-years-old in association with their menstrual period. Approximately 30% of cases are not associated with menses but occur in association with:

IV drug abuse	Nonsurgical traumatic wounds
Homosexuals	Parturition
Staphylococcal sepsis	Staphylococcal pneumonia
Surgical wound infections	

The toxins elaborated by *Staphylococcus aureus* are responsible for the clinical manifestations (TSST-1). There is a strong association between TSS and the recovery of *S. aureus* from vaginal cultures.

Broome CV: Epidemiology of toxic shock syndrome in the United States: Overview. Rev Infect Dis 11:S14–S21, 1989.

30. How is the diagnosis of toxic shock syndrome made?

The diagnosis is a clinical diagnosis based on the presence of certain signs and symptoms:

Definite TSS (all criteria must be present)
1. Temperature ≥ 38.9°C (102°F)
2. Rash (diffuse or palmar erythroderma) with desquamation of palms or soles 1–2 weeks after onset of illness.
3. Hypotension—manifested by one of the following:
   a. Systolic BP < 90 mmHg
   b. Orthostatic decrease in systolic BP > 15 mmHg
   c. Orthostatic dizziness or syncope
4. Clinical or laboratory abnormalities in three or more organ systems:
   a. Mucous membrane   e. Renal
   b. GI   f. Muscular
   c. Hepatic   g. Cardiovascular
   d. CNS

Probable TSS (at least 3 criteria with desquamation or at least 5 criteria without desquamation)
1. Temperature ≥ 38.9°C (102°F)
2. Diffuse or palmar erythroderma (rash)
3. Hypotension, orthostatic dizziness, or syncope
4. Myalgia
5. Vomiting, diarrhea, or both
6. Mucous membrane inflammation (conjunctivitis, pharyngitis, or vaginitis)
7. Clinical or laboratory abnormalities in two or more organ systems
8. Reasonable evidence for the absence of other causes of illness

Tofte RW, et al: Toxic shock syndrome in the United States: Evidence of a broad clinical spectrum. JAMA 246:2163–2167, 1981.

31. What is the significance of bacteremia or endocarditis due to *Streptococcus bovis*?

A strong association exists between lesions of the GI tract, particularly bowel carcinoma, and *S. bovis* bacteremia or endocarditis. Patients in whom this organism is identified should have a thorough evaluation of the GI tract.

32. How often is a current or past history of diarrhea evident in patients with amebic liver abscess?

Approximately one-third of patients with amebic liver abscess have a history of past or present diarrhea. The major presenting manifestations are those referable to the abscess itself or its extension and rupture into adjacent structures. *Entamoeba histolytica* is found in the stool in less than one-third of patients with an abscess.

33. Which part of the liver is most commonly involved with amebic liver abscess?

Amebic liver abscesses are most commonly single lesions involving the right superior or superior-posterior aspect of the liver.

34. Primary amebic meningoencephalitis due to *Naegleria fowleri* occurs predominantly in what epidemiologic setting?

Children or young adults who have been swimming, diving or water-skiing in small freshwater lakes, usually in the southern United States. The organism is associated with freshwater having heavy growths of algae and bacteria, probably resulting from high concentrations of sewage components in the water.

35. Why should aminoglycoside antibiotics be given with careful monitoring to patients with neuromuscular diseases such as myasthenia gravis?

Aminoglycoside antibiotics demonstrate neuromuscular blockade properties by inhibiting presynaptic release of acetylcholine and blocking postsynaptic receptors for acetylcholine. Patients with myasthenia gravis have shown increased sensitivity to the paralytic effects of these agents, as have patients simultaneously receiving other neuromuscular blockading agents (e.g., succinylcholine, D-tubocurare). The paralytic effects can be overcome with anticholinesterases and calcium.

Snavely SR, et al: The neurotoxicity of antibacterial agents. Ann Intern Med 101:92–104, 1984.

36. How can acute paralytic polio and Guillain-Barré syndrome be differentiated clinically?

	POLIO	GUILLAIN-BARRÉ
Fever	+	−
Acute illness	+	−
Signs of meningeal infection	+	−
Symmetrical paralysis	−	−
Motor loss	+	+
Sensory loss	Rare	80%
Pattern of progression of paralysis	No pattern	Ascending
Duration of progression of paralysis	3–4 days	Up to 2 weeks in stages

37. Name five different disease manifestations in humans secondary to the dimorphic fungus *Histoplasma capsulatum*.

1. Acute pulmonary histoplasmosis
2. Disseminated histoplasmosis
3. Mediastinal granuloma or fibrosis
4. Chronic cavitary pulmonary histoplasmosis
5. Histoplasmoma

38. Why does herpes simplex recur in small areas but varicella-zoster recurs in a dermatomal region?

Both herpes simplex (HSV) and varicella-zoster viruses (VZV) cause latent infections in human sensory nerve ganglia. However, the cells that are latently infected are different. HSV causes a latent infection of individual neuronal cells. With reactivation, infection does not spread well from cell to cell but does spread easily to the skin. Hence, only a small area of skin is involved during reactivation.

VZV, on the other hand, causes a latent infection in the satellite cells, and during reactivation, the infection readily spreads throughout the sensory ganglia. The virus then spreads to all areas of the sensory dermatome.

Croen KD, et al: Patterns of gene expression and sites of latency in human nerve ganglia are different for varicella-zoster and herpes simplex viruses. Proc Natl Acad Sci USA 85:9773–9777, 1988.

39. What sexually transmitted diseases commonly cause genital ulceration with regional adenopathy?

Syphilis   Genital herpes
Chancroid   Lymphogranuloma venereum
Granuloma inguinale (donovanosis)

Krockta WP, Barnes RC: Genital ulceration with regional adenopathy. Infect Dis Clin North Am 1:217–233, 1987.

40. What is hydrophobia? Why is it significant?

Patients with rabies encephalitis often have violent, jerky contractions of the diaphragm and accessory muscles of inspiration that are triggered by attempts to swallow liquids or other stimuli. Hydrophobia is pathognomonic of rabies.

41. What animal vectors are involved in human rabies?

Dogs account for > 90% of reported human cases of rabies in areas of the world where domestic rabies is not well controlled. Other domestic animals contribute 5–10% worldwide; these include cats, cattle, horses, sheep, and pigs. In the U.S., the principal vectors are wild mammals, including the striped skunk, raccoon, foxes, and insectivorous bats. Small rodents, birds, and reptiles are not known to be reservoirs of rabies.

Rupprecht CE: The ascension of wildlife rabies: A cause for public health concern or intervention? Emerging Infect Dis 1:107–114, 1995.

42. In which STD does the "groove sign" appear?

The "groove sign" is the occurrence of adenopathy above and below the inguinal ligament. Though it has been said to be pathognomonic of lymphogranuloma venereum, it is seen in only 15% or less of cases and also occurs in other infectious and neoplastic conditions.

Krockta WP, Barnes RC: Genital ulceration with regional adenopathy. Infect Dis Clin North Am 1:217–233, 1987.

43. How often does perinatal transmission of hepatitis B occur in offspring of women who are chronically hepatitis B surface antigen (HBsAg)-positive?

Women who are HBsAg-positive and hepatitis B e antigen (HBeAg)-positive transmit the virus to their offspring 50–70% of the time, whereas those who are HBsAg-positive but HBeAg-negative transmit it approximately 10% of the time. Neonates who acquire hepatitis B in the perinatal period tend to become chronic carriers and are at significantly increased risk for cirrhosis and hepatocellular carcinoma. These complications are potentially preventable with passive and active immunization of the infant.

44. What criteria are suggestive of UTI on the microscopic examination of a clean-catch urine specimen?

TYPE OF URINE	METHOD OF OBSERVATION	FINDING	INDICATION
Uncentrifuged	Hemocytometer	$\leq 10^3$ WBC/ml	Normal
		$> 10^4$ WBC/ml	Infection
	Low-power magnification (10 × objective)	> 2–3 WBC/field	Correlates with >10^4 WBC/ml

(*Table continued on next page.*)

TYPE OF URINE	METHOD OF OBSERVATION	FINDING	INDICATION
	High-power magnification (45 × objective)	1–2 WBC/field Bacteria WBC cast	≥ 10^5 WBC/ml ≥ 10^5 bacteria/ml Suggests renal involvement (pyelonephritis)
Uncentrifuged or centrifuged	High-power magnification	WBC cast RBC cast	(Same as above) Indicates glomerulonephritis

From Musher DM: Urinary tract infection. In Dupont H, Pickering L (eds.): Infectious Diseases Handbook. Menlo Park, CA. Addison-Wesley, 1986, p 450; with permission.

45. Which organisms are likely to cause a chronic UTI with urinary pH ≥ 7.5?

Urinary pH is elevated in chronic UTIs caused by organisms that are urease-producers. *Proteus* sp. are the most common organisms that cause this clinical presentation. Others include *Corynebacterium urealyticum, Staphylococcus saprophyticus, Ureaplasma urealyticum*, and *Providencia* sp. *Klebsiella* and *Serratia* sp. are rare causes.

O'Leary JJ, et al: The importance of urinalysis in infectious diseases. Hosp Physician 27:25–30, 1991.

46. Linear calcifications seen in the wall of the urinary bladder on a roentgenogram are indicative of what chronic infection?

Schistosoma haematobium infection may result in bladder wall calcifications due to the deposition of eggs in the submucosa and mucosa of the bladder. The consequent inflammatory response leads to scarring and calcium deposition.

47. Which antibiotics can be found in cyst fluid in patients with polycystic kidney disease?

Trimethoprim-sulfamethoxazole and chloramphenicol occur in significant concentrations in cyst fluid. Patients with polycystic disease and UTI may fail to improve with other antibiotics. Surgical aspiration or drainage of infected cysts may be necessary.

48. What factors are necessary for methenamine to function effectively as a urinary tract antiseptic?

Methenamine itself is not bactericidal but depends on hydrolysis, at an acid pH, to liberate ammonia and formaldehyde by the following reaction:

$$N_4(CH_2)_6 + 6H_2O \rightarrow 4NH_4^+ + 6HCHO$$

Formaldehyde is the bactericidal agent. For this reaction to work optimally, the urine pH needs to be < 7.0, and the hydrolysis needs sufficient time to occur, usually hours. Consequently, the drug is ineffective in patients with indwelling bladder catheters.

49. Which organism appears as delicate, weakly gram-positive, beaded filaments that also are acid-fast if 1% sulfuric acid is used to decolorize instead of acid-alcohol?

Nocardia species (e.g., *Nocardia asteroides*).

McNeil MM: The medically important aerobic actinomycetes: Epidemiology and microbiology. Clin Microbiol Rev 7:359–379, 1994.

50. What are the most common etiologic agents in the acute sinusitis syndrome?

Microbial Etiology of Acute Community-Acquired Antral Sinusitis

MICROBIAL AGENT	ADULTS (%)	CHILDREN (%)
Bacteria		
S. pneumoniae	31 (20–35)	36
H. influenzae (unencapsulated)	21 (6–26)	23
Mixed *S. pneumoniae* and *H. influenzae*	5 (1–9)	–

(*Table continued on next page.*)

Microbial Etiology of Acute Community-Acquired Antral Sinusitis (cont.)

MICROBIAL AGENT	ADULTS (%)	CHILDREN (%)
Bacteria (cont.)		
Anaerobic bacteria (*Bacteroides,*	6 (0–10)	–
Peptostreptococcus, Fusobacterium, etc.)		
S. aureus	4 (0–8)	–
S. pyogenes	2 (1–3)	2
M. catarrhalis	2	19
Gram-negative bacteria	0 (0–24)	2
Viruses		
Rhinovirus	15	–
Influenza virus	5	–
Parainfluenza virus	3	2
Adenovirus	–	2

Hamory BH: Etiology and antimicrobial therapy of acute maxillary sinusitis. J Infect Dis 139:197–202, 1979.

51. What percentage of patients with pneumococcal pneumonia also have bacteremia?
25–30%.

52. What are the radiographic changes associated with osteomyelitis?
1. Deep soft tissue swelling and obliteration of muscle planes (usually the earliest radiographic changes seen)
2. Periosteal reaction
3. Cortical irregularity
4. Rarefaction of bone
5. Sequestrum (devitalized area of bone following loss of vascular supply)
6. Involucrum (periosteal new bone formation in response to infection)

53. Which bacterial species usually causes osteomyelitis in patients with sickle cell disease?
Approximately 80% of cases of osteomyelitis complicating sickle cell disease are due to *Salmonella* species.

54. How reliable are sinus tract cultures for determining the etiologic agent of chronic osteomyelitis?
The likelihood that a sinus-tract isolate corresponds with an operative isolate is high if *Staphylococcus aureus* is the organism isolated from a sinus tract culture (78%); however, only 44% of sinus tract cultures from patients with biopsy-proven *S. aureus* osteomyelitis will yield this organism. The predictive values for the *Enterobacteriaceae, Pseudomonas aeruginosa*, and mixed cultures of *Streptococcus* species isolated from sinus tracts are < 50%, and only a small number of cultures from sinus tracts of patients with chronic osteomyelitis caused by these organisms will yield the causative pathogen.
Mackowiak PA, Jones SR, Smith JW: Diagnostic value of sinus tract cultures in chronic osteomyelitis. JAMA 239:2772–2775, 1978.

55. In a young, healthy patient who presents with *Pseudomonas aeruginosa* osteomyelitis of the calcaneus bone, what is the most likely cause of this disorder?
A puncture wound to the foot. Almost 90% of cases of osteomyelitis that result from puncture wounds to the feet are due to *P. aeruginosa*; the remaining 10% are due to various other gram-negative organisms, staphylococci, streptococci, and atypical mycobacteria.
Riley HD: Puncture wounds of the foot: Their importance and potential for complications. J Okla State Med Assoc 77:3–6, 1984.

56. Bacterial endophthalmitis secondary to penetrating trauma to the eye is associated with which pathogens?

S. epidermidis, *S. aureus*, streptococci	60%
Bacillus sp.	25%
Gram-negative rods	10%
Fungi	5%

Bacillus cereus causes a particularly fulminant form of the disease, with enucleation not uncommon. Given all the episodes of trauma that occur to the eye, secondary infection is relatively uncommon.

Davey RT Jr, et al: Post-traumatic endophthalmitis: The emerging role of *Bacillus cereus* infection. Rev Infect Dis 9:110–123, 1987.

57. Acute gastric anisakiasis results from what dietary habit?

Eating raw or smoked fish, most commonly mackerel. Symptoms consist of the acute onset of severe epigastric pain, nausea, and vomiting within 12 hours of ingestion. Treatment involves the endoscopic removal of the larvae.

Sugimachi K, et al: Acute gastric anisakiasis: Analysis of 178 cases. Arch Intern Med 253:1012–1013, 1985.

58. What is the most common cause of nonepidemic viral encephalitis in the U.S.?

Herpes simplex type 1, which causes a focal encephalitis.

59. Who should receive prophylaxis after exposure to persons with *Neisseria meningitidis* meningitis?

1. Household contacts

2. Individuals in closed populations, such as military barracks, nursery schools, college dormitories, and chronic care hospitals

3. Hospital personnel who have intimate exposure to infected patients (but not other personnel without such exposure)

60. Define fever of undetermined origin (FUO).

The classic definition of FUO as defined by Petersdorf and Beeson is:

1. Illness of > 3 weeks' duration: This eliminates any acute, self-limited illnesses.

2. Documented fever > 101°F or 38.3°C on several occasions

3. Uncertain diagnosis after 1 week in the hospital to allow completion of routine laboratory examinations

Petersdorf RG, Beeson PB: Fever of unexplained origin: Report of 100 cases. Medicine 40:1–29, 1961.

61. What are the major causes of FUO?

Causes of Fever of Undetermined Origin

I. Infection	II. Cancer
A. Generalized	A. Hematologic
1. Tuberculosis	1. Lymphoma
2. Histoplasmosis	2. Hodgkin's disease
3. Typhoid fever	3. Acute leukemia
4. Cytomegalovirus	B. Tumors with propensity to cause fever
5. Epstein-Barr virus	1. Hepatoma
6. Miscellaneous:	2. Renal cell carcinoma
a. Syphilis	3. Atrial myxoma
b. Brucellosis	
c. Malaria	III. Rheumatologic disorders
B. Localized	1. Rheumatoid arthritis
1. Infective endocarditis	2. Systemic lupus erythematosus
2. Empyema	3. Vasculitis

(*Table continued on next page.*)

Causes of Fever of Undetermined Origin (cont.)

B. Localized (cont.) 　3. Intra-abdominal infection 　　a. Peritonitis 　　b. Cholangitis 　　c. Abscess 　4. Urinary tract 　　a. Pyelonephritis 　　b. Perinephric abscess 　　c. Prostatitis 　5. Decubitus ulcer 　6. Osteomyelitis 　7. Thrombophlebitis	IV. Miscellaneous 　1. Drug-induced 　2. Immune complex (SLE, RA) 　3. Vasculitis 　4. Alcoholic hepatitis 　5. Granulomatous hepatitis 　6. Inflammatory bowel disease, 　　Whipple's disease 　7. Recurrent pulmonary emboli 　8. Factitious fever 　9. Undiagnosed

From Larson EB, et al: Fever of undetermined origin: Diagnosis and follow-up of 105 cases, 1970–1980. Medicine 61:269–292, 1982; with permission.

62. What types of reactions to penicillin may be predicted by skin testing prior to antibiotic use?

Skin testing is predictive of IgE-mediated reactions. Such reactions, including accelerated urticaria or anaphylaxis, occur with varying frequency depending on the skin test result. Among patients with a positive skin test, the frequency of these reactions varies from 10% in those without a previous history of penicillin allergy to 50–70% in those with a past history of penicillin allergy. In patients with a negative skin test, accelerated urticaria occurs in only 1% and anaphylaxis does not occur.

Skin test reactivity is not predictive of other types of reactions, such as serum sickness, maculopapular rash, exfoliative dermatitis, hemolytic anemia, or interstitial nephritis.

Sogn DD, et al: Results of the NIAID collaborative clinical trial to test the predictive value of skin testing with major and minor penicillin derivatives in hospitalized adults. Arch Intern Med 152:1025–1032, 1992.

63. What chest roentgenogram findings are very suggestive of thoracic actinomycosis?

1. Lesions extending through the chest wall
2. Involvement of adjacent lobes by transgression through an interlobar fissure
3. Periostitis or destruction of bones such as ribs or sternum adjacent to a pulmonary process
4. Vertebral destruction, with disc space sparing, due to extension from mediastinal or thoracic involvement.

64. Name a parasitic disease that mimics pulmonary tuberculosis (TB). How is it diagnosed?

The trematode lung fluke *Paragonimus westermani* can cause a pulmonary syndrome consistent with pulmonary TB. Chronic bronchitis, bronchiectasis, lung abscess, and pleural effusion are other clinical syndromes related to paragonimiasis. Examination of the sputum may show the characteristic operculated eggs.

Harinasuta T, et al: Trematode infections: Opisthorchiasis, clonorchiasis, fascioliasis, and paragonimiasis. Infect Dis Clin North Am 7:699–716, 1993.

65. What is a Simon focus?

During primary infection with *Mycobacterium tuberculosis*, apical and subapical pulmonary foci may undergo necrosis when delayed hypersensitivity develops. These foci then develop tiny calcific deposits, within which latent but viable mycobacteria persist. These foci can later reactivate.

66. What is Pott's disease?

Spinal tuberculosis. Percival Pott, an English surgeon, in 1779 first wrote the classic description of the disease that bears his name.

67. What are the clinical features of genitourinary tuberculosis?

Sterile pyuria	50%
Painless hematuria	40%
Fever	10%
Perinephric abscess	10%
Positive sputum culture	20–40%
Positive urine culture	80%

Christensen WI: Genitourinary tuberculosis: Review of 102 cases. Medicine 53:377–390, 1974.

68. What is Poncet's disease?

A polyarticular arthritis that occurs during active TB in which no infectious or other cause of the arthritis can be demonstrated. *Mycobacterium tuberculosis* cannot be isolated from the affected joint spaces. The disorder is felt to have an immunologic basis.

Dall L, et al: Poncet's disease: Tuberculous rheumatism. Rev Infect Dis 11:105–107, 1989.

69. Name the most important prognostic factor in tuberculous meningitis.

The patient's neurologic exam at clinical presentation appears to indicate the outcome. Patients who are stuporous or hemiplegic have a mortality rate around 80%, while patients with only meningismus and fever have a mortality rate around 5–9%. Patients with a more severe neurologic deficit should probably receive steroids.

Ogawa SK, et al: Tuberculous meningitis in an urban medical center. Medicine 66:317–326, 1982.

70. What is the differential diagnosis of eosinophilic meningitis?

- CNS infection caused by parasites (*Toxoplasma gondii, Trypanosoma* sp., *Trichinella spiralis, Toxocara canis, Toxocara cati, Taenia solium, Fasciola hepatica, Paragonimus westermani, Angiostrongylus cantonensis, Gnathostoma spinigerum*)
- *Mycobacterium tuberculosis*
- Fungi (*Coccidioides immitis, Histoplasma capsulatum*)
- Viruses (lymphocytic choriomeningitis virus)
- Rickettsiae
- Neoplasia (leukemia, lymphoma, meningeal tumors)
- Multiple sclerosis
- Hypereosinophilic syndrome
- Collagen vascular disease
- Allergic reaction to foreign body or direct instillation of drugs or contrast agent into the CSF
- Drug allergy (e.g., ibuprofen, ciprofloxacin)

Asperilla MO, et al: Eosinophilic meningitis associated with ciprofloxacin. Am J Med 87:589–590, 1989.

71. How many patients with tuberculous meningitis will have a positive PPD skin test?

The purified protein derivative PPD skin test is positive in 50–95% of patients with TB meningitis. Stated another way, the PPD is negative in up to 50% of patients with TB meningitis.

Ogawa SK, et al: Tuberculous meningitis in an urban medical center. Medicine 66:317–326, 1987.

72. Most cases of Rocky Mountain spotted fever (RMSF) occur in what region of the United States?

The south Atlantic states. Despite its name, few cases of RMSF occur in the Rocky Mountain states.

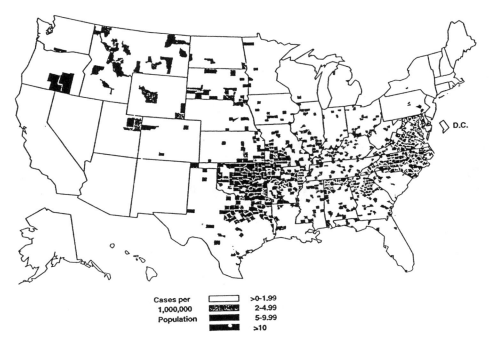

Cases per / 1,000,000 / Population
>0-1.99
2-4.99
5-9.99
>10

From Dalton MJ, et al: National surveillance for Rocky Mountain spotted fever, 1981–1992: Epidemiologic summary and evaluation of risk factors for fatal outcome. Am J Trop Med Hyg 52:405–413, 1995; with permission.

73. What are the major pulmonary syndromes associated with *Aspergillus* sp.? How are they treated?

1. **Allergic bronchopulmonary aspergillosis** (ABPA) occurs in patients with asthma who have eosinophilia, transient pulmonary infiltrates thought to be due to bronchial plugging, and elevated total serum IgE and IgG antibody to Aspergillus. Corticosteroids have been used to treat this disorder, although anecdotal reports suggest itraconazole may have a role.

2. **Aspergilloma** (fungus ball) results from colonization and growth of Aspergillus, usually within a preexisting pulmonary cavity. No specific treatment is usually given unless significant hemoptysis occurs, in which case surgical excision is performed.

3. **Invasive aspergillosis** usually occurs in individuals with profound granulocytopenia and is also being described more frequently in individuals with AIDS. Amphotericin B or one of the newer liposomal preparations, with or without surgical excision, is the therapy of choice.

4. **Chronic necrotizing aspergillosis** is a slowly progressive form of invasive aspergillosis that occurs in patients who have some underlying pulmonary disease (chronic obstructive pulmonary disease, sarcoidosis, pneumoconiosis, or inactive TB) or mild systemic immunocompromising illness (low-dose corticosteroids, diabetes mellitus, alcoholism). Patients have a chronic infiltrate that may slowly progress to cavitation or aspergilloma formation.

Latgé J-P: *Aspergillus fumigatus* and aspergillosis. Clin Microbiol Rev 12:310–350, 1999.

74. What is the Fitz-Hugh-Curtis syndrome? What organisms cause it?

The Fitz-Hugh-Curtis syndrome is a perihepatitis usually caused by either *Neisseria gonorrhoeae* or *Chlamydia trachomatis*. It is thought to occur by spread of organisms from the fallopian tubes to the surface of the liver. This should be considered one of the causes of right-upper-quadrant pain in young, sexually active persons. It occasionally has been reported in males, probably as a result of bacteremic spread.

75. Are fever patterns helpful in establishing the cause of fever?

There have been multiple classifications of fever patterns. For the most part, the pattern of fever is not helpful in establishing its cause. Two exceptions are fever secondary to cyclic neutropenia and fever secondary to malaria. Patients with cyclic neutropenia have fevers every 3 weeks, coincident with their neutropenia. Patients with malaria may have paroxysms of fever every 2 or 3 days, depending on the infecting parasite.

76. Which organisms most commonly cause infectious complications after a human bite?

Streptococci (alpha and group A β-hemolytic), *Staphylococcus aureus*, *Eikenella corrodens*, *Peptostreptococcus* sp., *Bacteroides* sp., and *Fusobacterium* sp. are the most common organisms cultured from human bite wounds.

Goldstein EJC: Bite wounds and infection. Clin Infect Dis 14:633–640, 1992.

77. Which other organisms should be considered after dog or cat bites?

Pasteurella multocida and *Capnocytophaga canimorsus* (DF-2). Several other pathogens have been transmitted after bites by these animals, including rabies, tularemia (cats), brucellosis (dogs), EF-4 (dogs), and blastomycosis (dogs).

Goldstein EJC: Bite wounds and infection. Clin Infect Dis 14:633–640, 1992.

78. What is the Jarisch-Herxheimer reaction?

It is a self-limited systemic reaction that occurs within 1–2 hours after the initial treatment of syphilis with antimicrobial agents. It is particularly common in patients treated for secondary syphilis but can occur when any stage is treated. The reaction consists of the abrupt onset of chills, fever, myalgias, tachycardia, hyperventilation, vasodilatation with associated flushing, and mild hypotension. It is probably due to the release of pyrogens from the spirochetes.

79. Which agents should be considered in the differential diagnosis of necrotizing pneumonia?

Staphylococcus aureus, aerobic gram-negative bacilli (excluding *Haemophilus influenzae*), and anaerobes. *Aspergillus* sp. and *Mycobacterium tuberculosis* may also cause this clinical picture.

80. What is typhlitis?

Typhlitis, also known as necrotizing enterocolitis or neutropenic enterocolitis, is a fulminate, necrotizing process that occurs in the GI tract of individuals with profound neutropenia. The disease is manifested by fever, abdominal pain and distention, rebound tenderness in the right lower quadrant, and diarrhea. Involvement of the cecum and terminal ileum is characteristic.

81. What is Blackwater fever?

Blackwater fever refers to the dark-colored urine associated with the clinical syndrome of acute and massive hemolysis seen during *Plasmodium falciparum* malaria. It may be etiologically related to the therapeutic use of quinine.

82. Which species of malaria is associated with the occurrence of febrile paroxysms every 72 hours?

Plasmodium malariae. The other species of malaria that infect humans—*P. vivax*, *P. ovale*, and *P. falciparum*—have 48-hour erythrocyte cycles and, therefore, a 48-hour fever pattern.

Hoffman SL: Diagnosis, treatment and prevention of malaria. Med Clin North Am 76:1327–1355, 1992.

83. Which species of malaria have exoerythrocytic stages from which late relapses may occur if treatment is not adequate?

Plasmodium vivax and *P. ovale* have exoerythrocytic stages in the liver. Relapse may occur months to years later.

Zucker JR, et al: Malaria: Principles of prevention and treatment. Infect Dis Clin North Am 7:546–567, 1993.

84. What causes "swimmer's itch"?

Schistosoma cercariae. Migratory birds, particularly ducks, harbor the adult worms and deposit the organism in freshwater, where snails become infected. Cercariae break out of the snails and penetrate the skin of warm-blooded animals. The cercariae are walled off and destroyed in the skin, which evokes an acute inflammatory response that results in the associated pruritus.

85. Where are Osler's nodes found? In what conditions are they seen?

Osler's nodes are small, painful, nodular lesions (2–15 mm in size) that usually appear in the pads of the fingers or toes. They may be seen in association with infective endocarditis (subacute), gonococcal infections, marantic endocarditis, hemolytic anemia, systemic lupus erythematosus, and intra-arterial catheters (distal to the cannulation site).

86. What organism is associated with the consumption of water chestnuts?

The intestinal fluke *Fasciolopsis buski*, which is endemic in the Far East and Southeast Asia. Infection occurs in individuals who ingest water chestnuts on which the metacercariae have encysted.

87. Extrusion of "sulfur granules" from a draining wound is characteristic of which infection?

Infections with *Actinomyces* sp. characteristically form external sinuses, which discharge "sulfur granules." These consist of conglomerate masses of branching filaments of the organism cemented together and mineralized by host calcium phosphate stimulated by tissue inflammation. They do not contain sulfur.

88. What is the causative agent of Whipple's disease?

Tropheryma whippelii, a gram-positive actinomycete that is not closely related to any other known bacterial genus. Whipple's disease is a multisystemic disorder characterized by migratory polyarthritis, diarrhea, malabsorption, weight loss, generalized lymphadenopathy, hyperpigmentation, and occasional neurologic abnormalities.

Relman DA, et al: Identification of the uncultured bacillus of Whipple's disease. N Engl J Med 327:293–301, 1992.

89. How often is the Gram stain likely to be positive in patients with bacterial meningitis?

The Gram stain of the CSF in patients with bacterial meningitis demonstrates the etiologic agent in most cases. The following table demonstrates the sensitivity of the Gram stain for each pathogen:

ORGANISM	POSITIVE (%)
Neisseria meningitidis	66%
Streptococcus pneumoniae	83%
Haemophilus influenzae	76%
Listeria monocytogenes	42%

90. Rhinocerebral mucormycosis occurs most commonly in what setting?

Rhinocerebral mucormycosis occurs almost exclusively in patients with diabetes mellitus, particularly when poorly controlled or with ketoacidosis. Occasional cases have been described in patients with hematologic neoplasms or renal insufficiency and in infants with severe diarrhea. The disease is characterized by black, necrotic lesions of the palate or nasal mucous membranes that rapidly involve the paranasal sinuses with extension into the brain. The organism has a particular predisposition to invade vascular structures.

Sugar AM: Mucormycosis. Clin Infect Dis 14(suppl):S126–S129, 1992.

91. The intermediate stage of which tapeworm causes the clinical syndrome of cysticercosis?

Cysticercus cellulosae is the intermediate stage of *Taenia solium*, the pork tapeworm, and causes the clinical syndrome of cysticercosis.

92. Why are anti-streptolysin O (ASO) antibodies of little help in the diagnosis of cutaneous infections by *Streptococcus pyogenes*?

The ASO response after skin infections is weak, probably because of inactivation of streptolysin O by skin lipids. Antibody responses to DNase B are brisk, as is the response to hyaluronidase. Antibodies to the latter two substances can be helpful in the serodiagnosis of streptococcal skin infections.

93. What is the most common cause of secondary pneumonia following illness due to influenza?

Streptococcus pneumoniae most commonly causes pneumonia after influenza virus infection. However, the incidence of pneumonia caused by *Staphylococcus aureus* is also increased, and so this agent must also be considered when treating a patient with this clinical syndrome.

94. What are the symptoms of scombroid fish poisoning? What causes it?

Scombroid, or histamine fish poisoning, is characterized by symptoms of a histamine reaction: flushing, headache, nausea, vomiting, abdominal cramps, diarrhea, and dizziness. It is thought to be due to histamine formed in the fish meat, in addition to the presence of substances that inhibit the degradation of histamine.

Mines D, et al: Poisonings: Food, fish, shellfish. Emerg Med Clin North Am 5:157–177, 1997.

95. What are the symptoms of ciguatera fish poisoning? What causes it?

Ciguatera fish poisoning is characterized by the onset of nausea, vomiting, diarrhea, abdominal cramps, and numbness or paresthesias of the structures of the oropharynx 1–6 hours following the ingestion of "poisoned" fish. Other symptoms may also be present, including shooting pains in the legs and pain in the teeth. It is caused by accumulation of ciguatoxin in the fish from the food chain. The source of the toxin in the food chain is a dinoflagellate (*Gambierdiscus toxicus*). The illness may last for days to months.

Underman AE, et al: Fish and shellfish poisoning. Curr Clin Top Infect Dis 13:203–225, 1993.

96. What diseases are associated with consumption of contaminated fish and shellfish?

Several viral, bacterial, and parasitic infections can result from ingestion of contaminated fish and shellfish. They include:

Hepatitis A	Norwalk virus gastroenteritis
Vibrio cholerae 0 group 1	*Vibrio cholerae* non-01
Vibrio parahaemolyticus	*Vibrio vulnificus*
Clostridium botulinum	*Giardia lamblia*
Diphyllobothriasis	Anisakiasis

In addition, disease due to seafood toxin consumption can occur:

Ciguatera poisoning	Paralytic shellfish poisoning due to *Gonyaulax* species
Scombroid poisoning	of dinoflagellates
Tetrodotoxication due to	Neurotoxic shellfish poisoning due to the toxic
eating puffer fish, *Fugu*	dinoflagellate, *Ptychodiscus brevis*

Eastaugh J, Shepherd S: Infectious and toxic syndromes from fish and shellfish consumption. A review. Arch Intern Med 149:1735–1740, 1989.

97. What is the significance of infection due to *Escherichia coli* O157:H7?

E. coli O157:H7 has emerged as a major cause of both sporadic cases and outbreaks of diarrheal disease in North America. Most outbreaks have been associated with the consumption of beef, most commonly undercooked ground beef. Other outbreaks have been associated with fecally contaminated drinking water supplies. It can cause either bloody or nonbloody diarrhea.

In addition, *E. coli* O157:H7 is responsible for most cases of hemolytic-uremic syndrome, a major cause of acute renal failure in children.

Boyce TG, et al: *Escherichia coli* O157:H7 and the hemolytic-uremic syndrome. N Engl J Med 333:364–368, 1995.

98. Which group of patients develops keratitis due to *Acanthamoeba*?

Acanthamoeba spp. cause a severe and difficult-to-treat keratitis in individuals who wear soft contact lenses. The incidence is much higher in those individuals who prepare their own saline solutions and also in persons who wear their lenses while swimming in lakes and swimming pools.

99. What causes acute hemorrhagic conjunctivitis?

Enterovirus 70 and coxsackie virus A24. It is characterized by ocular pain, swelling of the eyelids, and subconjunctival hemorrhage. The incubation period is 1 day, and the duration of illness is approximately 1 week. These facts distinguish it from adenovirus infection (epidemic keratoconjunctivitis), which has an incubation of 5–7 days and may have symptoms present for 2–3 weeks.

Syed NA, et al: Infectious conjunctivitis. Infect Dis Clin North Am 6:789–805, 1992.

100. What is the "hyperinfection" syndrome associated with *Strongyloides stercoralis*?

Hyperinfection syndrome due to *S. stercoralis* is the result of systemic dissemination by the filariform larval stage of the organism. This usually occurs in individuals who are immunocompromised, primarily due to defects in cell-mediated immunity. Patients present with abdominal pain, diarrhea, vomiting, shock, fever, cough, and decreased mental status. Bacteremia is a frequent accompanying event, usually with enteric organisms that are thought to accompany the larvae as they migrate through the bowel wall.

101. What is hepatitis C? Hepatitis E? Hepatitis G?

Hepatitis C and E are two of the non-A, non-B hepatitis viruses. **Hepatitis C** is due to an RNA virus and is spread in a manner similar to the hepatitis B virus (by the parenteral route). It is probably the major cause of transfusion-associated hepatitis.

Hepatitis E is also due to an RNA virus, but it is spread in a manner more like the hepatitis A virus (by the fecal-oral route). It is a significant cause of epidemic hepatitis in Asia and Africa and its severity is increased in pregnant women.

Hepatitis G is an RNA virus of global distribution that is transmitted parenterally. It causes a very mild acute hepatitis, rarely resulting in jaundice. Chronic hepatitis does occur.

Martin P, Friedman LS (eds): Viral hepatitis. Gastroenterol Clin North Am 23(3), 1994 (entire issue).

102. When does the window period occur during hepatitis B infection?

The window period occurs during acute infection when the patient no longer has detectable hepatitis B surface antigen (HBsAg). However, the patient will have antibody to the core antigen (anti-HBc) and should develop anti-HBsAg in the following month.

103. What preexisting or concurrent condition is necessary for the delta agent to cause infection in humans?

The delta agent is a defective RNA virus and is the causative agent of hepatitis D. It requires the presence of HBsAg for infection to occur, so it is seen as a coinfection with acute hepatitis B infection or as a superinfection in a chronic carrier of hepatitis B. It is generally spread by the parenteral route in the U.S., but other modes of spread seem to occur in other parts of the world.

Rizzetto M, et al: Delta hepatitis—present status. J Hepatol 1:187–193, 1985.

104. Which infection occurs in nursery workers who handle sphagnum moss?

Outbreaks of lymphocutaneous infection due to *Sporothrix schenckii* have occurred in nursery and forestry workers who handle seedlings packed in sphagnum moss. Disease has also been associated with contaminated hay, timbers, and thorny bushes, such as roses.

Coles FB, et al: A multistate outbreak of sporotrichosis associated with sphagnum moss. Am J Epidemiol 136:475–487, 1992.

105. What are the infectious causes of parotitis?

Acute Viral Parotitis	Acute Suppurative Parotitis
Mumps virus	*Staphylococcus aureus*
Influenza	*Streptococcus pneumoniae*
Parainfluenza types 1 and 3	Enteric gram-negative bacilli
Coxsackievirus A and B	*Haemophilus influenzae*
ECHO virus	*Actinomyces* sp.
Lymphocytic choriomeningitis	*Mycobacterium tuberculosis*
Anaerobic organisms	*Salmonella typhi*

106. What are the most common causes of infection in the first month following solid organ transplantation?

Infections in the first month following solid organ transplantation generally are not secondary to immunosuppression; they are the infections seen in most postoperative patients:

Pneumonia due to gram-negative bacilli, *Staphylococcus aureus*, or aspiration

Bacteremia (catheter-related)

Wound infections

Herpes simplex infections (usually reactivation)

Preexisting infections (e.g., strongyloidiasis, tuberculosis, or systemic mycoses)

107. What are the most common pathogens seen in months 2–6 following solid organ transplantation?

They are more typical of the pathogens seen in immunocompromised hosts:

Viruses	Others
Cytomegalovirus	Aspergillus
Epstein-Barr virus	Nocardia
Varicella-zoster virus	Toxoplasma
Papovavirus (BK and JC)	Cryptococcus
Adenovirus	*Pneumocystis carinii*
Herpes simplex virus	Legionella
Non-A, non-B hepatitis	*Listeria monocytogenes*

108. Which infectious diseases have been reported to be transmitted by blood transfusion?

The most common transmissible pathogens are viruses, but others have been implicated.

- Hepatitis A, hepatitis B, hepatitis D
- HIV-1, HIV-2, HTLV-1
- Syphilis
- Toxoplasmosis
- *Yersinia enterocolitica*
- Non-A, non-B hepatitis (including hepatitis C and G)
- Cytomegalovirus, Epstein-Barr virus
- Babesiosis
- Malaria
- American trypanosomiasis (Chagas' disease)

Berkman SA: Infectious complications of blood transfusion. Blood Rev 2:206–210, 1988.

109. What is a chagoma?

A chagoma (from Chagas) is the lesion caused by replication of *Trypanosoma cruzi* at the site of inoculation, i.e., at the site of the reduviid bug bite.

110. *Vibrio vulnificus* has been described primarily with which two clinical syndromes?

1. A cutaneous localized cellulitis after a localized inoculation

2. A high-mortality sepsis syndrome with bacteremia, usually occurring after raw-oyster ingestion and seen in immunocompromised patients, particularly cirrhotics.

111. What organism shares a common epidemiologic niche and the same tick vector as *Borrelia burgdorferi*?

Babesia microti, a protozoan that parasitizes human erythrocytes, shares some of the same geographic distribution as *B. burgdorferi* (Lyme disease). *Ixodes dammini [scapularis]* is the most important tick vector, with *Dermacentor variabilis* being a less frequent vector. Some of this same geographic distribution is also shared by the agent causing human granulocyte ehrlichiosis, for which *I. dammini* [*scapularis*] is also the vector. Consequently, it is theoretically possible to see infection with all three agents.

112. What infections are seen in individuals with cats?

Toxoplasmosis	Cat scratch disease (*Bartonella* sp.)
Hookworm	Pasteurellosis (usually bite wound)
Rabies	Toxocariasis (visceral larval migrans)
Strongyloidiasis	Tularemia
Dermatomycoses	

Elliot DL, et al: Pet-associated illness. N Engl J Med 313:985–995, 1985.

113. How do corticosteroids interfere with the immune system? What are the infectious consequences?

Corticosteroids predominantly influence cell-mediated immunity by interfering with mononuclear cell migration and bactericidal capacities. The consequences of this are increased numbers of infections with organisms that are normally controlled through cell-mediated immune mechanisms:

Viruses	**Bacteria**
Herpes simplex virus	*Legionella*
Varicella-zoster virus	*Salmonella*
Cytomegalovirus	*Mycobacterium*
JC virus	*Listeria monocytogenes*
Fungi	**Parasites**
Cryptococcus neoformans	*Strongyloides stercoralis*
Histoplasma capsulatum	*Toxoplasma gondii*
Coccidioides immitis	
Pneumocystis carinii	

114. What is the differential diagnosis for fever and pulmonary infiltrates in a patient with Hodgkin's disease?

Patients with Hodgkin's disease can become infected with the normal respiratory flora, such as *Streptococcus pneumoniae*, particularly following courses of chemotherapy. Classically, these patients are infected with organisms that are normally controlled by cell-mediated immunity. In addition, noninfectious entities such as tumor invasion, hemorrhage, radiation pneumonitis, and drug reactions have to be considered.

Rosenow EC III, et al: Pulmonary disease in the immunocompromised host. Mayo Clin Proc 60:473–487, 610–631, 1985.

115. Which infectious diseases are associated with fecal leukocytes?

Fecal polymorphonuclear leukocytes are seen with:

Shigella	Enteroinvasive *Escherichia coli*
Salmonella enteritidis	*Vibrio parahaemolyticus*
Clostridium difficile	*Campylobacter jejuni*
Entamoeba histolytica	

Fecal mononuclear leukocytes are seen with:

Salmonella typhi	*Yersinia enterocolitica*
Campylobacter fetus	

Guerrant RL: Principles and syndromes of enteric infection. In Mandell GL, et al (eds): Principles and Practice of Infectious Diseases. New York, Churchill Livingstone, 1995, pp 945–962.

116. Which infectious agents have been implicated in cervical carcinoma?

Cancer of the cervix behaves epidemiologically as if it were a sexually transmitted disease. Strong epidemiologic associations exist between cervical infections with herpes simplex virus and *Chlamydia trachomatis*, but the strongest association exists with infection with human papillomavirus. HPV types 16 and 18 have the strongest link with subsequent malignancy.

Paavonen J, et al: Cervical neoplasia and other STD-related genital and anal neoplasia. In Holmes KK, et al (eds): Sexually Transmitted Diseases, 2nd ed. New York, McGraw-Hill, 1990, pp 561–592.

117. What are the infectious causes of an eosinophilic pleural effusion?

1. Bacterial pneumonia (usually *Streptococcus pneumoniae*)
2. Fungi: *Cryptococcus neoformans, Histoplasma capsulatum, Coccidioides immitis*
3. *Mycobacterium tuberculosis*

Some authors feel that pleural fluid eosinophilia offers no help in differential diagnosis. Other common associations with eosinophils in the pleural fluid are spontaneous pneumothorax or repeated thoracenteses.

118. Name two types of bone marrow toxicity associated with the use of chloramphenicol.

1. Reversible bone marrow suppression due to inhibition of mitochondrial protein synthesis. It can be manifested by reticulocytopenia, anemia, leukopenia, or thrombocytopenia. Vacuolization of erythroid and myeloid precursors in the bone marrow occurs. This form of toxicity is dose related and seen most frequently in patients receiving 4 gm/day.

2. An idiosyncratic response, frequently manifested as an aplastic anemia. It is estimated to occur once in 24,500–40,800 patients who receive chloramphenicol. It may occur weeks to months after cessation of the drug.

119. Which viral illnesses are more severe in pregnancy?

Pregnant patients have been noted to have increased morbidity and/or mortality from varicella, influenza, hepatitis C, polio, and measles. Rubella, while associated with increased fetal defects, has not been noted to be more severe in pregnancy.

120. What is the significance of a methylthiotetrazole (MTT) side chain in certain cephalosporins? Which cephalosporins have one?

MTT side chains are associated with an increased risk of bleeding after antibiotic administration and with the occurrence of disulfiram-like reactions after ethanol ingestion. Cefamandole, cefoperazone, cefotetan, and moxalactam all have MTT side chains.

121. Other than allergy, what is the most important adverse effect of imipenem?

Seizures occur in up to 1% of patients on imipenem. Patients with a history of preexisting seizure disorder, recent head trauma, or chronic alcoholism are at increased risk. Seizures are also seen in patients with renal failure when the dose is not adjusted. Treatment consists of withdrawal of the drug and anticonvulsants.

Eng RHK, et al: Seizure propensity with imipenem. Arch Intern Med 149:1881–1883, 1989.

122. What are the two most important drug-drug interactions associated with ciprofloxacin?

1. Coadministration of ciprofloxacin with theophylline may result in increased theophylline levels and theophylline toxicity.

2. Magnesium- and aluminum-containing antacids decrease the bioavailability of ciprofloxacin, causing the peak serum levels to be in the subtherapeutic range.

Hendershot EF: Fluoroquinolones. Infect Dis Clin North Am 9:715–730, 1995.

123. Are any important drug-drug interactions associated with erythromycin?

Yes. Erythromycin alters the metabolism of a number of drugs, resulting in increased drug effect and possible toxicity. These drugs include:

Oral anticoagulants	Carbamazepine
Phenytoin	Corticosteroids
Cyclosporine	Theophylline
Digoxin	Ergot alkaloids

124. Describe the mechanisms of resistance to acyclovir.

Acyclovir triphosphate is a potent inhibitor of viral DNA polymerase. It enters the infected cell as acyclovir and is phosphorylated to a monophosphate by viral thymidine kinase (TK). Further phosphorylation is accomplished by cellular enzymes. The major mechanism of resistance is alteration in viral TK. Alterations in the DNA polymerase as a cause of resistance are much less common.

Whitley RJ, et al: Acyclovir: A decade later. N Engl J Med 327:782–789, 1992.

125. How frequently will a single stool smear be diagnostic in a patient with symptomatic giardiasis?

The diagnosis of giardiasis usually can be made by careful examination of the stool for trophozoites or cysts. The diagnosis is confirmed 50–70% of the time after only 1 stool examination and 90% of the time after examination of 3 stool specimens.

126. An immigrant from Mexico who presents with a seizure disorder and has multiple small ring-like lesions on a head CT scan is likely to have what disorder?

Neurocysticercosis. This is invasion of the CNS by the larval form of the pork tapeworm, *Taenia solium*. CT scans typically show cystic lesions that do not usually enhance with contrast and, in many cases, hydrocephalus. It is the most common cerebral parasitic infection in humans.

127. Name the etiologic agents of the STDs chancroid, lymphogranuloma venereum, and granuloma inguinale.

Chancroid	*Haemophilus ducreyi*
Lymphogranuloma venereum	*Chlamydia trachomatis*, serovars L1–3
Granuloma inguinale (donovanosis)	*Calymmatobacterium granulomatis*

128. What percentage of older patients with salmonella bacteremia will have an endovascular source of infection?

Approximately 25% of patients over age 50 will have an endovascular source. Salmonella organisms tend to "seed" abnormal tissues (e.g., hematomas, tumors, cysts, stones, and altered endothelium such as aortic aneurysms) during bacteremia.

129. Which organisms may be confused with *Listeria monocytogenes* on Gram stain or blood agar plates?

1. *Corynebacterium* spp.	4. *Streptococcus pneumoniae*
2. β-Hemolytic streptococci	5. *Erysipelothrix rhusiopathiae*
3. *Enterococcus*	6. *Lactobacillus* sp.

One should always make certain these organisms are not overlooked in clinical specimens submitted to the laboratory, especially spinal fluid.

Sen P, et al: Human listeriosis. Infect Med (May/June):204–215, 1987.

130. How is disease due to *Corynebacterium diphtheriae* produced?

Certain strains of *C. diphtheriae*, when infected by a lysogenic bacteriophage, produce a toxin that enters cells and interrupts protein synthesis, resulting in neuritis and myocarditis.

131. Infection with *Chlamydia psittaci* should be considered an occupational hazard for what group of individuals?

Petshop employees, pigeon fanciers, zoo workers, veterinarians, and poultry processors. It causes an atypical pneumonia.

132. Describe the serologic response to Epstein-Barr virus (EBV) infections.

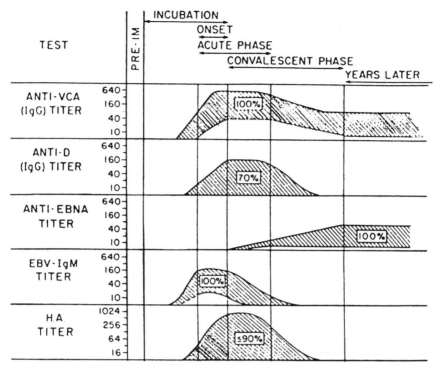

The typical sequence of serologic events following exposure to EBV. The incubation period ranges from 30–50 days. Antibody to viral capsid antigen (anti-VCA, difficult to detect in some labs) can be demonstrated at the time of clinical presentation and is diagnostic of acute infection. The EBV nuclear antigen (anti-EBNA) characteristically appears 3–4 weeks after the onset of clinical illness. Both the anti-VCA and anti-EBNA antibodies are present lifelong following infection. (HA, heterophile antibody; anti-D, antibody to early antigen) (From Schooley RT: Chronic fatigue syndrome: A manifestation of Epstein-Barr virus infection? In Remington JS, Swartz MN (eds): Current Clinical Topics in Infectious Disease, vol 9. New York, McGraw-Hill, 1988, pp 126–146; with permission.)

133. What is the differential diagnosis of infectious causes of monocytosis?

Infectious Causes	Noninfectious Causes
Tuberculosis	Myeloproliferative disorders
Epstein-Barr virus mononucleosis	Lymphomas
Rocky Mountain spotted fever	Solid tumors
Diphtheria	Gaucher's disease
Subacute bacterial endocarditis	Regional enteritis
Histoplasmosis	Ulcerative colitis
Typhus	Sprue
Brucellosis	Rheumatoid arthritis
Kala-azar	Systemic lupus erythematosus
Malaria	Polyarteritis nodosa
Syphilis	Post-splenectomy
Recovery from neutropenia	Sarcoidosis
Recovery from chronic infection	

From Calubiran O, et al: The significance of lymphocytes, monocytes, and platelets in infectious diseases. Hosp Physician 26:10–12, 1990, with permission.

134. What is the differential diagnosis of atypical lymphocytosis?

Disorders Associated with Atypical Lymphocytes

> 20% Atypical Lymphocytes	< 20% Atypical Lymphocytes	
Epstein-Barr mononucleosis	INFECTIONS	NON-INFECTIOUS CAUSES
Viral hepatitis	Varicella	Drug hypersensitivity reactions
CMV mononucleosis	Rubella	Drug fever
	Herpes simplex	Dermatitis herpetiformis
	Varicella-zoster	Radiation therapy
	Tuberculosis	Stress
	Brucellosis	Lead intoxication
	Smallpox	
	Babesiosis	
	Ehrlichiosis	
	Rubeola	
	Roseola infantum (HHV-6)	
	Influenza	
	Syphilis	
	Toxoplasmosis	
	Malaria	
	Rocky Mountain spotted fever	

From Calubiran O, et al: The significance of lymphocytes, monocytes, and platelets in infectious diseases. Hosp Physician 26:10–12, 1990; with permission.

135. Identify the sites and mechanisms of action of the various classes of antibiotics. Which are bactericidal and which are bacteriostatic?

Mechanism of Action of Antimicrobial Agents

CLASS	SITE OF ACTION	EFFECT	BACTERI-CIDAL	BACTERIO-STATIC
Penicillins, cephalosporins	Cell wall	Inhibit cross-linking of peptidoglycan, resulting in spheroplast formation	+	Occ.
Vancomycin	Cell wall	Block transfer of pentapeptide from cytoplasm to cell membrane	+	Occ.
Polymyxin B, colistin	Cytoplasmic membrane	Bind phospholipid and disrupt cell membrane	+	–
Aminoglycosides	Ribosome	Bind to 30S subunit, thereby inhibiting attachment of mRNA; also affects tRNA	+	–
Tetracyclines	Ribosome	Bind to 30S subunit and inhibit binding of tRNA	–	+
Chloramphenicol	Ribosome	Bind to 50S subunit and inhibit mRNA translation	Occ.	+
Erythromycin, clindamycin	Ribosome	Inhibit mRNA translation	Occ.	+
Rifampin	Nucleic acid synthesis	Impaired RNA formation by inhibiting DNA-dependent RNA-polymerase	+	Occ.
Metronidazole	Nucleic acid synthesis	Damages nucleic acid structure	+	–
Quinolones	Nucleic acid synthesis	Inhibit DNA gyrase	+	–
Sulfonamides	Nucleic acid synthesis	Competitive inhibition of paraamino-benzoic acid (PABA), thereby blocking formation of thymidine and purines	–	+

Occ. = occasionally (From Wyngaarden JB, Smith LH (eds): Cecil Textbook of Medicine, 18th ed. Philadelphia, W.B. Saunders, 1988, p 113; with permission.)

136. What is the MIC? MBC?

MIC—minimum inhibitory concentration: minimum concentration of a given antibiotic that will inhibit the growth of a given pathogen but will not kill it (usually expressed in μg/ml).

MBC—minimum bactericidal concentration: minimum concentration of a given antibiotic that will kill a given pathogen.

137. What causes hand-foot-mouth disease? Describe the clinical findings of this disease.

Hand-foot-mouth disease may be caused by a number of viruses in the picornavirus family. It has been most often associated with coxsackievirus A16, but outbreaks have also been attributed to coxsackieviruses A4, A5, A9, A10, B2, and B5 and enterovirus 71. It is characterized by an ulcerative exanthem, usually occurring on the buccal mucosa, which is followed by a vesicular exanthem on the hands and feet.

138. Discuss the epidemiologic aspects of *Penicillium marneffei* infection.

P. marneffei is endemic in Southeast Asia, particularly Vietnam, Thailand, Hong Kong, and the adjacent areas of China. Human disease almost always occurs as a disseminated infection in immunocompromised patients, and in recent years, most reported infections have been in patients with AIDS. Clinical manifestations include fever, anemia, weight loss, skin lesions, cough with pulmonary infiltrates, lymphadenopathy, and hepatomegaly.

Duong TA: Infection due to *Penicillium marneffei* an emerging pathogen: Review of 155 reported cases. Clin Infect Dis 23:125–130, 1996.

139. What are the diagnostic criteria for the chronic fatigue syndrome (CFS)?

According to the Centers for Disease Control and Prevention's consensus definition, in order to be diagnosed with CFS, a patient must have both of the following major criteria, and (1) at least 6 of the 11 symptom criteria and at least 2 of the 3 physical criteria or (2) they must have 8 or more of the symptom criteria:

Major criteria:

1. New onset of persistent or relapsing, debilitating fatigue or easy fatigability in a person who has no previous history of similar symptoms, that does not resolve with bedrest, and that is severe enough to reduce or impair average daily activity below 50% of the patient's premorbid activity level for a period of at least 6 months.

2. Other clinical conditions that may produce similar symptoms must be excluded by thorough evaluation based on history, physical exam, and appropriate laboratory findings.

Minor criteria:

A. Symptom criteria:
1. Mild fever (oral temperature 37.5–38.6°C, if measured by patient) or chills
2. Sore throat
3. Painful lymph nodes in the anterior or posterior cervical or axillary distribution
4. Unexplained generalized muscle weakness
5. Muscle discomfort or myalgia
6. Prolonged generalized fatigue after levels of exercise that would have been easily tolerated in the patient's premorbid state
7. Generalized headaches
8. Migratory arthralgia without joint swelling or redness
9. Neuropsychologic complaints including:
   a. Photophobia
   b. Transient visual scotomata
   c. Forgetfulness
   d. Excessive irritability
   e. Confusion
   f. Difficulty thinking
   g. Inability to concentrate
   h. Depression
10. Sleep disturbance (hypersomnia or insomnia)
11. Description of the initial symptom complex as initially developing over a period of a few hours to a few days

B. Physical criteria:
1. Low grade fever (oral temperature 37.6–38.6°C or rectal temperature 37.8–38.8°C)
2. Nonexudative pharyngitis
3. Palpable or tender anterior or posterior cervical or axillary lymph nodes, generally 2 cm in diameter

From Schooley RT: Chronic fatigue syndrome. In Mandell GL, Bennett JE, Dolin R (eds): Principles and Practice of Infectious Disease, 4th ed. New York, Churchill Livingstone, 1995, p 1306; with permission.

140. What precautions are needed when administering rifampin?

1. Rifampin has a significant first-pass effect after ingestion. Consequently, drug levels are optimal if the total daily dose is taken once instead of divided.

2. Rifampin stains secretions orange-red; individuals who wear soft contact lenses should be warned about staining of the lenses.

3. Rifampin reduces the serum concentration of a number of drugs because of its potent induction of hepatic microsomal enzymes, which may result in clinically important consequences:
- Decreased digoxin levels can result in decompensated heart failure.
- Decreased warfarin levels can result in inadequate anticoagulation.
- Exacerbation of hyperglycemia may result from decreased serum concentrations of oral hypoglycemic agents.
- Decreased efficacy of oral contraceptive agents may occur.
- Ketoconazole and itraconazole levels are substantially reduced.
- Thyroid replacement therapy may be inadequate due to decreased levels of L-thyroxine in patients with hypothyroidism.
- Rejection of solid organ transplants may result from decreased cyclosporine concentrations.
- Asthma or Addison's disease may relapse during glucocorticosteroid therapy.

Baciewicz AM, et al: Rifampin drug interactions. Arch Intern Med 144:1667–1671, 1984.

141. Which individuals are candidates for pneumococcal immunization?

Candidates for the Pneumococcal Vaccine

ADULTS
1. Immunocompetent adults at increased risk for pneumococcal disease or its complications because of chronic illnesses:

Cardiovascular disease	Diabetes mellitus	Cirrhosis
Pulmonary disease	Alcoholism	CSF leaks

2. Individuals ≥ 65 years old
3. Immunocompromised adults at increased risk for pneumococcal disease or its complications:

Anatomic or functional asplenia (including sickle cell anemia)	Lymphoma	Nephrotic syndrome
Hodgkin's disease	Multiple myeloma	Conditions associated with immunosuppression (e.g., organ transplantation)
	Chronic renal failure	

4. Adults with HIV infection, asymptomatic or symptomatic

CHILDREN
1. Children ≥ 2 years old with chronic illnesses specifically associated with increased risk for pneumococcal disease or its complications:

Anatomic or functional asplenia (including sickle cell anemia)	Nephrotic syndrome	Conditions associated with immunosuppression
	CSF leaks	

2. Children ≥ 2 years old with HIV infection, asymptomatic or symptomatic

SPECIAL GROUPS
1. Persons living in special environments or social settings with an identified increased risk of pneumococcal disease or its complications (e.g., certain Native American populations)

CDC: Prevention of Pneumococcal Disease. Recommendations of the Immunization Practices Advisory Committee. MMWR 46:10–13, 1997.

142. What is ecthyma gangrenosum?

Ecthyma gangrenosum consists of skin lesions that occur in association with gram-negative bacteremia, most commonly in neutropenic patients. *Pseudomonas aeruginosa* is the most commonly implicated bacteria, but other species have produced this lesion, including *Aeromonas hydrophila* and *Escherichia coli*. The lesions typically begin as painless erythematous macules which rapidly progress to papules and develop central vesicles or bullae. Eventually, they ulcerate to form gangrenous ulcers. The characteristic histologic appearance demonstrates large numbers of bacteria in and around blood vessels, but an absence of an inflammatory response.

143. Why is the use of astemizole, terfenadine, and cisapride absolutely contraindicated in individuals receiving itraconazole or ketoconazole?

Itraconazole and ketoconazole interfere with the metabolism of these three drugs, causing an elevation in their serum levels. This can lead to prolongation of the QT interval on the ECG, torsades de pointes, and even sudden cardiac death.

144. What animal is the reservoir for the agent causing the hantavirus pulmonary syndrome?

The deer mouse, *Peromyscus maniculatus*, is the reservoir for the Sin Nombre virus that causes the hantavirus pulmonary syndrome.

Childs JE, et al: Serologic and genetic identification of *Peromyscus maniculatus* as the primary rodent reservoir for a new hantavirus in the southwestern United States. J Infect Dis 169:1271–1280, 1994.

145. Which infection causes "owl's eye" of intranuclear inclusions in histopathologic specimens of involved tissues?

Cytomegalovirus infection produces a characteristic cytopathologic effect resulting in the "owl's eye" appearance of infected cells. Cytomegalic cells are large 25–35 mm cells and contain basophilic intranuclear inclusions that are frequently surrounded by a clear halo, producing the "owl's eye" effect.

146. Describe the spectrum of illness caused by *Bartonella* species.

Originally, *B. bacilliformis* was the only *Bartonella* species associated with human disease. Recently, however, the various organisms classified as *Rochalimaea* have been reclassified as *Bartonella*, and a number of different clinical syndromes are associated with these organisms:

1. *B. bacilliformis* infection manifests as 2 different syndromes:
   - Oroyo fever, in which patients experience fever, chills, diaphoresis, myalgias, arthralgias, and headaches. Generalized, nontender lymphadenopathy may occur. The patients develop hemolytic anemia, jaundice, and secondary infections.
   - Verruga peruana is a cutaneous, eruptive lesion that may or may not be preceded by Oroyo fever. The nodules appear usually over exposed parts of the body, but may involve mucous membranes and internal organs.
2. *B. quintana* is the causative agent of trench fever. Recently, a similar syndrome with endocarditis has been described in homeless men living in Seattle. *B. quintana* may also cause some of the same clinical manifestations as *B. henselae*.
3. *B. henselae* has been associated with several clinical presentations:
   - Cat-scratch disease, which most commonly presents as localized lymphadenopathy, but may have systemic findings such as hepatitis, encephalopathy, and neuroretinitis.
   - Bacillary angiomatosis, which occurs most commonly in immunocompromised patients (e.g., AIDS and organ transplant recipients). These neovascular, proliferative lesions may involve the skin, liver, spleen, bone, and brain.
   - Peliosis hepatis are blood-filled cystic structures that involve visceral organs, such as the liver, spleen, and lymph nodes.
   - A febrile, bacteremic syndrome that occurs most commonly in immunocompromised patients and may be relapsing.
4. *B. elizabethae* has been described in one patient with endocarditis.
5. *B. vinsonii* has not yet been associated with human disease.

147. What are the "flesh-eating" bacteria?

"Flesh-eating" bacteria is the term coined by the British press to describe invasive necrotizing infections caused by *Streptococcus pyogenes* (group A streptococci). These infections are characterized by aggressive soft-tissue infection, shock, adult respiratory distress syndrome, and renal failure. The mortality is 30–70%. The pathophysiology of these infections is thought to involve bacterial production of pyrogenic exotoxins, which function as superantigens to stimulate T-cell production of cytokines responsible for many of the clinical manifestations.

Stevens DL: Streptococcal toxic-shock syndrome: Spectrum of disease, pathogenesis, and new concepts in treatment. Emerging Infect Dis 1:69–78, 1995.

148. Which upper GI lesions are associated with *Helicobacter pylori*? Which are not?

LESION	ASSOCIATION WITH *H. PYLORI*
Peptic esophagitis	No association
Barrett's esophagitis	May colonize distal-most gastric epithelium in patients with gastric colonization
Chronic diffuse superficial gastritis	Nearly always associated
Type A (pernicious anemia) gastritis	Negative association
NSAID gastropathy	Negative or no association
Acute erosive gastritis (alcohol, aspirin, etc.)	No association
Gastric ulceration	Nearly universally observed in patients who are not ingesting NSAIDs or aspirin
Duodenal ulceration	Nearly universally associated with "idiopathic" lesions
Gastric adenocarcinoma	Associated with cancers of the body and antrum but not cardia
Gastric lymphoma	Strongly associated with MALT-type B-cell lymphomas

From Blaser MJ: *Helicobacter pylori* and related organisms. In Mandell GL, Bennett JE, Dolin R (eds): The Principles and Practice of Infectious Diseases, 4th ed. New York, Churchill Livingstone, 1995, p 1957; with permission.

149. Which conditions predispose patients to the development of cellulitis due to group A streptococci?

Cellulitis due to the group A streptococci (and sometimes B, C, or G) has been described in a number of clinical settings in which there has been **impairment of venous and lymphatic drainage**. These situations include:

- Extremities from which the saphenous vein has been harvested for CABG
- Following mastectomy with axillary lymph node dissection for breast cancer
- Following vulvectomy and inguinal lymphadenectomy for cancer of the vulva
- After regional lymph node dissection for melanoma
- Following traumatic injuries to extremities
- Following retroperitoneal lymph node dissections for genitourinary tumors

Simon MS, et al: Cellulitis after axillary lymph node dissection for carcinoma of the breast. Am J Med 93:543–548, 1992.

150. How long does it take for resolution of chest x-ray changes in patients who have been treated for pneumococcal pneumonia?

The great majority of patients who have been treated for *Streptococcus pneumoniae* pneumonia should have complete resolution of radiographic consolidation by 8–10 weeks. Findings such as volume loss, stranding, and pleural disease may take longer to resolve. Patients who are < 50 years old and do not have underlying alcoholism or preexisting airway disease will have earlier resolution.

151. In adults presenting with a sore throat, what clinical findings may suggest the possibility of infectious mononucleosis?

The presence of palatine petechiae, posterior auricular adenopathy, marked axillary adenopathy, or inguinal adenopathy substantially increases the possibility that the patient has infectious mononucleosis. If none of these findings is present, the chances are remote.

152. List the infectious causes of adrenal insufficiency.

Mycobacterium tuberculosis

Histoplasma capsulatum

Other fungi (*Cryptococcus neoformans, Coccidioides immitis, Sporothrix schenckii, Blastomyces dermatitidis, Paracoccidioides brasiliensis*)

Neisseria meningitidis (in Waterhouse-Friderichsen syndrome) and other organisms causing shock

In HIV infection, *Mycobacterium avium* complex and cytomegalovirus

Painter BF: Infectious causes of adrenal insufficiency. Infect Med 11:515–520, 1994.

153. What is the significance of *Clostridium septicum* infection?

There is a very strong association between *C. septicum* infection and underlying malignancy. Approximately 40% of cases will have a hematologic malignancy and 34% colorectal carcinoma. These patients frequently present with myonecrosis, often at sites distant from the presumed source of entry.

Kornbluth AA, et al: *Clostridium septicum* infection and associated malignancy: Report of 2 cases and review of the literature. Medicine 68:30–37, 1989.

154. How many blood cultures should be done for patients with suspected bacteremia or endocarditis in order to make a diagnosis?

If 20–30 ml of blood is drawn during each venipuncture (to be divided between 1 aerobic and 1 anaerobic blood culture bottle or between 2 aerobic bottles), one set of blood cultures will identify the offending pathogen approximately 91.5% of the time and two sets will be positive in > 99%. Consequently, two separate sets of blood cultures are normally recommended.

Smith-Elekes S, et al: Blood cultures. Infect Dis Clin North Am 7:221–234, 1993.

155. What is erythema nodosum leprosum?

This complication of therapy is seen in patients with the full lepromatous (LL) form of leprosy and most commonly occurs within the first year of treatment. It is manifested as nodular skin lesions that histopathologically resemble arthus-type reactions, with localized vasculitis in the veins and arteries characterized by PMN and eosinophilic infiltrates. It may also be associated with neuritis, polyarthritis and immune-complex glomerulonephritis.

Jacobson RR, et al: The diagnosis and treatment of leprosy. South Med J 69:979–985, 1976.

156. What infectious diseases result from human louse infestations?

The body louse, *Pediculus humanus humanus*, which is a strict human parasite, is responsible for transmission of 3 different bacterial species to humans. *Borrelia recurrentis* causes relapsing fever. *Bartonella quintana* is recognized as the cause of bacillary angiomatosis, bacteremia, trench fever, endocarditis and chronic lymphadenopathy, particularly among homeless individuals. *Rickettsia prowazekii* is the cause of epidemic typhus.

Raoult D, Roux V: The body louse as a vector of reemerging human diseases. Clin Infect Dis 29:888–911, 1999.

157. What organisms are responsible for most infections in patients with cystic fibrosis?

Chronic lung infection in patients with cystic fibrosis is usually caused by a limited number of organisms. *Staphylococcus aureus* and *Pseudomonas aeruginosa* are the most frequently isolated pathogens. *Burkholderia cepacia* is also commonly seen, particularly in adult patients with cystic fibrosis. Various other bacteria, including non-typeable *Haemophilus influenzae*,

Streptococcus pneumoniae and some of the *Enterobacteriaceae,* are occasionally isolated. The most important fungal pathogen is *Aspergillus fumigatus*, which causes allergic bronchopulmonary aspergillosis in this patient population.

Gilligan PH: Microbiology of airway disease in patients with cystic fibrosis. Clin Microbiol Rev 4:35–51, 1991.

158. What is xanthogranulomatous pyelonephritis?

Xanthogranulomatous pyelonephritis is a chronic infection of the renal parenchyma and surrounding tissues which occurs most commonly in the presence of renal lithiasis or urinary tract obstruction. It most commonly occurs in middle-age females and is usually due to *Proteus mirabilis* or *Escherichia coli.* The renal parenchyma becomes replaced by characteristic foamy histiocytes, which may also be found in urine cytologic specimens.

Goodman M, et al: Xanthogranulomatous pyelonephritis (XGP): A local disease with systemic manifestations. Medicine 58:171–181, 1979.

159. What are the various species of *Ehrlichia* that have been associated with human disease?

Four species of *Ehrlichia* have been recognized as causes of tick-borne zoonotic infections. The species that have been associated with human diseases include:

1. *Ehrlichia chaffeensis* cause human monocytic ehrlichiosis
2. *E. ewingii* has been identified as a cause of human granulocytic ehrlichiosis
3. *E. sennetsu* causes a mononucleosis-like illness in Japan and Malaysia
4. *E. canis* has been reported in one patient in Venezuela

Buller RS, et al: *Ehrlichia ewingii*, a newly recognized agent of human ehrlichiosis. N Engl J Med 341:148–155, 1999.

160. What is Lemierre's syndrome?

Lemierre's syndrome is suppurative thrombophlebitis of the internal jugular vein that results from acute oropharyngeal infection. This may lead to septic embolization, most often to the lungs. Anaerobic bacteria, particularly *Fusobacterium necrophorum*, are usually involved.

Sinave CP, Hardy GJ, Fardy PW: The Lemierre syndrome: Suppurative thrombophlebitis of the internal jugular vein secondary to oropharyngeal infection. Medicine 68:85–93, 1989.

161. What are bacterial superantigens and some diseases thought to be due to superantigen production?

Bacterial superantigens are a group of bacteria proteins that bind directly to the major histocompatibility complex class II molecule on antigen-presenting cells and cross-link the antigen-presenting cells with certain T-cell receptors. This results in polyclonal T-cell activation with elaboration of multiple different cytokines that are responsible for the clinical manifestations of the various related disorders. The diseases that have been implicated as being caused by superantigens are:

Staphylococcal toxic shock syndrome
Streptococcal toxic shock syndrome
Staphylococcal scalded skin syndrome
Staphylococcal food poisoning
Guttate psoriasis
Kawasaki syndrome
Atopic dermatitis

Schlievert PM: Role of superantigens in human disease. J Infect Dis 167:997–1003, 1993.

162. What are Koch postulates?

Koch postulates are criteria that were actually proposed by Henle and are used to establish a causal relation between a specific agent and a specific disease. The postulates are:

1. The agent must be present in every case of the disease.
2. The agent must be isolated from the diseased host and grown in pure culture.

3. The specific disease must be reproduced when a portion of the culture is inoculated into a healthy susceptible host.

4. The organism must be recovered again from the experimentally infected host.

163. What are the anatomic locations of wound infections due to dog and cat bites?

| | % OF PATIENTS | |
LOCATION OF WOUND	DOG BITE	CAT BITE
Hand	50	63
Thigh and/or leg	16	9
Face, scalp or neck	16	2
Shoulder, arm or forearm	12	23
Feet	4	3
Trunk	2	0

Talan DA: Bacteriologic analysis of infected dog and cat bites. N Engl J Med 340:85–92, 1999.

164. What are the identified risk factors associated with cases of acute hepatitis C infection?

RISK FACTOR	% OF CASES
Injection drug use	38
Other high risk/low socioeconomic status	44
Sexual/household	10
Transfusions	4
Occupational acquisition (healthcare)	2
Dialysis	1
None identified	1

Alter MJ: Epidemiology of hepatitis C in the west. Semin Liver Dis 15:5–14, 1995.

165. The use of medicinal leeches is associated with infection due to what organism?

Aeromonas hydrophila, which has the same freshwater habitat as the medicinal leech, *Hirudo medicinalis*, may complicate microvascular surgical infections where leeches are used because of their anticoagulant properties.

Abrutyn E: Hospital-associated infection from leeches. Ann Intern Med 109:356–358, 1988.

166. How does human disease due to *Dirofilaria immitis* usually present?

Dirofilaria immitis, the dog heartworm, usually presents as a solitary, noncalcified pulmonary nodule in humans. Because humans are an unsuitable host for this worm, larvae that mature in subcutaneous tissues after inoculation by infected mosquitoes enter veins and travel to the heart and act as emboli into the pulmonary arteries, resulting in infarcts.

Nicholson CP, et al: *Dirofilaria immitis*: A rare, increasing cause of pulmonary nodules. Mayo Clin Proc 67:646–650, 1992.

167. What are the various herpes viruses and what syndromes are they associated with?

HERPES VIRUS	CLINICAL SYNDROMES
Herpes simplex virus	Mucocutaneous lesions Encephalitis
Varicella zoster virus	Chickenpox Shingles

(*Table continued on next page.*)

HERPES VIRUS	CLINICAL SYNDROMES
Cytomegalovirus	Mononucleosis syndrome Meningoencephalitis, transverse myelitis, hepatitis, myocarditis, pneumonitis, esophagitis, colitis, and retinitis usually in immunocompromised individuals
Ebstein-Barr virus	Infectious mononucleosis Burkitt's lymphoma Nasopharyngeal carcinoma EBV-related lymphoproliferative syndromes
Human herpes virus 6	Roseola (exanthem subitum) and non-specific febrile illnesses in young children Mononucleosis-like syndrome in adults Encephalitis Hepatitis Opportunistic infections (interstitial pneumonitis) in immunocompromised individuals Possibly, chronic fatigue syndrome, lymphoproliferative disorders and histiocytic necrotizing lymphadenitis (Kikuchi's syndrome)
Human herpes virus 7	Possibly exanthum subitum-like illness, hepatitis and encephalitis
Human herpes virus 8	Kaposi's sarcoma Primary effusion (body cavity-based) lymphoma Castleman's disease
Herpes B virus	Myelitis and hemorrhagic encephalitis following primate bites and scratches

168. What are the most common medical presentations of factitious disorders?

PRESENTATION	NUMBER
Sepsis	12
Non-healing wounds	8
Fever	4
Electrolyte disorders	4
Purpura	2
Urinary tract infections	1
Thrombophlebitis	1
Anemia	1
"Multiple sclerosis"	1
"Acute myelogenous leukemia"	1
"Systemic lupus erythematosus"	1
Amenorrhea	1
Diarrhea	1
Feculent urine	1
Hypoglycemia	1
Erythema nodosa	1
Total	41

From Reich P, Gottfried LA: Factitious disorders in a teaching hospital. Ann Intern Med 99:240–247, 1983; with permission.

169. What are the six classic exanthems of childhood and their causes?

ORDER	EXANTHEMS	CAUSATIVE AGENTS
First	Rubeola (measles)	Measles virus
Second	Scarlet fever	*Streptococcus pyogenes*
Third	Rubella (German measles)	Rubella virus
Fourth	Filatow-Dukes' disease (variant of scarlet fever)	*Streptococcus pyogenes*
Fifth	Erythema infectiosum	Parvovirus B19
Sixth	Exanthem subitum (roseola)	Human herpes virus 6

170. What is the differential diagnosis of infectious causes of nodular lymphangitis?

Organisms That Can Cause Nodular Lymphangitis

COMMON CAUSES	UNUSUAL CAUSES	RARE CAUSES
Sporothrix schenckii	*Nocardia asteroides*	*Mycobacterium kansasii*
Mycobacterium marinum	*Mycobacterium chelonae*	*Blastomyces dermatitidis*
Nocardia brasiliensis	*Leishmania major*	*Coccidioides immitis*
Leishmania braziliensis		*Cryptococcus neoformans*
Francisella tularensis		*Histoplasma capsulatum*
		Streptococcus pyogenes
		Staphylococcus aureus
		Pseudomonas pseudomallei
		Bacillus anthracis
		Cowpox

From Kostman JR, DiNubile MJ: Nodular lymphangitis: A distinctive but often unrecognized syndrome. Ann Intern Med 118:883–888, 1993; with permission.

171. What is pigbel?

Pigbel, also known as enteritis necroticans, is a frequently fatal illness characterized by hemorrhagic, inflammatory, or ischemic necrosis of the jejunum. It usually occurs in developing countries and commonly affects individuals who ingest a voluminous meal after having been starved for a long period. It is caused by the β toxin produced by type C *Clostridium perfringens*.

Petrillo TM, et al: Enteritis necroticans (pigbel) in a diabetic child. N Engl J Med 342:1225–1253, 2000.

172. What types of infections occur principally in patients with diabetes mellitus?

Invasive otitis externa due to *Pseudomonas aeruginosa*
Rhinocerebral mucormycosis
Emphysematous cholecystitis
Emphysematous cystitis and pyelonephritis

Joshi N, et al: Infections in patients with diabetes mellitus. N Engl J Med 341:1906–1912, 2000.

173. What are infectious causes of hilar adenopathy?

BILATERAL HILAR ADENOPATHY	UNILATERAL HILAR ADENOPATHY
Tuberculosis	Tuberculosis
Histoplasmosis	Sporotrichosis
Coccidioidomycosis	Histoplasmosis
Varicella	Coccidioidomycosis
Epstein Barr virus	Tularemia
HIV	Pertussis
Rubeola	*Yersinia pestis*
Anthrax (inhalational)	Human herpes virus-6
Treponema pallidum	

From Cunha BA: Bilateral hilar adenopathy. Infect Dis Pract Clin 23:94–95, 1999; with permission.

174. What are the clinical manifestations of anthrax?

The clinical manifestations of anthrax are initiated after the introduction into the body of the endospores of the causative organism, *Bacillus anthracis*. The most common manifestations include:
- Cutaneous anthrax, which accounts for 95% of all anthrax in the United States.
- Gastrointestinal and oropharyngeal anthrax, which occur after ingestion of the endospores.
- Inhalational anthrax, which usually occurs after inhalation of the endospores which have contaminated animal hides or products.
- Anthrax meningitis, which occurs after bacteremic spread usually from a skin focus.

Dixon TC, et al: Anthrax. N Engl J Med 341:815–826, 1999.

175. What are the neurologic complications of Lyme disease?

The neurologic manifestations of Lyme disease are extremely variable and may include:
- Bell's palsy and other cranial neuropathies, particularly involving cranial nerves III, IV, and VI
- Radiculopathy that can involve any distribution
- Mononeuritis multiplex
- Aseptic meningitis, usually with a lymphocytic pleocytosis
- Encephalitis syndromes
- Transverse myelitis
- Demyelinating polyneuropathy

Finkel MF: Lyme disease and its neurologic complications. Arch Neurol 45:99–104, 1988.

176. What infections have been associated with eating raw seed sprouts?

Seed sprouts have been implicated as vehicles of transmission in outbreaks of foodborne illness due to *Bacillus cereus*, multiple different *Salmonella* serotypes and *Escherichia coli*, particularly O157:H7.

Taormina PJ, et al: Infections associated with eating seed sprouts: An international concern. Emerging Infect Dis 5:626–634, 1999.

177. Infection with what bacterial organism is the most frequently reported antecedent event before the development of Guillain-Barré Syndrome?

Approximately 1 in 2000 infections due to *Campylobacter jejuni* may be complicated by the development of Guillain-Barré Syndrome.

Allos BM, et al: *Campylobacter jejuni* strains from patients with Guillain-Barré syndrome. Emerg Infect Dis 4:263–268, 1998.

178. What microbial agents are traditionally considered as potential biologic warfare agents?

Bacillus anthracis	Viral encephalitides (e.g., Venezuelan equine
Brucella suis	encephalitis)
Coxiella burnetii	Viral hemorrhagic fevers (e.g., Lassa fever, Rift Valley
Francisella tularensis	fever, Crimean Congo hemorrhagic fever, Ebola,
Smallpox virus	Marburg)
Yersinia pestis	

Kortepeter MG, Parker GW: Potential biological weapons threats. Emerging Infect Dis 5:523–527, 1999.

BIBLIOGRAPHY

1. Fields BN, Knipe DM (eds): Field's Virology, 3rd ed. New York, Lippincott-Raven, 1996.
2. Guerrant RL, Walker DH, Weller PF (eds): Tropical Infectious Diseases. Philadelphia, Churchill Livingstone, 1999.
3. Mandell GL, Bennett JE, Dolin R (eds): Principles and Practice of Infectious Diseases, 5th ed. New York, Churchill Livingstone, 2000.
4. Merigan TC Jr, Bartlett JG, Bolognesi D: Textbook of AIDS Medicine, 2nd ed. Baltimore, Williams & Wilkins, 1999.
5. Rubin RH, Young LS (eds): Clinical Approach to Infection in the Compromised Host, 2nd ed. New York, Plenum Publishers, 1988.

5. GASTROENTEROLOGY

Rhonda A. Cole, M.D.

Indigestion is charged by God for enforcing morality on the stomach.
Victor Hugo
Les Miserables

A good digestion turneth all to health.
George Herbert
The Temple

GASTROINTESTINAL (GI) BLEEDING

1. List the five ways in which GI bleeding presents.

1. Hematemesis: vomiting of blood. The blood may be a fresh, bright red or look like coffee grounds.

2. Melena: black, tarry, foul-smelling stool.

3. Hematochezia: bright red blood per rectum, blood mixed with stool, bloody diarrhea, or clots.

4. Occult GI blood loss: normal-appearing stool that is hemoccult-positive.

5. Symptoms only: syncope, dyspnea, angina, palpitations, or shock.

2. Describe the initial approach to the patient who presents with acute GI bleeding.

In any patient presenting with acute GI bleeding, there are three key words: resuscitation, resuscitation, and resuscitation! The initial approach should include a rapid assessment to gauge the urgency of the situation, especially whether the patient is hemodynamically stable or unstable (blood pressure and signs of orthostasis must be assessed). Venous access should be obtained with a large-bore IV cannula, and fluids such as normal saline should be begun immediately. Blood should be obtained for a complete blood count, clotting studies, platelets, routine chemistry, and type and cross-match.

Clearly, the urgency of management depends on the results of the initial assessment. If the patient appears hemodynamically stable with minor bleeding, further management can be undertaken electively. If there are signs of an acute, life-threatening bleed and an unstable condition, aggressive resuscitation and evaluation for the source must be undertaken immediately. A nasogastric (NG) tube should be placed to assess for evidence of an upper GI source and, if present, to document the rapidity of bleeding. Close monitoring of vital signs and urinary output in an intensive care setting is imperative. The patient also must be monitored for signs of concomitant heart, lung, renal, or CNS disease.

A good rule of thumb is that blood transfusions should be given as quickly as the patient has lost blood. For example, if the patient presents with massive hematochezia and is hemodynamically compromised, packed red blood cells (PRBCs) should be given as quickly as possible. If, on the other hand, the patient presents with iron deficiency anemia, hemoccult positive stools, and stable vital signs, he or she may not require blood transfusions.

Once the patient has been stabilized, a search can be carried out to localize the source of bleeding and perform any indicated endoscopic therapy.

The presence of a GI bleed should be confirmed by inspecting the stool for melena or hematochezia and the NG tube aspirate for blood. The site of bleeding frequently can be determined from the patient's complaints. Upper GI bleeding often presents with hematemesis combined with melena; hematochezia with a negative NG aspirate suggests a lower GI source.

3. What is the mortality rate for GI bleeding?

Despite the advances in therapeutic endoscopic intervention, the mortality rate for GI bleeding remains ~10% overall and ranges from 5% to 15%.

4. What are the common causes of upper GI bleeding?

1. Duodenal and gastric ulcers
2. Esophageal or gastric varices in cirrhotic patients
3. Mallory-Weiss tears (most commonly seen in alcoholics or patients with forceful vomiting)
4. Erosive gastritis as a result of nonsteroidal anti-inflammatory drugs (NSAIDs) or intubation in the intensive care unit (ICU)
5. Esophagitis

5. What questions addressed in the history and physical examination help to identify the source of an upper GI bleed?

1. Does the patient have a history of prior bleeding episodes?
2. Does the patient have a family history of diseases that cause bleeding?
3. Does the patient have superimposed illnesses that may lead to bleeding, such as cirrhosis, carcinoma, coagulopathy, a known connective tissue disorder, or amyloidosis?
4. Has the patient had prior surgery of the intestinal tract, such as gastric surgery for peptic ulcer or placement of an arterial bypass graft?
5. Is the patient an alcoholic or does he or she take ulcerogenic drugs, such as aspirin or NSAIDs?
6. Has the patient recently had a caustic ingestion?
7. Was the bleeding episode preceded by abdominal pain, dyspepsia, or retching?
8. Has the patient had recent nosebleeds?

6. Is examination of the skin helpful in identifying the source of an upper GI bleed?

The skin examination may suggest a potential source if certain stigmata are present. Lymphadenopathy or abdominal masses may suggest sources for intra-abdominal pathology.

Skin Findings in Conditions That Cause GI Bleeding

DISEASE	ASSOCIATED SKIN FINDINGS
Peutz-Jeghers syndrome	Pigmented macules on lips, palms, soles
Malignant melanoma	Melanoma
Hereditary hemorrhagic telangiectasias	Telangiectasias on lips, mouth, palms, soles (Osler-Weber-Rendu syndrome)
Blue rubber bleb nevus	Dark blue soft nodules
Bullous pemphigoid	Oral and skin bullae
Neurofibromatosis	Café-au-lait spots, axillary freckles, neurofibromas
Cronkhite-Canada syndrome	Alopecia; hyperpigmentation of creases, hands, and face
Cirrhosis	Spider angiomata, Dupuytren's contracture
Neoplasm	Acanthosis nigricans
Kaposi's sarcoma	Cutaneous Kaposi's sarcoma
Ehlers-Danlos syndrome	Skin fragility, keloids, paper-thin scars
Pseudoxanthoma elasticum	Yellow "chicken fat" papules and plaques in flexural areas
Turner's syndrome	Webbing of neck, purpura, skin nodules

From Berger T, Silverman S: Oral and cutaneous manifestations of gastrointestinal disease. In Sleisenger MH, Fordtran JS (eds): Gastrointestinal Disease, 5th ed. Philadelphia, W.B. Saunders, 1994, pp 268–285, with permission.

7. When should endoscopy be performed in upper GI bleeding?

Endoscopy is the procedure of choice in an active GI bleed. It allows clinical decisions to be made about further therapy for the bleeding lesion. Endoscopy is usually performed within the first 24–72 hours after admission. The timing depends in some respects on the stability of the patient and whether bleeding continues. Patients who show evidence of ongoing bleeding despite resuscitative efforts should have emergent endoscopy during resuscitation to define the source and institute endoscopic therapy. If the bleeding has stopped, elective endoscopy can be done after full resuscitation has been achieved.

Contraindications to endoscopy include suspected perforation, impending cardiopulmonary arrest, and an uncooperative patient.

8. Which patients are at high risk for continued bleeding and should undergo emergency (immediate) upper GI endoscopy?

Elderly patients (age > 60)

Patients with fresh blood per NG tube or rectum

Patients who remain hemodynamically unstable despite aggressive resuscitative measures

Patients who rebleed during the same hospital admission

Patients who have multiple comorbid illnesses, such as cardiac disease, liver disease, diabetes, etc.

Silverstein FE, et al: The national ASGE survey on upper gastrointestinal bleeding: II. Clinical prognostic factors. Gastroint Endosc 27:80, 1981.

9. What are the common causes of lower GI bleeding?

Hemorrhoids are the most common cause but rarely present with massive bleeding that requires hospitalization.

Diverticulosis accounts for a significant percentage of cases. Diverticular bleeding may occur from either the right or left colon.

Angiodysplasia or **vascular ectasias** are one of the more common well-recognized causes in older patients. They are commonly found in the cecum and ascending colon.

Neoplasms of the large bowel usually present with chronic occult bleeding but occasionally bleed acutely.

Other **less common causes** include Meckel's diverticulum, ischemic or inflammatory bowel disease, solitary ulcers of the cecum and rectum, and aortoenteric fistulas.

10. Describe the diagnostic approach to a patient with lower GI bleeding.

A complete **history** and **physical examination** may yield important information about the source of the bleeding. A history of hemorrhoids, inflammatory bowel disease, preceding crampy abdominal pain (suggesting ischemia), and painless faucet-like bleeding (suggesting a diverticular source) may be key findings.

Low-lying lesions, such as hemorrhoids, anal fissures, rectal ulcers, colitis, or rectal tumors, can be identified easily with **flexible sigmoidoscopy** or **proctoscopy**. The next diagnostic test is **colonoscopy**, unless the bleeding is too massive to allow preparation and examination. (Whether the colon should be cleansed for colonoscopy in patients with lower GI tract bleeding remains controversial. In any case, in cases of severe lower GI tract bleeding with no preparation it is impossible to determine the level of bleeding because blood, clots, and other debris are found scattered throughout the colon.)

If the bleeding site is localized at colonoscopy, local **endoscopic therapy** may be undertaken to achieve hemostasis of certain lesions. If only diverticulosis is found, it is unlikely that the endoscopist will be able to localize the specific diverticulum that bled, but the value of the procedure is to rule out other lesions at the bleeding site and to help localize the area if surgery must be performed.

With bleeding too rapid to perform colonoscopy or with a negative colonoscopy despite continued brisk bleeding, **arteriography** should be the next step. With active bleeding (0.5–1 ml/min), arteriography may reveal the site and localize it to the right or left colon or small bowel, helping to direct the surgeon for resection. In addition, the radiologist may be able to institute therapy by selective infusion of vasopressin or embolization of the bleeding vessel.

If the bleeding rate is too slow to yield a positive arteriogram, a **radionuclide bleeding scan** using 99mTc–sulfur colloid may be an effective means of detecting ongoing bleeding (0.1 ml/min). The technetium **"tagged" RBC scan** can detect even slower rates of bleeding, and the scan can be repeated at a later time if the initial scan is negative. Most radiologists perform an RBC scan before arteriography to aid in localizing the site for injection of blood vessels.

Any patient with a lower GI bleed in whom an obvious source cannot be found should have a diagnostic **upper GI endoscopy** to rule out an upper tract source. This should be done before any surgical procedure. Nearly 20% of all "lower GI" bleeding actually has its source in the upper tract.

11. Does melena indicate a right-sided colonic source and hematochezia a left-sided source?

Usually. The color of stool depends on colonic transit time. If the stool remains in contact with bacteria that degrade hemoglobin, the resulting stool is melenic. Although right-sided lesions are usually associated with melena (dark, tarry stools) and left-sided lesions with hematochezia (passage of bright red blood per rectum), the opposite also can be seen. Therefore, the evaluation of a patient with hematochezia must include examination of the proximal colon.

Cuellar RE, et al: Gastrointestinal trace hemorrhage. Arch Intern Med 150:1381, 1990.

12. What distinguishes melena from black-colored stool?

The smell. Melenic stool is black and tarry and has a distinguishable smell. Once you smell it, you will never forget it. Stools are simply black-colored and not melenic if they lack the characteristic pungent, foul smell.

13. What impact do NSAIDs have on the GI tract and bleeding?

The traditional NSAIDs exert their anti-inflammatory and analgesic effects by inhibiting cyclooxygenase (COX) 1 and 2. COX-1 is responsible for producing the protective prostaglandins of the GI tract, which in summation lessen the chances that ulcerogenic drugs such as NSAIDs will result in erosions or ulcers. Traditional NSAIDs increase the potential of developing ulcers (gastric > duodenal) as well as the risk of bleeding from NSAID-induced ulcers. There is a 2–4% risk of developing a bleeding ulcer each year that a patient is chronically maintained on NSAIDs.

Singh G: Recent considerations in nonsteroidal anti-inflammatory drug gastropathy [review]. Am J Med 105(Suppl 1B): 31S–38S, 1998.

14. What GI lesions may be seen with chronic NSAID use?

UPPER GI	SMALL INTESTINE	COLON
Subepithelial petechial hemorrhages	Ulcers	Colitis
Erosions	Strictures	Ulcers
Ulcers	Diaphragms	Strictures
Stomach > duodenum	Enteropathy	Diverticular bleeding
Bleeding		
Stomach >> duodenum		? Collagenous colitis
Perforations/obstruction		Relapse of inflammatory bowel
Esophageal erosions/ulcers		disease

Cryer B, Kimmey MB: Gastrointestinal side effects of nonsteroidal anti-inflammatory drugs. Am J Med 105(1B):20S–30S, 1998.

15. What are the major benefits of the COX-2–specific NSAIDs?

Gastrointestinal safety! The two FDA-approved COX-2–specific NSAIDs—rofecoxib (Vioxx) and celecoxib (Celebrex)—have been documented in multiple, large-scale, placebo-controlled trials to have a much lower risk of producing GI toxicity. Rofecoxib diminishes the incidence of bleeding from peptic ulcers, perforations, and ulcers by > 50+%. Celecoxib produces a statistically less significant reduction than rofecoxib. With the added GI safety profile, studies are under way to assess the use of COX-2–specific NSAIDs in the management of other disease states in which the use of traditional NSAIDs has been limited by GI side effects. Of note, the COX-2– specific agents are no more effective as anti-inflammatory or analgesic agents than traditional NSAIDs.

Bombardier C, et al: Comparison of upper GI toxicity of refecoxib and naproxen in patients with rheumatoid arthritis. N Engl J Med 343:1520–1528, 2000.

Silverstein FE, Faigh G, Goldstein JL, et al: Gastrointestinal toxicity with celecoxib vs nonsteroidal anti-inflammatory drugs for osteoarthritis and rheumatoid arthritis. The CLASS study: A randomized controlled trial. JAMA 284:1247–1255, 2000.

16. What are the possible causes of esophageal varices?

Elevation of pressure in the hepatic portal system leads to the development of varices. The normal portal venous pressure (~10mmHg) increases to > 20mmHg in portal hypertension. The causes of portal hypertension are classified as presinusoidal, sinusoidal and postsinusoidal. The most common cause in the Western world is alcohol-related cirrhosis.

Presinusoidal: portal vein thrombosis, splenic vein thrombosis, primary biliary cirrhosis, schistosomiasis.

Sinusoidal: cirrhosis, idiopathic.

Postsinusoidal: congestive heart failure, constrictive pericarditis, hepatic vein thrombosis (Budd-Chiari syndrome), veno-occlusive disease.

17. Which two factors determine whether esophageal varices will bleed?

Portal pressure and variceal size. The portal-to-hepatic vein pressure gradient must be > 12 mmHg (normal = 3–6 mm Hg) for varices to develop. Beyond this level, there is poor correlation between portal pressure and likelihood of bleeding. The best predictor of impending variceal hemorrhage is size. When varices reach a diameter > 5 mm, they are more likely to rupture and bleed. At any given pressure, the wall of a large varix is under greater tension than the wall of a small varix and must be thicker to withstand the pressure.

18. How do you treat a patient with bleeding esophageal varices?

In patients with suspected bleeding varices, the first line of therapy after **volume resuscitation** and blood transfusion is **upper GI endoscopy**. While the patient is awaiting endoscopy, an intravenous infusion of **octreotide** (Sandostatin) should be initiated to lower portal pressure. In many instances, octredotide is highly effective in stopping or slowing bleeding until endoscopy can be performed. The objectives of endoscopic therapy are to control acute bleeding, minimize therapy-induced complications, and prevent rebleeding.

Upper GI endoscopy should be done as soon as possible to document the site of bleeding and to perform either **endoscopic esophageal sclerotherapy** (EST) or **esophageal band ligation** (EVL) if the bleeding site is found to be variceal. In EST, the endoscopist injects a sclerosing solution into and around the bleeding varix; this results in rapid occlusion of the varix by thrombus or perivariceal edema so that active bleeding ceases in 80–90% of patients. In EVL, tiny rubber bands are used to ensnare varices, causing strangulation and eventual sloughing and obliteration. Currently EVL is the preferred endoscopic method of treating esophageal varices.

If sclerotherapy or ligation is unsuccessful, the next step is **balloon tamponade** of the bleeding varices using a Sengstaken-Blakemore tube. The next step is a **transjugular intrahepatic portosystemic shunt** (TIPS) performed by an interventional radiologist (see figure on following page). **Surgery** (either a portosystemic shunt or esophageal transection) is the last resort because the mortality rate is > 50% when shunts are performed emergently.

19. What is Dieulafoy's lesion?

Dieulafoy's lesion (exulceratio simplex) is an uncommon cause of massive GI bleeding. A large submucosal artery erodes through the mucosa without overlying ulceration or other obvious mucosal damage. Dieulafoy's lesion has the potential to bleed profusely but intermittently; thus, it is easily missed at endoscopy unless it is actively bleeding. In most cases, Dieulafoy's lesion is located in the proximal stomach within 6 cm of the gastroesophageal junction, but it may occur in

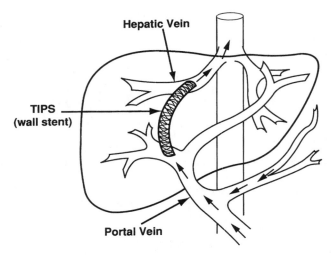

The TIPS procedure involves placement of a metallic wire stent between the hepatic and portal veins. (From McNally PR (ed): GI/Liver Secrets. Philadelphia, Hanley & Belfus, 1996, with permission.)

the antrum, duodenum, jejunum, colon, and rectum. Treatment is initially endoscopic thermal co-agulation or injection sclerotherapy. Surgical wedge resection remains the definitive management.

Dy NM, et al: Bleeding from the endoscopically identified Dieulafoy lesion of the proximal small intes-tine and colon. Am J Gastroenterol 90:108, 1994.

20. What are the major features of Meckel's diverticulum?
• Incidence: 1–3% of the population
• Usually found within 100 cm of the ileocecal valve
• Cause of 50% of cases of lower GI bleeding in children
• Rare cause for bleeding in patients older than 40 years
• Gastric mucosa is present in approximately 40%

21. How is Meckel's diverticulum diagnosed?
^{99m}Technetium scan is positive in about 75% of patients. An alternative is arteriography. Other studies are unrevealing.

22. In the patient who has undergone multiple unsuccessful evaluations for localization of recurrent occult GI bleeding, what test needs to be performed?
In patients who have had multiple upper GI endoscopies, colonoscopies, barium studies, RBC scans and arteriograms but the source of blood loss remains elusive, the test that needs to be per-formed is enteroscopy. The source of bleeding is most likely arteriovenous malformations (or an-giodysplasias), which usually hide in the small intestine. Of particular note, before a patient undergoes enteroscopy the hemoglobin should be 10 or higher to aid in detecting these tiny vessels.

LIVER AND HEPATITIS

23. What are the differences between hepatitis A, B, and C?
Hepatitis A, called infectious hepatitis, is easily spread by the fecal/oral route. The hepatitis A virus (HAV) causes a short-lived, benign, acute hepatitis that is not followed by chronic liver disease. IgG antibodies to HAV remain positive for life. To determine if the hepatitis is acute, one must look for IgM antibodies in the serum.

Hepatitis B, called serum hepatitis, is contracted by contact with blood or other bodily se-cretions from an infected patient, usually through a break in the skin or use of a contaminated needle. Unlike hepatitis A, hepatitis B may cause chronic disease and cirrhosis. It also predisposes to hepatocellular carcinoma (hepatoma). A carrier state is possible in which patients demonstrate persistent hepatitis B surface antigenemia (HBsAg) without clinically evident disease and are able to transmit the disease.

Hepatitis C previously was included in the non-A, non-B hepatitis category. It is the form of hepatitis most commonly contracted from blood transfusion. It also is the most common viral cause of chronic liver disease and increases the patient's risk for developing hepatoma (hepatocellular carcinoma). The most widely available marker of disease is anti-hepatitis C virus (HCV), which denotes chronic infection. HCV-RNA can be used to determine the level of disease activity and to measure response to therapy.

24. Which of the hepatitides is of major health concern?

Hepatitis C. It is estimated that as many as 1 in 10 persons are at risk for this potentially chronic liver disease for which there is currently no cure. More than 50% of people who have served in the U.S. armed forces are positive for hepatitis C, making the illness a priority in the federal health system. The frequency of complications associated with HCV infection is expected to triple within the next 20 years. This corresponds to a 61% increase in the incidence of cirrhosis, a 68% increase in the incidence of hepatocellular carcinoma, a 279% increase in decompensated liver disease, and a 528% increase in the demand for liver transplantation. At least one-third of all infected people have no known risks for this potentially debilitating illness.

Viral Hepatitis Guide for Practicing Physicians. Cleve Clin J Med 67(Suppl 1), 2000.

Sarbah SA, Younossi Z: Hepatitis C: An update on the silent epidemic. J Clin Gastroenterol 30:125–143, 2000.

25. How is HAV transmitted?

HAV typically is transmitted through contaminated water supplies and is most common in developing countries with poor hygiene and inadequate sanitation. Transplacental or perinatal transmission of the virus has not been documented. Homosexual men have a higher prevalence of antibodies to HAV, which suggests possible sexual transmission.

26. Describe the symptoms and duration of hepatitis A. How is it diagnosed and treated?

The symptoms of hepatitis A are relatively nonspecific and are similar to those of any cause of hepatitis: anorexia, fatigue, malaise, right-upper-quadrant abdominal discomfort, and jaundice. The duration of illness tends to vary, but most patients recover within 4 weeks of the onset of clinical disease.

Hepatitis A can be diagnosed by the detection of HAV-specific IgM in the blood; this antibody is present in all symptomatic patients. Treatment is purely supportive, and no antiviral agent accelerates recovery.

27. What are the recommendations for hepatitis A vaccination?

Children older than 2 years who are at risk, travelers to endemic areas, military personnel and others with occupational exposure, intravenous drug abusers, people with high-risk sexual practices, Native Americans and Alaskans (ethnic groups with high rates of HAV), people in communities with outbreaks of HAV, and patients with clotting factor disorders and chronic liver disease.

HAV (Havrix) vaccine

Children 2–18 years old: 360 EL.U/0.5 cc, 2 doses 1 month apart; then 0.5 cc 6–12 months after primary series.

Adults: 720 EL.U/0.5 cc, 1 dose; then 0.5 cc 6–12 months after primary series.

Vaqta (inactivated hepatitis A vaccine)

Children 2–17 years old: 25 U/0.5 cc, 1 dose, then 0.5 cc, 1 dose 6–18 months after primary dose.

Adults: 50 U/cc, 1 dose, then 50 U/cc, 1 dose, 6 months after primary dose.

Cleveland Clinic Journal of Medicine Viral Hepatitis Guide for Practicing Physicians. Clevel Clin J Med 67(Suppl 1), 2000.

28. What is the usual serologic response after naturally acquired hepatitis B infection?

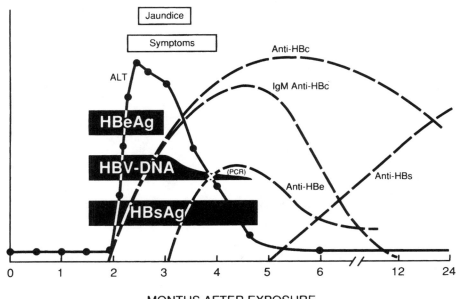

MONTHS AFTER EXPOSURE

Clinical and serologic course of a typical case of acute hepatitis B. HBsAg, hepatitis B surface antigen; HBeAg, hepatitis B e antigen; DNA-p, DNA polymerase; HBV-DNA, hepatitis B virus DNA; ALT, alanine aminotransferase (SGPT); anti-HBC, antibody to hepatitis B core antigen; anti-HBe, antibody to HBeAg; anti-HBs, antibody to HBsAg. (From Hoofnagle JH: Acute viral hepatitis. In Mandell GL, et al (eds): Principles and Practice of Infectious Diseases, 4th ed. New York, Churchill Livingstone, 1995, p 1143, with permission.)

29. Which serologic marker indicates protection in a person who has completed the hepatitis B vaccine protocol?

The currently available hepatitis B vaccine is composed only of HBsAg and induces an antibody response only to HBsAg. The anti-HBsAg response correlates well with protection against HBV infection. Of healthy persons vaccinated by the IM route, 95% develop protection against HBV.

30. How should you treat a healthcare worker with a recent (< 48 hour) needlestick exposure to hepatitis B?

The worker should receive hepatitis immunoglobulin (HBIg), 0.06 ml/kg IM, as soon as possible and within 7 days of exposure. If the worker has not previously received the hepatitis B vaccine, the vaccination program should be initiated with the usual three doses—the first dose within 14 days after exposure and again at 1 and 6 months.

31. Can HCV be sexually transmitted?

Yes. Probably about 15% of all cases result from sexual transmission, although in most cases the risk of transmission is thought to be low. In studies of monogamous relationships there was no transmission over > 20 years, but the risk increases with multiple partners and the presence of sexually transmitted diseases. There are currently no formal recommendations for barrier protection for monogamous partners, but safe-sex practices are strongly recommended.

32. How effective is treatment of hepatitis C?

Treatment options for chronic hepatitis C are limited to 3 drug classes: interferons, antiviral nucleoside analogs (ribavirin, lamivudine, famciclovir), and nonnucleoside antiviral drugs (amantidine and rimantadine). None of these achieves a curative rate of even 50%. Monotherapy with interferon has been quite disappointing with a response rate of ~15–20%, although treating patients for a minimum of 12 months slightly improved these results. Most trials have shown that combination therapy with interferon alfa-2b and ribavirin (Rebetron) is more effective than any other therapy. Length of treatment is a minimum of 6 months with monitoring of HCV-RNA, which is the most reliable indicator of response to therapy.

Maddrey WC: Safety of combination interferon alfa-2b/ribavirin therapy in chronic HCV-relapsed and treatment-naïve patients. Semin Liver Dis 19(Suppl 1):67–75, 1999.

Zdilar D, et al: Hepatitis C, interferon alfa, and depression. Hepatology 31:1207–1211, 2000.

33. How is hepatitis D virus (delta virus) transmitted?

The hepatitis D virus (HDV) is a very small RNA virus that contains a defective genome and requires HBsAg to become pathogenic. Infection may occur under two circumstances:

1. In conjunction with simultaneous infection with hepatitis B in a previously unexposed patient (coinfection)

2. In chronic carriers of HBsAg (superinfection)

Hepatitis D is diagnosed by detecting IgM antibody to HDV in acute serum or an increase in IgG antibody to HDV in convalescent serum.

34. What is hepatitis E? Hepatitis G?

Hepatitis E virus causes enterically (fecal-oral) transmitted non-A, non-B hepatitis. It is endemic to Southeast and Central Asia, Africa, and Mexico but is rare in the U.S. It is also responsible for large epidemics of acute hepatitis. It is possible that zoonotic HEV infection may occur in areas where animal hosts are abundant, including pig farming areas in the U.S. This illness is particularly severe in pregnant women, in whom mortality rates from acute liver failure may reach 20%.

Hepatitis G is an RNA virus that is transmitted primarily through blood and blood products. It frequently occurs as a coinfection with hepatitis C or other hepatitis viruses as a result of common modes of transmission. Currently no data support any role for hepatitis G in chronic or serious liver disease.

35. When should patients with acute viral hepatitis be hospitalized?

Older age	Pregnancy
Underlying systemic illnesses	Underlying chronic hepatitis of another etiology
Encephalopathy	Social problems that may result in loss of follow-up
Ascites	Worsening PT or bilirubin with improving transaminases
Bilirubin >15 mg/dl	= fulminant hepatic failure
Hypoglycemia	Volume depletion or inability to hold any fluids down
Prothrombin time (PT) >15 sec	Albumin < 3mg/dl

36. What three disorders may result in very high transaminases (> 1000)?

Ischemia, viral hepatitis, and drug-induced hepatitis.

37. What causes chronic liver disease?

Viral hepatitis B, C and D	Drug-induced hepatitis
Wilson's disease	Autoimmune hepatitis
Alcohol	Alpha$_1$ antitrypsin

NUTRITION

38. Name the six common vitamins and trace minerals and the clinical manifestations of their respective deficiency states.

Thiamine	Beriberi, muscle weakness, tachycardia, heart failure
Niacin	Pellagra, glossitis
Vitamin A	Xerophthalmia, hyperkeratosis of skin

Vitamin E	Cerebellar ataxia, areflexia
Zinc	Hypogeusia, acrodermatitis
Chromium	Glucose intolerance

39. Name the two most common nutritional deficiencies in patients with intestinal disease.

Deficiencies of folate and calcium. When the small bowel is diseased, intestinal loss of calcium is excessive, and the rate of bone resorption is insufficient to maintain serum calcium. Severe folate deficiency most often is associated with chronic alcoholism, celiac sprue, tropical sprue, and blind loop syndrome. Minor deficiencies can be found in Crohn's disease and following partial gastrectomy. Because folate absorption is largely completed in the upper small intestine, malabsorption is worse in disorders that affect the upper gut. However, any intestinal disorder accompanied by a decrease in dietary intake or rapid transport may result in folate deficiency.

40. An elderly white man presents with profound peripheral neuropathy and a markedly low serum B$_{12}$. Physical examination reveals an abdominal scar consistent with previous laparotomy, but the patient does not remember what kind of surgery was done. What two possible operations may result in B$_{12}$ deficiency? Why?

1. **Gastrectomy.** Vitamin B$_{12}$ absorption starts in the stomach. The vitamin binds to intrinsic factor and R-proteins produced in the stomach. In the duodenum, the R-proteins are hydrolyzed off the vitamin B$_{12}$ in the presence of an alkaline environment, which then allows further binding of B$_{12}$ with intrinsic factor. Vitamin B$_{12}$ cannot be absorbed unless it is bound to intrinsic factor. If the patient's stomach was completely or partially removed, he would have insufficient intrinsic factor.

2. **Terminal ileal resection.** The patient may have had Crohn's disease and undergone resection of a large portion (> 100 cm) of terminal ileum, the site of absorption of the vitamin B$_{12}$–intrinsic factor complex.

Both mechanisms of deficiency are easily treated with supplemental intramuscular vitamin B$_{12}$ injections.

41. What is the most common disorder of carbohydrate digestion in humans?

Lactase deficiency. Lactase-deficient adults retain 10–30% of intestinal lactose activity and develop symptoms (diarrhea, bloating, and gas) only when they ingest sufficient lactose. Symptoms result when the colonic bacteria metabolize lactose to methane, carbon dioxide, and short-chain fatty acids.

42. After avoiding dairy products, the patient reports resolution of symptoms. Does this confirm the diagnosis of lactose deficiency?

No. The diagnosis cannot be made simply by advising the patient to avoid dairy products for 2 weeks to determine if the altered bowel habits revert to normal, because many patients who respond to such manipulations are not lactose-deficient. The diagnostic test of choice is the lactose hydrogen breath test.

43. What are medium-chain triglycerides (MCTs)? In which intestinal diseases are they used as therapy?

MCTs are lipids containing only medium-length fatty acid chains (C6–C12). They are absorbed differently from long-chain triglycerides, which are more common in the diet. MCTs can be absorbed intact by enterocytes and pass directly into the portal circulation. Patients with a variety of small intestinal diseases—short bowel syndrome, biliary obstruction, and pancreatic insufficiency—absorb MCTs more efficiently than long-chain triglycerides.

44. Outline the fundamental principles of total parenteral nutrition (TPN).

1. Patients generally require 25–35 kcal/kg for maintenance.
2. The optimal calorie/nitrogen ratio appears to be ~160 cal/gm N.
3. The average adult requires ~30 ml water/kg body weight/day.

4. IV lipid emulsions are a suitable source of nonprotein calories that contribute to conservation of body protein. A regimen in which calories are supplied by both dextrose solution and lipid emulsions, with fat providing 20–30% of the total calories, appears to be the most effective form of parenteral nutrition.

45. What are the most common complications of TPN? How are they treated?

The most common complications are related to catheter placement and management. Examples include infections, thrombosis, nonthrombotic occlusion, and other mechanical complications during line placement. Catheter-related complications can be minimized by maintaining strict and reproducible technique as well as meticulous line care.

In prolonged TPN, especially when excessive carbohydrate calories are given, patients frequently develop liver tenderness and transaminase elevations. The increased liver values are thought to reflect hepatic steatosis. Abnormal levels of aspartate aminotransferase (AST) and alanine aminotransferase (ALT) should return to normal when TPN is discontinued. If TPN is continued, one should decrease the dextrose infusion and increase the amount of fat calories.

A complication of long-term (home) TPN is metabolic bone disease, which is similar to osteomalacia and osteoporosis. The addition of acetate or phosphate may offset the urinary calcium losses and restore positive calcium balance in these patients.

An increased incidence of cholecystitis and cholelithiasis related to gallbladder stasis is seen in patients on TPN.

46. Which vitamin deficiencies may develop in a patient maintained on long-term TPN (> 6 mo) containing only sodium, potassium, chloride, bicarbonate, glucose, and amino acids?

This TPN solution clearly is lacking in vitamins and trace minerals. In a matter of weeks, the patient would be expected to develop deficiencies in magnesium, zinc, essential fatty acids, and water-soluble vitamins (with the exception of B_{12}). Over several months, vitamin K and copper deficiencies would develop. Over a period of years, deficiencies in the fat-soluble vitamins A and D as well as selenium, chromium, and vitamin B_{12} would result.

CANCER

47. When should screening for colorectal cancer (CRC) begin?

In asymptomatic people with normal risk, screening should begin at age 50.

48. What are appropriate methods for colon cancer screening?

Beginning at age 50 every person should have a digital rectal examination (DRE) and fecal occult blood testing (FOBT). If the test is positive the patient should be referred for examination of the entire colon. Examination of the colon can be obtained either by an air contrast barium enema (ACBE), followed by flexible sigmoidoscopy to complete a thorough examination of the colon, or by colonoscopy with biopsy/removal of any abnormal lesions.

49. What is the gold standard for colon cancer screening?

The gold standard is colonoscopy. Only at colonoscopy is one able to perform polypectomy (removal of polyps) and/or biopsy of abnormal lesions or masses. If a person at normal risk undergoes colonoscopy at age 50 and the findings are normal, he or she does not require another colonoscopy for 7–10 years, unless symptoms develop.

50. What are the risk factors for CRC?

- Colon cancer in a first-degree relative < 60 years old
- Familial adenomatous polyposis (FAP)
- Dietary factors
  Low intake of fiber, fruits, vitamins E and C, beta carotene, calcium
  High intake of fat, meat, animal protein

- Cancer family syndrome
- Chronic ulcerative colitis that affects the left colon more than the right
- Hereditary nonpolyposis colon cancer (HNPCC)
- Lynch syndrome I or Lynch syndrome II
- Personal history of uterine, endometrial, or breast cancer
- Personal history of CRC or adenomatous polyp > 1cm
- Advanced age (> 80 years old)

51. Describe the natural history of CRC.

Much evidence indicates that all colon cancers develop from a polyp. The adenoma-adenocarcinoma sequence is believed to be the underlying mechanism. A mutation in the adenomatous polyposis coli (APC) gene on chromosome 5 occurs in at least 60% of spontaneous colon cancers. These mutations result in abnormalities of adhesion, migration, and replication, thereby leading to the growth of a microadenoma, which over time becomes larger and potentially malignant. It takes an average of 7 years for a polyp to develop into a cancer, allowing ample time for screening and prevention. Yet colon cancer is the second most frequent cause of cancer death in the U.S.

52. What is the significance of an adenomatous polyp?

Adenomatous polyps are neoplastic polyps found most often in the colon; they give rise to symptoms only when they become large. Often they are detected incidentally on colonoscopic exam or barium enema. Their importance relates to their malignant potential; nearly all colonic carcinomas arise from adenomatous polyps. Approximately 75% of adenomatous polyps are tubular adenomas, 15% are tubulovillous adenomas, and the rest are villous adenomas. Villous tumors are more likely to be malignant than tubular adenomas. Other factors that relate to malignant potential include tumor size > 1 cm, degree of cellular atypia, and number of polyps present.

Adenomatous polyps should be removed with endoscopic polypectomy. Affected patients should undergo colonoscopy at routine intervals so that additional polyps may be removed before they progress to malignancy.

53. What is the recommended follow-up if a polyp is detected on screening colonoscopy?

Follow-up depends upon the pathology of the polyp:

Hyperplastic polyps	No follow-up (no malignant potential unless the polyp is > 2 cm)
Adenomatous polyps	Every 3 years until negative; then every 5 years
Villous polyps	Every 1–2 years until negative; then every 5 years

54. A patient presents with an "apple core" lesion in the sigmoid colon, which on biopsy is found to be adenocarcinoma. Which tests should be included in the routine preoperative evaluation?

If carcinoma is detected by either radiographs or sigmoidoscopy, a full colonoscopic exam should be done because of the high incidence of synchronous lesions. Half of patients with a single cancer of the colon have additional polyps, which may require modification of treatment.

Endoscopic ultrasound (EUS) is fast becoming the gold standard for preoperative staging. The accuracy of EUS in experienced hands is > 90%, and the information gained allows the surgeon to plan well the surgical approach.

Preoperative serum carcinoembryonic antigen (CEA), liver aminotransferases, and alkaline phosphatase tests should be ordered. If the preoperative CEA is elevated, it usually falls to a normal level postoperatively if all tumor has been removed. Patients with a rising CEA level after total resection should be suspected of having a recurrence. Elevated AST and ALT levels suggest clinically silent liver metastases, and an elevated alkaline phosphatase may point to bone metastases.

An abdominal CT scan should be performed with and without contrast to exclude clinically silent liver metastases. The presence of metastases does not prevent palliative surgery, but it does affect postoperative therapy.

55. Are there any options for chemoprevention of colon cancer?

Yes. Currently the use of NSAIDs in chemoprevention of colon cancer is an area of intense research. Studies have consistently found that the regular use of NSAIDS is associated with a reduced risk of colon cancer (regular use = 4 days /week for 3+ months). The preventive effect probably resuls from COX-2 inhibition. Celecoxib (Celebrex), a COX-2–selective NSAID, has been approved by the FDA for use in familial adenomatous polyposis (FAP). It reduces the number of adenomatous polyps in this syndrome. Ongoing studies with rofecoxib (Vioxx) the only other FDA-approved COX-2–selective NSAID, are showing similar results. In the not too distant future it is likely that these and other COX-2–selective agents may be prescribed to aid in preventing colon cancer in patients at increased risk.

Smalley W et al: Use of nonsteroidal anti-inflammatory drugs and incidence of colorectal cancer. Arch Intern Med 159:161–166, 1999.

56. Name the most common malignant neoplasms of the small intestine.

Adenocarcinoma	45%
Carcinoid	34%
Leiomyosarcoma	18%
Lymphoma	3%

57. What are the most common benign neoplasms of the small intestine?

Adenoma > leiomyoma > lipoma.

INFLAMMATORY BOWEL DISEASE

58. Explain the differential diagnosis in a young patient with Crohn's disease of the ileum who presents with right-upper-quadrant discomfort and jaundice.

In the patient with inflammatory bowel disease (IBD) who presents with jaundice, the diagnostic considerations include pericholangitis, sclerosing cholangitis, choledocholithiasis, and primary hepatocellular disease. Pericholangitis is a histologic finding representing inflammatory changes of the small bile ductules and may be one end of the spectrum of sclerosing cholangitis. Sclerosing cholangitis is focal narrowing and inflammation of the intra- and extrahepatic biliary tree. These diseases have been reported only with IBD affecting the colon and are much more common with ulcerative colitis than with Crohn's colitis.

A more likely consideration is choledocholithiasis. Patients with longstanding ileal disease or ileal resection are unable to resorb bile salts and therefore have a diminished bile salt pool. This results in supersaturation of bile with cholesterol with subsequent precipitation of cholesterol crystals and gallstone formation. With these possibilities in mind, the patient should be evaluated for extrahepatic duct obstruction or hepatocellular disease.

59. How do Crohn's disease and ulcerative colitis differ?

Distinguishing Features of Ulcerative Colitis and Crohn's Disease

	CROHN'S DISEASE	ULCERATIVE COLITIS
Symptoms	Pain is more common; bleeding is uncommon	Diarrhea with a bloody-mucosal discharge, cramping
Location	Can affect the GI tract from mouth to anus	Limited to colon
Pattern of colonic involvement	Skip lesions	Continuous involvement, rectum always involved
Histology	Transmural inflammation, granulomas, focal ulceration	Mucosal inflammation, crypt abscesses, crypt distortion

Table continued on following page

Distinguishing Features of Ulcerative Colitis and Crohn's Disease (Continued)

	CROHN'S DISEASE	ULCERATIVE COLITIS
Radiologic	Terminal ileal involvement, deep ulcerations, normal haustra between involved areas, strictures, fistulas	Rectum involved, shortened colon, absence of haustra (lead-pipe sign)
Complications	Obstruction, fistulas, abscesses, kidney stones, gallstones, B_{12} deficiency	Bleeding, toxic megacolon, colon cancer

60. What are the pathologic gold standards for differentiating between Crohn's disease and ulcerative colitis?

The finding of a granuloma = Crohn's disease. The finding of crypt abscesses = ulcerative colitis. These findings are documented in fewer than one-third of patients but, when present, are believed to be pathognomonic of these diseases.

61. Are patients with Crohn's disease at increased risk for the development of GI cancers?

Yes, although the increased risk is less well documented with Crohn's disease than with ulcerative colitis. The overall relative risk is believed to be as high as 10-fold above the risk in the general population. Crohn's disease also increases the risk for carcinoma of the small bowel.

62. What are complications of IBD?
- Colon cancer
- Nutritional deficiencies
- Failure to thrive in children
- Intestinal perforation or stricture
- Toxic megacolon
- Cytomegalovirus colitis

63. What are the extraintestinal manifestations of IBD?

Arthritis, ankylosing spondylitis, sacroiliitis, osteoporosis, erythema nodosum, pyoderma gangrenosum, aphthous ulcers, iritis, uveitis, episcleritis, fatty liver, gallstones, pericholangitis, sclerosing cholangitis, cholangiocarcinoma, kidney stones, venous thrombosis, weight loss, hypoalbuminemia, anemia, vitamin and electrolyte abnormalities.

ULCERS

64. What are the two major functions of acid secretion in the stomach?

1. Acid activates the enzyme pepsin by converting pepsinogen to pepsin, initiating the first stages of protein digestion.

2. Acid serves as an antibacterial barrier to protect the stomach from colonization.

65. How does the pathogenesis of duodenal and gastric ulcers differ?

Duodenal ulcer disease, with a peak incidence in young adults, has frequent recurrences over a period of 10–20 years. The precise pathogenesis is not completely understood but has been associated with the following:
- *Helicobacter pylori* infection in > 90% of cases. Recurrence rates are dramatically reduced after eradication of the bacteria.
- Increased acid secretion that correlates with an increased number of parietal cells in the gastric mucosa.
- Increased responsiveness of the parietal cells of the stomach to stimulation factors, such as food, gastric acid, or histamine.
- Increased vagal activity.

Gastric ulcer disease, with a peak incidence in the elderly, is not associated with these factors. Patients have normal or even decreased gastric acid secretion. Gastric ulcers probably develop because of a change in the mucosal resistance to the acid. NSAIDs play a prominent role in the etiology of gastric (more than duodenal) ulcer disease.

66. What are the five major indications for peptic ulcer surgery?

1. **Intractability** relates to symptoms, not to delayed healing. The diagnosis of intractability requires clinical confirmation that an ulcer is responsible for the patient's symptoms.

2. **Hemorrhage.** Surgery to control bleeding is occasionally necessary but carries a high mortality rate. It should be considered in patients who require a large-volume blood transfusion (6–8 units/24 hr) to correct losses, who have one or more rebleeding episodes in the hospital, or who have persistent bleeding requiring transfusion over 48–72 hours in the hospital.

3. **Perforation** requires immediate surgery.

4. **Penetration** represents erosion of an ulcer through the entire thickness of the wall of the stomach or intestine without leakage of digestive contents into the peritoneal cavity. The diagnosis is usually suggested by a change in symptoms, and treatment is surgical if complicated penetration exists.

5. **Obstruction.** Gastric outlet obstruction occurs in 2% of all patients with ulcer disease. Standard therapy has been surgical, but endoscopic balloon dilatation of the stenotic pylorus may be another possibility.

67. What are the reasons for recurrent ulcers in patients who have undergone previous ulcer surgery?

• Untreated *H. pylori* infection
• NSAID use
• Incomplete vagotomy
• Adjacent nonabsorbable suture that acts as an irritant
• "Retained antrum" syndrome, in which antral tissue left behind at surgery produces a continued source of gastric production
• Antral G-cell hyperplasia (uncommon)
• Zollinger-Ellison syndrome (gastrinoma)
• Gastric cancer

Other factors that may contribute to recurrent ulcers but have not necessarily been implicated as primary causes include smoking, enterogastric reflux (bile acid reflux), primary hyperparathyroidism, and gastric bezoar.

68. What are the most common causes of peptic ulcer disease in order of frequency?

1. *H. pylori* infection (duodenal >> gastric)
2. Traditional NSAIDs (gastric >> duodenal)
3. Hyperacidity states (e.g., Zollinger-Ellison syndrome)

69. What is *H. pylori* infection?

H. pylori infection is the most infectious disease worldwide. It is estimated that 1 in 10 persons are infected. This microaerophilic spiral bacterium inhabits the mucus layer of the stomach. It is associated with the development of peptic ulcer disease in up to 90+% of patients with duodenal ulcers. Although millions are infected only ~10% develop peptic ulcer disease.

70. Which diseases are strongly associated with *H. pylori* infection?

Peptic ulcer disease (duodenal >> gastric)
Chronic active gastritis
MALToma (mucosa-associated lymphoid tissue)
Gastric carcinoma

71. What methods are used to test for *H. pylori*?

• Urea breath test (UBT)
• Serology (enzyme-linked immunosorbent assay [ELISA] IgG)

- Endoscopy with biopsy or with rapid urease testing (RUT)
- Urine, fecal, or salivary detection of *H. pylori* (still undergoing validation but less sensitive and specific)

The most sensitive and specific tests are the UBT and endoscopy with biopsy/RUT. Both tests have sensitivity and specificity > 95%. The major difference is that endoscopy is obviously an invasive test. The serologic tests can determine infection but cannot be used to follow a patient for documentation of cure because titers may remain high for several months to years. The best test for follow-up is either UBT or endoscopy.

72. What is the treatment for *H. pylori* infection?

Over 60 treatment regimens have been used. Triple therapy (two antibiotics plus a proton pump inhibitor) is the gold standard, resulting in eradication of > 90% of the organism. At present no regimen results in 100% cure. It is prudent to know the resistance rates to antibiotics in the population of patients being treated so that adjustments may be made. In addition, no resistance to bismuth has yet been documented. The following is a typical *H. pylori* regimen (eradication rate of 90–95%):

Clarithromycin, 250 mg (2 tablets orally twice daily)

Amoxicillin, 500 mg (2 tablets orally twice daily)

Lansoprazole, 30 mg orally twice daily; omeprazole, 20 mg orally twice daily; or rabeprazole (20 mg twice daily)

73. What is the most common presenting sign of peptic ulcer disease in the elderly?

Melena. The majority of patients are asymptomatic until they present with GI bleeding. A fatal hemorrhagic event may be the first sign of an ulcer in the elderly. Of note, a high percentage of elderly are at risk as a direct result of the use of traditional NSAIDs. Elderly people who ingest NSAIDs account for the majority of patients who succumb to GI bleeding.

74. What is the clinical triad of the Zollinger-Ellison syndrome (ZES)?

Gastric acid hypersecretion, severe ulcer disease of the upper GI tract as a direct result of acid hypersecretion, and a non-β cell tumor of the pancreas that secretes the hormone gastrin (gastrinoma). The other common feature of ZES is diarrhea, which may precede the diagnosis of ZES by many years. The diagnosis should be suspected in patients with a compatible clinical history and gastric acid hypersecretion.

PANCREATITIS

75. What are the most common causes of acute pancreatitis in the U.S.?

Acute pancreatitis is due to choledocholithiasis, ethanol abuse, or idiopathic causes in 90% of cases in the U.S. Most patients who previously were believed to have idiopathic pancreatitis have been found to have diminutive gallstones (microlithiasis) as the cause. In the private hospital setting, 50% of patients with acute pancreatitis have gallstones (gallstone pancreatitis). In public hospitals, up to 66% of first episodes are caused by excessive alcohol consumption.

Marshall JB: Acute pancreatitis: A review with emphasis on new developments. Arch Intern Med 153:1185, 1993.

76. Which drugs can cause acute pancreatitis?

Strongest association: asparaginase, azathioprine, 6-mercaptopurine, ddI, pentamadine

Analgesics: acetaminophen, piroxicam, (?) NSAIDs

Diuretics: furosemide, thiazides, metolazone

Antibiotics: sulfonamides, tetracyclines, erythromycin

Anti-inflammatory agents: salicylates, 5-ASA products, sulfasalazine, corticosteroids, cyclosporine

Toxins: ethanol, methanol

Hormones: estrogens, oral contraceptive pills (OCPs)

Others: octreotide, cimetidine, ranitidine, valproic acid, ergotamine, methyldopa, zalcitabine, isotretinoin

77. List Ranson's criteria for the prognosis in acute pancreatitis.

Ranson initially published prognostic criteria for acute pancreatitis in 1974. They are still used today. When there are fewer than three positive signs, the patient has mild disease and an excellent prognosis. The mortality rate is 10–20% with 3–5 signs and 50% with 6 or more signs.

Prognostic Criteria in Acute Pancreatitis

ON ADMISSION	IN INITIAL 48 HOURS
Age > 55 yr	Hematocrit decrease > 10%
White blood cell count > 16,000/mm^3	Blood urea nitrogen increase > 5 mg/dl
Serum lactate dehydrogenase > 350 IU/L	Serum calcium < 8 mg/dl
Blood glucose > 200 mg/dl	Partial pressure of oxygen in arterial blood < 60 mmHg
AST > 250 IU/L	Base deficit > 4 mEq/L
	Estimated fluid sequestration > 6 L

Ranson JH: Etiologic and prognostic factors in human acute pancreatitis: A review. Am J Gastroenterol 77:633, 1982.

78. What are the causes of an increase in serum amylase?

Several conditions other than acute pancreatitis can cause an increase in serum amylase:

Macroamylasemia

Renal failure

Mesenteric infarction

Parotitis

Burns

Cholecystitis

Endoscopic retrograde cholangiopancreatography (ERCP)

Perforated peptic ulcer disease

Ruptured ectopic pregnancy

Diabetic ketoacidosis

Peritonitis

Tumors of pancreas, salivary glands, ovary,
  lung, prostate

Pancreatitis complications (pseudocyst, abscess,
  ascites)

79. What are Cullen's and Grey Turner's signs?

These signs are associated with acute hemorrhagic pancreatitis:

Cullen's sign: ecchymotic discoloration in the umbilicus

Grey Turner's sign: ecchymotic discoloration around the flanks

80. How is gallstone pancreatitis treated?

Gallstone or biliary pancreatitis refers to acute pancreatitis resulting from choledocholithiasis. Most patients are elderly, appear seriously ill, and have a bilirubin > 3.0 mg/dl and amylase >500 IU. Imaging studies such as ultrasound document dilated biliary ducts or the presence of cholelithiasis in most patients. The initial management is conservative therapy with IV antibiotics, nothing per mouth (NPO), and close monitoring. Patients who do not respond within 48 hours are deemed to have severe pancreatitis and ERCP is performed. ERCP can document the offending stone and provide definitive therapy, such as sphincterotomy with stone removal. After resolution of the acute symptoms, the patient should undergo a cholecystectomy, as the recurrence rate is > 35% within 6–8 weeks after the index attack.

Fan ST, et al: Early therapy of acute biliary pancreatitis by endoscopic papillotomy. N Engl J Med 328:228, 1993.

VASCULAR DISEASE

81. What is intestinal angina?

When occlusive vascular disease, usually atherosclerosis, affects two of the three major arteries supplying the gut, it may be associated with a syndrome of intermittent, cramping, midabdominal pain commonly called intestinal angina. Symptoms worsen during eating, often causing patients to lose weight simply by avoiding meals or eating small meals. The diagnosis is facilitated by angiography, which documents significant stenosis of vessels. Treatment for patients with a significant gradient across the stenosis is surgical bypass, endarterectomy, or percutaneous transluminal angioplasty.

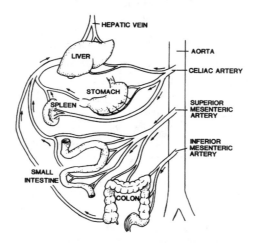

Major splanchnic organs and blood vessels. (From McNally PR (ed): GI/Liver Secrets. Philadelphia, Hanley & Belfus, 1996, with permission.

82. Which two colonic segments are most commonly involved in ischemic colitis? Why?

Ischemic colitis most commonly occurs in the regions lying in the "watershed" areas between two adjacent arterial supplies. These are the **splenic flexure**, which lies between the inferior and superior mesenteric arteries, and the **rectosigmoid junction**, which lies between the inferior mesenteric and interior iliac arteries.

Brandt LJ, et al: Colonic ischemia. Surg Clin North Am 72:203, 1992.

83. What are the classic signs and symptoms of ischemic colitis?

1. Sudden onset of mild, crampy, left-sided abdominal pain
2. Painless hematochezia within 24 hours of onset of pain

DIARRHEA

84. What differentiates osmotic from secretory diarrhea? Give examples of each.

Osmotic diarrhea is caused by ingestion of excessive amounts of a poorly absorbable but osmotically active solute. Commonly implicated substances include mannitol or sorbitol (seen in patients chewing large quantities of sugar-free gum), magnesium sulfate (Epsom salt), and some magnesium-containing antacids. Carbohydrate malabsorption also may cause osmotic diarrhea through the action of unabsorbed sugars (lactulose). Clinically, osmotic diarrhea stops when the patient fasts (or stops ingesting the poorly absorbable solute).

Secretory diarrhea involves a disruption of normal bowel function. Small intestinal epithelial cells normally secrete less than they absorb, ultimately leading to a net absorption of fluid and electrolytes. If this process is interrupted by a pathologic process that stimulates increased secretion or inhibits absorption, secretory diarrhea may result. Causes of secretory diarrhea include enterotoxin-mediated secretion, as with *Vibrio cholerae* and enterotoxigenic *Escherichia coli* infection; hormone production by tumors such as VIPomas; and use of laxatives containing phenolphthalein. Unabsorbed bile acids and fatty acids also may induce colonic secretion and diarrhea.

Fedorak RN, et al: Basic investigation of a patient with diarrhea. In Field M (ed): Textbook of Diarrheal Diseases. New York, Elsevier, 1991, pp. 191–218.

85. Which three diagnostic features can distinguish secretory from osmotic diarrhea?

1. The stool osmolar gap is < 50 mOsm/kg in secretory diarrhea but > 50 mOsm/kg in osmotic diarrhea. Normal stool osmolality is ~290 mOsm/kg.

2. Secretory diarrhea is typically unrelated to ingested foods or solutes and persists during a 24–72-hour fast, whereas osmotic diarrhea stops when ingestion of the offending solute ends.

3. Patients with a pure secretory diarrhea do not have WBCs, RBCs, or fat in the stool.

86. What are the two basic mechanisms by which bacteria cause infectious diarrhea? Give examples of each type.

1. **Enterotoxigenic.** Bacteria adhere to the mucosa and then secrete an enterotoxin that stimulates epithelial cell secretion. Examples include enterotoxigenic *E. coli* (ETEC) and *V. cholerae.*

2. **Enteroinvasive.** Organisms adhere to epithelial cells in preparation for invasion of the mucosa. Many of the invasive organisms also release toxins that stimulate secretion by the intestinal cell, but by a mechanism that does not involve activation of adenylate cyclase. Organisms that invade the mucosa and result in diarrhea include *Salmonella* spp., *Shigella* spp., enteroinvasive *E. coli* (EIEc), *Campylobacter* spp., and *Yersinia* spp.

The toxigenic bacteria do not induce visible changes in the intestinal mucosa during infection. In contrast, mucosal damage, inflammatory infiltrate, and ulceration are commonly seen with the invasive organisms. For this reason, fecal leukocytes are typically present in infections with enteroinvasive organisms, whereas few or no WBCs are seen in the stool of patients infected with enterotoxigenic organisms.

87. What organisms are responsible for bacillary dysentery?

The term *dysentery* refers to a diarrheal stool that contains inflammatory exudate (pus) and blood. Bacillary dysentery refers to infectious diarrhea caused by invasive pathogens, most commonly *Shigella, Salmonella,* and *Campylobacter* spp. and enteroinvasive or enterohemorrhagic *E. coli.*

88. A 50-year-old woman complains of 6–8 loose stools per day for 1 month. The cause is not immediately evident after a careful history and physical exam. What diagnostic tests should be performed at this stage?

If performed early in the disease course, a complete blood count, serum chemistry profile, and urinalysis may help to pinpoint the likely causes of diarrhea. For example, the patient who has an anemia with a very high mean corpuscular volume may be suspected of having malabsorption and diarrhea based on the presence of ileal disease and inability to absorb vitamin B_{12}.

Basic stool studies, including bacterial culture and sensitivity, Sudan stain for fat, Wright's stain for WBCs, test for occult blood, and a phenolphthalein test for the presence of laxative ingestion, are simple and quickly obtainable tests that may give valuable results.

Proctosigmoidoscopy is an important part of the examination in most patients with chronic and recurrent diarrhea. Examination of the rectal mucosa may reveal pseudomembranes seen with antibiotic-associated diarrhea, discrete ulceration typical of amebiasis, or a diffusely inflamed granular mucosa seen in ulcerative colitis. Biopsy specimens can be obtained through the scope for histologic examination, and fresh stool samples can be collected for cultures.

89. When do you become concerned about diarrhea?

Age > 70	Immunocompromised patient
> 6 stools per day	Abdominal cramps
Tenesmus	Fever
Dysentery	GI bleeding
Hypotension or tachycardia	Signs of severe dehydration: dry mucous membranes
Oliguria	and poor skin turgor

90. What is travelers' diarrhea? How do you prevent it?

Travelers' diarrhea is a common term given to the onset of diarrhea in patients who have traveled to other countries, usually in the third world, where the enteric flora are different. Eighty percent of the cases of travelers' diarrhea are caused by bacteria that can be transmitted via a fecal-oral route. Travelers should carefully select, handle, and prepare food and dairy products. Everything should be washed thoroughly and freshly cooked. Commercially bottled water, carbonated beverages, and beer are safe – but ice is not! Medical prophylaxis includes either of the following regimens:

Bismuth subsalicylate, 2 tablets 4 times/day
Trimethoprim-sulfamethoxazole, 1 ds tablet/day
Ciprofloxacin, 500 mg/day (or one of the other fluoroquinolones)

91. How does the time of onset of illness relate to the possible causes of food poisoning?

ONSET	SYMPTOMS AND SIGNS	AGENTS
<1 hr	Nausea, vomiting, abdominal cramps	Heavy metal poisoning (copper, zinc, tin, cadmium)
< 1 hr	Paresthesias	Scrombroid poisoning, shellfish poisoning, Chinese restaurant syndrome (MSG), niacin poisoning
1–6 hr	Nausea and vomiting	Preformed toxins of *Staphylococcus aureus* and *Bacillus cereus*
2 hr	Delirium, parasympathetic hyperactivity, hallucinations, disulfiram reaction, or gastroenteritis	Toxic mushroom ingestion
8–16 hr	Abdominal cramps, diarrhea	In vivo production of enterotoxins by *Clostridium perfringens* and *B. cereus*
6–24 hr	Abdominal cramps, diarrhea, followed by hepatorenal failure	Toxic mushroom ingestion (*Amanita* spp.)
16–48 hr	Fever, abdominal cramps, diarrhea	*Salmonella* and *Shigella* spp., *Clostridium jejuni*, invasive *Escherichia coli*, *Yersinia enterocolitica, Vibrio parahemolyticus*
16–72 hr	Abdominal cramps, diarrhea	Norwalk agent and related viruses, enterotoxins produced by *Vibrio* spp., *E. coli*, and occasionally *Salmonella* and *Shigella* spp., and *C. jejuni*
18–36 hr	Nausea, vomiting, diarrhea, paralysis	Food-borne botulism
72–100 hr	Bloody diarrhea without fever	Enterotoxigenic *E. coli*, most frequently serotype O157:H7
1–3 wk	Chronic diarrhea	Raw milk ingestion

Mandell GL, et al (eds): Principles and Practice of Infectious Diseases, 4th ed. New York, Churchill Livingstone, 1995, with permission.

NONHEPATITIS LIVER DISEASE

92. List the common causes of jaundice in pregnant patients.
- Viral hepatitis A, B, C, and E (accounts for 50%)
- Acute fatty liver of pregnancy
- HELLP syndrome (**h**emolysis, **e**levated **l**iver enzymes, **l**ow **p**latelets)
- Toxemia (preeclampsia or eclampsia)
- Cholestasis of pregnancy
- Cholelithiasis/choledocholithiasis
- Drug-induced liver disease

93. Describe the two predominant forms of alcoholic liver injury. Which one may progress to cirrhosis?

Mild alcoholism impairs the excretion of triglyceride from hepatocytes, resulting in the typical fatty liver with fat globules in parenchymal cells. The fatty liver of alcoholism generally causes hepatomegaly and minimal elevations in aminotransferases. Jaundice is rarely seen unless the disease progresses to severe hepatocellular failure.

The more severe form of alcoholic liver injury is alcoholic hepatitis, characterized by focal necrosis of liver cells. Clusters of neutrophils and Mallory bodies (clumps of hyaline) can be seen on liver biopsy. The lesions of alcoholic hepatitis characteristically occur in the center of the lobule and are accompanied by fibrosis. In its severe form, manifestations include marked jaundice and transaminase elevations (up to 10 times normal), which may be accompanied by impaired synthesis of coagulation proteins leading to a prolonged prothrombin time. Typically, in alcoholic hepatitis, unlike viral hepatitis, the AST is greater than the ALT and the AST:ALT ratio is > 2:1. Alcoholic hepatitis may progress to cirrhosis. Alcohol abuse is the most frequent cause of cirrhosis in the U.S.

94. What are Child-Pugh's Criteria for the staging of the patient with cirrhosis?

PARAMETER	SCORE 1	SCORE 2	SCORE 3
Albumin	> 3.5	2.8–3.5	< 2.8
Bilirubin	< 2.0	2.0 - 3.0	> 3.0
Prolongation of PT	< 4 sec	4–6 sec	> 6 sec
Ascites	Absent	Moderate	Massive
Encephalopathy	None	Moderate (controlled by diuretics)	Severe
Child's Score:	A = 5-6	B = 7–9	C = > 9

PT = prothrombin time.

95. What are the clinical manifestations of liver disease and their pathogenetic basis?

SIGN/SYMPTOM	PATHOGENESIS	LIVER DISEASE
Constitutional		
Fatigue, anorexia, malaise, weight loss	Liver failure	Severe acute or chronic hepatitis Cirrhosis
Fever	Hepatic inflammation or infection	Liver abscess Alcoholic hepatitis Viral hepatitis
Fetor hepaticus	Abnormal methionine metabolism	Acute or chronic liver failure
Cutaneous		
Spider telangiectasias, palmar erythema	Altered estrogen and androgen metabolism	Cirrhosis
Jaundice	Diminished bilirubin excretion	Biliary obstruction Severe liver disease
Pruritus		Biliary obstruction
Xanthomas/xanthelasma	Increased serum lipids	Biliary obstruction/cholestasis
Endocrine		
Gynecomastia, testicular atrophy, diminished libido	Altered estrogen and androgen metabolism	Cirrhosis
Hypoglycemia	Decreased glycogen stores and gluconeogenesis	Liver failure

Table continued on following page

SIGN/SYMPTOM	PATHOGENESIS	LIVER DISEASE
Gastrointestinal		
RUQ abdominal pain	Liver swelling, infection	Acute hepatitis
		Hepatocellular carcinoma
		Liver congestion (heart failure)
		Acute cholecystitis
		Liver abscess
Abdominal swelling	Ascites	Cirrhosis, portal hypertension
GI bleeding	Esophageal varices	Portal hypertension
Hematologic		
Decreased RBCs, WBCs, and/or platelets	Hypersplenism	Cirrhosis, portal hypertension
Ecchymoses	Decreased synthesis of clotting factors	Liver failure
Neurologic		
Altered sleep pattern, subtle behavioral changes, somno-lence, confusion, ataxia, asterixis, obtundation	Hepatic encephalopathy	Liver failure, portosystemic shunting of blood

RUQ = right upper quadrant, RBCs = red blood cells, WBCs = white blood cells.
From Andreoli TE, et al: Cecil Essentials of Medicine, 2nd ed. Philadelphia, W.B. Saunders, 1990, p 312, with permission.

96. A patient with known cirrhosis of the liver presents with massive swelling of his abdomen. A fluid wave can be elicited on examination of the abdomen by striking one flank and feeling the transmitted wave on the opposite flank. What is the appropriate diagnostic procedure at this point?

After the diagnosis of new-onset ascites is made on physical exam, all patients should undergo abdominal paracentesis and ascitic fluid analysis. A small amount of fluid is aspirated from the midline of the abdomen between the umbilicus and pubis with a small-gauge needle. The most important tests to order are the albumin and cell count.

The serum albumin value should be measured within a few hours of the paracentesis to ensure accuracy. Ascitic fluid with a serum:ascitic fluid albumin gradient (S-A AG) > 1.1 gm/dl is designated as **high-gradient ascites**, whereas ascitic fluid with values < 1.1 gm/dl is designated as **low-gradient ascites**. Diseases usually associated with high-gradient ascites include portal hypertension (i.e., cirrhosis), congestive heart failure, constrictive pericarditis, inferior vena cava obstruction, hypoalbuminemia, Meigs' syndrome, myxedema, fulminant hepatic failure, nephrotic syndrome (occasionally), and mixed ascites. Low-albumin gradient ascites is commonly seen with peritoneal neoplasms, pancreatic ascites, tuberculosis, nephrotic syndrome, ascites due to bowel obstruction or infarction, and ascites in connective tissue diseases. The terms high-albumin gradient and low-albumin gradient should replace the terms transudative and exudative in the description of ascites.

A large number of RBCs in the fluid or grossly bloody ascites suggests neoplasm. An ascitic fluid and WBC count > 500/ml is strongly suggestive of a peritoneal infection or an inflammatory process. Other tests to be ordered in the appropriate clinical settings include cytologic examination, lactic dehydrogenase, specific tumor markers, glucose, and cultures for bacteria, mycobacteria, and fungi.

Friedman LS, et al: Work-up of the patient with ascites. Hosp Med 31:11, 1995.

97. What pathogenetic mechanisms are responsible for ascites formation in patients with cirrhosis?

Ascites forms when there is a disturbance in the normal balance between the formation and reabsorption of peritoneal fluid in the direction of net formation. Factors that lead to this imbalance in cirrhotic patients are as follows:

1. Increased hydrostatic pressure in the portal circulation due to increased resistance to flow through the cirrhotic liver favors net leakage of fluid into the extravascular space.

2. Increased renal sodium and water retention due to:
   a. Secondary hyperaldosteronism
   b. Increased antidiuretic hormone (ADH) release

3. Impaired hepatic and splanchnic removal of lymphatic fluid due to elevated hepatic sinusoidal pressure.

4. Decreased intravascular oncotic pressure due to decreased hepatic protein (albumin and others) synthesis.

5. Increased plasma vasopressin and epinephrine levels with resultant vasomotor changes.

98. What are the routine tests ordered on a sample obtained from a paracentesis?

RBC count, cell differential, Gram stain, culture and sensitivity, protein, albumin, and glucose.

99. List the treatments available for ascites.

1. Sodium restriction to 22 mEq/day (0.5 gm NaCl)
2. Removal by paracentesis
3. Fluid restriction, if dilutional hyponatremia occurs
4. Diuretic agents, if dietary restriction does not suffice
   a. Potassium-sparing agents: spironolactone, triamterene
   b. Loop diuretics: furosemide, ethacrynic acid, bumetanide
5. TIPS
6. Peritoneovenous (LeVeen) shunts
7. Extracorporeal ultrafiltration
8. Liver transplantation

Runyon BA: Care of patients with ascites. N Engl J Med 330:337, 1995.

100. How common is drug-induced liver disease?

More than 600 medicines have been reported to cause liver injury. Drug-induced liver disease accounts for 2–5% of hospital admissions for jaundice in the U.S. and 10–20% of cases of fulminant liver failure. Acetaminophen and alcohol are the two most common offending agents.

101. How is acetaminophen toxic to the liver? At what dose?

Acetaminophen is toxic to the liver only when taken in excessive doses or when the protective detoxifying pathway in the liver is overwhelmed. Accumulation of the toxic metabolic, N-acetyl-p-benzoquinone, is responsible for death of hepatocytes. Hepatotoxicity of acetaminophen occurs in nonalcoholic patients at doses > 7.5 gm. A potentially lethal effect is seen with ingestion of > 140 mg/kg (10 gm in a 70-kg man). Chronic alcoholics are at greater risk of acetaminophen injury due to alcohol induction of the cytochrome P450 system and attendant malnutrition and low levels of glutathione. Glutathione is an intracellular protectant naturally found in the hepatocyte. Acetaminophen is the second most common cause of death from poisoning in the United States.

102. What are the indications for liver transplantation?

Advanced cirrhosis	Fulminant hepatic failure
Metabolic liver disease	Cholestatic disorders
Alcoholic liver disease	Hepatic malignancies

103. What is hereditary hemochromatosis (HHC)?

Most patients with HHC are never correctly diagnosed. It is as common as sickle cell disease, affecting an estimated 500,000 to 1,000,000 patients of all races. It is a disorder characterized by inappropriately high iron absorption due to abnormal allele(s) on chromosome 6. Patients with HHC absorb twice as much iron per day (2–4 gm) compared with normal people (1–2 gm), which over time accumulates in the liver and heart and affects other body systems. In the past the classic triad of HHC was bronze skin, diabetes, and hepatomegaly. Currently the disease is diagnosed by documentation of increased iron stores, exclusion of other causes of iron overload, and identification of a familiar pattern of iron overload.

104. What is the best radiologic test for diagnosing HHC?

Magnetic resonance imaging (MRI) offers the best noninvasive method for estimating hepatic iron content. In the MRI of the abdomen, the liver of patients with HHC has an intensity level resulting in a bright color compared with the other organs as a result of the increased iron stores. MRI has still not replaced liver biopsy and quantitative iron stores, but this finding on MRI has been found to be an accurate assessment of hepatic iron overload.

ESOPHAGEAL DISEASE

105. Describe the approach to treatment of gastroesophageal reflux disease (GERD).
  1. **Dietary and lifestyle changes**
     a. Postural therapy
        • Elevate head of bed 6–8 inches
        • Avoid lying down after eating; remain upright for at least 2 hours after eating (most important lifestyle change)
     b. Limit intake of foods and drink that reduce lower esophageal sphincter (LES) pressure:
• Fatty foods	• Peppermint
• Acidic foods	• Caffeine
• Onions	• Alcohol
• Chocolate	• Tomato-based sauces and foods
     c. Avoid medications that reduce LES pressure:
• Theophylline	• Calcium channel blockers
• Nitrates	• Anticholinergic agents
• Tranquilizers	• β-Adrenergic agonists
• Progesterone	
     d. Stop smoking
     e. Decrease the size of meals
     f. Weight reduction (if obese)
  2. **Antisecretory agents** (H_2 antagonists)
  3. **Proton pump inhibitors** (omeprazole, lansoprazole, rabeprazole, pantoprazole, and esomeprazole) are the most potent single agent for treating severe reflux esophagitis; they act to increase the pH of gastric contents and heal erosive esophagitis.
  4. **Procedures** designed to restore LES competence or prevent reflux (endoscopic or surgical)

Katzka DA: Treatment of GERD: Lifestyle modifications. Pract Gastroenterol 24(8):14–32, 2000.

Sachs G: Biologic considerations in the selection of antisecretory therapy. PPI Revol 2(2):1–7, 2000.

106. What are the atypical manifestations of GERD?

Atypical chest pain	Adult onset asthma
Recurrent bronchitis or aspiration pneumonia	Vocal cord tumors or polyps
Dysphonia	Laryngitis
Recurrent or chronic cough	

107. What is Barrett's esophagus? How should patients be managed?

Barrett's esophagus is a complication that develops in patients with longstanding reflux peptic esophagitis. It represents a unique reparative process in which the original squamous epithelial cell lining of the esophagus is replaced by a metaplastic columnar-type epithelium. In most adults, this epithelium resembles intestinal mucosa, complete with goblet cells. When the lower esophagus is lined by this columnar-type epithelium, it is termed Barrett's esophagus.

The clinical significance lies primarily in the malignant potential of Barrett's esophagus. There is an increased risk (30–125 higher than in the general population) of esophageal adenocarcinoma arising in the Barrett's epithelium. The actual incidence is unknown, but the average is about 10%. Currently adenocarcinoma of the junction, which primarily arises from Barrett's epithelium, is the fastest growing GI cancer among white men in the U.S.

The management of Barrett's esophagus is the same as the treatment of GERD. Acid suppression with proton pump inhibitors in high doses controls symptoms and heals esophageal damage. Although the inflammatory changes associated with Barrett's epithelium can be healed, once Barrett's epithelium has developed, the process cannot be reversed by any form of antireflux therapy. Ongoing trials are evaluating such techniques as photodynamic therapy, endoscopic mucosal resection, and laser surgery for the eradication of Barrett's esophagus, but to date nothing has proved to be 100% curative.

108. Is routine surveillance for esophageal cancer necessary in patients with Barrett's esophagus?

The benefits of periodic endoscopic screening for dysplasia have not been demonstrated. Endoscopic surveillance and four-quadrant biopsies of each 2-cm segment of the esophagus at 1–2 year intervals are advocated by most experts.

109. Name the three types of esophageal dysphagia. How can a patient's history be used to distinguish among them?

1. **Transfer**—pathologic alteration in the neuromotor mechanism of the oropharyngeal phase. Patients give a history of difficulty in swallowing liquids, whereas solids pass normally. Such patients may have stroke, myasthenia gravis, amyotrophic lateral sclerosis, or botulism.

2. **Transit**—abnormal peristalsis and LES function. Transit dysphagia is due to motor disorders in which the primary peristaltic pump of the esophagus fails. Motor disorders often begin with dysphagia to both solids and liquids. They are commonly seen in such entities as achalasia and scleroderma. Dysphagia that worsens on ingesting cold liquids and improves with warm liquids suggests a motor disorder.

3. **Obstructive**—mechanical narrowing of the esophagus. Obstructive dysphagia may be due to intrinsic lesions blocking the esophagus (e.g., peptic strictures, esophageal webs, carcinoma) or to extrinsic lesions (e.g., mediastinal tumors) compressing the esophagus. It typically presents as dysphagia to solid food and may progress to include liquids. Patients usually give a history of eating only soft foods, chewing foods longer, and avoiding steak, apples, and fresh bread. Solid-food dysphagia associated with a long history of heartburn and regurgitation suggests a peptic stricture. If the bolus can be dislodged by repeated swallowing or drinking water, a motor disorder is usually the cause.

After a thorough history and physical examination, the initial diagnostic step is a barium swallow. The barium swallow is then quickly followed by an upper GI endoscopy.

110. What is achalasia?

Achalasia is the best-known motor disorder of the esophagus. Its usual onset is in patients aged 25–60 years, with an equal frequency in men and women. Its symptoms include dysphagia (solids and liquids), regurgitation of undigested foods, heartburn, and chest pain. The diagnosis can be made by esophageal manometry, which yields the following characteristic findings:

- Loss of peristalsis (absolute requirement)
- Failure of the LES to relax
- Increased LES pressure

111. What is the most frequent form of infectious esophagitis? How does it present?

The most frequent form of infectious esophagitis is candidal esophagitis. Most fungal infections occur in immunocompromised patients, especially those with AIDS, but they are also seen in patients with less obvious immune defects (e.g., diabetics, malnourished elderly, alcoholics, patients taking antibiotics or steroids). The symptoms include painful swallowing (odynophagia), retrosternal pain, dysphagia, fever, and bleeding. Physical examination may reveal oral thrush.

Sutton FM, et al: Infectious esophagitis. Gastrointest Endosc Clin North Am 4:713, 1994.

112. Which drugs are commonly implicated as causes of pill-induced esophagitis?

Doxycycline	Tetracycline	Slow-release potassium chloride
Ascorbic acid	Quinidine	Aspirin
NSAIDs	Ferrous sulfate	

113. How are 24-hour pH monitoring, esophageal manometry, and endoscopy used to assess patients with suspected esophageal disease?

24-Hour ambulatory pH monitoring of the esophagus provides a temporal profile of acid reflux events and acid clearance and correlates these events with symptoms. Specific variables measured include the number of reflux episodes in 24 hours, acid clearance times from the esophagus, and esophageal exposure to acid. These values can be determined while the patient is in the upright or recumbent position. This is the gold standard test for documenting or excluding GERD and determining whether atypical GERD symptoms are a result of acid reflux. Anyone who undergoes surgery for GERD must have a 24-hour pH probe and esophageal manometry.

Esophageal manometry is useful in evaluating patients with noncardiac chest pain and a history suggestive of esophageal motor disorder, achalasia, or esophageal reflux disease.

Endoscopy provides a direct view of the esophageal mucosa and allows directed biopsy when necessary. Endoscopy and biopsy are necessary to make a definitive diagnosis of many esophageal diseases (e.g., malignancy). The benefits of endoscopy include the ability to perform therapeutic intervention such as biopsy, cytology, brushing, dilations, and stent placement.

114. What is nocturnal acid breakthrough?

Nocturnal acid breakthrough or occasional acid breakthrough is arbitrarily defined as a drop in intragastric pH < 4 for 1 hour or longer during the night. This phenomenon appears to be histamine-mediated because patients with symptomatic nocturnal acid breakthrough experience more relief with an H_2 blocker than with a proton pump inhibitor. Many believe that this phenomenon is a not an actual disease, because it is a normal physiologic response to have a decrease in intragastric pH after midnight.

Robinson M. Clinical relevance and management of 'occasional acid breakthrough' on proton pump inhibitor therapy. Pract Gastroenterol 24:55–57, 2000.

Peghini PL, et al: Understanding nocturnal acid breakthrough on proton pump inhibitors. Pract Gastroenterol 24:60–67, 2000.

115. What is the differential diagnosis of dyspepsia?

Peptic ulcer disease (PUD)	Nonerosive esophageal reflux disease (NERD)
GERD	Biliary tract disease: cholelithiasis, cholecystitis
Nonulcer dyspepsia (NUD)	Cancer
Pancreatitis	

MALABSORPTION

116. What causes Whipple's disease?

Whipple's disease is a systemic disease that may affect almost any organ system of the body, but in most cases, it involves the small intestine. The causative agent is the bacterium *Tropheryma whippelii*. Patients present with intestinal malabsorption, weight loss, diarrhea, abdominal pain, fever, anemia, lymphadenopathy, and arthralgias. Nervous system symptoms, pericarditis, or endocarditis also may be present.

The pathologic feature is infiltration of involved tissues with large glycoprotein-containing macrophages that stain strongly positive with a periodic acid–Schiff stain. This diagnosis is most often made by biopsy of the small intestine. One can also see characteristic rod-shaped, gram-positive bacilli that are not acid-fast.

117. How is Whipple's disease treated?

Effective treatment includes prolonged antibiotic therapy, usually with double-strength trimethoprim/sulfamethoxazole given for a minimum of 1 year. Repeat intestinal biopsy should document the disappearance of the Whipple bacillus before therapy is discontinued. Relapses are not uncommon and are treated for a minimum of 6–12 months. Patients allergic to sulfonamides should receive parenteral penicillin.

118. In a small-bowel biopsy, the mucosa shows flat villa with markedly hyperplastic crypts. What is this disease?

Celiac sprue, also called gluten enteropathy, is an allergic disease characterized by malabsorption of nutrients secondary to the damaged small intestinal mucosa. The responsible antigen is gluten, a water-insoluble protein found in cereal grains such as wheat, barley, oats, and rye. Withdrawal of gluten from the diet results in complete remission of both clinical symptoms and mucosal lesions. Although this disease is present worldwide, the distribution varies; the highest prevalence is in western Ireland.

119. What is dermatitis herpetiformis? How does it relate to celiac sprue?

Dermatitis herpetiformis is a pruritic skin condition that also may be reversed with dietary therapy (gluten restriction). It is characterized by papulovesicular lesions in a symmetrical distribution on the elbows, knees, buttocks, face, scalp, neck, and trunk. Although most patients with celiac sprue do not develop skin lesions of dermatitis herpetiformis, patients with dermatitis herpetiformis usually have the sprue-like mucosal lesion in the small bowel. The two diseases appear to be distinct entities that respond to the same dietary restrictions. Unlike the intestinal disease, the skin lesions can be treated with the antibiotic dapsone, with a clinical response within 1–2 weeks.

120. What is the blind-loop syndrome?

The blind-loop syndrome is a constellation of symptoms and laboratory abnormalities that include malabsorption of B_{12}, steatorrhea, hypoproteinemia, weight loss, and diarrhea. These symptoms are attributed to overgrowth of bacteria within the small intestine and have been associated with a number of diseases and surgical abnormalities. The common link between these conditions is abnormal motility of a segment of small intestine, resulting in stasis. Therapy, which is aimed at reducing bacterial overgrowth, consists of antibiotics and, when feasible, correction of the small intestinal abnormality that led to the condition.

121. Describe the pathophysiologic mechanisms that can lead to fat malabsorption.

Normal fat absorption requires all phases of digestion to be intact. The process begins with secretion of pancreatic lipase and colipase. These enzymes are activated intraluminally and require an optimal pH of 6–8. Both enzymes are necessary for triglyceride hydrolysis in the duodenum. Any disorder that causes deficiencies of pancreatic enzyme secretion or leads to an acidic intraluminal environment can lead to fat malabsorption.

The products of triglyceride hydrolysis (i.e., fatty acids and monoglycerides) then must be solubilized by bile salts to form micelles, which are subsequently absorbed by the small intestinal epithelium. Any disorder that interrupts the enterohepatic circulation or secretion of bile salts may impair micelle formation and therefore result in fat malabsorption.

If the intestinal epithelial cell is in some way diseased, monoglyceride absorption and processing into chylomicrons for transport out of the small intestine may be impaired, leading to fat malabsorption. Disease of the intestinal lymphatics with impaired chylomicron transport has also been reported to result in fat malabsorption.

122. Which diseases can affect fat absorption?

- Chronic pancreatitis
- Cystic fibrosis

- Pancreatic carcinoma
- Postgastrectomy syndrome
- Biliary tract obstruction
- Terminal ileal resection or disease
- Cholestatic liver disease
- Intestinal epithelial disease, such as Whipple's disease, sprue, eosinophilic gastroenteritis
- Lymphatic disease, such as abetalipoproteinemia, intestinal lymphangiectasia, lymphoma, and tuberculous adenitis
- Small bowel bacterial overgrowth (bile salts are deconjugated and inactivated by bacteria)
- Zollinger-Ellison syndrome (low intraluminal pH)

Weber SA: Malabsorption: An overview. In Lindner AE (ed): Mediguide to Gastrointestinal Disease, vol. 6. Philadelphia, American Society of GI Endoscopy, 1995, p 1.

123. Which conditions are associated with or may result in small bowel bacterial overgrowth?

Any abnormality of the small intestine that results in local stasis or recirculation of intestinal contents is likely to be associated with marked proliferation of intraluminal bacteria. The gold standard for diagnosing bacterial overgrowth is culture in the upper small bowel of > 100,000 cfu/ml. Associated disorders include:

1. Gastric proliferation of bacteria, as seen in hypochlorhydric or achlorhydric states, particularly in combination with motor or anatomic disturbances.

2. Small intestinal stagnation associated with anatomic alterations after surgery, such as afferent loop syndrome after a Billroth II procedure.

3. Duodenal and jejunal diverticulosis, particularly as seen in scleroderma.

4. Surgically created blind loops, such as end-to-side anastomoses.

5. Chronic low-grade obstruction secondary to small intestinal strictures, adhesions, inflammation, or carcinoma.

6. Motor disturbances of the small intestine, such as scleroderma, idiopathic pseudo-obstruction, or diabetic neuropathy.

7. Abnormal communication between the proximal small intestine and the distal intestinal tract, as seen in gastrocolic or jejunocolic fistulas or resection of the ileocecal valve.

8. Immunodeficiency syndromes such as AIDS, primary immunodeficiency states, and malnutrition.

124. How does bacterial overgrowth of the small bowel result in fat malabsorption?

The bacterial enzymes deconjugate intraluminal bile salts to free bile acids, which are unable to solubilize monoglycerides and free fatty acids into micelles for absorption by the epithelial cells. The result is impaired absorption of fat and fat-soluble vitamins.

125. What constitutes a normal fecal fat concentration?

The typical U.S. diet consists of 100–150 gm of fat per day. Fat absorption is extremely efficient, and most of the ingested fat is absorbed with very little excretion into the stool. The average fecal fat concentration for the normal person is 4–6 gm/day, ranging to an upper limit of normal of approximately 7 gm.

126. What is steatorrhea? How is it detected?

Patients with steatorrhea, or increased excretion of fecal fat, may have up to 10 times this amount in the stool. To detect steatorrhea, a 72-hour stool sample is collected while the patient is on a defined dietary fat intake of > 100 gm/day. Chemical analysis of the stool collection measures the amount of fat. This test is highly reliable but neither specific nor sensitive in determining the etiology of steatorrhea.

Weber SA: Malabsorption: An overview. In Lindner AE (ed): Mediguide to Gastrointestinal Disease 6:1, 1995.

OBSTRUCTION

127. Name the four most common causes of mechanical small bowel obstruction (SBO) in adults.
1. Adhesions (approximately 74%)
2. Hernias (8%)
3. Malignancies of the small bowel (8%)
4. Inflammatory bowel disease with stricture formation

128. What historical and physical clues may help to determine the location of the obstruction in SBO?

The patient with mechanical SBO typically presents with crampy, intermittent abdominal pain occurring in paroxysms, 4–5 minutes apart. Proximal obstruction presents in a more acute fashion, with vomiting as a prominent complaint. The vomiting is typically bilious and nonfeculent, and pain occurs at short-spaced intervals. Abdominal distention may be minimal or absent if the location is high in the small bowel.

Distal obstruction may have a more insidious onset of symptoms. Vomiting is often present but is a less prominent complaint. When present, the vomiting is often feculent. Pain occurs at longer-spaced intervals compared with that seen in proximal SBO. The lower the blockage, the more likely there is to be abdominal distention due to accumulation of fluid and gas in the intestine.

129. What findings on the plain film x-ray suggest an SBO?

Plain abdominal x-rays in SBO usually reveal abnormally large quantities of gas in the bowel. This gas can be identified as small intestinal gas by the presence of the valvulae conniventes, which usually occupy the entire transverse diameter of the small bowel. This feature can be distinguished from colonic haustral markings, which occupy only a portion of the diameter of the bowel. In addition, loops of small bowel are most commonly located in the more central portion of the abdomen, whereas colonic gas is usually seen in the periphery of the x-ray film. In the patient with classic mechanical SBO, there is minimal or no colonic gas. The upright or decubitus abdominal film reveals multiple air-fluid levels with distended loops of small bowel resembling inverted Us.

130. Is surgery necessary in all patients with SBO?

In most circumstances, the best therapy for mechanical SBO is surgical correction of the obstruction. The timing of the operation depends on the following three factors: (1) the duration of obstruction and the severity of fluid, electrolyte, and acid-base abnormalities; (2) the improvement of vital organ function (i.e., management of concomitant cardiac and pulmonary disorders); and (3) the risk of strangulation. Because the mortality rate of SBO associated with strangulation is high, operative intervention should be performed early in the course.

In certain patients, however, a short trial of conservative, nonoperative management is appropriate. Patients in the immediate postoperative period may respond to simple nasogastric (NG) suction. Similarly, patients with obstruction caused by disseminated intra-abdominal carcinomatosis, Crohn's disease, radiation strictures, or adhesions following previous surgery may improve with simple management and NG suction. If conservative medical therapy is used, the patient should show continuous improvement during the first 12–24 hours of therapy. If not, surgical relief of the obstruction should be performed.

131. What seven entities may cause small bowel ileus?

Paralytic ileus is a relatively common disorder and occurs when neural, humoral, and metabolic factors combine to stimulate reflexes that inhibit intestinal motility. The result is small bowel and/or colonic distention due to intestinal muscle paralysis. The seven common causes of paralytic ileus are:
1. Abdominal surgery
2. Peritonitis
3. Generalized sepsis

4. Electrolyte imbalance (especially hypokalemia)
5. Retroperitoneal hemorrhage
6. Spinal fractures
7. Pelvic fractures.

Drugs such as phenothiazines and narcotics inhibit small bowel motility and also may contribute to paralysis. Treatment consists of NG suction to relieve distention and IV fluids to replace losses, followed by correction of the underlying disorder.

132. What conditions may aggravate or be associated with colonic pseudo-obstruction?
1. Trauma (nonoperative) and surgery (gynecologic, orthopedic, urologic)
2. Inflammatory processes (pancreatitis, cholecystitis)
3. Infections
4. Malignancy
5. Radiation therapy
6. Drugs (narcotics, antidepressants, clonidine, anticholinergics)
7. Cardiovascular disease
8. Neurologic disease
9. Respiratory failure
10. Metabolic disease (diabetes, hypothyroidism, electrolyte imbalance, uremia)
11. Alcoholism

133. Name the most common cause of gastric outlet obstruction.
Peptic ulcer disease.

134. In what clinical setting are bezoars likely to be seen?
Bezoars are clusters of food or foreign matter that have undergone partial digestion in the stomach, fail to pass through the pylorus into the small bowel, and form a mass in the stomach. Bezoars may be composed of hair (trichobezoars) or, more commonly, plant matter (phytobezoars). They may become quite large and can present with abdominal mass, gastric outlet obstruction, attacks of nausea and vomiting, and peptic ulceration. Factors important in the formation of bezoars include the amount of indigestible materials in the diet (pulpy, fibrous fruit or vegetables such as oranges), the quality of the chewing mechanism, and loss of pyloric function, which limits the size of food particles that may enter the duodenum.

Saeed ZA, et al: A method for the endoscopic retrieval of trichobezoars. Gastrointest Endosc 39:698, 1993.

BILIARY TRACT DISEASE

135. How prevalent is asymptomatic cholelithiasis in adult Americans over age 40? How many ultimately develop symptoms?
Forty percent of Americans over age 40 have gallstones, and 10–30% of these become symptomatic at some point.

136. Is surgery indicated for asymptomatic cholelithiasis?
Elective surgery is generally not indicated. It has been previously recommended that elective cholecystectomy be performed in diabetic patients with asymptomatic cholelithiasis, but evidence suggests that such patients have a higher complication rate from elective cholecystectomy.

137. Which U.S. ethnic groups have the highest prevalence of cholesterol gallstone formation?
American Indians and Mexican-Americans.

138. What percentage of gallstones are radiopaque?
Pigment gallstones, which account for 20–30% of gallstones in the U.S., are often radiopaque and can be seen on plain radiographs of the abdomen. Cholesterol gallstones, which account for 70–80%, are radiolucent.

139. What are the types of gallstones?

Cholesterol	70-80% of all stones in Western countries; risks are female gender, obesity, age over 40, and multiparity
Pigmented	20–30%
Black	Calcium bilibrubinate; risks are cirrhosis, chronic hemolytic syndromes
Brown	Calcium salts can form de novo stones in bile ducts; associated with infections of biliary system

140. Describe the therapeutic approach to the patient with cholangitis who has previously undergone cholecystectomy.

Bacterial cholangitis is a life-threatening illness that requires urgent intervention with immediate drainage of the common bile duct and relief of the obstruction. Treatment can be performed via endoscopic retrograde cholangiopancreatography (ERCP) or percutaneous transhepatic cholangiogram (PTC). The advantages of ERCP include the ability to treat the primary disease process using sphincterotomy, with removal of common bile duct stones or placement of an internal drain, and avoidance of the morbidity associated with percutaneous external drainage. Nonoperative therapy using ERCP and endoscopic drainage in patients with cholangitis has a mortality rate of only 1–2%, whereas in the setting of emergency surgery the mortality rate is as high as 40%. Elective surgery can be done later, if needed, and is associated with a lower mortality than surgery in the acute setting.

141. What is Charcot's triad?

Right-upper-quadrant pain, jaundice, and fever. This triad is present in ~50% of patients with bacterial cholangitis.

142. In the initial diagnostic evaluation of a patient with suspected obstructive jaundice, which diagnostic tests are available? How do they compare?

The cause of jaundice can be determined in many cases from **clinical data** and **routine laboratory tests**. The only special study that is routinely useful in the early evaluation of obstructive jaundice is an **ultrasound scan** of the gallbladder, bile ducts, and liver. Ultrasound is fairly specific for detecting gallstones and ductal dilatation (which signifies ductal obstruction). However, a negative scan does not prove the absence of stones or obstruction, because the sensitivity of ultrasound in detecting obstruction is only about 90%.

Abdominal CT is fairly sensitive for detecting ductal dilatation and can be useful in localizing the site of ductal obstruction. A CT scan is less able to detect stones of the gallbladder and common bile duct than ultrasound, but it is better able to image mass lesions and to evaluate the pancreas.

MRI and **magnetic retrograde cholangiopancreatiography** (MRCP) are fast becoming more useful as diagnostic tools in the evaluation of obstructive jaundice. MRCP can reveal the size of the ducts and document presence of stones, although it has not supplanted ultrasound. At present neither of these imaging studies is widely available.

Endoscopic ultrasound (EUS) is an excellent noninvasive method of assessing patients with obstructive jaundice. It can image the entire pancreaticobiliary system and document the presence of tumors, stones, or strictures. More advanced EUS systems are equipped to guide biopsies and obtain tissue samples via fine needle aspiration (FNA). The primary limitation of EUS is that it is not yet widely available.

Liver biopsy in patients with extrahepatic ductal obstruction is not routinely useful. It may reveal evidence of cholestasis and cholangitis but does not help to determine the cause. A liver scan using technetium sulfur colloid is of very little value in jaundiced patients.

143. If the bile ducts are dilated on the ultrasound or CT scan, what is the next step?

The next step should include an evaluation to determine the cause of the obstruction and an attempt to relieve the obstruction and provide drainage. The two modalities that can achieve these ends are endoscopic retrograde cholangiopancreatography (ERCP) and PTC.

ERCP is a relatively simple procedure if a trained endoscopist is available. The common bile duct is cannulated endoscopically and dye is injected, yielding a cholangiogram. If bile duct stones, biliary stricture, or an obstructive lesion is seen, a variety of therapeutic maneuvers can be performed during ERCP, including sphincterotomy with stone removal, dilatation of the stricture, or placement of a biliary stent or nasobiliary catheter.

PTC offers similar advantages, but it adds the additional morbidity and discomfort of percutaneous needlestick and the possibility of external biliary drainage after the procedure. The overall risk of both procedures is fairly low, and they compare favorably in effectiveness.

IRRITABLE BOWEL SYNDROME

144. What makes the diagnosis of irritable bowel syndrome (IBS)?
The criteria for diagnosing IBS were refined in 1998 and are termed the Rome II Criteria. IBS is defined as a functional bowel disorder characterized by at least 3 months, which do not have to be consecutive, in the past 12 months of abdominal discomfort or pain that has 2 or 3 of the following features:

Relief with defecation

Onset associated with a change in frequency of stool

Onset associated with a change in form or appearance of stool

Thompson WG, et al: Functional bowel disorders and functional abdominal pain. Gut 45(Suppl 2): 1143–1147, 1999.

145. When should you suspect organic disease instead of IBS?

New onset of symptoms in an elderly patient

Pain that interferes with normal sleep patterns

Weight loss

Anemia

Blood in the stools

Pain on awakening from sleep

Diarrhea that awakens the patient

Fever

Steatorrhea

Physical examination abnormalities

American Gasroenterological Association: Irritable bowel syndrome: A technical review for practice guideline development. Gastroenterology 112:2120–2137, 1997.

146. What is the differential diagnosis of IBS?

Psychiatric disorders: depression, anxiety, somatization

Diabetes

Scleroderma

Inflammatory bowel disease

Chronic pancreatitis

Postgastrectomy syndromes

Medications

Hypothyroidism

Lactose malabsorption

Endocrine disorders

Celiac sprue

Infectious diarrhea

Drossman DA: Review article: An integrated approach to the irritable bowel syndrome. Aliment Pharmacol Ther 13(Suppl 2):3–14, 1999.

BIBLIOGRAPHY

1. Barkin JS, O'Phelan CA (eds): Advanced Therapeutic Endoscopy, 3rd ed. New York, Raven Press, 1997.
2. Brandt LJ (ed): Clinical Practice of Gastroenterology. New York, Churchill Livingstone, 1999.
3. Huang ES, Tang WHW, Lee DS, et al (eds): Internal Medicine Handbook for Clinicians: Resident Survival Guide. Philadelphia, Scrub Hill Press, 2000.
4. Lyman BE, Croft CL (eds): Gastrointestinal Disease in Primary Care, Philadelphia, Lippincott Williams & Wilkins, 2000.
5. Rhodes JM, Tsai HH (eds): Clinical Problems in Gastroenterology. London, Mosby-Wolfe, 1995.
6. Sleisenger MH, Fordtran JS (eds): Gastrointestinal Disease: Pathophysiology, Diagnosis, and Management, 6th ed. Philadelphia, W.B. Saunders, 1997.
7. Tytgat GNJ, Classen M, Waye JD, Nakazawa S: Practice of Therapeutic Endoscopy, 2nd ed. London, W. B. Saunders, 2000.
8. Yamada T (ed): Textbook of Gastroenterology, 3rd ed. Philadelphia, J.B. Lippincott, 1998.
9. Zakim D, Boyer TD (eds): Hepatology: A Textbook of Liver Disease, 3rd ed. Philadelphia, W.B. Saunders, 1996.
10. Zollo AJ (ed): Medical Secrets, 2nd ed. Philadelphia, Hanley & Belfus, 1997.

6. ONCOLOGY

Teresa G. Hayes, M.D., Ph.D., and Mary Anne Doherty, M.D.

> *While there are several chronic diseases more destructive to life than cancer, none is more feared.*
>
> Charles H. Mayo (1865–1939)
> *Annals of Surgery 83:357, 1926*

GENERAL ISSUES

1. How is carcinogenesis defined?

Carcinogenesis is the alteration of normal cells into malignant cells. It is almost always a multistage evolution of genetic and epigenetic alterations that eventuates in cells that escape the normal growth constraints of the host.

2. One of the risk factors for cancer is the genetic background of the patient. What are the known genetically related mechanisms of neoplasia?

Four broad categories of genes can influence the origin and progression of neoplasia:

1. **Oncogenes:** These are genes in humans and other animals that have the capacity to transform normal cells into malignant ones. These genes, acquired at conception or mutated during life, make the patient susceptible to cancer by virtue of altering or impairing several processes:

    a. Production of nuclear transcription factors that control cell growth (e.g., *myc*).

    b. Signal transduction within cells (e.g., *ras*).

    c. Interaction of growth factors and their receptors (e.g., *her/neu*).

More than 100 different oncogenes have been identified, but only some of these have been associated with human cancers exclusively. Mutations convert proto-oncogenes to oncogenes by amplification, translocation, and point mutation.

2. **Tumor suppressor genes:** Mutations of these genes must occur in both alleles to cause loss of function and thus affect tumor growth. Multiple tumor suppressor genes have been identified (e.g., *p53* and *rb*), and these are found in many different types of cancers. These mutations are the basis of the inherited predispositions to cancers and are inherited in the heterozygous state.

3. **Regulators of cell death:** The cell death genes are involved in the programmed death (**apoptosis**) of cells no longer needed by the body. Mutation in one of these genes (e.g., *bcl-2*) allows cells to live that should have died, causing excess accumulation of cells. Activation of the **telomerase** gene, which controls cell senescence, is thought to cause cells to become immortal by turning off the normal aging process.

4. **Mutator genes:** Genes such as hMSH2 and hMLH1 are responsible for ensuring the fidelity of the DNA duplication process. When the gene products subsequently fail to function, the mutation rate increases and inherited predispositions to cancers are observed. The tumor suppressor genes and oncogenes are thought to be the target of the faulty DNA editing process.

3. Besides genetic predisposition, what are some environmental "causes" of cancer?

Examples of Carcinogens

Social agents—tobacco, alcohol

Occupational exposures—arsenic, benzene, CCl_4, chromium, combustion by-products (engine exhaust), polycyclic hydrocarbons (coal byproducts)

(Table continued on next page.)

Examples of Carcinogens (cont.)

Ionizing radiation—UV-B (sunlight), mining, others

Dietary factors—aflatoxin B, high-fat diet, nitrates/nitrites (converted endogenously to nitrosamines), smoked foods

Foreign body reactants—asbestos fiber

Chronic inflammation—ulcerative colitis

Infectious agents—Epstein-Barr virus, hepatitis B and C viruses, human papillomavirus, human T-lymphotropic virus, *Helicobacter pylori*

Iatrogenic agents—cancer chemotherapeutic drugs, DES, estrogens, Thoratrast

---

4. Are there "protective" factors?

- Diets high in antioxidants, including many fruits and vegetables (such as tomatoes and broccoli), are felt to protect against cancer development by scavenging for free radicals.
- Some vitamins may modify the effect of chemical carcinogenesis: vitamin A (which promotes the differentiation of epithelial tissues), vitamin C (which blocks the formation of n-nitrosocarcinogens from nitrite and secondary amines), and vitamin E (which is a free-radical scavenger).

5. Which cancers tend to cluster in families?

The common cancers (breast, endometrial, colon, prostate, lung, melanoma, and stomach) have a 2–3 times increased risk of development in first-degree relatives. This may be due to hereditary factors, shared exposures to environmental carcinogens, chance associations, or a combination of all three.

- The familial clustering of breast cancer may be due, in about 5–10% of cases, to a genetic locus (BRCA1 or BRCA2, others) that is predictive of familial breast and ovarian cancer.
- In the **Lynch** syndrome, cancer family adenocarcinomatosis, there is an autosomal dominant pattern of predisposition to nonpolyposis colorectal cancer, as well as an increased incidence of other cancers, including endometrial, ovarian, breast, stomach, small intestine, pancreatic, urinary tract, and biliary tract.
- The **Li-Fraumeni** syndrome is a familial cancer syndrome with an autosomal dominant pattern of inheritance in which there is a varied spectrum of mesenchymal and epithelial tumors, and multiple primary neoplasms in children and young adults. The gene for this cancer (p53) is located on the short arm of chromosome 17.
- Multiple endocrine neoplasia **(MEN) type 1**, associated with a gene on chromosome 11, causes parathyroid, pituitary, and islet cell tumors.
- **MEN type 2** has two phenotypes: medullary thyroid carcinoma, pheochromocytoma, and parathyroid hyperplasia in the A type, and medullary thyroid carcinoma, pheochromocytoma, marfanoid habitus, and mucosal neuromas in type B. The gene for MEN 2A is on chromosome 10.

6. How are tumor markers used in diagnosing and treating cancer?

Tumor markers include enzymes, hormones, gene loci, and oncofetal antigens that are associated with particular tumors. The markers reflect the presence of the tumor or the quantity of the tumor (tumor burden). Many cancers do not produce markers, and those tumors that are known to produce markers may sometimes fail to do so, particularly if they are very poorly differentiated. Some of the markers, such as prostate specific antigen (PSA) and alpha-fetoprotein (AFP), are highly sensitive, highly specific, and of high predictive value. Others, such as lactic dehydrogenase (LDH) or carcinoembryonic antigen, are nonspecific and may be elevated in many conditions besides malignancies. The most important use of these markers is in following the effects of therapy on tumor burden and in detecting recurrent disease after initial therapy.

7. Which are the four most common tumor markers? How are they used?

1. **Carcinoembryonic antigen (CEA).** CEA is a glycoprotein of 200,000 daltons that is found in gastrointestinal mucosal cells and pancreaticobiliary secretions. Elevations occur with breaks in the mucosal basement membrane by a tumor but can also occur in smokers, and with cirrhosis, pancreatitis, inflammatory bowel disease, and rectal polyps. CEA is most useful in monitoring the activity of disease in recurrent colorectal cancer.

2. **Prostate specific antigen (PSA).** PSA is a serine protease found only in the prostate, whose normal function is liquefaction of seminal gel. The serum level of PSA may be elevated in any type of prostate disease, including benign prostatic hypertrophy, prostatitis, and prostate cancer. However, high levels of PSA, especially in patients with small volume prostates, are a strong indicator of probable prostate cancer.

3. **Alpha-fetoprotein (AFP).** AFP is an α-globulin of 70,000 daltons that is made by the yolk sac and liver of the human fetus. It is elevated in hepatomas and certain germ cell neoplasms and has been found to be a very sensitive marker for disease activity. Although AFP is rather nonspecific and can be elevated in acute viral and chronic hepatitis, very high levels correlate with the presence of these malignancies.

4. **Human chorionic gonadotropin (HCG).** HCG is a glycoprotein normally secreted by the trophoblastic epithelium of the placenta. It is used as a sensitive and specific marker for germ cell tumors of the testes and ovary and extragonadal presentations of these tumors.

8. List the principles used in formulating combination chemotherapy regimens.

Principles of Combination Chemotherapy

1. Drugs used should have activity against the tumor.
2. Drugs should be selected with dissimilar toxicities.
3. Drugs with different mechanisms of action should be used.
4. Several cycles of therapy, with adequate biological effect, should be used before determining efficacy.
5. Recovery time of normal tissues should be allowed before starting the next cycle.

9. What are the mechanisms of drug resistance of tumors to chemotherapeutic agents?

Mechanisms of Drug Resistance in Chemotherapy

1. Intrinsic cytokinetic or biochemical resistance
2. Impaired transport of the drug into the cell, or active extrusion from the cell
3. Altered drug affinity for the target enzyme
4. Amplification of genes
5. Membrane alterations from overproduction of high-weight glycoproteins

10. What are the toxic effects of chemotherapy?

The most common immediate effects are nausea and vomiting, which vary in presence and degree with the type of drug. Some medications, such as cisplatin, are very emetogenic, whereas others, like fludarabine, are unlikely to cause emesis.

The most dangerous adverse effect is myelosuppression. Leukopenia predisposes to acute and serious infections; thrombocytopenia predisposes to bleeding; and anemia may worsen other problems, such as chronic obstructive pulmonary disease and atherosclerotic cardiovascular disease.

Toxicities of Chemotherapeutic Agents

DRUG	ACUTE TOXICITY	DELAYED TOXICITY
Bleomycin (Blenoxane)	Nausea/vomiting, fever, hypersensitivity reactions	**Pneumonitis/pulmonary fibrosis**,* rash and hyperpigmentation, stomatitis, alopecia, Raynaud's, cavitating granulomas
Carboplatin (Paraplatin)	Nausea/vomiting	**Myelosuppression**,* peripheral neuropathy (uncommon), hearing loss, hemolytic anemia, transient cortical blindness
Chlorambucil (Leukeran)	Seizures, nausea/vomiting	**Myelosuppression**,* pulmonary infiltrates and fibrosis, leukemia, hepatic toxicity, sterility
Cisplatin (Platinol)	Nausea/vomiting, anaphylactic reaction	**Renal damage**,* ototoxicity, myelosuppression, hemolysis, $\downarrow Mg^+$/ Ca^{2+}/K^+, peripheral neuropathy, Raynaud's, sterility
Cyclophosphamide (Cytoxan)	Nausea/vomiting, anaphylaxis, facial burning with IV administration, visual blurring	**Myelosuppression**,* alopecia, hemorrhagic cystitis, sterility, lung infiltrates/fibrosis, $\downarrow Na^+$, leukemia, bladder cancer, SIADH
Cytarabine (ara-C)	Nausea/vomiting, diarrhea, anaphylaxis	**Myelosuppression**,* oral ulceration, conjunctivitis, hepatic damage, fever, pulmonary edema, neurotoxicity (high dose), rhabdomyolysis, pancreatitis with asparaginase
Dacarbazine (DTIC)	Nausea/vomiting, diarrhea, anaphylaxis, pain on administration	**Myelosuppression**,* cardiotoxicity,* alopecia, flulike syndrome, renal impairment, hepatic necrosis, facial flushing, paresthesias, photosensitivity, urticarial rash
Daunorubicin (Cerubidine)	Nausea/vomiting, diarrhea, red urine, severe local tissue necrosis on extravasation, transient ECG changes, anaphylactoid reaction	**Myelosuppression**,* cardiotoxicity,* alopecia, stomatitis, anorexia, diarrhea, fever and chills, dermatitis in previously irradiated areas, skin and nail pigmentation
Doxorubicin (Adriamycin)	Nausea/vomiting, red urine, severe local tissue necrosis on extravasation, diarrhea, fever, transient ECG changes, ventricular arrhythmia, anaphylactoid reaction	**Myelosuppression**,* cardiotoxicity,* alopecia, stomatitis, anorexia, conjunctivitis, acral pigmentation, dermatitis in previously irradiated areas, acral erythrodysesthesia, mucositis
Etoposide (VP16)	Nausea/vomiting, diarrhea, fever, hypotension, allergic reaction	**Myelosuppression**,* alopecia, peripheral neuropathy, mucositis and hepatic damage with high doses, leukemia
Floxuridine (FUDR)	Nausea/vomiting, diarrhea	**Oral and GI ulceration**,* **myelosuppression**,* alopecia, dermatitis, hepatic dysfunction with infusion
Fluorouracil (5-FU)	Nausea/vomiting, diarrhea, hypersensitivity, photosensitivity	**Oral and GI ulcers**, **myelosuppression**,* diarrhea, ataxia, arrhythmias, angina, hyperpigmentation, handfoot syndrome, conjunctivitis, CHF

(*Table continued on next page.*)

Toxicities of Chemotherapeutic Agents (cont.)

DRUG	ACUTE TOXICITY	DELAYED TOXICITY
Gemcitabine (Gemzar)	Fatigue, nausea and vomiting	**Bone marrow depression**, especially thrombocytopenia; edema; pulmonary toxicity; anal pruritus
Ifosfamide (Ifex)	Nausea/vomiting, confusion, nephrotoxicity, metabolic acidosis, **cardiac toxicity with higher dose***	**Myelosuppression**,* **hemorrhagic cystitis**,* alopecia, SIADH, neurotoxicity
Irinotecan (Camptosar)	Nausea and vomiting, diarrhea, fever	**Diarrhea, anorexia**, stomatitis, bone marrow depression, alopecia, abdominal cramping
Mechlorethamine (nitrogen mustard)	Nausea/vomiting, local reaction and phlebitis	**Myelosuppression**,* alopecia, diarrhea, oral ulcers, leukemia, amenorrhea, sterility
Methotrexate	Nausea/vomiting, diarrhea, fever, anaphylaxis, hepatic necrosis	**Oral/GI ulceration**,* **myelosuppression**,* hepatic toxicity, renal toxicity, **pulmonary infiltrates and fibrosis**,* osteoporosis, conjunctivitis, alopecia, depigmentation
Mitoxantrone (Novantrone)	Blue-green sclera and pigment in urine, nausea/vomiting, stomatitis	**Myelosuppression**,* cardiotoxicity, alopecia, white hair, skin lesions, hepatic damage, renal failure
Paclitaxel (Taxol), docetaxel (Taxotere)	Hypersensitivity, hypotension, nausea, pain on extravasation	**Myelosuppression**,* alopecia, peripheral neuropathy, rash and edema (docetaxel)
Vinblastine (Velban)	Nausea/vomiting, local reaction and phlebitis with extravasation	**Myelosuppression**,* alopecia, stomatitis, loss of DTRs, jaw pain, muscle pain, paralytic ileus
Vincristine (Oncovin)	Local reaction with extravasation	**Peripheral neuropathy**,* alopecia, mild myelosuppression, constipation, paralytic ileus, jaw pain, SIADH

* Dose-limiting effects.
Drugs of choice for cancer chemotherapy. Med Lett 42:83–92, 2000.

11. Which chemotherapeutic drugs are associated with cardiotoxicity?

Cardiotoxicity is most frequently associated with **doxorubicin** (Adriamycin), which causes a progressive loss of cardiac muscle cells. In previously normal hearts, this toxicity is dose-related and does not become clinically important until a total dose of approximately 450 mg/m^2 is administered. In patients with already compromised cardiac function, this toxicity may occur at lower dosages. Cardiac radionuclide gated wall motion studies (multiple-gated acquisition [MUGA] scans) or echocardiograms measuring ejection fraction are used to monitor changes in cardiac function.

12. Define the term neoadjuvant therapy.

Neoadjuvant therapy means treatment with chemotherapy is given prior to definitive surgery or radiotherapy. This differs from adjuvant therapy, in which the tumor has been grossly removed by surgery and chemotherapy is administered afterwards to prevent recurrence. Patients given neoadjuvant therapy often have large or fixed tumors, and the idea is to shrink these tumors to make subsequent surgical removal or radiotherapy easier and more effective.

13. What are radiosensitizers?

Radiosensitizers are chemical agents that increase the sensitivity of cells in vitro to radiation and are usually classified as non-hypoxic cell sensitizers. This class of compounds includes drugs such as halogenated pyrimidine nucleoside analogs, 3-amino-benzamide, diamide, and various platinum compounds, among others. Radiosensitization by these compounds may be mediated by a variety of mechanisms, none of which is precisely known. However, it is often assumed that effects on the induction and/or repair of radiation-induced damage may be involved.

14. Define the term tumor doubling time.

Tumor doubling time refers to the time required for the tumor to double in size. The doubling time of cancers varies greatly among cancers. Tumors may be ranked with respect to the doubling time.

Tumor Doubling Times for Common Cancers

Primary lung cancer	
Adenocarcinoma	21 weeks
Squamous cell carcinoma	12
Small cell carcinoma	11
Breast cancer	
Primary	14
Lung metastases	11
Soft-tissue metastases	3
Colorectal cancer	
Primary	90
Lung metastases	14

From Tannock IF, Hill RP (eds): The Basic Science of Oncology, 2nd ed. New York, McGraw Hill, 1992, p 155; with permission.

15. How is the doubling time of tumors calculated from chest x-rays?

The doubling time of tumors can be roughly calculated from chest x-rays by measuring the diameter of the lesion (assuming it is approximately spherical) and calculating its volume with the formula: volume = $4/3 \ \pi r^3$, where π is *pi* and r is the radius of the lesion. After the volume is calculated on two separate occasions, doubling time can be extracted from a plot of volume versus time.

This calculation assumes very simple growth kinetics and the absence of other factors affecting the growth, which is rarely, if ever, the case. Tumor cell populations exhibit a reduction in net fractional growth rate with increasing population size. The Gompertz equation describes this slowing of growth with size and takes into account various other factors, such as decreasing blood supply with increasing size of tumor.

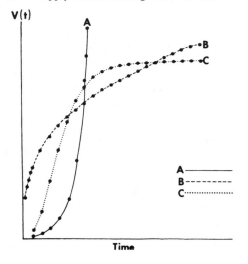

A, Exponential tumor growth curve; *B*, cube-root function growth curve; *C*, tumor growth curve from the Gompertz equation. (From Silver RT, et al: Some new aspects of modern cancer chemotherapy. Am J Med 63:772–787, 1977, with permission.)

COMPLICATIONS OF CANCER

16. What are the causes of anemia in cancer patients?

The anemia may be secondary to blood loss due to bleeding from tumors or gastritis from the use of nonsteroidal anti-inflammatory agents such as aspirin. It may also be caused by hemolysis (which may be secondary to antibodies associated with the tumor), disseminated intravascular coagulation (DIC), sepsis, or related to a paraneoplastic syndrome in cases of cancer of the pancreas or prostate.

Anemia also can be caused by bone marrow suppression by chemotherapy or marrow involvement by the tumor. Anemia of chronic disease is common in cancer patients, and the diagnosis is made when no other cause of anemia can be found and plasma iron is < 60 mg/dl, total iron binding capacity (TIBC) is 100–250 mg/dl, and ferritin is > 60 ng/ml. The hematocrit is generally 25–30%. An inadequate erythropoietin response to the anemia and an inadequate response to treatment with recombinant human erythropoietin have been demonstrated in some patients.

17. What are the predisposing factors, organisms, and sources for infection in cancer patients?

Predisposing factors for infection in cancer patients include defects in cellular and humoral immunity, organ compromise due to tumor-related obstruction, chemotherapy-related granulocytopenia, disruption of mucosal (e.g., respiratory and alimentary tract) and integumental surfaces, iatrogenic procedures or placement of prosthetic devices, central nervous system dysfunction, and hyposplenic or postsplenectomy states.

Organisms currently accounting for the majority of infections in cancer patients are the gram-positive organisms, especially the coagulase-negative staphylococci, *Staphylococcus aureus*, and streptococci. Infections with gram-negative Enterobacteriaceae (*Klebsiella*, *Enterobacter*, *E. coli*, and *Pseudomonas* sp.) have declined since the early 1980's. Fungal organisms found in infected cancer patients include *Aspergillus*, *Candida* sp., and *Cryptococcus*. The most common viral infections found in cancer patients are herpes simplex and varicella-zoster.

The vast majority of infections originate from the patients' own endogenous flora. **Sources** of infection in neutropenic cancer patients include the lungs, urinary tract, skin, upper aerodigestive tract (mouth, skin, teeth), central nervous system, rectum, perirectum, biopsy sites, and the GI tract (appendicitis, cholecystitis, perforations). Cultures should include blood, urine, sputum, and, if appropriate, stool, pleural fluid, and peritoneal fluid.

18. Which tumors spread to bone most commonly? Are these lesions osteoblastic or osteolytic?

Cancers of the lung, breast, kidney, prostate, and thyroid, as well as multiple myeloma and malignant melanoma, spread to bone most commonly. Renal cell carcinoma and multiple myeloma tend to be purely lytic, prostate carcinoma tends to be mainly blastic, and the others are mixed. The most frequently involved bones are the spine, ribs, pelvis, and long bones. Tumors that are lytic are most often associated with hypercalcemia, whereas blastic metastases are rarely associated with this complication. The pain of bone metastases is characterized by a dull, aching discomfort that is worse at night and may improve with physical activity.

19. Which tumors metastasize to the lungs?

Most types of tumors can metastasize to the lungs. Therefore, the more common the tumor, the more commonly it is found to have spread to the lung (e.g., breast cancers). Although they also can spread to the lungs, GI cancers tend to first metastasize locally and to the liver before pulmonary involvement is seen. Those tumors that spread via the bloodstream, such as sarcomas, renal cell carcinoma, and colon cancer, tend to produce nodular lung lesions. Those that spread via lymphatic routes, such as cancers of the breast, pancreas, stomach, and liver, often manifest a pattern of lymphangitic spread.

20. What are the symptoms of intracranial metastases?

Headache occurs in up to 50% of patients with intracranial metastases. It is classically described as occurring early in the morning, disappearing or decreasing after arising, and often being associated with nausea and/or projectile vomiting. Other symptoms include focal signs, such as unilateral weakness, numbness, seizures, or cranial nerve abnormalities. Nonfocal complaints such as mental status changes or ataxia may be seen. The diagnosis is made by contrast enhanced CT or MRI of the brain. Treatment consists of decreasing intracranial pressure with steroids, followed by radiotherapy. Surgery is sometimes used in patients with single intracranial lesions.

21. What are the signs and symptoms of malignant pericardial effusion?

The presentation of malignant pericardial effusion can resemble heart failure, with dyspnea, peripheral edema, and an enlarged heart on chest x-ray. However, the dyspnea is often out of proportion to the degree of pulmonary congestion seen on the x-ray. Kussmaul's sign, or jugulovenous distention with inspiration, and pulsus paradoxus of > 10 mmHg with distant heart sounds are clues to the presence of a pericardial effusion. Confirmation of the clinical diagnosis is made by echocardiogram or CT scan. Malignant effusions are usually exudates and are often hemorrhagic. Cytology is helpful if positive but does not exclude cancer if negative.

Treatment is dependent on the patient's condition but should include drainage of the fluid for diagnostic as well as therapeutic reasons. A nonsurgical approach is preferred, with catheter drainage followed by sclerosis of the pericardium, sometimes with a sclerosing agent such as doxycycline. Other approaches include subxiphoid pericardiectomy, balloon pericardiectomy, pericardial window, and pericardial stripping for patients with prolonged life expectancy.

22. What are the presenting symptoms and signs of spinal cord compression?

Ninety-five percent of cancer patients with spinal cord compression present with back pain. Other symptoms include lower extremity weakness, bowel or bladder incontinence, or increased deep tendon reflexes in the lower extremities. The diagnosis is made by magnetic resonance imaging (MRI) or by myelography with computed tomography, which will demonstrate a blockage of the spinal canal. Treatment is directed first at relieving spinal cord swelling and pain, using high dose steroids and adequate pain medication. However, definitive treatment must be carried out emergently to prevent further neurological deterioration, which may be irreversible. Radiotherapy and/or surgery should be initiated immediately.

The most common tumors causing cord compression are lung cancer, breast cancer, prostate cancer, carcinoma of unknown primary, lymphoma, and multiple myeloma. The most common site of cord compression is the thoracic spine, followed by the lumbosacral spine and the cervical spine.

23. Which tumors are associated with nonbacterial thrombotic endocarditis?

Also known as **marantic endocarditis**, this paraneoplastic syndrome is associated with **mucinous adenocarcinomas**, most commonly of the lung, stomach, or ovary, but has been described in other types of cancers as well. It is revealed by the appearance of embolic peripheral or cerebral vascular events causing arterial insufficiency, encephalopathy, or focal neurologic defects. Heart murmurs are often not present. Echocardiograms are often negative, and the diagnosis is usually made post mortem. Treatment with anticoagulants or antiplatelet drugs has been tried with little success.

24. What are the tumor-related causes of hypercalcemia?

Causes of increased calcium in cancer patients are:

1. **Lytic bone metastases**, which release calcium into the bloodstream. This is the most common cause in solid tumors with bony metastases.

2. **Humoral hypercalcemia of malignancy** (HHM) has been demonstrated in patients without bony metastases. Cancers associated with this syndrome secrete a non-PTH substance with activity similar to parathyroid hormone. HHM is associated most commonly with squamous cell cancers of the lung, esophagus, or head and neck, but can also be found in renal cell carcinoma, transitional cell carcinoma of the bladder, and ovarian carcinoma.

3. Formerly known as **osteoclast activating factor**, osteolytic substances such as interleukin 1 (IL-1), IL-6 and TNFα (lymphotoxin) have been shown to cause hypercalcemia in plasma cell dyscrasias.

4. **Vitamin D metabolites** are produced by some lymphomas. These promote intestinal calcium absorption.

25. What is the tumor lysis syndrome?

When rapidly growing tumors are effectively treated with chemotherapy, breakdown products of tumor lysis are released into the vascular system in large amounts. This may cause hyperkalemia, hyperuricemia, hyperphosphatemia, and hypocalcemia. Renal failure may result from the hyperuricemia. This complication is usually seen within a few hours to days following the treatment of tumors such as acute leukemia, Burkitt's lymphoma, and occasionally other rapidly dividing lymphomas. It is rarely, if ever, seen with solid tumors, but has been described in small cell carcinoma of the lung.

Treatment is the same as for renal failure, with vigorous hydration, dialysis if necessary, and appropriate treatment of electrolyte disorders. Preventive treatment with intravenous hydration and allopurinol given before the chemotherapy is the best course.

26. Which medications are commonly used for severe cancer pain?

Narcotic Analgesics for Severe Cancer Pain

	EQUI-ANALGESIC DOSE (MG*)		DURATION (HR)	PLASMA HALF-LIFE (HR)	COMMENTS
Morphine	IM	10	4–6	2–3.5	Standard for comparison. Also available in slow release tabs, rectal suppositories, and elixirs
	oral, SL	60	4–7	2–3.5	
Oxycodone	oral	30	3–5	–	Available as 5 mg dose in combination with aspirin or acetaminophen; also available alone in slow release form
Hydromorphone	IM	1.5	4–5	–	Available as rectal suppository; potent; very high street abuse potential
	oral	7.5	4–6	2–3	
Methadone	oral	20		15–30	Good oral potency; requires careful titration to avoid drug accumulation
Fentanyl	transdermal	2.5	72	13–22	For long-term control of chronic pain; good for patients who can't swallow; also available in oral transmucosal form

* Relative potency of drugs, as compared with morphine, for severe pain.
Modified from Foley KM: The treatment of cancer pain. N Engl J Med 313:84–95, 1985.

27. What are the commonly used medications for mild to moderate cancer pain?

Oral Non-narcotic and Narcotic Analgesics for Mild to Moderate Cancer Pain

	EQUI-ANALGESIC DOSE (MG*)	DURATION (HR)	PLASMA HALF-LIFE (HR)	COMMENTS
Aspirin	650	4–6	3–5	Standard for non-narcotic comparisons; GI and hematologic effects limit use
Acetaminophen	650	4–6	1–4	Weak anti-inflammatory effects; safer than aspirin; limited use in liver failure

(*Table continued on next page.*)

Oral Non-narcotic and Narcotic Analgesics for Mild to Moderate Cancer Pain (cont.)

	EQUI-ANALGESIC DOSE (MG*)	DURATION (HR)	PLASMA HALF-LIFE (HR)	COMMENTS
Codeine	30–60	4–6	3	Biotransformed to morphine; available in combination with non-narcotic analgesics; may cause constipation and nausea
Hydrocodone	5–10	4–8	4	Also has antitussive activity
Ibuprofen	400	4–6	2–4	Monitor for renal effects; GI side effects can limit use in cancer patients. Good for treatment of bony pain from metastases

* Relative potency of drugs, as compared with aspirin, for mild to moderate pain.
Modified from Foley KM: The treatment of cancer pain. N Engl J Med 313:84–95, 1985.

28. What are the neuromuscular complications of cancer?

SITE	PARANEOPLASTIC SYNDROME	AUTOANTIBODIES (ASSOCIATED CANCER)
Brain and cranial nerves	Paraneoplastic cerebellar degeneration	anti-Yo (GYN cancer) anti-Hu (SCLC) anti-Tr (HD) anti-Ri (breast cancer)
	Opsoclonus-myoclonus	anti-Ri (breast cancer)
	Carcinoma associated retinopathy	anti-recoverin (SCLC)
	Optic neuritis	
	Limbic encephalitis	anti-Hu (SCLC)
	Brainstem encephalitis	anti-Hu (SCLC)
Spinal cord	Myelitis	anti-Hu (SCLC)
	Subacute motor neuronopathy	anti-Hu (SCLC)
	Motor neuron disease/ALS	anti-Hu (rarely)
	Necrotizing myelopathy	
	Stiff-man syndrome	anti-amphiphisin (breast, SCLC)
Peripheral nerves and dorsal root ganglia	Subacute or chronic sensorimotor neuropathy	
	Acute polyradiculopathy (GBS)	
	Neuropathy associated with plasma cell dyscrasias	Anti-MAG
	Brachial neuritis	
	Mononeuritis multiplex	
	Sensory neuronopathy	
	Autonomic neuronopathy	
Neuromuscular junction	Lambert-Eaton myasthenic syndrome	Anti-VGCC
	Myasthenia gravis	Acetylcholine receptor Ab
Muscle	Dermatomyositis/ polymyositis	
	Acute necrotizing myopathy	
	Carcinoid myopathy	
	Neuromyopathy	
	Neuromyotonia	Ab to potassium channels

These syndromes frequently occur together as part of paraneoplastic encephalomyelitis/sensory neuronopathy with anti-Hu antibody. GYN = gynecologic; SCLC = small cell lung cancer; HD = Hodgkin's disease; MAG = myelin associated glycoprotein; Ab = antibody; VGCC = voltage-gated calcium channel; GBS = Guillain-Barré syndrome,
Schiff D, et al: Neurologic emergencies in cancer patients. Neurol Clin 16:449–481, 1998, with permission.

GASTROINTESTINAL AND LIVER CANCERS

29. Summarize the risk factors for esophageal cancer.

Squamous cell cancer of the esophagus occurs in the 40–60 year age group and is seen mainly in men. It is more common in blacks and in Far Eastern countries. Risk factors include:

- Geography: Africa, China, Russia, Japan, Scotland, and the Caspian region of Iran have an increased incidence
- Nonwhite male population
- Excessive alcohol use
- Excessive tobacco use
- Native Bantu beer (southern Africa)
- Chronic hot beverage ingestion
- Lye ingestion: > 30% of cases develop esophageal cancer
- Tylosis: > 40% of cases develop esophageal cancer
- Achalasia
- Plummer-Vinson syndrome
- Nontropical sprue
- Oral and pharyngeal cancer
- Occupational exposure to asbestos, combustion products, ionizing radiation
- Other occupational exposure: waiters, bartenders, metal workers, and construction workers
- Decreased dietary intake of fruits and vegetables throughout adulthood

Adenocarcinoma of the esophagus in a younger population without the traditional risk factors has been associated with chronic esophagitis, reflux disease, and Barrett's esophagus. The incidence of esophageal adenocarcinoma has greatly increased over the last decade. Adenocarcinoma of the esophagus is now more prevalent than squamous cell carcinoma in the United States and western Europe, with most tumors located in the distal esophagus and esophagogastric junction.

Devesa SS, et al: Changing patterns in the incidence of esophageal and gastric carcinoma in the United States. Cancer 83:2049–2053, 1998.

30. How does esophageal cancer present?

Presenting Symptoms of Esophageal Carcinoma

Dysphagia: first with solids, then with liquids	Occult GI bleeding	Choking
	Aspiration pneumonia	Hoarseness
Weight loss	Cough	Chest pain on swallowing
Regurgitation	Fever	GERD

31. How should esophageal cancer be treated?

Treatment depends largely on the patient and his or her physical condition at the time of presentation. The only curative procedure is surgery. However, fewer than half of the patients are operable at the time of presentation, and of these, only one-half to two-thirds have tumors that are resectable. Radical radiation therapy has been tried in selected patients, but the 5-year survival rates are < 15%. Local recurrence is reported in about 50% of these patients, and toxicity is high, with complications of radiation pneumonitis, aspiration, tracheoesophageal fistulas, mediastinal perforations, radiation myelitis, hemorrhage, and constrictive pericarditis reported.

Several studies are investigating the use of chemotherapy in combination with radiotherapy either alone or prior to surgery. To date, encouraging responses have been noted, but no definite increase has been seen in long-term survival.

32. List the risk factors for gastric cancer.

Precursor conditions

Chronic atrophic gastritis and intestinal
  metaplasia

Genetic and environmental factors

Family history of gastric cancer
Blood type A

Precursor conditions (cont.)
Pernicious anemia
Partial gastrectomy for benign disease
Helicobacter pylori infection
Ménétrier's disease
Gastric adenomatous polyps
Barrett's esophagus

Genetic and environmental factors (cont.)
Hereditary nonpolyposis colon cancer syndrome
Low socioeconomic status
Low consumption of fruits and vegetables
Consumption of salted, smoked, or poorly
    preserved foods
Cigarette smoking

In addition, the role of oncogenes and tumor suppressor genes is being elucidated. Allelic deletions of the *MCC*, *APC*, and p53 tumor-suppressor genes have been reported in 33, 34, and 64% of gastric cancers, respectively. Gastric cancer rarely involves mutations in the *ras* oncogene. Disparities between mutations associated with the intestinal and diffuse types of gastric cancers may account for their different natural histories.

33. What are the symptoms at the time of diagnosis of patients with gastric cancer?

Symptoms at the Time of the Initial Diagnosis among 18,365 Patients with Gastric Cancer

SYMPTOMS	FREQUENCY (%)
Weight loss	61.6
Abdominal pain	51.6
Nausea	34.3
Anorexia	32.0
Dysphagia	26.1
Melena	20.2
Early satiety	17.5
Ulcer-type pain	17.1
Lower-extremity edema	5.9

Fuchs CS, et al: Gastric carcinoma. N Engl J Med 333:32–41, 1995.

34. What are the risk factors, signs, and symptoms of pancreatic cancer?

Risk Factors for Pancreatic Cancer

- Smoking (2–3 times increased risk)

- Diet high in calories, fat, and protein, low in fruits and vegetables

- Diabetes mellitus

- Chronic pancreatitis

- Surgery for peptic ulcer disease

- Heredity: syndromes such as familial pancreatic cancer, hereditary pancreatitis, familial adenomatous polyposis syndrome, familial atypical multiple mole melanoma syndrome (hereditary dysplastic nevus syndrome), BRCA2, and Peutz-Jeghers syndrome

- Occupational exposure to 2-naphthylamine and petroleum products (>10 yr increases risk to 5:1), DDT

- Males > females

- Blacks > whites

Evans DB, et al: Cancer of the pancreas. In DeVita, et al (eds): Cancer: Principles and Practice of Oncology, 6th ed. Philadelphia, Lippincott Williams & Wilkins, 2001.

Signs and Symptoms of Pancreatic Cancer Based on Tumor Location

	HEAD	BODY/TAIL
Symptoms		
Weight loss	92%	100%
Jaundice	82%	7%
Pain	72%	87%
Anorexia	64%	33%
Nausea	45%	43%
Vomiting	37%	37%
Weakness	35%	43%
Signs		
Jaundice	87%	13%
Palpable liver	83%	—
Palpable gallbladder	29%	—
Tenderness	26%	27%
Ascites	19%	20%

Adapted from Moossa AR, et al: Tumors of the pancreas. In Moossa AR, et al (eds): Comprehensive Textbook of Oncology, 2nd ed. Baltimore, Williams & Wilkins, 1991, p 964, with permission.

35. Which tests are most useful in diagnosing pancreatic cancer?

TEST	DIAGNOSTIC YIELD (VARIOUS SERIES)
CA19-9 level > 200 U/ml	97%
CT scan of abdomen	83–94%
ERCP*	94%
Angiography	90%
Ultrasound of abdomen	75–90%
MRI of abdomen	NA

* ERCP = endoscopic retrograde cholangiopancreatography.
Forsmark CE, et al: Diagnosis of pancreatic cancer and prediction of unresectability using the tumor-associated antigen CA19-9. Pancreas 9:731–734, 1994.

After a radiographic diagnosis of a mass is made, percutaneous or open biopsy may be done. In various series, a positive cytologic diagnosis has been obtained in 87–100% of cases.

36. Describe the diagnostic and staging evaluation for patients suspected of having pancreatic cancer.

Helical CT and gadolinium-enhanced MRI have largely replaced ERCP as diagnostic modalities for suspected carcinoma of the pancreas. These techniques allow accurate depiction of local tumor extent, involvement of adjacent vascular structures, and distant metastases. If a lesion in the pancreas is seen, CT-guided fine needle aspirate can confirm the diagnosis of malignancy. Additional staging includes routine laboratory studies, chest x-ray, and other tests as directed by the history and physical. If there is bone pain or elevated alkaline phosphatase, then bone scan should be done.

Low, RN: Magnetic resonance imaging of the abdomen: Applications in the oncology patient. Oncology 14(6 suppl 3):5–14, 2000.

37. What are the risk factors for hepatocellular carcinoma?

Underlying cirrhosis from any cause appears to be the most important risk factor for the development of hepatocellular carcinoma. The evidence available indicates that chronic infection with **hepatitis B or C viruses** is the major etiologic agent for human hepatocellular carcinoma, since it causes development of cirrhosis. Macronodular cirrhosis is found in 85% of patients with hepatocellular carcinoma, and it is theorized that this is a result of the chronic infection with the virus, which may occur as early as the perinatal stage.

There are extensive studies of **aflatoxins** in human foods in Africa that suggest a quantitative relationship between average human aflatoxin consumption and the incidence of hepatocellular carcinoma around the world. In a small proportion of hepatocellular carcinomas, the cause appears to be related to other factors, including other hepatotropic viruses, tobacco, alcohol, other chemicals, mycotoxins, and hepatic parasites. The relative importance of these factors seems to vary among populations.

38. List the common presenting features of primary tumors of the liver.

Common Presenting Features of Primary Liver Tumors

Asthenia	85–90%
Hepatomegaly	50–100%
Abdominal pain	50–70%
Jaundice	45–80%
Fever	9.5%

Hepatomas also can present in many unusual ways, including:
• Hemoptysis, secondary to pulmonary metastases
• Rib mass, secondary to bony metastasis
• Encephalitis-like picture, secondary to brain metastasis
• Heart failure, secondary to cardiac metastasis and thrombosis of the inferior vena cava
• Priapism, secondary to soft-tissue metastasis
• Bone pain and pathologic fractures, secondary to bony metastases

39. What are the systemic manifestations of hepatocellular carcinoma?
Hepatoma
 Endocrine
  Erythrocytosis   Hypercalcemia
 Nonendocrine
  Hypoglycemia   Hyperlipidemia
  Porphyria cutanea tarda Dysfibrinogenemia
  Cryofibrinogenemia   Alphafetoglobulin synthesis
  Osteoporosis
Hepatoblastoma
 Precocious puberty   Hemihypertrophy
 Cystinuria
Margolis S, et al: Systemic manifestations of hepatoma. Medicine 51:381–390, 1972.

40. Which environmental factors are thought to be related to the development of colon cancer?
There are abundant epidemiologic data to support the link between environmental factors and colorectal cancer:
 1. The disease is more frequent among upper socioeconomic classes living in urban areas.
 2. There is a direct correlation with calorie consumption, dietary fat, oil, and meat protein.
 3. A direct correlation is seen between mortality from coronary artery disease and mortality from colorectal cancer.
 4. Migrant groups tend to assume the incidence rates of their new environments.
 5. Burkitt noted many years ago that in South Africa the low incidence of large bowel cancer was correlated with a diet high in roughage. However, more recent studies did not confirm that high fiber diets reduce the incidence of colon cancer. Others have correlated a diet high in cruciferous vegetables with a lower incidence of this cancer.
 6. Regular use of non-steroidal anti-inflammatory drugs (NSAIDs), especially aspirin, significantly decreases the risk of developing colorectal cancer.
Nevertheless, as with all epidemiologic data, confounding factors not identified may be significant.

41. Besides environmental factors, are there other risk factors associated with the development of colon cancer?

Up to 25% of patients with colorectal cancer have a **family history** of the disease, suggesting the involvement of a genetic factor or factors. Genes so far identified for their involvement in colorectal carcinogenesis are K-*ras*, *APC*, *DCC*, *hMSH2*, *hMLH1*, *hPMS1*, and p53.

Two clinical types of cancer are seen. **Familial adenomatous polyposis, Gardner's syndrome**, and **hereditary nonpolyposis colorectal cancer** are autosomal dominant syndromes: the first two account for < 1% of all colorectal cancers, and the last for 6–15%. Hereditary nonpolyposis colorectal cancer is a familial cancer syndrome that differs in natural history and genetic characteristics from sporadic colorectal cancer.

Familial polyposis coli is characterized by thousands of adenomatous polyps throughout the large bowel. If left untreated, cancer will develop in all patients with this syndrome. The cancer will usually manifest under age 40. The more common nonpolyposis syndrome also involves the proximal large bowel. The median age at presentation is < 50 years, and patients with a strong family history should be intensively screened.

Nonenvironmental Risk Factors in Colorectal Cancer

Age	> 40 in symptomatic patients
Associated disease	Ulcerative colitis
	Granulomatous colitis
	Peutz-Jeghers syndrome
	Familial polyposis syndrome
Past history	Colon cancer or polyps
	Female genital or breast cancer
Family history	Juvenile polyps
	Colon cancer or polyps
	Familial polyposis syndrome

Winawer S: Early diagnosis of colorectal cancer. Curr Conc Oncol March/April 1981, p 8.

42. Compare the TNM and Dukes classification systems for colon cancer. Give the 5-year survivals.

Colon Cancer Classification and Five-Year Survivals

	TNM				5-YR
STAGE	T	N	M	DUKES	SURVIVAL
Stage 0	T0: no evidence of tumor	N0	M0	—	
Stage I	T1: invades submucosa	N0	M0	A	> 90%
Stage I	T2: invades muscularis propria	N0	M0	B1	85%
Stage II	T3: through wall into serosa	N0	M0	B2	70–75%
Stage II	T4: invades other organs or structures, or perforates visceral peritoneum	N0	M0	B2	70–75%
Stage III	Any T	N1:1–3 regional nodes positive	M0	C1: invades muscularis, positive nodes	30–65%
Stage III	Any T	N2: ≥ 4 regional nodes positive	M0	C2: through wall, positive nodes	30–65%
Stage IV	Any T	Any N	M1	D	< 5%

43. What are the presenting symptoms of colon cancer?

The presenting symptoms depend on the location of the lesion. Lesions in the **ascending colon**, where the stool is still quite liquid, do not present with mass effects. However, these tumors frequently ulcerate, leading to chronic blood loss, and patients present with symptoms of anemia or with guaiac-positive stools on screening tests. In the **transverse bowel**, the stool is more concentrated and formed, so that symptoms of obstruction such as abdominal cramping, abdominal pain, or perforation may bring the patient to the attention of the physician. Cancers in the **rectosigmoid** present with tenesmus, narrowing of the stool, and hematochezia.

44. What are the uses and limitations for carcinoembryonic antigen (CEA) level testing?

CEA is an antigen produced by many colon cancers. It cannot be used for screening because it usually (85% of cases) is normal in patients with stage I disease, those who are most amenable to curative surgery. It has also been found to be elevated in cancers of the stomach, pancreas, breast, ovary, and lung and with various nonmalignant conditions such as alcoholic liver disease, inflammatory bowel disease, heavy cigarette smoking, chronic bronchitis, and pancreatitis.

Testing should be done preoperatively in patients undergoing resection for colon cancer, so that the data can be used to follow the course of the disease and treatment. CEA returns to normal in 30–45 days after complete resection of tumors producing it. Thus, postoperative measurement should not be made prior to this time. If a preoperative elevated level that returns to normal after surgery subsequently becomes elevated, it is a very reliable indicator of tumor recurrence. CEA can also be used as a marker for response to chemotherapy.

45. How is chemotherapy used in the treatment of colon cancer?

Chemotherapy has two roles in its treatment. The first, and broader, role is in the treatment of **metastatic disease**, where the agents most commonly used are 5-fluorouracil (5-FU), leucovorin, and irinotecan (CPT-11), alone or in combination. Response rates in metastatic disease are in the range of 20–40%.

The second use of chemotherapy is in an **adjuvant setting**. Patients who were treated with 5-fluorouracil and leucovorin after curative-intent resections of stage III colon cancer were found to have reduced recurrence rate and death rate compared to non-treated controls, and this is now considered standard postoperative therapy for stage III patients. In patients with stage II disease, treatment can be given to patients at high risk for recurrence, as judged by pathologic features of the resected specimens. Tumor vaccines and other immunotherapy are currently under investigation.

46. What is the mechanism of action of 5-fluorouracil (5-FU), and what are its side effects?

5-FU is a potent inhibitor of thymidylate synthetase. Thymidylate synthetase binds strongly to 5-fluorodeoxyuridylate, one of the metabolites of 5-fluorouracil. Without thymidylate synthesis, tumor cells cannot form dTMP, a precursor of DNA synthesis.

Side effects of 5-FU include myelosuppression, cerebellar ataxia, dacryocystitis, angina, mucositis, diarrhea, and hyperpigmentation.

PROSTATE CANCER

47. What tests are available for the diagnosis and staging of prostate cancer? How do their results correlate with the stage?

Diagnostic Evaluation and Staging of Prostate Cancer

	HISTOLOGY OF PROSTATE BIOPSY SPECIMEN	URINARY SYMPTOMS	NONINVASIVE ASSESSMENT OF METASTATIC DISEASE				
STAGE			SAP	PSA	BONE SCAN	PELVIC CT SCAN	SURGICAL LN SAMPLING
I	Incidental histologic finding in 5% or less of resected tissue, well differentiated	Compatible with BPH	N	Often ↑	—	—	Usually not performed

(Table continued on next page.)

Diagnostic Evaluation and Staging of Prostate Cancer (cont.)

STAGE	HISTOLOGY OF PROSTATE BIOPSY SPECIMEN	URINARY SYMPTOMS	NONINVASIVE ASSESSMENT OF METASTATIC DISEASE				SURGICAL LN SAMPLING
			SAP	PSA	BONE SCAN	PELVIC CT SCAN	
II	Incidental histologic finding in > 5% of resected tissue, or tumor not well differentiated, or palpable nodule confined to prostate	Compatible with BPH	N	Often ↑	—	—	+ in 8–25% (indicating stage IV disease)
III	Extends through prostate capsule	Present	N	Usually ↑	—	—	+ in 40–50% (indicating stage IV disease)
IV	Invades other organs or metastatic	Present	Often ↑	Usually ↑	±	±	+ in 95% of patients with elevated SAP

SAP, serum alkaline phosphatase; PSA, prostate specific antigen; LN, lymph node; BPH, benign prostatic hypertrophy; ↑, elevated; –, negative, +, positive.

48. What is the currently used staging system for prostate cancer?

TNM Classification of Prostate Cancer

Primary Tumor

TX	Cannot be assessed
TO	No evidence of primary tumor
T1	Clinically inapparent, not palpable or visible by imaging
T1a	Incidental histologic finding in ≤ 5% of resected tissue
T1b	Incidental histologic finding in > 5% of resected tissue
T1c	Identified by needle biopsy (e.g., because of elevated PSA values)
T2	Confined to the prostate
T2a	Involves one lobe
T2b	Involves both lobes
T3	Extends through the prostatic capsule
T3a	Extracapsular extension (unilateral or bilateral)
T3b	Seminal vesicle invasion
T4	Fixed or invades adjacent structures other than seminal vesicles: bladder neck, external sphincter, rectum, levator muscles and/or pelvic wall

Regional lymph nodes

NX	Cannot be assessed
NO	No regional lymph node metastasis
N1	Metastasis to regional lymph node or nodes

Distant metastases

MX	Cannot be assessed
MO	None
M1	Distant metastases
M1a	Nonregional lymph node (or nodes)
M1b	Bone (or bones)
M1c	One or more other sites

(Table continued on next page.)

TNM Classification of Prostate Cancer (cont.)

Stage Grouping

I	T1aN0M0, grade 1
II	T1aN0M0, grade 2–4
	T1b-c, T1, T2; N0M0, any grade
III	T3N0M0, any grade
IV	T4 or N1 or M1, any grade

American Joint Committee on Cancer: Cancer Staging Manual, 5th ed., Philadelphia, Lippincott-Raven, 1997.

49. What is the long-term survival of patients with prostate cancer?

Survival in Prostate Cancer by Stage

TNM STAGE	5 YEAR SURVIVAL (%)
I	92
II	94
III	91
IV	32–48

50. How are the prostatic acid phosphatase and prostatic specific antigen (PSA) used in the treatment of prostate cancer?

Prostatic specific antigen is a glycoprotein found in the ductular epithelium of normal and malignant prostate tissue. Serum levels reflect the volume of the prostate and therefore may be elevated in large benign prostates as well as in tumors. PSA can be a useful immunohistochemical marker when the primary site of tumor is occult. It is currently used as a screening method. The America Cancer Society and the American Urological Association recommend yearly rectal exam and PSA in men age > 50 or age > 40 for high-risk groups (blacks, strong family history).

Acid phosphatases are enzymes that hydrolyze esters of orthophosphoric acid in an acid milieu. One of these, the **prostatic acid phosphatase**, may be found to be elevated in the majority of patients with advanced or stage IV prostatic cancer, and its level correlates with the disease activity. It may be used as a marker for treatment response. It is not useful as a screening test in early-stage disease and is a much less sensitive marker than PSA.

51. How do the TNM and AUA staging systems relate?

TNM		AUA	
T0	No evidence of primary tumor	A	No palpable lesion
T1a	Incidental histologic finding in ≤ 5% of resected tissue	A1	Focal
T1b	Incidental histologic finding in >5% of resected tissue	A2	Diffuse
T1c	Identified by needle biopsy (e.g., because of elevated PSA values) but not palpable or visible by imaging		
T2	Tumor present clinically or grossly, limited to gland	B	Confined to prostate
T2a	Involves one lobe	B1	Small, discrete nodule
T2b	Involves both lobes	B2	Large or multiple nodules or areas
T3	Extends through prostatic capsule	C	Localized to periprostatic area
T3a	Extracapsular extension (unilateral or bilateral)	C1	No involvement of seminal vesicles, < 70 gm

(Table continued on next page.)

TNM		AUA	
T3b	Seminal vesicle invasion	C2	Involvement of seminal vesicles, > 70 gm
T4	Fixed or invades adjacent structures other than seminal vesicles: bladder neck, external sphincter, rectum, levator muscles and/or pelvic wall		
N1	Metastasis to regional lymph node or nodes	D1	Pelvic lymph node metastasis or urethral obstruction causing hydronephrosis
M1	Distant metastases	D	Metastatic disease
M1a	Nonregional lymph node (or nodes)	D2	Bone or distant lymph node or soft tissue metastasis
M1b	Bone (or bones)		
M1c	One or more other sites		

American Joint Committee on Cancer: Cancer Staging Manual, 5th ed., Philadelphia, Lippincott-Raven, 1997.

52. What are the effects and mechanisms of the various androgen-deprivation therapies for prostate cancer?

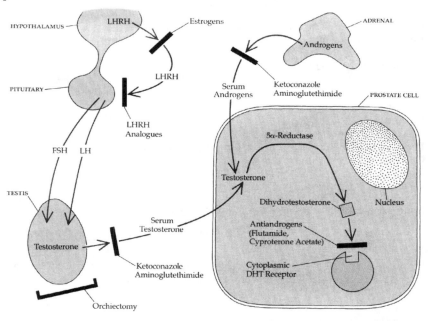

Androgen deprivation, which prevents the trophic influence of testosterone on the prostate in advanced prostate carcinoma, can be effected in a variety of ways. Estrogens such as diethylstilbestrol (DES) inhibit the release of luteinizing hormone-releasing hormone (LHRH) from the hypothalamus, thus diminishing the release of follicle-stimulating hormone (FSH) and luteinizing hormone (LH) from the anterior pituitary and reducing the signal that stimulates testosterone production by the testes. LHRH analogues such as leuprolide initially stimulate but ultimately inhibit the release of FSH and LH from the anterior pituitary and thus have an estrogen-like effect. The testes, which produce most of the testosterone, can be removed by orchiectomy. Ketoconazole and aminoglutethimide inhibit a variety of steroid synthetic pathways, including those that produce androgens in the testes and adrenal glands. In the prostate cells, testosterone is converted into dihydrotestosterone (DHT) by the enzyme 5a-reductase. Antiandrogens such as flutamide, cyproterone acetate, and certain progestational agents block the binding of DHT to its cytoplasmic receptor. (From Rubenstein E, Federman DD (eds): Scientific American Medicine. New York, Scientific American, 1993, p 12(IXA):8; with permission.)

53. What is appropriate therapy for prostate cancer at each stage?

Therapy for Prostate Cancer by Stage

STAGE	THERAPY
I	Watchful waiting, radical prostatectomy, external-beam radiation therapy, TURP if needed for BPH symptoms
II	Radical prostatectomy, external-beam radiation therapy, brachytherapy, watchful waiting for selected patients
III	Radiation therapy ± hormonal therapy (under study), radical prostatectomy with pelvic lymphadenectomy, watchful waiting for selected patients
IV	For urinary obstruction, transurethral prostatectomy (TURP) or radiation therapy For asymptomatic patients, endocrine manipulation or close observation Hormonal therapy for symptomatic disease Palliative radiation therapy for symptomatic areas Chemotherapy for disease refractory to hormonal therapy

BPH, benign prostatic hypertrophy.

GENITOURINARY CANCERS

54. List the risk factors for the development of bladder cancer.

Environmental factors

Occupational hazards
  Workers in dye industry
  Hairdressers
  Painters
  Leather workers
Geographic
Endemic schistosomiasis

Self-ingested toxins
  Tobacco
  Phenacetin
  Artificial sweeteners (possibly)
Miscellaneous
  Alkylating agent (cyclophosphamide)

Previous cancers, especially those of the uroepithelial tract

Cytogenetic abnormalities

Presence of the Ha-*ras* oncogene
Alterations in the 53 suppressor gene

Methylation of the *myc* oncogene
Abnormalities on chromosomes 1, 5, 7, 9, 11, 17

55. What are the most common causes of isolated hematuria?

Major Causes of Isolated Hematuria

TYPE OF BLEEDING	CAUSES
Glomerular bleeding	Mild forms of glomerulonephritis: IgA nephropathy, hereditary nephritis, thin basement membrane disease, postinfectious glomerulonephritis Long-distance running
Extraglomerular renal bleeding	Pelvic calculi Hypercalciuria Carcinoma: renal cell, transitional cell (esp. with analgesic abuse) Sickle cell trait or disease Cystic diseases: polycystic kidney disease, medullary sponge kidney Coagulation disorders: hemophilia, anticoagulation therapy Trauma Vascular malformation Venereal diseases: emboli, vasculitis

(Table continued on next page.)

Major Causes of Isolated Hematuria (cont.)

TYPE OF BLEEDING	CAUSES
Extrarenal bleeding	Ureters: calculi Bladder: catheterization, carcinoma, infection caused by common bacteria or *Mycobacterium tuberculosis*, cyclophosphamide Prostate: hypertrophy, carcinoma Urethra: trauma, urethritis

From Rubenstein E, Federman DD (eds): Scientific American Medicine. New York, Scientific American, 1993, 10:III:10.

56. How does renal cell cancer present?

Presenting Signs and Symptoms of Renal Cell Cancer

Classic triad	9%	Anemia	21%
Gross hematuria		Tumor calcification on x-ray	13%
Abdominal mass		Symptoms from metastases	10%
Pain		Fever	7%
Hematuria	59%	Asymptomatic when diagnosed	7%
Abdominal mass	45%	Erythrocytosis	3%
Pain	41%	Hypercalcemia	3%
Weight loss	28%	Acute varicocele	2%

From Skinner DG, et al: Diagnosis and management of renal cell carcinoma: A clinical and pathologic study of 309 cases. Cancer 28:1165, 1971, with permission.

Despite the classic triad of presenting features, renal cell cancer has been called "the internist's tumor" due to its various unusual presentations. These include amyloidosis, hypercalcemia, hypertension, hepatopathy without liver metastases, enteropathy, heart failure, and immune complex glomerulonephritis, among others.

57. What is the prognosis for renal cell cancer?

Survival depends on stage as well as grade of the tumor:

STAGE	5-YEAR SURVIVAL (%)	
I	Confined to the renal parenchyma, ≤ 7 cm in greatest dimension	76–88%
II	Confined to the renal parenchyma, > 7 cm in greatest dimension	65%
III	Involves the renal vein, inferior vena cava, or regional lymph nodes	35%
IV	Invades beyond Gerota's fascia or distant metastases	5–9%

GRADE	5-YEAR SURVIVAL (%)	
I	Highly differentiated tumors, sharply demarcated from surrounding tissue	100%
IIA	Moderately differentiated tumors, locally well circumscribed but not necessarily provided with capsule	59%
IIB	Moderately differentiated tumors, poorly circumscribed but not diffusely infiltrating or markedly polymorphous and mitotic	36%
III	Poorly differentiated, markedly polymorphous tumors that are diffusely infiltrating. Tumors with abundant growth in capillary vessels	0%

American Joint Committee on Cancer: Cancer Staging Manual, 5th ed., Philadelphia, Lippincott-Raven, 1997.

58. What treatments are available for advanced stage renal cell cancer? How effective are they?

There are few effective therapies for advanced stage renal cell cancer. Some data suggest a hormonal influence in these tumors, theorized to be related to the embryonic origins of the tissue.

Megestrol acetate has been used with variable success, mainly resulting in responses of 10–15%. A few **chemotherapeutic agents** have been slightly active, with response rates in the same range as the hormonal treatments. The most commonly used agent is vinblastine. Currently, biological response modifiers such as interferon, interleukins, tumor necrosis factor, and activated lymphocytes are being used; under strict selection criteria, overall response rates of 15–30% have been achieved, but some durable responses occur. The most effective therapy is early diagnosis and surgery.

59. How common is testicular cancer in the U.S.?

Testicular cancer is responsible for approximately 1.1% of all cancers in U.S. males. The majority of these are in patients 29 to 35 years of age, with 6,900 new cases annually. The incidence of testicular cancer is higher in those patients with cryptorchidism, Klinefelter's syndrome, and testicular feminization syndrome.

The etiology of this cancer is unknown, but age, genetic influences, repeated infection, radiation, and possible endocrine abnormalities have been suggested. Cytogenetic markers associated with germ cell cancer of the testes include the presence of isochromosome 12p. When present in multiple copies, a poorer prognosis is indicated.

Greenlee RT, et al: Cancer Statistics, 2000. CA Cancer J Clin 50:7–33, 2000.

60. What are the presenting features of testicular cancer?

Tumors that present locally are detected as a mass in the scrotum. The mass is often painless, although pain is noted in about 25% of reported cases. When the tumor has already spread (5–15%), symptoms of metastases to the lungs and liver are seen. Other diagnostic possibilities of a scrotal mass include epididymitis, hydrocele, inguinal hernia, hematocele, hematoma, testicular torsion, spermatocele, varicocele, and gumma.

61. Which pathological types are most commonly seen among testicular cancers?

Current Pathologic Classification of Germinal Tumors of the Testes

HISTOLOGY	FREQUENCY
Tumors of one histologic type	
Seminoma (germinoma)	
Typical	35%
Anaplastic	4%
Spermatocytic	1%
Embryonal carcinoma	20%
Teratoma	10%
Choriocarcinoma	1%
Tumors of mixed histologic type	
Embryonal carcinoma and teratoma (teratocarcinoma)	24%
Other combinations	5%

62. What are the stages of testicular cancer and their relation to overall survival?

Stages of Testicular Cancer

I	No lymph node involvement or distant metastases
II	Regional lymph node metastasis
III	Distant metastasis to nonregional lymph nodes, lungs, or other sites

The stages are further subdivided based on the results of serum lactic dehydrogenase (LDH) and tumor marker studies (alpha-fetoprotein and beta human chorionic gonadotropin). Survival can no longer be determined on the basis of stage but is much more dependent on the response to therapy. In patients who respond, the survival curves plateau at about 90%.

63. How should testicular cancer be treated?

Transinguinal orchiectomy is performed in all patients with testicular carcinoma. This serves to make the pathologic diagnosis and is the treatment for stage I cancer.

For **pure seminoma**, limited cases are treated with radiation to the retroperitoneal nodes, or close observation followed by radiation if there is relapse. Disseminated disease is treated with combination chemotherapy.

For **nonseminomatous tumors**, retroperitoneal lymphadenectomy is most commonly done. If nodes are positive, patients may be treated with 2–4 cycles of adjuvant chemotherapy.

For patients with **stage III disease**, or earlier stage disease with bulky mediastinal or retroperitoneal masses, three to four courses of chemotherapy are given, followed by resection of any residual disease.

Tumor markers—alpha-fetoprotein (AFP) and human chorionic gonadotropin (HCG)—are followed for evidence of recurrent disease. These are quite sensitive for the presence of disease, although normal values do not rule out disease.

64. List the possible long-term effects of therapy for testicular cancer.
1. Impotence
2. Infertility
3. Renal dysfunction
4. Raynaud's phenomenon
5. Hearing loss
6. Generalized vascular disorders (acute myocardial infarction, deep venous thrombosis, stroke)
7. Leukemia

65. Describe the extragonadal germ cell syndrome.

The extragonadal germ cell syndrome is characterized by germ cell tumors found in the mediastinum, retroperitoneum, or pineal gland in relatively young males, with elevated HCG or AFP, and marked elevation of lactic dehydrogenase (LDH). These patients often respond to treatment with chemotherapy developed for testicular cancer. It is very important that a careful search for an occult testicular primary be carried out, since the testis is thought to be a relative sanctuary from the effects of chemotherapy. Ultrasound evaluation is useful in this setting.

LUNG CANCER

66. What is the most common cause of cancer death in the U.S. today, excluding skin cancer?

Lung cancer. See cancer incidence percentages in the figures below.

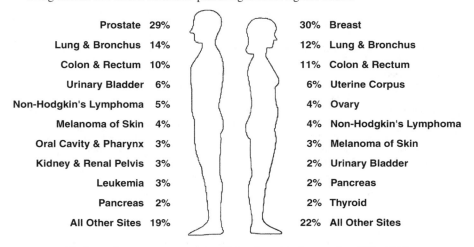

Prostate	29%			30%	Breast
Lung & Bronchus	14%			12%	Lung & Bronchus
Colon & Rectum	10%			11%	Colon & Rectum
Urinary Bladder	6%			6%	Uterine Corpus
Non-Hodgkin's Lymphoma	5%			4%	Ovary
Melanoma of Skin	4%			4%	Non-Hodgkin's Lymphoma
Oral Cavity & Pharynx	3%			3%	Melanoma of Skin
Kidney & Renal Pelvis	3%			2%	Urinary Bladder
Leukemia	3%			2%	Pancreas
Pancreas	2%			2%	Thyroid
All Other Sites	19%			22%	All Other Sites

Estimated new cancer cases—10 leading sites by gender, U.S., 2000.
* Excludes basal and squamous cell skin cancers and in situ carcinomas except urinary bladder.
Percentages may not total 100% due to rounding.

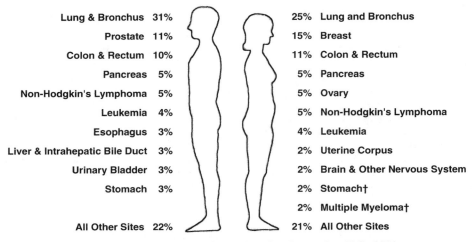

Lung & Bronchus	31%			25%	Lung and Bronchus
Prostate	11%			15%	Breast
Colon & Rectum	10%			11%	Colon & Rectum
Pancreas	5%			5%	Pancreas
Non-Hodgkin's Lymphoma	5%			5%	Ovary
Leukemia	4%			5%	Non-Hodgkin's Lymphoma
Esophagus	3%			4%	Leukemia
Liver & Intrahepatic Bile Duct	3%			2%	Uterine Corpus
Urinary Bladder	3%			2%	Brain & Other Nervous System
Stomach	3%			2%	Stomach†
				2%	Multiple Myeloma†
All Other Sites	22%			21%	All Other Sites

Estimated cancer deaths—10 leading sites by gender, U.S., 2000.
* Excludes in situ carcinomas except urinary bladder.
† These two cancers both received a ranking of 10; they have the same projected number of deaths and contribute the same percentage. Percentages may not total 100% due to rounding.
From CA Cancer J Clin 50:7–33, 2000, with permission.

67. What are the common presenting signs and symptoms of lung cancer?

Common Signs and Symptoms of Lung Cancer

---

1. *Symptoms secondary to central or endobronchial growth of the primary tumor:*

Cough	Dyspnea from obstruction
Wheeze and stridor	Pneumonitis from obstruction (fever, productive cough)
Hemoptysis	

2. *Symptoms secondary to peripheral growth of the primary tumor:*

Pain from pleural or chest wall involvement	Dyspnea on a restrictive basis
Cough	Lung abscess syndrome from tumor cavitation

3. *Symptoms related to regional spread of the tumor in the thorax by contiguity or by metastasis to regional lymph nodes:*

Tracheal obstruction	Esophageal compression with dysphagia
Recurrent laryngeal nerve paralysis with hoarseness	Phrenic nerve paralysis with elevation of the hemidiaphragm and dyspnea
Sympathetic nerve paralysis with Horner's syndrome	C8 and T1 nerve compression with ulnar pain and Pancoast's syndrome
Superior vena cava syndrome from vascular obstruction	Pericardial and cardiac extension with resultant tamponade, arrhythmia, or cardiac failure
Lymphatic obstruction with pleural effusion	Lymphangitic spread through the lungs with hypoxemia and dyspnea

4. *Symptoms due to distant metastases or systemic effects:*

Bone pain	Hemiparesis
Painful lymphadenopathy	Weight loss
Hypercalcemia	Fatigue, malaise

Modified from Cohen MH: Signs and symptoms of bronchogenic carcinoma. In Straus MJ (ed): Lung Cancer. Clinical Diagnosis and Treatment, 2nd ed. New York, Grune & Stratton, 1983, pp 97–111, with permission.

68. What are the accepted and proposed risk factors for lung cancer?
- **Cigarette smoking** causes 85% of lung cancers in men. In women, lung cancer has surpassed breast cancer as the leading cause of cancer death. Passive smoking (side-stream smoke) also increases the risk of lung cancer, causing 25% of the lung cancers seen in nonsmokers.
- **Radon exposure** increases the risk of lung cancer, especially in smokers, who have a 10-fold higher risk. An estimated 25% of lung cancer in nonsmokers and 5% in smokers is attributed to radon daughter exposure in the home.
- **Marijuana smoking** increases the risk of lung cancer in smokers.
- **Emphysema**, which develops in smokers, is associated with an increased risk.
- **Other agents**: Bis-chloromethylether, arsenic, nickel, ionizing radiation, asbestos, chromates

69. Which chromosomal defects are associated with lung cancer?
Deletion of 3p (usually 3p14–23) is found in virtually all cases (93%) of small cell lung cancer (SCLC, both classic and variant), in 100% of bronchial carcinoids, and 25% of non-SCLC.

Also seen are absent or reduced expression of the *rb* gene at 13q14, increased production of the c-*jun* oncogene product, and constitutive expression of c-*raf*-1 gene on 3p25. More than 50% of all lung cancers contain a mutation of the *p53* tumor suppressor gene. A *ras* family oncogene is mutated in about 20% of non-SCLC, but not in SCLC.

Various tumor markers can be used to assess prognosis. Elevated levels of CA-125, expression of blood group antigen A in tumor cells, expression on tumor cells of the carbohydrate antigen H/Le^y/Le^b, activation of the K-*ras* oncogene, increased expression of p186*neu* have all been associated with poorer prognosis of patients with lung cancer.

70. Which tests are used for the evaluation of suspected lung cancer?
The primary evaluation should include a chest x-ray and sputum cytology. If the expectorated sputum cytology is negative, bronchoscopy with biopsy, percutaneous biopsy, or thoracoscopy may be done. Preoperative evaluation includes CT scanning of the chest and upper abdomen to evaluate for mediastinal and hilar nodes and for liver and/or adrenal metastases. Pulmonary function tests and mediastinoscopy should be done if surgical resection is considered. Routine hematology and biochemical tests may suggest the presence of bone marrow or liver metastases, and screening for the presence of brain metastases can be done using CT or MRI. Elevated alkaline phosphatase with normal liver CT suggests bony metastasis, and a bone scan should be done.

71. Which paraneoplastic syndromes are associated with lung cancer?

Paraneoplastic Syndromes in Lung Cancer

1. Systemic symptoms
  Anorexia-cachexia (31%)
  Fever (21%)
  Suppressed immunity
	5. Neurologic-myopathic
	  Lambert-Eaton syndrome (SCLC)
	  Peripheral neuropathy
	  Subacute cerebellar degeneration

2. Endocrine (12%)
  Ectopic PTH: hypercalcemia (epidermoid)
    SIADH (SCLC)
  Ectopic secretion of ACTH: Cushing's syndrome
	Cortical degeneration
	  Polymyositis
	  Retinal blindness
	6. Cutaneous

3. Skeletal
  Clubbing (29%)
  Hypertrophic pulmonary osteoarthropathy:
    periostitis (1–10%) (adenocarcinoma)
	Dermatomyositis
	  Acanthosis nigricans
	7. Hematologic (8%)
	  Anemia

4. Coagulation-thrombotic
  Migratory thrombophlebitis, Trousseau's syndrome: venous thrombosis
  Nonbacterial thrombotic endocarditis: arterial emboli; DIC: hemorrhage
	Granulocytosis
	  Leukoerythroblastosis
	8. Renal (1%)
	  Nephrotic syndrome
	  Glomerulonephritis

Cohen MH: Signs and symptoms of bronchogenic carcinoma. In Straus, MJ (ed): Lung Cancer. Clinical Diagnosis and Treatment. New York, Grune & Stratton, 1977, pp 85–94.

72. Describe the TNM staging system for lung cancer.

TNM Classification for Lung Cancer

TX	Primary tumor cannot be assessed, or tumor proven by presence of malignant cells in sputum or bronchial washings but not visualized by imaging or bronchoscopy
T0	No evidence of primary tumor
Tis	Carcinoma in situ
T1	Tumor 3 cm or less, surrounded by lung or visceral pleura, not in main bronchus
T2	Tumor > 3 cm; or involves main bronchus, 2 cm or more distal to the carina; or invades visceral pleura; or associated with atelectasis or obstructive pneumonitis that extends to the hilar region but does not involve the entire lung
T3	Tumor of any size that directly invades any of the following: chest wall (including superior sulcus tumors), diaphragm, mediastinal pleura, parietal pericardium; or tumor in the main bronchus less than 2 cm distal to the carina but without involvement of the carina; or associated atelectasis or obstructive pneumonitis of the entire lung
T4	Tumor of any size that invades: mediastinum, heart, trachea, great vessels, esophagus, vertebral body, carina; separate tumor nodule(s) in the same lobe, or tumor with a malignant pleural effusion
N0	No regional lymph node metastasis
N1	Metastasis to ipsilateral peribronchial and/or ipsilateral hilar lymph nodes and intrapulmonary nodes including involvement by direct extension of primary tumor
N2	Metastasis to ipsilateral mediastinal and/or subcarinal node(s)
N3	Metastasis in contralateral mediastinal, contralateral hilar, ipsilateral or contralateral scalene or supraclavicular lymph node(s)
M0	No distant metastasis
M1	Distant metastasis, including separate tumor nodule(s) in a different lobe (ipsilateral or contralateral)

	STAGE GROUPING	5 YEAR SURVIVAL (%)
IA	T1N0M0	61
IB	T2 N0M0	38
IIA	T1N1M0	34
IIB	T2N1M0, T3N0M0	24
IIIA	T1–2 N2M0, T3 N1–2M0	13
IIIB	Any T N3M0, T4 Any N M0	5
IV	Any T Any N M1	1

Mountain CF. Revisions in the international system for staging lung cancer. Chest 111:1710–1717, 1997.

73. Which drugs and other treatment modalities are used to manage small cell lung cancer?

Because of early hematogenous spread and the fact that 30% of patients present with limited unresectable stage III disease, chemotherapy (using etoposide, cisplatin, and other combinations) and radiotherapy are used. These combinations in limited stage disease have resulted in complete remission rates of 40–60%, median survival of 16–24 months, and five year survivals of 5–10%. Radiotherapy to the brain remains somewhat controversial, and timing, dose, and long term complications continue to be argued.

74. How effective is the treatment of advanced stage (IV) small cell lung cancer?

Patients with advanced stage small cell lung cancer often have good partial responses to chemotherapy, but the responses are not durable. Median survival for patients with extensive disease who respond to treatment is 6–12 months. However, this is a significant improvement over the survival of untreated patients, which is measured in weeks.

75. What is the superior vena cava (SVC) syndrome? What is its significance in lung cancer?

SVC syndrome results when the flow of blood in the SVC is obstructed due to thrombosis within the vessel or compression of the vein externally. Seventy-five to 85% of the cases are due to compression by a tumor, with lung cancer, especially SCLC, accounting for up to 80% of these. Lymphoma and other mediastinal malignancies account for the remaining cases.

Although obstruction of the vena cava has been considered a life-threatening **oncologic emergency**, only rarely does it progress to cause laryngeal edema, seizures, coma, and death. Usually, patients present with dyspnea, face and arm edema, a sense of fullness in the head, and cough. Collateral circulation often develops, leading to the finding of prominent veins over the neck and chest and limiting the severity of symptoms.

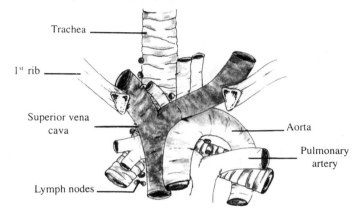

Anatomy of the superior vena cava

From Wood, ME, Bunn PA Jr: Hematology/Oncology Secrets. Philadelphia, Hanley & Belfus, 1994, p 240; with permission.

76. How is non-small cell lung cancer treated?

The first decision to be made is whether the patient is a candidate for resection. If the patient is medically able to undergo resection, then it should be performed only if the following are *not* present:

1. Distant metastases
2. Malignant pleural effusion
3. Superior vena cava obstruction
4. Involvement of supraclavicular, cervical, or contralateral mediastinal nodes
5. Recurrent laryngeal nerve paralysis
6. Involvement of the tracheal wall, or mainstem bronchus < 2 cm from the carina
7. Small cell carcinoma histology

Recent evidence suggests that in stage IIIA disease (large tumor or involvement of mediastinal nodes), preoperative chemotherapy and radiotherapy significantly improve survival. If patients are not able to undergo surgery and they do not have small cell cancer, then combined chemotherapy and radiotherapy are indicated. The only contraindication to radiation therapy is the presence of such bulky disease that treatment would compromise remaining lung tissue. In higher stage disease, systemic chemotherapy or palliative care are options, depending on the performance status of the patient.

77. What are the acute and long-term complications of chemotherapy and radiotherapy used in the treatment of lung cancer?

Acute	Long term
Tumor lysis syndrome	Neurologic damage with resultant:
Myelosuppression predisposing to:	Confusion
Infection	Episodic hemiparesis
Bleeding	Ataxia
Anemia	Progressive organic brain syndrome
Renal toxicity (cisplatin)	Leukemia
Peripheral neuropathy (cisplatin,	Second primary carcinomas and sarcomas
taxanes, vinorelbine)	Pulmonary fibrosis
Radiation pneumonitis and esophagitis	Constrictive pericarditis

78. What are the presenting symptoms of head and neck cancer?

SITE	SYMPTOMS
Oral cavity: lips, buccal mucosa, alveolar ridge, retromolar trigone, floor of mouth, hard palate, anterior $\frac{2}{3}$ of tongue	Mass, ulcer, leukoplakia, bleeding, pain, loose teeth, earache, trismus, halitosis
Larynx: supraglottic (false cords, arytenoid), glottic (true vocal cords), subglottic	Hoarseness, bleeding, sore throat, thyroid cartilage pain
Pharynx: nasopharynx, oropharynx, soft palate, uvula, tonsil, base of tongue, hypopharynx, pyriform sinus	Sore throat, earache, epistaxis, nasal voice, dysphagia, masses, hearing loss, blood-streaked saliva
Maxillary sinus	Sinusitis, epistaxis, headache
All sites	Bleeding (oral or nasal), neck nodes, pain at site of tumor or referred pain

79. What are the risk factors for squamous cell cancer of the head and neck area?

Tobacco is the most significant contributing factor to the development of head and neck cancers. Nine of ten patients with cancer in this area are smokers. Snuff dipping and tobacco chewing are also causally related to the development of oral cancer. Smokers have an increased mortality related to head and neck cancer once it has been diagnosed, showing a 2-fold increase in mortality over nonsmokers.

Alcohol is also strongly correlated with the development of head and neck cancer. About half the patients with these cancers have cirrhosis, and three quarters drink alcohol excessively.

Another factor is poor dental hygiene. Woodworkers have an increased incidence of nasopharyngeal cancer. Syphilitic glossitis predisposes to tongue cancer, and nickel compounds to nasal sinus cancer. The Epstein-Barr and herpes simplex type I viruses have been implicated in up to 15% of new cases.

80. Describe the evaluation and initial staging of patients with head and neck cancer.

Initial staging of head and neck cancer includes a thorough **triple endoscopy** of upper and lower airway and upper aerodigestive tract, with biopsy of any suspicious lesions. Measurement and biopsy, if indicated, of any cervical or supraclavicular nodes should be performed. A **CT scan** of the area contributes to the determination of the extent of disease. If elements of the routine blood counts and biochemical profile are abnormal, a bone scan and/or CT scan of the liver may be done. If there is a history of alcohol abuse, liver scans in the face of abnormal liver function tests are useful only if there is hepatomegaly.

The most common sites of metastases of these tumors are local lymphatics, followed by lung metastases. Bone metastases occur in about 15% of the patients. Brain metastases are rare and are seen mainly in patients with nasopharyngeal cancer. It is also important to remember that second primaries in the aerodigestive tract are not uncommon. Depending on tobacco and alcohol history, another cancer, of the head and neck, esophagus, or lung, may be seen in up to 20% of patients at some time in the course of their disease.

81. Currently, what is the most appropriate treatment of head and neck cancer?

Traditionally, head and neck cancers have been treated primarily with surgery, usually involving extensive and radical dissection, and often accompanied by postoperative radiotherapy. Radiotherapy also was used for recurrences that were no longer amenable to surgery. However, the current trend is to treat with **multimodality therapy**, using chemotherapy, either in combination with radiotherapy or prior to surgery or radiotherapy. The optimum combination of these agents and modalities has not yet been determined, and trials are ongoing. One problem is that the natural history of these tumors is quite divergent, meaning results will vary depending on the patient mix. Stopping smoking and alcohol consumption, combined with the use of retinoic acid derivatives, may be helpful in preventing the occurrence of second primary cancers in the head and neck region.

82. Which chemotherapeutic agents are used in the treatment of squamous cell cancers of the head and neck? How effective are they?

Several agents are effective, and include cisplatin and 5-fluorouracil infusions, paclitaxel, carboplatinum, methotrexate, bleomycin, and mitomycin C. Response rates for these agents vary from 25–80%, depending on the agent, schedule, tumor type, previous treatment, and performance status. Combination chemotherapy regimens usually show higher initial response rates but have yet to show an increase in survival rates.

BREAST CANCER

83. What are the current recommendations for screening for breast cancer?

There are currently several sets of recommendations from the various specialty organizations whose members are engaged in breast cancer screening. These are as follows:

Recommended Frequency of Screening for Breast Cancer

ORGANIZATION	AGE > 50		AGE < 50	
	MAMMOGRAM	BREAST EXAM	MAMMOGRAM	BREAST EXAM
American Cancer Society	Annual	Annual	Age 40–49, annual	Age 40–49, annual Age 20–39, every 3 years
National Cancer Institute	Annual	With every periodic physical exam	Starting at age 40, every 1-2 years*	With every periodic exam
American College of Obstetricians and Gynecologists	As determined by woman's doctor		Age 35–50, baseline*	Age 35–50, exams recommended
American College of Radiology	Annual	Annual	Age 40-49, annual	
American College of Physicians	Age 50–59, on "routine" basis Age ≥ 60, as determined by doctor and patient	—	Not recommended	
U.S. Preventive Services Task Force	Age 50–69, annual	Age 50–69, annual	Not recommended	Age 40–49, annual

* Mammography recommended more frequently for women with high risk factors.

In addition, it is important for the primary care physician to identify high-risk patients who may have a mutation in a dominant breast cancer susceptibility gene. Such families have a history of breast or ovarian cancer in as many as half of all female relatives, with early age of onset and/or bilateral or multifocal disease. These patients have been shown to have a high incidence of the *BRCA1* and *BRCA2* genes on chromosome 17 and 13, respectively. Patients with these gene mutations have been shown to have a cumulative lifetime risk of breast cancer ranging up to 87%.

84. How is the diagnosis of breast cancer established?
By tissue examination. This may be done by percutaneous fine needle aspirate, with or without x-ray direction, or by incisional or excisional biopsy. While mammograms are essential in screening and localizing tumors, up to 15% of breast cancers may not be seen on mammogram, and the diagnosis cannot be made definitively without tissue confirmation. Any clinically suspicious mass must be biopsied.

85. At what age does the incidence rate of breast cancer peak?

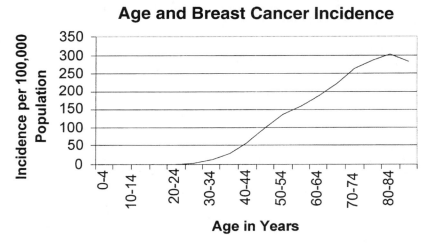

Annual age-specific incidence rates of breast cancer, 1993–1997. From: SEER Cancer Statistics Review, 1973–1997, http://seer.cancer.gov/Publications/CSR1973_1997/breast.pdf

86. What are the risk factors for breast cancer?
1. **High risk factors** (associated with a 3× or more increase)
   a. Age (> 40 years old)
   b. Previous cancer in one breast
   c. Breast cancer in a first- or second-degree family member
   d. History of multiple breast biopsies
   e. Parity: nulliparous, or first pregnancy after age 31 years
   f. Lobular carcinoma in situ
   g. Gene mutations: *BRCA1*, *BRCA2*, *hMSH2*, *hMLH1*, *hPMS1*, *p53*, others.
   h. Radiation exposure to chest wall during childhood or adolescence
2. **Intermediate risk** (1.2 to 1.5× risk)
   a. Early menarche or late menopause
   b. Oral estrogens
   c. History of cancer of the ovary, uterus, or colon
   d. Alcoholic beverages (?)
   e. Obesity

87. What can women do to reduce their risk of breast cancer?

Recent studies have shown that for women at high risk for breast cancer due to a previous personal history of breast cancer, first-degree family members with breast cancer, and other factors, the use of tamoxifen can reduce the occurrence of new breast cancers by about half. Some women who are known to carry the *BRCA1* or *BRCA2* gene mutations choose to undergo prophylactic simple mastectomies, which reduce the incidence of breast cancer by about 90%.

Vogel VG: Breast cancer prevention: A review of current evidence. CA 50:156–170, 2000.

88. What are the poor prognostic factors in primary breast cancer?

1. Estrogen or progesterone receptors negative
2. Positive HER-2/neu oncogene
3. Premenopausal patient
4. Large tumor size
5. Positive axillary nodes
6. Local skin involvement
7. Fixed axillary nodes
8. Distant metastasis
9. Aneuploidy and high cathepsin D
10. Nuclear grade 3 (poor)
11. High S-phase fraction

89. Describe the appropriate treatment of local-regional breast cancer.

Although there is no single "right" way to treat localized breast cancer, and a great deal of controversy exists, the following guidelines are available:

Stage I—"Lumpectomy" with axillary dissection and radiation; or modified radical mastectomy. **Lumpectomy/radiotherapy** is used if cosmesis is important, complete excision is possible, and > 6000 rads can be delivered to the tumor bed. **Modified radical mastectomy** is used if cosmesis is unimportant, lesion size is large relative to breast size, or radiotherapy is not technically possible.

Stage II—**Modified radical mastectomy** with postoperative chemotherapy and/or hormonal therapy, depending on estrogen and progesterone receptor status of the tumor and menopausal status of the patient.

Stage III—**Modified radical mastectomy** with postoperative chemotherapy and/or hormonal therapy, depending on estrogen and progesterone receptor status of the tumor and menopausal status of the patient, followed by local radiotherapy. For very large or fixed tumors that are initially deemed to be inoperable, preoperative chemotherapy or hormonal therapy may render such cancers surgically removable.

Stage IV—**Systemic chemotherapy** or **hormone therapy**, depending on hormone receptor status, reserving surgery and radiotherapy for local control.

90. How is adjuvant therapy used in the management of breast cancer?

Current Recommendations for the Use of Adjuvant Systemic Therapy in Breast Cancer

	PREMENOPAUSAL	POSTMENOPAUSAL
Node negative: *		
ER or PR negative	Chemotherapy	Chemotherapy
ER or PR positive	Chemotherapy + TAM, ovarian ablation or LHRH agonist	Tamoxifen ± chemotherapy
Node positive: **		
ER or PR negative	Chemotherapy	Chemotherapy
ER or PR positive	Chemotherapy + TAM, ovarian ablation or LHRH agonist	Tamoxifen ± chemotherapy

* Adjuvant treatment is recommended for patients with poor prognosis tumors: tumor size > 2 cm, poor nuclear grade, high S phase fraction. ** Adjuvant treatment is recommended for all patients. ER = estrogen receptor; PR = progesterone receptor; TAM = tamoxifen; LHRH = luteinizing hormone-releasing hormone

In addition, postoperative chest wall and regional lymph node radiation therapy is given to patients considered to be at high risk for local recurrence. Risk factors for local recurrence include 4 or more positive axillary nodes, extracapsular nodal extension, large primary tumors and positive or very close tumor resection margins.

91. Which agents are used in the treatment of metastatic breast cancer? How effective are they?

Among the most effective chemotherapy agents for breast cancer are adriamycin, epirubicin, paclitaxel (Taxol), taxotere, vinorelbine, cyclophosphamide, methotrexate, fluorouracil, capecitabine, and prednisone. These agents are used singly or in combination in the treatment of advanced or metastatic breast cancer. If the tumor overexpresses the *Her/neu* oncogene, trastruzumab (Herceptin) may be added to improve the effectiveness of chemotherapy.

Overall induction response rates range from 55–65%. Median survival times are 14 to 18 months. The survival rates depend more on the site of the metastatic disease than on the treatment, with visceral disease faring more poorly than bony or soft tissue metastases. Most patients receive more than one treatment regimen, since the median time to failure of most programs is about 6 months.

For bony or soft tissue metastases in patients with estrogen or progesterone receptor positive breast cancer, hormonal agents such as tamoxifen, anastrazole, or LHRH agonists (in premenopausal women) can be used for effective palliation lasting many months.

GYNECOLOGIC CANCERS

92. What are the current recommendations for screening carcinoma of the cervix?

Recommendations concerning periodic screening of women in the U.S. using Pap* smears have been developed for the various risk groups. **Low-risk** groups are those women who have never had sexual activity, have had a hysterectomy for nonmalignant reasons, or have reached the age of 60 and have never had a positive Pap smear. **High-risk** patients are those who are sexually active early, have had many partners, or are in low socioeconomic groups.

The American Cancer Society and the American College of Obstetricians and Gynecologists (ACOG) recommend that asymptomatic women over 18 years of age and those under age 18 who are sexually active have annual screening for at least three years. Following this, some recommend they be screened every 2–3 years until age 65, while others suggest yearly screening as long as the patient is sexually active. High-risk patients should be screened yearly.

* From Papanicolaou-Traut smear.

93. What is the appropriate management of a patient with an abnormal Pap smear?

An abnormal Pap smear should lead to colposcopy and/or biopsy. If **carcinoma in situ** or **dysplasia** is found, cryotherapy, laser therapy, cone biopsy, or hysterectomy should be performed, depending on the size and extent of the lesion.

If **invasive cancer** is found on biopsy, a metastatic workup is indicated. Stage I disease is treated with radical hysterectomy or radiation therapy, whereas all other stages are further evaluated with a CT scan. If the para-aortic nodes are enlarged, a needle biopsy should be done. Those with a positive biopsy are treated with pelvic radiation therapy and concurrent chemotherapy. If nodes are normal on the CT scan or if the needle biopsy is negative, then laparotomy with para-aortic node biopsies should be considered to determine the actual state of the nodes. If the biopsy is positive, then treatment should proceed as for other positive-node biopsies. If it is negative, treatment is external beam radiotherapy followed by intracavitary radioactive implants.

94. Which studies are used in the staging of carcinoma of the cervix?

Pelvic exam
Biochemical profile
Chest x-ray
CT scan or MRI (MRI is preferred)
Lymphangiograms may be useful in selected cases
Cystoscopy and proctosigmoidoscopy for advanced disease

95. What are the 5-year survival rates, relative to stage, for carcinoma of the cervix?

STAGE	DESCRIPTION	5-YEAR SURVIVAL
I	Tumor strictly confined to the cervix	89–100%
II	Tumor extends beyond the uterus but not to the pelvic wall The tumor involves the vagina but not the lower third	67%
III	Tumor extends to the pelvic wall, and/or involves the lower third of the vagina, and/or causes hydronephrosis or nonfunctioning kidney	53%
IV	Tumor extends beyond the true pelvis, or has involved the bladder or rectal mucosa, or has distant metastases	5–24%

96. How is carcinoma of the cervix treated?

STAGE	TREATMENT
IA	Total or radical hysterectomy, conization or intracavitary radiation
IB, IIA	External-beam pelvic irradiation combined with 2 or more intracavitary applications; radical hysterectomy with bilateral pelvic lymphadenectomy ± postoperative total pelvic irradiation plus chemotherapy; radiation therapy plus chemotherapy with cisplatin or cisplatin/5-FU for patients with bulky tumors
IIB, III, IVA	Radiation therapy plus chemotherapy: intracavitary radiation and external-beam pelvic irradiation combined with cisplatin or cisplatin/fluorouracil chemotherapy
IVB	Chemotherapy with agents such as cisplatin, paclitaxel, ifosfamide-cisplatin, or irinotecan. Radiotherapy may be used for palliation

Cervical Cancer, PDQ® Treatment Statements for Health Professionals, National Cancer Institute. See their Internet site http://cancernet.nci.nih.gov/

97. Name the risk factors for carcinoma of the endometrium.
1. Infertility
2. Obesity
3. Failure of ovulation
4. Dysfunctional bleeding
5. Prolonged estrogen use
6. Diabetes mellitus
7. Hypertension
8. Polycystic ovaries
9. Familial cancer syndrome (Lynch)
10. Tamoxifen use

98. What are the 5 year survival rates for the various grades and stages of endometrial cancer?

Grades and Stages of Endometrial Cancer

	DESCRIPTION	5-YEAR SURVIVAL
Grade		
I	Differentiated	81%
II	Intermediate	74%
III	Undifferentiated	50%
Stage		
I	Tumor confined to the corpus	92%
II	Tumor involves the corpus and cervix	78%
III	Tumor extends outside the corpus, but not outside the true pelvis (may involve the vaginal wall or the parametrium but not the bladder or rectum)	42%
IV	Tumor involves the bladder or rectum or extends outside the pelvis, or has distant metastases	14%

99. Name the risk factors for ovarian cancer.
• Nulliparity or low parity
• Presence of basal cell nevus syndrome
• Family history of ovarian cancer or ovarian cancer syndromes
• Gonadal dysgenesis (46XY type)
• History of breast, endometrial or colon cancer
• Asbestos exposure
• Presence of Peutz-Jeghers Syndrome
• Use of fertility drugs (?)

NIH Consensus Development Panel on Ovarian Cancer: Ovarian cancer: Screening, treatment, and follow-up. JAMA 273:491–497, 1995.

100. What is the appropriate use of the CA-125 antigen?
CA-125 serum tumor marker is an antigenic determinant detected by radioimmunoassay and is elevated in 80% of epithelial ovarian cancers. Because it is elevated in only half of patients with stage I cancers and is elevated in a significant proportion of healthy women and women with benign disease, it is not a sensitive or specific screening test. In high-risk patients or in patients suspected of having an ovarian cancer, it should be used in conjunction with bimanual rectovaginal pelvic examination and transvaginal ultrasonography. It is also useful as a marker of disease recurrence after surgical resection of ovarian cancer.

101. List the paraneoplastic syndromes associated with ovarian cancer.
1. Neurologic:
   Peripheral neuropathy
   Organic brain syndrome
   AML-like syndrome
   Cerebellar ataxia (anti-Yo
      paraneoplastic cerebellar
      degeneration)
   Cancer-associated retinopathy
   Opsoclonus-myoclonus
2. Cross-matching of blood antigens
3. Cushing's syndrome
4. Hypercalcemia
5. Thrombophlebitis
6. Dermatomyositis
7. Palmar fasciitis and polyarthritis

102. What are the 5-year survival rates for the various stages of carcinoma of the ovary?

STAGE		5-YEAR SURVIVAL
I	Growth limited to the ovaries	84%
II	Growth involving one or both ovaries with pelvic extension	63%
III	Tumor involving ovaries with peritoneal implants outside the pelvis and/or positive retroperitoneal or inguinal nodes	29%
IV	Distant metastases	17%

103. What is the treatment for advanced stage ovarian cancer?
Patients with stage III epithelial ovarian cancers are first treated with surgery, consisting of total abdominal hysterectomy and bilateral salpingo-oophorectomy with omentectomy and de-bulking of as much gross tumor as possible. This is followed by intravenous chemotherapy with cisplatin or carboplatin combined with taxol or cyclophosphamide. Patients with stage IV disease are given combination chemotherapy. The survival benefit of surgical debulking in patients with stage IV extra-abdominal disease is not yet known.

104. What is a molar pregnancy?
Molar pregnancies refer to a group of benign and malignant gestational trophoblastic neoplasms. The most malignant of these is choriocarcinoma, which prior to the advent of chemotherapy

was invariably fatal within 1 to 2 years. The most common variant, hydatidiform mole, occurs in only 1 in 2000 pregnancies in the U.S.

105. What is the therapeutic classification of a molar pregnancy?
1. Molar pregnancy
   a. Pre-evacuation
   b. Post-evacuation
2. Persistent or retained mole (after 8 weeks)
3. Nonmetastatic trophoblastic disease
   a. No histologic evidence of choriocarcinoma
   b. Choriocarcinoma
4. Metastatic trophoblastic disease
   a. No histologic evidence of choriocarcinoma
   b. Choriocarcinoma (low risk)
   c. Choriocarcinoma (high risk)

From Rutledge F, et al (eds): Gynecologic Oncology. New York, John Wiley, 1976, p 145, with permission.

LYMPHOMAS

106. What are some unusual epidemiological features of Hodgkin's disease?
The epidemiology of Hodgkin's disease is scientifically intriguing, suggesting an infective agent. It occurs more frequently in individuals from small families and in children raised in hygienic, isolated environments. DNA from the Epstein-Barr virus and other human herpesviruses has been found in a significant proportion of cases of Hodgkin's disease. Genetic predisposition, as well as infective agents, could explain the increased incidence in some families. Hodgkin's disease is more common in some tropical countries and in the Middle East in children < 10 years.

Jarrett RF, MacKenzie J: Epstein-Barr virus and other candidate viruses in the pathogenesis of Hodgkin's Disease. Semin Hematol 36:260–269, 1999.

107. What are the "favorable" lymphomas?
MALT (mucosa-associated lymphoid tissue) lymphomas involving the stomach have an extremely good prognosis, and can frequently be cured by antibiotics alone.

The low-grade (or "favorable") lymphomas of the Rappaport classification are:
    Diffuse, well-differentiated lymphocytic
    Nodular, poorly differentiated lymphocytic
    Nodular, mixed lymphocytic-histiocytic

They are described as favorable because their natural history is characterized by a relatively long survival, indolent course, and easy response to minimal therapy. However, the low-grade lymphomas generally present in stage III or IV, and are usually incurable.

108. What are the "unfavorable" lymphomas? What is their prognosis?
The unfavorable, or high grade, non-Hodgkin's lymphomas are:
    Large cell immunoblastic
    Lymphoblastic
    Burkitt's

Although these types of lymphoma are very aggressive in their biologic behavior, they are potentially curable with chemotherapy. Many of the other types of non-Hodgkin's lymphoma (nodular histiocytic, diffuse poorly differentiated lymphocytic, diffuse mixed lymphocytic and histiocytic, and diffuse large cell) are called intermediate grade, as their aggressiveness and responsiveness to treatment are intermediate between the low-grade and high-grade lymphomas.

Mantle cell lymphoma, CNS lymphomas and lymphomas associated with HIV infection are particularly difficult to treat, the latter due to the immunocompromised status of the host.

109. Which cytogenetic abnormalities are associated with lymphomas?

Recurrent chromosomal aberrations have been found to correlate with certain histologic types of lymphoma:

1. A translocation between chromosome 18 and 14 (involving the *bcl-2* oncogene on chromosome 18 and the heavy chain immunoglobulin gene on chromosome 14) is found in 85% of patients with follicular lymphomas.

2. A translocation between chromosomes 8 and 14 is found in 85% of patients with small noncleaved cell (Burkitt's or non-Burkitt's) lymphoma. The remaining 15% of patients have 2:8 or 8:22 translocations. These three translocations place the *c-myc* oncogene on chromosome 8 next to the immunoglobulin heavy chain (chromosome 14) or light chain (chromosomes 2 and 22) genes.

110. How are lymphomas staged?

Stage I	Single node region or single extranodal site
Stage II	Two or more node regions, same side of diaphragm
Stage III	Nodal disease above and below diaphragm
Stage IV	Disseminated extranodal disease

Additional designations:

S	Splenic involvement
E	Localized extranodal involvement
A	Absence of constitutional symptoms
B	Presence of ≥10% weight loss in preceding 6 months, fever and/or night sweats

111. How does the natural history of Hodgkin's disease compare with that of non-Hodgkin's lymphomas?

	HODGKIN'S DISEASE	NON-HODGKIN'S LYMPHOMAS
Age	Bimodal: 5–34 and > 50	Median age 50
Symptoms	B symptoms are more common in older age and higher state; in mixed cellularity and lymphocyte depleted, may have severe symptoms with minimal nodes	B symptoms uncommon unless patient has a very high tumor burden
Signs:		
↑ Nodes	Seen > 90% at presentation	Least common in histiocytic type
Waldeyer's	Uncommon	30% in some series
Cervical	65%	10–20%
Mediastinal	10%	2–3%
Abdominal	Retroperitoneal	Mesenteric
Extranodal	3%	Up to 60% in histiocytic
GI	4%	20–40%
CNS	Uncommon except in immunocompromised	Common, esp. lymphocytic
Pleural effusion	From obstruction due to mediastinal nodes	Chylous

112. What are the 5-year survival rates relative to histologic type of the non-Hodgkin's lymphomas?

HISTOLOGIC TYPE	FIVE YEAR SURVIVAL (%)
Anaplastic large T/null cell	77
Marginal zone B-cell, MALT	74
Follicular, all grade	72

(Table continued on next page.)

HISTOLOGIC TYPE	FIVE YEAR SURVIVAL (%)
Lymphoplasmacytoid	59
Marginal zone B cell, nodal	57
Small lymphocytic (CLL)	51
Primary mediastinal large B-cell	50
High-grade B cell, Burkitt's-like	47
Diffuse large B-cell	46
Mantle cell	27
Precursor T-lymphoblastic	26
Peripheral T-cell, all types	25
Burkitt's	4

The Non-Hodgkin's Lymphoma Classification Project: A clinical evaluation of the International Lymphoma Study Group classification of non-Hodgkin's lymphoma. Blood 89:3909–3918, 1997.

113. Which infectious agents are associated with the development of lymphoma?

Several types of infections are thought to be causative agents of non-Hodgkin's lymphoma, including hepatitis C virus, Epstein-Barr virus in Burkitt's lymphoma, human T cell lymphotropic virus (HTLV I) in T cell leukemia-lymphoma, and *Helicobacter pylori* in mucosa-associated lymphoid tissue (MALT) lymphoma. Epstein-Barr virus genomes are also found in many cases of Hodgkin's disease.

114. Which cancers are associated with AIDS? How is their incidence changing with the use of highly active antiretroviral therapy?

Kaposi's sarcoma, non-Hodgkin's lymphoma, and cervical cancer are all AIDS-defining conditions. The rates of Hodgkin's disease and anal carcinoma are also significantly increased in some populations of AIDS patients. The incidence of Kaposi's sarcoma has been falling over time. Although the absolute number of cases is falling in most (but not all) series, non-Hodgkin's lymphoma accounts for an increasing proportion of AIDS-defining illness.

Grulich AE: Update: Cancer risk in persons with HIV/AIDS in the era of combination antiretroviral therapy. The AIDS Reader 10:341–346, 2000.

115. What phenotype is most highly associated with the development of melanoma?

Typical physical characteristics of patients with melanoma are fair skin, reddish hair, and freckles. Familial melanoma families have been described in which > 25% of the kindred are affected with a vertical distribution of disease. There is an early age of onset, from the third to fourth decades. The incidence of multiple primary melanomas is increased, as is the presence of atypical nevi (B-K moles or familial atypical multiple melanoma [FAMM] with melanocyte dysplasia). However, there is a superior overall survival, possibly related to earlier detection. Ocular melanoma is also seen in this group of patients. The gene for the dysplastic nevus syndrome/familial melanoma is located on chromosome 1.

116. Where does melanoma metastasize?

Melanoma can metastasize anywhere in the body, including lungs, liver, and bones. It is one of the few cancers that can cross the placenta and spread to a developing fetus. It often metastasizes to the bowel, where it causes obstruction and bleeding. Lesions seen on barium dye studies are ulcerated with a central crater and a surrounding heaped-up border, causing the barium to pool in a "target" configuration.

BIBLIOGRAPHY

1. American Joint Committee on Cancer: Cancer Staging Manual, 5th ed. Philadelphia, Lippincott-Raven, 1997.

2. Calabresi P, Schein PS (eds): Basic Principles and Clinical Management of Cancer, 2nd ed. New York, Macmillan, 1993.
3. Casciato DA, Lowitz BB (eds): Manual of Clinical Oncology, 3rd ed. Boston, Little, Brown, 1995.
4. DeVita T Jr, Hellman S, Rosenberg SA (eds): Cancer: Principles and Practice of Oncology, 6th ed. Philadelphia, Lippincott Williams & Wilkins, 2001.
5. Haskell CM: Cancer Treatment, 4th ed. Philadelphia, W.B. Saunders, 1995.
6. Holland JF, Frei E, et al (eds): Cancer Medicine, 4th ed. Baltimore, Williams & Wilkins, 1997.
7. National Cancer Database, 1985–1995. http://www.facs.org/index.html
8. National Guideline Clearinghouse. http://www.guideline.gov/index.asp
9. PDQ Cancer Information Summaries. http://cancernet.nci.nih.gov/index.html
10. SEER Cancer Statistics Review, 1973–1997. http://seer.cancer.gov/Publications/
11. Tannock IF, Hill RP (eds): The Basic Science of Oncology, 3rd ed. New York, McGraw- Hill, 1998.

7. NEPHROLOGY

Sharma S. Prabhakar, M.D.

Bones can break, muscles can atrophy, glands can loaf, even the brain can go to sleep without immediately endangering our survival; but should the kidneys fail . . . neither bone, muscle, gland nor brain could carry on.

Homer W. Smith (1895–1962)
From Fish to Philosopher, Ch. 1

Too much attention has been paid to the excretory offices of the kidney to the neglect of its conservative services.

John P. Peters
Yale Journal of Biology & Medicine, 1953

ASSESSMENT OF RENAL FUNCTION

1. What is the glomerular filtration rate (GFR)?

Glomerular filtrate is the ultrafiltrate of plasma that exits the glomerular capillary tuft and enters the Bowman's capsule to begin the journey along the tubule of the nephron. It is the initial step in the formation of urine. The volume of this filtrate formed per unit time is called the glomerular filtration rate (GFR) and is usually expressed in ml/min.

2. How is the GFR measured clinically? Describe the rationale.

The GFR is measured indirectly with a marker substance contained in glomerular filtrate, which is then excreted in the urine. The amount of this substance leaving the kidney (urinary mass excretion) must equal the amount of marker substance entering the kidney as glomerular filtrate; it must not be reabsorbed, secreted, or metabolized after entering the kidney tubule. Then, the volume of glomerular filtrate, represented by the urinary mass excretion of the marker substance, can be calculated by dividing the urinary mass excretion of the marker substance by the concentration of the substance in the glomerular filtrate.

The marker substance is chosen so that its concentration in the glomerular filtrate is equal to its concentration in the plasma, i.e., the substance is freely filterable across the glomerular capillary. Therefore, the amount of substance X entering the kidney equals the GFR multiplied by the plasma concentration of the substance (P_x). Likewise, the amount of the substance leaving the kidney in the urine equals the urinary concentration of the substance (U_x) multiplied by the urine flow in ml/min (V). Therefore, the formula for calculating GFR using our marker substance X becomes:

$$GFR \times P_x = U_x V$$

or

$$GFR = U_x V / P_x$$

A stable plasma concentration of the substance (steady-state situation) is required to make the above equation useful.

3. Name two marker substances used to measure GFR.

The polysaccharide **inulin** is often used in laboratory determinations of GFR. However, it requires constant intravenous infusion, making it somewhat impractical for routine clinical use in patients. **Creatinine** is used as a marker substance in clinical settings.

4. Why is creatinine used as a marker substance for GFR determinations in clinical settings?

Creatinine is an endogenous substance, derived from the metabolism of creatine in skeletal muscle, that fulfills almost all of the requirements for a marker substance: it is freely filterable, not metabolized, and not reabsorbed once filtered. There is a small amount of tubular secretion that makes the creatinine clearance a slight overestimate of the GFR, but this overestimate becomes quantitatively important only at low levels of GFR.

Creatinine is released from muscle at a constant rate, resulting in a stable plasma concentration. The creatinine clearance is commonly determined from a 24-hour collection of urine. This time period is used to average out the sometimes variable creatinine excretion that may occur hour to hour. Creatinine is easily measured, making it a nearly ideal marker for GFR determination.

5. Can the completeness of a 24-hour urine collection be judged?

Since total creatinine excretion in the steady state is dependent on muscle mass, day-to-day creatinine excretion remains fairly constant for an individual and is related to lean body weight. In general, men excrete 20–25 mg creatinine/kg body weight/day, whereas women excrete 15–20 mg/kg/day. Therefore, a 70-kg man excretes ~1400 mg creatinine/day. Creatinine excretion levels measured on a 24-hour urine collection that are substantially less than the estimated value suggest an incomplete collection.

6. What is the relationship between the plasma creatinine concentration and GFR?

Because creatinine production and excretion remain constant and equal, the amount of creatinine entering and leaving the kidney remains constant. Thus:

$$GFR \times P_{Cr} = U_{Cr} \times V = constant$$

or

$$GFR = (1/P_{Cr}) \times constant$$

Creatinine excretion remains constant as GFR declines until the GFR reaches very low levels. Therefore, the GFR is a function of the reciprocal of the plasma creatinine concentration.

7. Does a given plasma creatinine concentration reflect the same level of renal function in different patients?

Not necessarily. Remember that creatinine production is directly proportional to muscle mass, and that the plasma creatinine concentration (P_{Cr}) is determined in part by creatinine production. Examination of the creatinine clearance (Ccr) for an 80-kg man compared to that of a 40-kg woman, assuming both individuals have P_{Cr} of 1.0 mg/dl (0.01 mg/m), shows the following:

For the 80-kg man, creatinine excretion should be:

$$80 \text{ kg} \times 20 \text{ mg/kg/day} = 1600 \text{ mg/day} = 1.11 \text{ mg/min}$$

$$GFR = (1.11 \text{ mg/min})/(0.01 \text{ mg/ml}) = 111 \text{ ml/min}$$

For the 40-kg woman, creatinine excretion should be:

$$40 \text{ kg} \times 15 \text{ mg/kg/day} = 600 \text{ mg/day} = 0.42 \text{ mg/min}$$

$$GFR = (0.42 \text{ mg/min})/(0.01 \text{ mg/ml}) = 42 \text{ ml/min}$$

This demonstrates that the same P_{Cr} can represent markedly different GFRs in different individuals. The difference in creatinine excretion is related to differences in muscle mass, which are related to lean body weight and age. The following formula was devised to provide a rough estimate of the GFR in situations where a measured Ccr is not immediately available:

$$Ccr = (140-[Age \times Lean \text{ body wt in kg}])/(P_{Cr} \times 72)$$

If we use this formula to estimate the GFR of the above individuals and assume an age of 50 years for each, we get a GFR of 100 for the man and 50 for the woman. These estimates are in the range of those determined previously and serve to illustrate the relative differences in the GFR calculated for two individuals with the same P_{Cr}. Recognizing this fact and using this formula to estimate GFR could prevent a serious error when selecting the dose of a drug that is excreted by the kidneys.

8. How does the blood urea nitrogen (BUN) relate to the GFR?

BUN is excreted primarily by glomerular filtration. Its level in the plasma tends to vary inversely with GFR. BUN, however, is a much less ideal marker of GFR than is creatinine. Its production may not be constant, in that it varies with protein intake, liver function, and catabolic rate. In addition, urea can be reabsorbed once filtered into the kidney, and this reabsorption increases in conditions with low urine flow, such as volume depletion. This latter circumstance is one cause of a high (> 15:1) BUN:creatinine ratio in plasma. Thus, creatinine is the better marker for GFR. But the plasma level of BUN can be used along with the Ccr to indicate the presence of certain states, such as volume depletion.

9. What is the difference between clearance and excretion?

Urinary **excretion** of a substance is simply the total amount of a substance excreted per unit of time. It is usually expressed in mg/min. **Clearance** expresses the efficiency with which the kidney removes a substance from the plasma. It is the volume of plasma that would have to be completely cleared of a substance per unit of time that accounts for the amount of that substance appearing in the urine per unit of time. It is expressed in volume per unit of time, usually ml/min.

For example, substance (X) having plasma concentration (P_x) of 1.0 mg/ml, urine concentration (U_x) of = 10 mg/ml, and urine flow (V) of 1.0 ml/min has the following clearance:

$$Cl_x = (U_x/P_x) \times V = (10 \text{ mg/ml} \times 1 \text{ ml/min})/1.0 \text{ mg/min} = 10 \text{ ml/min}$$

The calculated clearance of 10 ml/min indicates that the amount of substance X appearing in the urine is the same as if 10 ml of plasma were completely cleared of the substance and excreted in the urine each minute. The urinary excretion of X is 10 mg/min, but this measurement does not indicate the efficiency with which the substance is removed from the plasma.

10. How does measurement of urinary protein excretion help in the evaluation of renal disease?

Normal urinary protein excretion is < 150 mg/day, with albumin constituting < 50% of this protein. Failure of the tubules to reabsorb the normally filtered small-molecular-weight (MW) proteins leads to **tubular proteinuria**. This occurs in diseases that affect tubular function, and the proteins are almost entirely of smaller MW rather than albumin.

Glomerular proteinuria occurs when the normal glomerular barrier to the passage of plasma proteins is disrupted. This results in variable quantities of albumin and sometimes larger MW proteins spilling into the urine.

Quantitatively, tubular proteinuria is usually < 1 g/24 hr, and glomerular proteinuria is usually > 1 g/24 hr. When the proteinuria is > 3.5 g/1.73 m^2 body surface area, it is said to be in the **nephrotic range**. Significant degrees of proteinuria (> 150 mg/day) could indicate intrinsic renal disease. Quantification and characterization of the proteinuria are useful in detecting not only the presence of renal disease but also in determining involvement of the tubule, glomerulus, or both.

11. What information can be gained from examining urine sediment?

Urine sediment is normally almost cell-free, is usually crystal-free, and contains a very low concentration of protein (< 1+ by dipstick). Examination of this sediment is a very important part of the workup of any patient with renal disease. The examination should be performed by the physician prior to diagnostic or therapeutic decisions. The information obtained must be correlated with all other aspects of the patient's history, physical examination, and laboratory database. The examination can provide evidence of many conditions, including renal inflammation (cells, protein), infection (WBCs, bacteria), stone disease (crystals), and systemic diseases (bilirubin, myoglobin, hemoglobin, etc.).

ACUTE RENAL FAILURE

12. What is acute renal failure (ARF)?

ARF is a syndrome of many etiologies characterized by a sudden decrease in renal function leading to a compromise in the kidney's ability to regulate normal homeostasis. This inability is multifactorial. The kidney is unable to maintain the content and volume of the extracellular fluid or perform its routine endocrine functions. In most cases, ARF is a potentially reversible process.

13. Why is it important to distinguish acute from chronic renal failure (CRF)?
- The clinical manifestations of ARF are generally more severe than those associated with CRF.
- Unlike CRF, a cause for ARF can usually be identified and must be addressed to prevent further kidney or other organ damage.
- ARF is a potentially reversible disorder if the causative factor or factors are identified and corrected, and appropriate supportive care must be given to optimize the chances for recovery of renal function.

14. What is meant by oliguria?
Oliguria refers to a urine volume that is inadequate for the normal excretion of the body's metabolic waste products. Since the daily load of metabolic products amounts to approximately 600 mOsm and the maximal urine concentrating ability of the human kidney is about 1200 mOsm/kg H_2O, there is a minimal obligate urine volume of 500 ml/day for most individuals. Therefore, a 24-hour urine volume of **< 500 ml/day** is said to represent oliguria. When associated with ARF, oliguria portends a poorer prognosis than does nonoliguric ARF.

15. What is anuria? Why is it important to distinguish it from oliguria?
Anuria refers to a 24-hour urine volume of < 100 ml. It denotes a severe reduction in urine volume that is commonly associated with obstruction, renal cortical necrosis, or severe acute tubular necrosis (ATN). It is important to make the distinction between oliguria and anuria so that these diagnostic entities will be considered and appropriate therapy planned.

16. Describe the diagnostic work-up for a patient with ARF.
From an etiological standpoint, ARF can be divided into three categories: prenal, renal, and postrenal failure. This approach is important because pre- and postrenal causes of ARF can often be corrected rather quickly, and if corrected, further renal injury can frequently be avoided. Placement into the renal category should lead to a search for the agents, factors, or processes that may have resulted in acute renal injury, such as acute tubular necrosis. This approach not only aids in diagnosis but also leads to the appropriate therapy.

17. What are some common causes of ARF in the U.S.?
A. Prenal
  1. True volume depletion
     a. GI losses (vomiting, diarrhea, bleeding)
     b. Renal losses (diuretics, osmotic diuresis [glucose], hypoaldosteronism, salt-wasting nephropathy, diabetes insipidus)
     c. Skin or respiratory losses (insensible losses, sweat, burns)
     d. Third-space sequestration (intestinal obstruction, crush injury or skeletal fracture, acute pancreatitis)
  2. Hypotension (shock)
  3. Edematous states (heart failure, hepatic cirrhosis, nephrosis)
  4. Selective renal ischemia (hepatorenal syndrome, NSAIDs, bilateral renal artery stenosis, calcium channel blockers)
B. Renal causes
  1. Postischemic (all causes of severe prerenal disease, esp. particularly hypotension)
  2. Nephrotoxins
     a. Drugs and exogenous toxins
        Common: Aminoglycoside antibiotics, radiocontrast media, cisplatin, NSAIDs
        Rare: Cephalosporins, rifampin, amphotericin B, polymyxin B, methoxyflurane, acetaminophen overdose, heavy metals (mercury, arsenic, uranium), carbon tetrachloride, EDTA, tetracyclines

   b. Heme pigments
      Rhabdomyolysis (myoglobinuria)
      Intravascular hemolysis (hemoglobinuria)
   C. **Postrenal causes**
      1. Obstruction due to strictures, stones, malignancies, prostatic enlargement

18. What is meant by prerenal failure?

This syndrome refers to a decrease in renal function resulting from a decrease in renal perfusion. The decrease in renal perfusion leads to functional changes within the kidney, which in turn compromise the kidney's ability to perform its homeostatic functions. This disorder is potentially correctable by addressing the factors leading to renal hypoperfusion. In severe cases, renal hypoperfusion can be severe enough and prolonged enough to result in structural damage, and hence can lead to the "renal" category of ARF. Therefore, it is important that the prerenal syndrome be identified and corrected promptly.

19. What is acute tubular necrosis (ATN)?

ATN is a syndrome with multiple etiologies that is characterized by structural and functional damage of the renal tubules and a functional decrease of glomerular function. If the patient survives, ATN is self-limited, with most patients recovering renal function within 8 weeks. It is most commonly caused by ischemia, but there are a multitude of other causes.

20. How can the use of urinary indices help to distinguish prerenal failure from ATN?

Patients with prerenal azotemia have intact tubular function. The kidney, in this setting, is attempting to minimize solute and water excretion in an effort to preserve extracellular fluid volume. By contrast, the tubules of patients with ATN do not properly recover solutes and water that have been filtered into the kidney. Thus, the urine of patients with prerenal azotemia typically reveals:

   1. Low urinary sodium concentration (< 20 mEq/l)
   2. Low fractional excretion of sodium (< 1.0%)
   3. Low free-water excretion (high urine osmolality > 500 and high urine specific gravity > 1.015).

By contrast, the urinary indices of patients with ATN reveal the kidney's relative inability to reabsorb sodium (urinary Na > 40 mEq/l and fractional Na excretion of > 3.0%) and to reabsorb water (urine osmolality < 350 mOsm/l and urine specific gravity < 1.010). Remember that there is considerable crossover between renal and prerenal failure with regard to these indices, and hence no value absolutely indicates one or the other diagnosis. The indices should be used along with other data (i.e., history, physical examination) to arrive at a clinical impression.

21. What is meant by the fractional excretion of sodium (FE_{Na+})? What is its relevance to the diagnosis of ARF?

FE_{Na+} is calculated by using the following equation:

$$FE_{Na+} = (U_{Na+} \times P_{Cr} \times 100)/(P_{Na+} \times U_{Cr})$$

where U_{Na+} and P_{Na+} = urinary and plasma sodium concentrations (in mEq/L) and U_{Cr} and P_{Cr} = urinary and plasma creatinine in mg/dl.

An FE_{Na+} value < 1% favors prerenal states, whereas a value > 1% indicates intrarenal states or ATN. The test is more accurate than urinary Na measurement in this differentiation. However, it should be noted that an FE_{Na+} < 1% is occasionally reported for various causes of ARF other than prerenal states.

It is also to be noted that an intact sodium reabsorptive capacity is necessary for the use of this test. Thus, in conditions such as underlying chronic renal disease, hypoaldosteronism, diuretic therapy, or metabolic alkalosis with bicarbonaturia, the FE_{Na+} will be inappropriately high despite the presence of volume depletion.

22. List the four classic phases of ARF.

- The **initial stage** is usually not recognized clinically and represents the period of exposure to the insult.
- The classic **oliguric phase** is characterized by oliguria, but patients in this phase are commonly nonoliguric. During this phase, the deterioration in renal function becomes evident.
- The **diuretic phase** is characterized by a gradual increase in urine volume, often to very high levels. It is thought to represent movement of filtrate through tubules which have yet to completely recover their absorptive function.
- The **recovery phase** is characterized by the gradual return of glomerular function.

23. What are the indications for dialysis in ARF?

Definite Indications for Dialysis in ARF

1. Uncontrollable hyperkalemia
2. Fluid overload with pulmonary edema
3. Uremic pericarditis
4. Uremia encephalopathy (seizures, coma)
5. Bleeding diathesis due to uremia
6. Refractory metabolic acidosis (HCO_3^- < 10 mEq/l)
7. Severe azotemia (BUN > 100 mg/dl, serum Cr > 10 mg/dl).

24. Is the mortality in ARF significant?

The overall mortality in ARF is very high (40–60%) despite the availability of dialysis. The mortality is worse in the subcategory of patients with a history of surgery or trauma. The prognosis is better in the absence of respiratory failure, bleeding, or infection and also in patients with nonoliguric ATN. ARF occurring in the obstetric setting also has a better prognosis, with only a 10–20% mortality.

25. Under what clinical situations do angiotensin-converting enzyme (ACE) inhibitors lead to ARF?

In bilateral renal artery stenosis and renal artery stenosis of the single kidney or transplant kidney. It is believed that ARF under these conditions is mediated by ACE inhibitor-induced poststenotic dilatation of efferent arterioles and consequent reduction of glomerular hydrostatic pressure. In normal persons, this effect is offset by dilatation of afferent sites and maintenance of GFR. In the recent past, there have been reports of reversible renal failure in patients with chronic essential hypertension treated with ACE inhibitors. In these patients with severe nephrosclerosis, GFR depends on angiotensin-induced efferent arteriolar constriction. In patients with decreased effective renal blood flow, as in congestive heart failure, cirrhosis, or nephrosis, systemic hypotension and effective arteriolar dilatation caused by ACE inhibitors result in ARF.

Toto RD, et al: Reversible renal insufficiency due to angiotensin converting enzyme inhibitors in hypertensive nephrosclerosis. Ann Intern Med 115:513–519, 1991.

26. How frequently does nephrotoxicity due to exposure to radiocontrast agents occur?

The incidence of contrast-induced renal failure is variable. Most retrospective studies report an incidence of < 1%, whereas most prospective studies reported an incidence of 4–70% depending on the patient population studied. In one of the more recent prospective studies, the frequency was 12%.

Hou SH, et al: Hospital acquired renal insufficiency: A prospective study. Am J Med 74:243–248, 1983.

27. What are the important risk factors for radiocontrast-associated ARF?

Risk Factors for Contrast-induced ARF

1. Azotemia (Cr > 1.5 mg/dl)	6. Uric acid > 8.0 mg/dl
2. Albuminuria > 2+	7. Multiple radiologic studies
3. Hypertension	8. Solitary kidney
4. Age > 60 yrs	9. Contrast medium > 2 ml/kg
5. Dehydration	10. Multiple myeloma with renal insufficiency

Berns AS et al: Nephrotoxicity of contrast media. Kidney Int 36:730–40, 1989, with permission.

28. What are the pathogenetic factors responsible for ARF with contrast dyes?
1. Hemodynamic changes
2. Osmolality
3. Proteinuria
4. Tubular obstruction
5. Allergic and immunologic reactions
6. Enzymuria
7. Direct toxicity
8. Altered glomerular permeability

Cronin RE: Southwestern Internal Medicine Conference: Renal failure following radiologic procedures. Am J Med Sci 298:342–356, 1989.

29. Do patients with myeloma have an increased risk of ARF with use of radiocontrast agents?
For several years, multiple myeloma was believed to be an important risk factor for radiocontrast-agent-induced ARF. However, several large studies have noted a prevalence of < 5%. In the absence of preexisting renal failure or proteinuria, multiple myeloma by itself is unlikely to predispose to ARF following exposure to radiocontrast media. Considering the high prevalence of renal disease in patients with myeloma, avoidance of radiocontrast agents is still recommended.

CHRONIC RENAL FAILURE

30. List the stages of progressive renal failure.
1. Reduced renal reserve
2. Renal insufficiency
3. Renal failure
4. Uremic syndrome
5. End-stage renal disease (ESRD)

Patients with normal renal function have nephron mass in excess of that necessary to maintain a normal GFR. Thus, with progressive loss of renal mass, that lost initially is the **renal reserve**, which is not reflected by a rise of BUN and creatinine or in a disturbance of homeostasis.

If the progression continues, this stage is followed by **renal insufficiency**, which is associated with mild elevation of BUN and creatinine and very mild symptoms, including nocturia and easy fatigability.

With further progression, **renal failure** ensues. This stage is characterized by apparent abnormalities of renal excretory function, including disturbances in water, electrolyte, and acid-base metabolism.

Continued worsening of renal function is followed by the **uremic syndrome**, which includes multiple dysfunction of major organ systems in addition to the abnormalities of excretory function described.

Finally, **ESRD** appears, at which time the remaining renal function is unable to sustain normal body function. Renal replacement therapy (dialysis or transplantation) is required.

31. How do the remaining intact nephrons adapt in the diseased kidney?
When nephron mass is lost, the remaining intact (functioning) nephrons compensate to maintain the same excretory function performed by the normal kidney. The individual nephrons accomplish this task by increasing the GFR and excretion of salt and water compared to levels when

there was a full contingent of functioning nephrons. The increased excretory function is accomplished by reducing reabsorption of filtered salt and water, often resulting in polyuria and nocturia.

32. The compensatory mechanisms can help to maintain near-normal excretion for the diseased kidney with a reduced GFR. What is the major disadvantage these patients suffer with respect to excretory function when compared to patients with normal renal function?

Patients with chronic renal insufficiency have a reduced ability to respond to changes in intake with appropriate changes in excretory function. For example, if a person with normal renal function suddenly increases salt intake, the kidney quickly adjusts its function, allowing for increased excretion of salt which returns total body salt to or toward normal. The remaining functioning nephrons of persons with decreased GFR are chronically excreting a higher salt load and are thus much closer to their maximum salt-excreting ability. Hence, these patients are less able to adjust to an increased salt intake by increasing salt excretion.

At the opposite extreme, the remaining nephrons of the patient with a decreased GFR are less able to reduce their high salt excretion to compensate for a reduction in salt intake. These patients are more at risk of becoming salt-depleted in response to salt restriction than are patients with normal renal function.

33. Explain the "trade-off" concept of progressive renal disease.

This concept refers to compensatory mechanisms intended to alleviate the renal abnormalities resulting from compromised renal function, leading to adverse consequences in other organ systems. For example, the hyperphosphatemia and hypocalcemia occurring with progressive renal insufficiency result in increased parathyroid hormone secretion in an attempt to increase phosphate excretion and increase serum calcium levels. This secondary hyperparathyroidism has the desired effect on calcium and phosphate but leads to increased bone resorption and the bone disease called osteitis fibrosa cystica.

34. Why is the renal potassium excretory ability usually well-maintained down to very low (10–15 ml/min) levels of GFR in patients with progressive CRF?

As is the case for salt excretion, the remaining intact nephrons significantly increase potassium excretion such that the level of excretion per nephron is much higher than when there was a full contingent of nephrons. This allows for a total renal K excretion that is nearly normal. In addition, there is evidence that the extrarenal K excretion, especially by the colon, is increased in patients with CRF. By these mechanisms, patients with a significant decrease in GFR are unlikely to be hyperkalemic purely as a result of chronic renal insufficiency. In this clinical situation, if hyperkalemia is seen, consideration should be given to acute rather than chronic renal insufficiency, hormonal disorders (i.e., hyporenin hypoaldosteronism), or tubular disorders (i.e., obstructive uropathy).

35. Name the common causes of CRF.

The major causes of CRF found in patients entering the end-stage renal disease (ESRD) program in the U.S. are listed below. Note that diabetes and hypertension together account for about two-thirds of ESRD cases.

Common Causes of Chronic Renal Failure

Diabetes mellitus	31%
Hypertension	27%
Glomerulonephritis	13%
Polycystic kidney disease and other interstitial diseases	4%
Obstructive uropathy	5%
Others	20%

Alfrey AC, et al: Chronic renal failure. In: Schrier RW (ed): Renal and Electrolyte Disorders, 5th ed. Boston, Lippincott-Raven Co., 1997, p 508, with permission.

36. How does protein restriction affect the progression of CRF?

Many studies in animals and humans have shown that dietary protein restriction slows the progression of CRF. In diabetics, several studies show that protein restriction retards the progression of CRF. Nutritional status should be monitored regularly, regardless of the protein intake prescribed, to ensure that patients do not become malnourished.

For patients with a moderate loss of renal function (GFR 25–55 ml/min), there are no conclusive data that a low-protein diet is beneficial. In such patients, it is recommended to prescribe a standard protein diet (> 0.8 g/kg/day), unless there is evidence of progression of renal insufficiency, at which time a protein intake of 0.8 g/kg/day is indicated. For patients with more severe CRF (GFR 13–25 ml/min), dietary protein restriction to 0.6 g/kg/day delays progression in compliant patients. In a recent multicenter prospective study involving nondiabetic patients, further dietary protein restriction to < 0.6 gm/kg/day did not confer additional benefit.

Klahr S, et al: Modification of diet in renal disease study group. N Engl J Med 330:877–884, 1994.

37. What are the postulated mechanisms of the hypertension commonly observed in patients with renal disease?

Most patients with renal disease have an expanded extracellular fluid volume that is felt to contribute to hypertension. Other contributing mechanisms that have been postulated include stimulation of the renin-angiotensin system and increased catecholamines.

38. Do ACE inhibitors have renal protective effects in diabetics?

Yes. Sufficient data now exist supporting the use of ACE inhibitors, especially in diabetic patients with clinical or subclinical renal involvement, to retard the progression of diabetic nephropathy (both in terms of proteinuria as well as renal failure). A recent, large-scale, multicenter, prospective study concluded that captopril treatment was associated with a 50% reduction in the risk of death, dialysis, or transplantation in diabetics, an effect independent of blood pressure control. It is therefore recommended to initiate therapy with ACE inhibitors in patients with IDDM who have either microalbuminuria (30–300 mg/day in at least 2 of 3 measurements) or overt albuminuria (> 300 mg/day). ACE inhibitor therapy should be instituted in these circumstances regardless of the presence of hypertension or renal failure.

Lewis EJ, et al: The effect of angiotensin converting enzyme inhibition on diabetic nephropathy. N Engl J Med. 329:1456–1462, 1993.

39. What is meant by uremia?

Uremia refers to a symptom complex that results from severe renal insufficiency. It is characterized by some degree of dysfunction of most organ systems of the body.

DIALYSIS

40. What are the indications for dialysis in a patient with CRF?

Dialytic therapy should be started when conservative management fails to maintain the patient in reasonable comfort. Usually, dialysis is required when the GFR drops to 5–10 ml/min. It is both unnecessary and risky to adhere to strict biochemical indications. Broadly speaking, the development of uremic encephalopathy, neuropathy, pericarditis, and bleeding diathesis are indications to start dialysis immediately. Fluid overload, congestive heart failure, hyperkalemia, metabolic acidosis, and hypertension uncontrolled by conservative measures are also indications for starting patients on dialysis therapy.

41. What is dialysis disequilibrium syndrome? How do you prevent it?

Dialysis disequilibrium syndrome is a neurologic complication that tends to occur during initiation of dialysis. It occurs in the first few dialyses and is characterized by nausea, vomiting, confusion, psychosis, and seizures. These symptoms occur toward the end of dialysis or afterward, when the dialysis has been particularly rapid. The syndrome is attributed to increased hydrogen ion concentration in the brain due to differential diffusion of CO_2 and HCO_3^- across the blood-brain barrier, leading to the generation of idiogenic osmoles and the development of cerebral edema. This complication is prevented by a gradual increase of dialysis time and blood flow rate, the use of slower dialyzers, and the use of high dialysate sodium.

42. Which clinical manifestations of uremia (CRF) can be improved with dialysis? Which ones worsen?

Improve	Persist	Develop or worsen
Uremic encephalopathy	Renal osteodystrophy	Dialysis dementia
Seizures	Hypertriglyceridemia	Nephrogenic ascites
Pericarditis	Amenorrhea and infertility	Dialysis pericarditis
Fluid overload	Peripheral neuropathy	Dialysis bone disease
Electrolyte imbalances	Pruritus	Accelerated atherosclerosis
GI symptoms	Anemia	Carpal tunnel syndrome
Metabolic acidosis		(amyloid-related)
		Risk of hepatitis

43. Which poisons and toxins are dialyzable?

The toxins that can be removed by hemodialysis include alcohols (ethanol, methanol, ethylene glycol), salicylates, heavy metals (Hg, As, Pb), and halides. In addition, hemoperfusion successfully removes barbiturates, sedatives (meprobamate, methaqualone, glutethimide), acetaminophen, digoxin, procainamide, quinidine, and theophylline.

44. What is the principal contraindication for starting chronic dialysis?

The presence of potentially reversible abnormalities. These include volume depletion, urinary tract infection, urinary obstruction, hypercatabolic state, uncontrolled hypertension, hypercalcemia, nephrotoxic drugs, and low cardiac output state.

45. What is chronic ambulatory peritoneal dialysis (CAPD)? What are its indications?

CAPD is a manual form of peritoneal dialysis, usually performed by the patient, in which 1–2 liters of dialysate fluid are infused into the peritoneal space through a Tenckhoff catheter and then drained after a dwell time of 4–6 hours. The exchanges are repeated 4–5 times a day. CAPD is indicated in any patient with ESRD. It is the treatment of choice for diabetics with severe peripheral vascular disease, since they are at increased risk in hemodialysis. This method provides for more independence and mobility, and it should be offered to all young patients leading active lives. The contraindications include blindness, severe disabling arthritis, colostomy, poor motivation, and quadriplegia.

46. What are the common complications of CAPD?

Mechanical: Pain, bleeding, leakage, inadequate drainage, intraperitoneal catheter loss, abdominal wall edema, scrotal edema, incisional hernia, other hernia, intestinal hematoma, intestinal perforation

Infections, inflammation: Bacterial or fungal peritonitis, tunnel infection, exit-site infection, diverticulitis, sterile peritonitis, eosinophilic peritonitis, sclerosing peritonitis, pancreatitis

Cardiovascular: Acute pulmonary edema, fluid overload, hypotension, arrhythmia, cardiac arrest, hypertension

Pulmonary: Basal atelectasis, aspiration pneumonia, hydrothorax, respiratory arrest, decreased FVC

Neurologic: Convulsion, ? dialysis disequilibrium syndrome

Metabolic: Hyperglycemia, hyperosmolar nonketotic coma, postdialysis hypoglycemia, hyperkalemia, hypokalemia, hypernatremia, hyponatremia, metabolic alkalosis, protein depletion, hyperlipidemia, obesity

47. Name the common causes of death in dialysis patients.

Despite important technical developments, the mortality in dialysis patients remains significant—about 15% in the first year. The most common cause of death is cardiovascular failure, with hypotension and diabetes as important predisposing factors. Sepsis is the next leading cause of death, followed by bleeding complications, cerebrovascular accidents, pericardial effusion with tamponade, trauma (accidents), suicide, and others.

48. What are the causes of peritonitis in a patient on peritoneal dialysis?

Peritonitis is an important complication of CAPD. The frequency of infection has decreased considerably since this dialysis method was introduced, to about 1 episode every 18–24 patient months. This decrease is mainly due to the addition of a Luer-Lok adapter between the catheter and tubing and institution of monthly tubing changes. Causative organisms include *Staphylococcus epidermidis* and *S. aureus* (70%), gram-negative organisms (20%), and fungi and tuberculosis (5%).

49. How do you treat peritonitis in a patient on peritoneal dialysis?

The empiric treatment of acute peritonitis involves short lavage (2–3 exchanges drained rapidly), followed by 4 exchanges of 2 liters/day containing antibiotic coverage for both the common gram-positive and gram-negative organisms. 1000 units of heparin is added to each 2 liters if the fluid is fibrinous. If the chosen antibiotic(s) is removed by peritoneal dialysis (i.e., aminoglycosides), the antibiotic must be added to the dialysate at a concentration comparable to the desired trough level in the serum to minimize removal of the drug(s). Appropriate changes in antibiotics can be made after sensitivity patterns are available. Treatment is stopped 1 week after the first negative culture.

50. Discuss developments in the treatment of anemia of CRF.

The most important development is the use of recombinant human erythropoietin (EPO). Studies since 1987 have documented the efficacy of this agent in improving the anemia and minimizing the need for blood transfusion. More importantly, the importance of correcting the iron deficiency in these patients by not only restoring the iron stores but also decreasing the requirements of the more expensive erythropoietin has been recognized.

Eschbach JW, et al: Recombinant human erythropoietin in anemic patients with end stage renal disease: Results of a phase III multicenter clinical trial. Ann Intern Med 111:992–1000, 1989.

51. What is dialysis bone disease?

The bone disease in uremic patients does not necessarily improve after initiation of chronic dialytic therapy. In fact, additional factors are added that promote and complicate osteodystrophy. For instance, exposure to aluminum (as phosphate binders or, less commonly, in dialysate) superimposes a form of osteomalacia on secondary hyperparathyroidism.

Sherrard DJ, et al: The spectrum of bone disease in end stage renal failure—an evolving disorder. Kidney Int 48:436–442, 1993.

52. What is dialysis-associated amyloidosis?

Long-term dialytic therapy is associated with accumulation and deposition of amyloid fibrils containing β_3-microglobulins. It usually manifests after 5–7 years of chronic dialytic therapy and is seen in most patients after 10 years of dialysis. Clinically, it manifests as asymptomatic lytic bone lesions, carpal tunnel syndrome (often bilateral), tenosynovitis, scapulohumeral periarthritis, and destructive arthropathy. No satisfactory preventive measures are available.

Koch KM: Dialysis related amyloidosis. Kidney Int 41:1416–1429, 1992.

53. How does dialysis-induced hypoxemia develop?

A fall in P_aO_2 of 5–35 mmHg is a frequent and important complication of hemodialysis. It occurs in up to 90% of patients on dialysis and resolves within 1–2 hours after discontinuation of dialysis. This fall is clinically insignificant in the routine dialysis patient but important in people with preexisting respiratory compromise.

The pathogenesis is multifactorial and depends in part on the type of hemodialysis (acetate versus bicarbonate). It is important to remember the CNS-controlled ventilation is normally inhibited by hypocarbia (decreased $PaCO_2$) and alkalemia. Acetate dialysis removes CO_2 gas from the plasma, causing hypocarbia and depressed ventilation. Bicarbonate dialysis causes alkalemia (especially if the dialysate bicarbonate is > 35 mEq/l) due to diffusion of the bicarbonate into the patient and subsequent depressed ventilation. In addition, the cuprophane membrane of the artificial kidney can activate complement, leading to leukoagglutination in the pulmonary capillaries. This causes diffusion abnormalities, widening of the alveolar-arterial O_2 gradient, and hypoxemia. It is less common now with the advent of dialyzers using newer synthetic membranes.

Bregman H, et al: Complications during hemodialysis. In Daugirdas JT, Ing TS (eds): Handbook of Dialysis. Boston, Little, Brown, 1994.

PROTEINURIA/NEPHROTIC SYNDROME

54. What factors normally inhibit entry of plasma proteins into the glomerular ultrafiltrate?
The glomerular barrier is functionally a filter whose pores are of a given size and lined by negatively charged particles. Consequently, the features of a given plasma protein that limit its entry into the glomerular ultrafiltrate include large size (MW), negative charge, and noncompact configuration.

55. Describe the four general mechanisms by which abnormally increased urinary protein excretion (> 150 mg/day) occurs.
The four general mechanisms are glomerular, tubular, overflow, and secretory.

1. **Glomerular proteinuria** occurs as a result of damage to the glomerular filtration barrier (in glomerulonephritis), leading to excessive leakage of plasma proteins into the glomerular ultrafiltrate.

2. **Tubular proteinuria** occurs when there is suboptimal reabsorption of the normally filtered protein as a result of renal tubular disease. It is this recovery of the small amount of normally filtered protein (usually ~2 g/day) that allows for the normal urinary excretion of < 150 mg/day of protein.

3. **Overflow proteinuria** results from disease states that lead to excessive levels of plasma proteins (such as in multiple myeloma). The proteins are filtered and overload the reabsorptive capacity of the renal tubules.

4. **Secretory proteinuria** describes the proteinuria that occurs because of the addition of protein to the urine after glomerular filtration. The protein may come from the renal tubules (as with Tamm-Horsfall protein from the ascending limb of the loop of Henle) or from the lower GU tract.

56. What conditions are associated with heavy proteinuria despite severe reduction in GFR?
Heavy proteinuria is generally indicative of glomerular disease. In most glomerular diseases, proteinuria tends to decrease with diminishing GFR as the filtration of proteins also tends to decrease. However, in certain conditions, such as diabetic nephropathy, amyloidosis, focal glomerulosclerosis, and probably reflex nephropathy, proteinuria (often in the nephrotic range) persists despite severely diminished GFR.

57. A 23-year-old white man has 1.2 g of proteinuria in 24 hours. His urinalysis and other laboratory studies are otherwise normal. What is the differential diagnosis?
Significant (> 0.5 g/24 hr) but nonnephrotic (< 3.5 g/24 hr) proteinuria can be seen in the following conditions:
1. **Benign orthostatic proteinuria**
2. **Idiopathic glomerular disease (esp. in early stages)**
   Focal glomerulosclerosis   Membranous nephropathy
   IgA nephropathy   Amyloidosis

3. **Systemic diseases**
   Diabetic nephropathy   Congestive heart failure
   Essential hypertension   Febrile states

58. The commonly available urinary dipstick is most sensitive to which urinary protein?
Albumin. Excretion of even large amounts of some nonalbumin proteins (such as Bence-Jones proteins) will not be evident on this screening test. A more sensitive quantitative test, such as sulfosalicylic acid, must be used to recognize the presence of nonalbumin urinary proteins. Electrophoresis can then be used to identify the specific protein(s).

59. At what age does orthostatic proteinuria most commonly occur? What is its prognosis?
This term refers to excessive urinary protein excretion that occurs only when standing and normalizes when recumbent. It occurs most commonly in **adolescents** and carries an excellent long-term prognosis. It usually resolves spontaneously.

60. Define nephrotic syndrome.
This syndrome is a symptom complex resulting from various etiologies and characterized by heavy proteinuria (usually > 3.5 g/day), generalized edema, and lipiduria with hyperlipidemia. Because all the other features are a consequence of marked proteinuria, some authorities restrict the definition of "nephrosis" to heavy proteinuria alone.

61. What is the nephritic syndrome?
The nephritic syndrome is a renal disorder that results from diffuse glomerular inflammation. It is characterized by the sudden onset of gross or microscopic hematuria, decreased GFR, low urine output (oliguria), hypertension, and edema. It can result from many different etiologies but is traditionally represented by postinfectious glomerulonephritis following infections with certain strains of group A β-hemolytic streptococci.

62. What are the various causes of an acute nephritic syndrome?
  Postinfectious glomerulonephritis
   Poststreptococcal glomerulonephritis
   Postinfectious (nonstreptococcal) glomerulonephritis
   Bacterial: Pneumococci, *Klebsiella*, staphylococci, gram-negative rods, meningococci,
     secondary syphilis, brucellosis, *Leptospira*, *Mycoplasma*, *Salmonella*
   Viral: Varicella, infectious mononucleosis, mumps, measles, hepatitis B, coxsackievirus
   Rickettsial: Rocky Mountain spotted fever, typhus
   Parasitic: *Falciparum* malaria, toxoplasmosis, trichinosis
  Idiopathic glomerular diseases
   Membranoproliferative glomerulonephritis
   Mesangial proliferative glomerulonephritis
   IgA nephropathy
  Multisystem diseases
   Systemic lupus erythematosus (SLE)
   Henoch-Schönlein purpura
   Essential mixed cryoglobulinemia
   Infective endocarditis
  Miscellaneous
   Guillain-Barré syndrome
   Postirradiation of renal tumors

63. Which four categories of diseases cause the idiopathic nephrotic syndrome?
   Minimal change disease   Membranous nephropathy
   Focal and segmental glomerulosclerosis   Proliferative glomerulonephritides

64. What is the most common cause of nephrotic syndrome in children? In adults?
Children: minimal change disease (also called lipoid nephrosis or nil lesion)
Adults: diabetes mellitus and idiopathic membranous nephropathy among primary glomerular diseases

65. In evaluating patients with nephrotic syndrome, which disease must you rule out before considering the syndrome to be due to a primary renal disease? Why?
The general disease categories to be ruled out include:
• Drugs that may result in excessive urinary protein excretion (gold, penicillamine)
• Systemic infections: e.g., hepatitis B and C, HIV, malaria
• Neoplasia (lymphomas)
• Multisystem collagen vascular diseases (SLE)
• Diabetes (nephropathy is classically associated with nephrotic syndrome)
• Heredofamilial diseases, such as Alport's syndrome.

The distinction between the above causes and primary renal disease is important for a number of reasons. Diagnostically, identification of some of these processes may help to identify the renal lesion without the need for a renal biopsy (as in diabetes). Therapeutically, treatment of such disorders may involve simple discontinuation of the offending agent (such as a drug). Management may need to be directed at a systemic disease (infection) rather than at the renal lesion itself.

66. Name the common complications of the nephrotic syndrome.
1. **Edema and anasarca**
2. **Hypovolemia** with acute prerenal and/or parenchymal renal disease. In the nephrotic syndrome, decreased effective arterial blood volume can lead to various degrees of renal underperfusion, resulting in renal failure in severe cases.
3. **Protein malnutrition** due to massive protein losses in excess of dietary replacement.
4. **Hyperlipidemia**, which raises the risk of atherosclerotic cardiovascular disease.
5. **Increased susceptibility to bacterial infection**, which often involves the lungs, meninges (meningitis), and peritoneum. Common organisms include *Streptococcus* (including *S. pneumoniae*), *Haemophilus influenzae*, and *Klebsiella* sp.
6. **Proximal tubular dysfunction,** which may lead to Fanconi syndrome with urinary wasting of glucose, phosphate, amino acids, uric acid, potassium, and bicarbonate.
7. **Hypercoagulable state** manifested by an increased incidence of venous thrombosis, particularly in the renal vein. The mechanism may in part involve urinary loss of factors that normally inhibit clotting.

67. Are the syndromes of nephritis and nephrosis mutually exclusive?
No. Some forms of glomerular diseases are characteristically nephrotic in their presentation (e.g., nil lesion). On the other hand, some aggressive forms of proliferative glomerulopathies present as nephritic syndrome. Some others manifest mixed features.

Interrelationship of Morphologic and Clinical Manifestations of Glomerular Injury

	Nephrosis	
Minimal change glomerulopathy	++++	
Membranous glomerulopathy	+++	
Focal glomerulosclerosis	++	+
Mesangioproliferative glomerulopathy	++	++
Membranoproliferative glomerulopathy	++	+++
Proliferative glomerulonephritis	+	+++
Acute diffuse proliferate glomerulonephritis	+	++++
Crescentic glomerulonephritis		++++
		Nephritis

Adapted from Mandal AK, et al: Diagnosis and Management of Renal Disease and Hypertension. Philadelphia, Lea & Febiger, 1988, p 248, with permission.

68. A 62-year-old man with nephrotic syndrome is found to have no systemic etiology. What is the differential diagnosis?

As opposed to that seen in children, minimal lesion on renal biopsy in an elderly patient warrants an extensive search to rule out underlying malignancy, especially lymphomas (both Hodgkin's and non-Hodgkin's) and other solid tumors (such as renal cell carcinoma). One-third of elderly patients with membranous nephropathy have underlying malignancy (colon, stomach, or breast).

NEPHROLITHIASIS

69. What three mechanisms are believed important in determining the development of nephrolithiasis?

Urinary tract stones occur in a wide variety of diseases and as a consequence of a variety of physiologic and pathologic processes. The three mechanisms currently thought to contribute to urinary stone formation are:
1. Precipitation-crystallization from supersaturated solutions
2. Absence of inhibitors of stone formation normally present in urine
3. Presence of a macromolecular matrix

Precipitation of a substance to form stones depends on many factors, including solubility, concentration, and urine characteristics (i.e., pH). Normal constituents of urine that inhibit stone formation include citrate, pyrophosphate, and magnesium. Reduced concentrations of these substances are felt to contribute to stone formation. Protein matrix contributes to the formation, growth, and/or aggregation of stones. This matrix derives in part from renal tubular epithelial cells and from the uroepithelium.

70. What are the common constituents of urinary stones in the U.S.?

Calcium oxalate	35%
Calcium apatite	35%
Magnesium ammonium phosphate (struvite)	18%
Uric acid	6%
Cystine	3%

71. How does urine pH affect urinary stone formation?

In general, an alkaline urine pH favors precipitation of inorganic stones—calcium phosphate (which undergoes rearrangement into hydroxyapatite) and magnesium ammonium phosphate (struvite). An acid pH favors precipitation of organic stones—uric acid and cystine. Urine pH has little effect on calcium oxalate solubility and therefore little influence on formation of these stones.

72. Which factors predispose to the formation of magnesium ammonium phosphate (struvite) stones?

Alkaline urine pH and high concentrations of urinary ammonia lead to supersaturation of this substance. This environment is created by the presence of urea-splitting bacteria (commonly *Proteus, Pseudomonas, Klebsiella,* and *Staphylococcus*), which contain the enzyme urease and convert urea to ammonia and CO_2.

73. Which common metabolic conditions predispose to the formation of urinary stones?
- **Idiopathic hypercalciuria** is present in approximately 50% of stone-forming patients in the U.S. It is divided into absorptive (due to excessive GI absorption of calcium) and renal (due to renal leak of calcium) types.
- **Hyperuricosuria** (with and without gout) is present in approximately 30% of stone-formers. Increased uric acid excretion can also contribute to the formation of calcium-containing stones.
- **Hyperoxaluria** of various causes is present in about 15%.

- **Low urinary citrate excretion** is present in about 50% and can contribute to stone formation in most states.

Less common causes include chronic UTI, primary hyperparathyroidism, cystinuria, and distal renal tubular acidosis. Typically, more than one of the above conditions is present in a stone-forming patient.

74. Name the three common sites in the genitourinary tract where urinary stones are retained and obstruct urine flow.

The ureteropelvic junction, the mid-ureter as it crosses the iliac artery, and the ureterovesical junction.

75. What are the consequences of urinary obstruction by a stone?

A stone acutely lodged in the GU tract can cause severe, colicky pain that radiates toward the lower abdomen and genital area. In women who have children, the pain is often described as more severe than the pain of labor. The increased pressure inside the collecting system decreases the net pressure for glomerular filtration, resulting in a decreased GFR. The resulting urinary stasis predisposes to infection.

All of these problems correct toward normal if the stone passes or is removed from the urinary tract within a few days. If the obstruction becomes chronic, permanent renal injury can ensue, with an irreversible reduction in GFR and chronic dilatation of the collection system. This dilated collecting system is less efficient in delivering urine to the bladder (because of compromised peristalsis), predisposing to urinary stasis and infection.

76. How should you manage the patient with acute urinary tract obstruction due to a stone?

Most stones pass spontaneously in a few hours to days. Supportive management with analgesics and oral fluids will usually suffice. Such patients should have serum chemistries done to document the degree of renal dysfunction (if any) and an imaging procedure (intravenous, pyelography, renal ultrasound, etc.) to locate the stone and estimate its size in order to help determine the possible need for surgical intervention. Once the acute phase ends with exit of the stone, evaluation should be aimed at identifying the condition that led to the formation of the stone, which will lead to a protocol for long-term management.

77. Are patients often successful in recovering stones that are passed at home?

A reasonable percentage will recover stone material from their urine. However, laboratory analysis is usually not readily available, and the approach to management is more often empirical than based on analysis of recovered stones.

78. What conservative, nonmedical management is recommended for patients with a propensity to form renal stones?

In general, such patients should maintain a dilute urine, which can be accomplished by a high intake of hypotonic fluids. Recovery and characterization of stones, if possible, help to diagnose the predisposing condition and guide management.

Except for the oxalate stones, whose formation is not much influenced by urine pH, maintenance of an acid urine inhibits the formation of inorganic stones (calcium apatite, struvite) and maintenance of an alkaline urine inhibits formation of organic stones (uric acid, cysteine). Increasing the urinary concentration of natural inhibitors (citrate, pyrophosphate, magnesium) can limit aggregation and growth of crystals.

79. What drugs are useful in managing these patients?

More specific management depends on the predisposing condition:

- Absorptive hypercalciuria can be managed by reducing dietary calcium (type 2 only) or by using cellulose sodium phosphate, which binds intestinal calcium and prevents its absorption (type 1), or the diuretic thiazide, which promotes renal calcium absorption.

• Renal hypercalciuria can also be treated with thiazides.
• Primary hyperparathyroidism should be treated with parathyroidectomy.
• Uricosuric states resulting from the overproduction of uric acid should be treated with allopurinol, or with potassium citrate if patients have hyperuricosuria associated with calcium oxalate stones.
• Conditions associated with excessive intestinal oxalate absorption can be treated with a low oxalate diet and use of magnesium or calcium salts, which bind oxalate and inhibit its reabsorption.
• Cystinuria can be managed conservatively (i.e., dilute or alkaline urine) or with penicillamine (increases the solubility of cysteine) if the conservative measures are ineffective.
• Patients with struvite stones must have their UTIs treated with antibiotics and may also be given the urease inhibitor acetohydroxamic acid.

80. What are the three forms of lithotripsy?

Litho-(stone or calculus) *tripsy* (crushing) is a way of breaking up stones by use of shock waves or ultrasound and may serve as an alternative to operation or cystoscopy for the removal of stones in the kidney and urinary tract. The three forms now available clinically are:
1. Extracorporeal shock-wave lithotripsy
2. Percutaneous ultrasonic lithotripsy
3. Endoscopic ultrasonic lithotripsy

URINARY TRACT OBSTRUCTION

81. List the common causes of ureteric obstruction in adults.

Renal stones	Blood clot
Prostatic, bladder, or pelvic malignancy	Pregnancy
Retroperitoneal lymphoma, metastasis, or fibrosis	Stricture
Accidental surgical ligation	

82. How do unilateral and bilateral obstructions differ in their effects on the GFR?

Unilateral obstruction does not necessarily lead to a clinically measurable decrease in GFR, but bilateral obstruction quite often does. In patients with normal renal function, unilateral obstruction with complete obliteration of ipsilateral function will force recruitment of the nephron reserve of the unaffected, contralateral kidney, resulting in no changes or only small changes in total GFR. Relatively large reductions in functioning nephron mass (about 40%) are necessary to elicit an appreciable rise in the plasma creatinine (P_{Cr}) concentrations when baseline renal function is normal (P_{Cr} 0.8–1.2 mg/dl). The relatively small change in GFR, in patients with normal baseline renal function who are subjected to unilateral obstruction, likely will not be reflected by a rise in P_{Cr}.

The response is different for patients with baseline renal insufficiency. Such patients have already lost their reserve nephron mass and are likely using compensatory mechanisms to maintain their GFR. Unilateral obstruction in such patients may result in a significant fall in GFR and is more likely to be associated with a rise in P_{Cr}.

Bilateral obstruction leads to a decreased GFR in patients with both normal and abnormal renal function.

83. Describe the differences in clinical presentation between acute and chronic obstruction of the urinary tract.

Partial or complete obstruction of the urinary tract compromises urine passage whether it is acute or chronic. Nevertheless, the urinary findings and clinical consequences differ depending on the duration of the obstruction. After release of an **acute (< 24 hrs) obstruction**, there is commonly a decrease in excretion of sodium, potassium, and water. This results in excretion of a urine low in sodium and with increased osmolarity, a situation also seen with volume depletion.

In contrast, release of **chronic obstruction** commonly results in increased excretion of sodium and water and decreased excretion of acid (with urinary loss of bicarbonate) and potassium. These abnormalities can lead to volume depletion, free-water deficit (reflected by hypernatremia), and hyperkalemic non-anion-gap metabolic acidosis.

84. What abnormalities of tubular function can occur with chronic obstruction?

Chronic obstruction affects primarily distal rather than proximal nephron functions, including reabsorption of sodium and water and secretion of acid and potassium. The decreased **water** reabsorption results from decreased responsiveness of the collecting tubule to antidiuretic hormone (ADH), yielding a form of nephrogenic diabetes insipidus. The **acid** secretory defect results in incomplete bicarbonate recovery from the urine and a non-anion-gap metabolic acidosis. The **potassium** secretory defect results in potassium retention and hyperkalemia. Therefore, obstructive nephropathy is a common cause of hyperkalemic, hyperchloremic, non-anion-gap metabolic acidosis. These abnormalities usually resolve after correction of the obstruction but may require weeks or months to do so.

85. Which components of polyuria (postobstructive diuresis) are seen immediately after correction of chronic obstruction?

The patient with obstruction and compromised renal function accumulates solute and water that are ordinarily excreted by the normally functioning kidney. Correction of the obstruction results in appropriate excretion of the accumulated urea, NaCl, and water in an effort to return the volume and content of the extracellular fluid to normal. This polyuria is physiologic. However, a minority of such patients will have a pathologic polyuria, resulting from poor salt and/or water reabsorption. These abnormalities commonly resolve within a few hours but may last for days.

86. How do you tell if the postobstructive polyuria is physiologic or pathologic?

Usually the polyuria is physiologic, but the patient must be observed. Pathologic polyuria may occur because of either salt or water loss (or both). Pathologic salt loss will be reflected by continued excretion of a large amount of urinary sodium in the setting of volume depletion. Pathologic water loss will be reflected by excretion of large volumes of dilute urine in the face of rising serum osmolality. In pathologic polyuria, appropriate fluid replacement therapy should be instituted. If replacement is instituted during the physiologic polyuria, one will "chase" the patient's volume status such that the polyuria will continue as a result of the fluids being administered.

87. What are some complications of urinary tract obstruction?

In addition to the decrease in GFR and the potential tubular abnormalities, the resulting urinary stasis can predispose to infection, renal stones, and papillary necrosis. The salt and water retention can lead to hypertension.

88. What is "functional" obstruction of the urinary tract?

This refers to abnormalities that compromise the exit of urine from the kidney in the absence of anatomic obstruction of the outflow tract. Two examples of an atonic bladder and vesicoureteral reflux are:

An **atonic bladder** is unable to empty itself completely and hence contains urine, continuously yielding a higher than normal hydrostatic pressure. This high bladder pressure is transmitted via the ureters and may cause the abnormalities described above.

Patients with **vesicoureteral reflex** have retrograde flow of urine into the ureter and/or kidney during voiding. This occurs because of an incompetent vesicoureteral valve. The transmitted pressure is felt to contribute to the renal abnormalities. Both of these conditions also predispose to infection.

89. How is the diagnosis of lower urinary tract obstruction (LTO) made?

The history, clinical setting, and the laboratory findings provide important clues:

- A palpable urinary bladder on examination is strong evidence for LTO or an atonic bladder.
- The distended bladder as well as hypertrophied kidneys can sometimes be demonstrated on plain abdominal x-rays.
- A post-void residual urine of > 100 ml obtained on Foley catheter insertion is supportive of LTO.
- Renal ultrasound is a relatively sensitive, noninvasive procedure that is commonly used to investigate the possibility of LTO.
- Retrograde pyelography (selective catheterization and insertion of contrast dye into both ureters via cystoscopy) is occasionally necessary when the above studies do not yield a diagnosis and clinical suspicion remains strong for obstruction. Intravenous pyelograms (IVPs) should be avoided due to the risk of additional renal injury from the contrast dye.
- Abdominal CT scan is helpful but is more expensive than ultrasound.
- Radionuclide renal scans suggest LTO when there is prompt uptake of the dye with prolonged excretion.

GLOMERULAR DISORDERS

90. What is a primary glomerulopathy?

Primary glomerular disease (or primary glomerulopathy) denotes a heterogeneous group of kidney diseases in which the glomeruli are the predominantly involved elements. Extrarenal involvement, if present, is usually secondary to consequences of the glomerular insult. Most of these disorders are idiopathic. The cardinal manifestations of the primary glomerular disorders are proteinuria, hematuria, alterations in GFR, and salt retention leading to edema, hypertension, and pulmonary congestion.

91. Which clinical syndromes are manifested by the primary glomerulopathies?

The clinical features of the primary glomerulopathies appear in various combinations in any given glomerular disorder and present as one of the following clinical syndromes:

1. **Acute glomerulonephritis** (AGN): An acute illness of abrupt onset characterized by variable degrees of hematuria, proteinuria, decreased GFR, and fluid and salt retention. It is usually associated with an infectious agent and tends to resolve spontaneously.

2. **Nephrotic syndrome:** An illness of insidious onset characterized primarily by heavy proteinuria of usually > 3.5 g/day in an adult and usually associated with hypoalbuminemia, lipidemia, and anasarca.

3. **Chronic glomerulonephritis:** A vague illness of insidious onset characterized primarily by progressive renal insufficiency, with a protracted downhill course of 5–10 years' duration. Varying degrees of proteinuria, hematuria, and hypertension are present.

4. **Rapidly progressive glomerulonephritis** (RPGN): A clinical disorder of rather subacute onset but with rapid progression to renal failure and no tendency toward spontaneous recovery. Patients are usually hypertensive, hematuric, and oliguric.

5. **Asymptomatic urinary abnormalities:** Patients have microscopic hematuria and/or proteinuria (usually < 3 g/day) but with no clinical symptoms.

92. Which strains of streptococci cause poststreptococcal glomerulonephritis (PSGN)? What factors determine the nephritogenicity?

Only certain serotypes of group A (β-hemolytic) streptococci are nephritogenic. Type 12 is the most common type, but types 1, 2, 3, 18, 25, 49, 55, 57, and 60 are also nephritogenic. In contrast, all strains of streptococci can cause acute rheumatic fever, which is why the incidence of nephritis differs from that of rheumatic fever in outbreaks of streptococcal infection.

The M-protein in streptococci is poorly linked to nephritogenicity. Recent evidence indicates that nephritogenicity is more closely related to endostreptosin, a cell membrane antigen. Other streptococcal cytoplasmic antigens and autologous antigens also have been implicated.

93. Describe the typical urine sediment from a patient with PSGN. Does a normal urinalysis rule out this diagnosis?

The urinalysis in PSGN is characterized by a nephritic sediment (see Question 91), high specific gravity, and nonselective proteinuria. The proteinuria is < 3 g/day in > 75% of patients, although proteinuria in the nephrotic range is occasionally seen. Pyuria is often noted, indicating glomerulitis. Hematuria is almost always present in either gross (smoky urine) or microscopic form. Red cell casts, if present, are very diagnostic. Dysmorphic erythrocytes are found in abundance. However, a benign urinary sediment does not rule out acute PSGN if clinical features are suggestive. In some cases, biopsy studies have confirmed PSGN.

94. What is the prognosis in acute PSGN? What are the poor prognostic signs?

In children, the immediate and late prognosis is quite favorable in both epidemic and sporadic cases. A diuresis occurs in 1 week, and serum creatinine returns to normal in 3–4 weeks. The mortality in acute cases is < 1%, and chronic sequelae are uncommon. Microscopic hematuria may last 6 months, and proteinuria may persist for as long as 3 years in 15% of patients. The factors indicating a poor prognosis include persistent heavy proteinuria, extensive crescents or atypical humps in initial biopsy, and severe disease in the acute phase requiring hospitalization.

In adults, the prognosis is good in epidemic forms but less predictable in sporadic cases. Severe impairment of renal function at the onset, persistent proteinuria, elderly age, and crescent formation on biopsy are poor prognostic factors.

95. How do you treat hypertension associated with acute PSGN?

Fluid and salt retention are the basis for hypertension in PSGN. Therefore, loop diuretics, such as furosemide, are very useful. Potassium-sparing diuretics are to be avoided. Other antihypertensives are rarely indicated. When needed, vasodilators such as hydralazine, diazoxide, and nitroprusside are most useful. Plasma renin activity levels are often decreased, and hence β-blockers and ACE inhibitors are less useful alone but may be used in conjunction with vasodilators. Clonidine, methyldopa, or nifedipine can also be used.

96. What is rapidly progressive glomerulonephritis (RPGN)? Is it synonymous with crescentic nephritis?

The term RPGN is used to denote the clinical syndrome associated with rapid and progressive deterioration of renal function, often terminating, if untreated, in ESRD within a period of weeks to months. Histologically, it is characterized by extensive glomerular crescent formation, in most cases involving over 75% of glomeruli. The cells of the crescents are thought to be derived from blood-borne monocytes.

RPGN is strictly a clinical expression, whereas crescentic nephritis denotes the histologic picture in such patients. Several primary glomerulopathies demonstrate variable degrees of crescent formation, but they do not progress rapidly as in RPGN.

97. How does routine urinalysis help in the evaluation of a primary glomerular disease?

In glomerular disease, the urinary sediment usually conforms to one of three different forms:

Nephrotic	Nephritic	Chronic
Heavy proteinuria	Red cells	Less proteinuria and hematuria
Free fat droplets	Red cell casts	Broad, waxy casts
Oval fat bodies	Variable proteinuria	Pigmented granular casts
Fatty casts	Frequent white cell and	
Variable hematuria	granular cells	

Schreiner GE: The identification and clinical significance of casts. Arch Intern Med 99:356–369, 1957.

98. What are the renal manifestations of HIV disease?

The most common chronic renal disease from HIV infection is a type of focal glomerulosclerosis, the so-called HIV nephropathy. Typically, nephrotic proteinuria, large echogenic kidneys, minimal or modest hypertension, and rapidly progressive renal failure characterize the disease. Dialysis is well tolerated; however, the mean survival is less than 1 year in patients with full-blown AIDS. Transplantation is contraindicated in HIV nephropathy. The other renal manifestations include hyponatremia, hyperkalemia (often secondary to adrenal disease or hyporenin hypoaldosteronism), hypouricemia, and acute renal failure, often due to anti-HIV medications.

99. How is a patient with recurrent hematuria evaluated?

The first step is to exclude urinary stones and other structural lesions such as tumors of the upper and lower urinary tract. This may involve renal imaging and urinary instrumentation. The presence of dysmorphic erythrocytes or red cell casts helps to distinguish glomerular bleeding from lower tract bleeding. Glomerular bleeding accounts for recurrent hematuria in over a quarter of patients below age 40 years. The main causes of recurrent isolated glomerular hematuria include IgA nephropathy or Berger's disease (the most common primary glomerulopathy worldwide), thin basement membrane nephropathy, and idiopathic hypercalciuria. Demonstration of the first two entities may require renal biopsy.

100. What is Berger's disease?

Berger's disease is primary IgA nephropathy. It is the most common type of primary glomerulopathy worldwide and is characterized by recurrent episodes of painless hematuria, often gross, and presence of RBC casts in urine. Hypertension and proteinuria are often minimal or modest. Only 25% of the patients progress to end stage renal disease.

RENAL BONE DISEASE

101. What is Bricker's "trade-off" hypothesis?

Early in the course of renal failure, the kidney fails to excrete phosphorus, leading to a transient and often undetectable rise in serum phosphorus. This tends to lower the serum ionized calcium temporarily, leading to stimulation of parathyroid hormone (PTH) secretion. The increased levels of PTH reduce tubular reabsorption of phosphate, leading to phosphate excretion and thereby tending to normalize the serum calcium and phosphorus levels. However, this is occurring at the expense of an elevated PTH level. With further declines in renal function, the serum phosphorus tends to rise, and the whole cycle is repeated.

With advancing renal failure, these changes tend to keep serum calcium and phosphorus levels below normal at the expense of increasing serum PTH levels. The serum level of PTH is increased in an attempt to normalize serum phosphate and calcium levels, but the "trade-off" is the bone disease caused by the elevated PTH levels (osteitis fibrosa cystica). This is the so-called "trade-off" hypothesis propounded by Neil Bricker and is the basis for the secondary hyperparathyroidism seen in renal failure.

102. List the three major bone histologic subtypes found in renal osteodystrophy.

Osteitis fibrosa cystica, which is a result of high bone turnover (bone changes due to secondary hyperparathyroidism), **osteomalacia**, and, occasionally, **osteosclerosis**. With better management of patients with ESRD, the long-term course of renal bone disease and its clinical features have changed, and newer entities have emerged. Adynamic or aplastic bone disease or low bone turnover has become a fairly common bone disease. Aluminum accumulation causes osteomalacia, which is one cause of adynamic bone disease. Decreased vitamin D, diabetes, and iron accumulation are other factors associated with adynamic bone disease.

103. What is the role of aluminum in renal bone disease?

Recent evidence has shown that aluminum accumulation in the bone is a major factor in causing osteomalacia and anemia in patients with CRF and in those on dialysis. After the dialysate concentration of aluminum was lowered to insignificant amounts, it became obvious that oral ingestion of aluminum in the form of aluminum-containing phosphate binders was an important cause of aluminum-related bone disease. Orally ingested aluminum can accumulate over time to levels significant enough to cause aluminum bone disease. The mechanism of the aluminum effect on bone is believed to be due to deposition of the metal along the mineralization front, leading to interference with mineralization. In addition, aluminum may impair the function of osteoblasts.

104. Why will a patient with CRF and marked hypocalcemia often fail to manifest tetany?
Tetany is a clinical manifestation of severe hypocalcemia in adults. Ionized calcium is decreased in the presence of alkalemia, so that tetany usually manifests only in the presence of an alkalemic pH. The degree of ionization is favorably increased by the acidemia seen in CRF, the result being that the ionic calcium is usually not reduced enough to cause tetany. However, if the acidosis is excessively treated with alkalizing agents, tetany may become manifest.

105. How do you manage secondary hyperparathyroidism in patients with chronic renal failure?
The cornerstone of treatment of secondary hyperparathyroidism involves measures to reduce serum parathormone levels. This is accomplished by use of vitamin D analogues. However, this should not be attempted before the serum phosphorus level is normalized or the product of calcium and phosphorus is lowered to less than 70. The most commonly used vitamin D preparation is calcitriol (1,25 dihydroxycholecalciferol) either orally or intravenously. More recently other analogues of vitamin D such as 19-nor-cholecalciferol (Zemplar) and 1α calcidiol (Hectoral) have been successfully used and are claimed to be less hypercalcemic.

106. Does bone disease improve with dialysis or renal transplantation?
Renal osteodystrophy is not always improved with dialytic therapy. Indeed, the symptoms may worsen or progress because a number of additional factors are introduced that either directly or indirectly influence the severity of renal bone disease, including the aluminum content of dialysate, heparin administration, and administration of large amounts of acetate.
In patients who undergo renal transplantation, the uremic bone disease improves to a great extent. Increased osteoclastic and osteoblastic activities are noted within a few weeks after transplantation. However, in some patients, osteoporosis and the effects of secondary hyperparathyroidism may persist for as long as 1–2 years. In addition, steroid therapy may be responsible for osteoporosis and osteonecrosis that complicate the later phases of the post-transplant period. Another abnormality that may develop in the post-transplant phase is a renal phosphate leak, which if severe may contribute to osseous abnormalities.

RENAL TRANSPLANTATION

107. When should renal transplantation be considered?
Renal transplantation is indicated in all patients with ESRD who need some form of renal replacement therapy.

108. What are some important contraindications?
Absolute contraindications

Reversible renal disease	Active infection
Recent malignant disease	Active glomerulonephritis
Presensitization to donor Class I major transplantation antigens	AIDS

Relative contraindications

Fabry's disease	Oxalosis
Advanced age	Psychiatric problems
Presence of anatomic urologic abnormality	Iliofemoral occlusion
	Chronic active hepatitis

109. What are the donor-selection criteria in living-related transplantation?

Donors should have a normal physical examination, be under age 65, and have the same ABO blood group as the recipient (or be type O). An angiogram is necessary to exclude the presence of multiple or abnormal renal arteries, because such abnormalities make the surgery prolonged and difficult. In general, the left kidney is preferred because of the longer renal vein. Some relative contraindications for kidney donation include severe hypertension, diabetes mellitus, HIV positivity, active medical illness, urologic abnormalities, persistently abnormal urinalyses, and family history of nephritis, polycystic kidney disease, or other renal disease.

110. What factors are considered important in evaluating suitability of a cadaver kidney?

The donor should have been free of neoplastic or infectious disease, preferably under 60 years of age, and have had good urine output and a normal serum creatinine before death. Urinalyses should be normal, and urine cultures should be negative. The kidney should be transplanted as early after harvesting as possible. The graft function tends to be worse after 24 hours following harvesting. Of course, the donor should be free of infection with hepatitis B virus and HIV.

111. Give the current survival figures for renal transplant recipients in the U.S.

The l-year patient survival rate for living-related renal transplantation is now around 95–100%, and for cadaveric transplantation, about 90%. With cyclosporine therapy, graft survivals are 90% and 80%, respectively, for living and cadaveric kidney transplants.

DIABETIC RENAL DISEASE

112. What is the incidence of renal involvement in diabetes mellitus?

CRF is an important cause of morbidity and mortality in all diabetics. Diabetes contributes up to 50% of all cases of ESRD in the U.S. Among type I diabetics, 40–60% develop CRF between 10–30 years after onset of diabetes. Although about one-third of type II diabetics develop proteinuria, only 4% develop nephrotic syndrome and 6% develop ESRD. However, due to the large number of type II diabetics, they constitute the majority of diabetics on dialysis. The difference between the behavior of types I and II diabetes is probably dependent on the age of onset of the disease.

113. What is the earliest evidence of renal involvement in diabetes mellitus?

The earliest renal changes in diabetes consist of an increase in GFR of 25–50% and a slight enlargement of the kidney that persists for 5–10 years. At this stage, there may be a slight increase in albumin excretion rate (microalbuminuria), but the total protein excretion remains in the normal range.

114. Why is diabetic nephropathy associated with large kidneys?

Diabetic nephropathy is one of the causes of CRF associated with normal-sized or large kidneys. Renal size is increased early in the course of diabetic renal disease and involves hypertrophy and hyperplasia. Elevated levels of growth hormone, often seen with uncontrolled hyperglycemia, are incriminated in this renal hypertrophy. However, the exact etiology remains unknown.

115. Are patients with microalbuminuria more likely to develop overt renal disease?

The course of diabetic nephropathy is characterized by a preclinical phase, followed by a clinical phase. The clinical phase starts with the appearance of proteinuria on urine dipstick. Even in the preclinical phase, there is an increased amount of albumin excretion over the normal (20–40 mg/min), measurable by sensitive radioimmunoassays. Studies indicate that patients with this "microalbuminuria" are more likely to develop overt diabetic nephropathy than those who do not exhibit microalbuminuria.

116. What is the most important factor influencing the course of diabetic nephropathy?

Hypertension. In the proteinuria phase, 50–75% of all diabetics develop hypertension, and by the time they reach ESRD, almost all diabetics have hypertension. In the proteinuric phase, if hypertension is controlled, the rate of decline of GFR can be decreased from 1 ml/min/mo to 0.39 ml/min/mo.

Parving et al: Early aggressive anti-hypertensive treatment in diabetic nephropathy. Am J Kidney Dis 22:188–195, 1993.

117. What maneuvers are renoprotective in diabetic nephropathy?

Control of blood pressure, blood sugar levels, and dietary protein restriction have all been shown to decrease proteinuria and retard the progression of renal failure. More recently, angiotensin converting enzyme (ACE) inhibitors have been shown to accomplish the same, even in normotensive diabetic subjects. There is preliminary evidence that angiotensin receptor blockers also accomplish the same objective.

118. How do you treat hypertension in diabetes mellitus?

Many studies have shown that calcium channel blockers and ACE inhibitors are very well-tolerated and effective in diabetes. **ACE inhibitors** should be the first-line agents in therapy for hypertension in DM. Shortly after ACE inhibitors are started, serum creatinine and potassium should be monitored to detect patients who develop hyperkalemia or an abrupt reduction in GFR. If no adverse effects are seen for at least 2 weeks, ACE inhibitors can be safely continued.

ACE inhibitors have been shown in recent large-scale clinical trials to reduce proteinuria and slow the progression of CRF in diabetes. It is unclear whether **calcium channel blockers** are as effective as ACE inhibitors in achieving these objectives, but they are effective in controlling the blood pressure in renal failure. β-blockers may be effective, but their effects on the lipid profile and need for dose modification in renal failure and dialysis make them less desirable. Other agents, while being effective, may not offer any advantages over ACE inhibitors or calcium channel blockers.

119. Do diabetics with renal failure tolerate dialysis as well as nondiabetics?

Several years ago, it was thought that diabetics were not good candidates for dialytic therapy, because about 80% of diabetics with ESRD who were placed on hemodialysis died in the first year. Over the last 15 years, results have improved significantly. One recent report indicates a 1-year survival of 85% and a 3-year survival of 60% in diabetics on hemodialysis. However, even today, diabetics tend to do poorly compared to nondiabetics. Their 3-year survival is 20–30% less, and their mortality is 2.25 times higher than that of nondiabetics. Atherosclerotic cardiac disease is the most common cause of death, with infections a close second.

120. Does diabetic nephropathy recur following renal transplantation?

Histologic lesions typical of diabetic renal disease appear in kidneys transplanted into diabetics in as early as 1–3 years. However, clinical deterioration of kidney function attributable to these lesions is uncommon.

121. What is pseudodiabetes of uremia?

In nondiabetics with CRF, there is a peripheral resistance to the action of endogenous insulin, resulting in hyperglycemia. If a glucose tolerance test is performed, the resulting curve resembles that of diabetes. This phenomenon is called pseudodiabetes of uremia. The absence of fasting hyperglycemia and the typical changes of diabetic retinopathy distinguish this pseudodiabetes from diabetic uremia.

122. Can meticulous control of blood sugar levels prevent diabetic renal disease?

The hyperfiltration and hypertrophy seen early in the course of diabetic nephropathy can be corrected with insulin treatment. Strict glycemic control can reverse the elevated GFR and renal hypertrophy and also can decrease the spontaneous or exercise-induced microalbuminuria seen in the preclinical phase. Intensive control of blood sugar is recommended in all type I diabetics. The goal is to maintain a blood glucose level within or close to the normal range while avoiding hypoglycemic attacks. These goals frequently require 2–3 insulin injections per day or use of an insulin pump with close monitoring of blood glucose levels. However, once overt nephropathy begins and progressive renal insufficiency ensues, the benefit of tight glycemic control is still observed, although less pronounced than in the preclinical phase.

Diabetes Control and Complications Trial (DCCT) research group: The effects of intensive treatment of diabetes on the development and progression of long-term complications in insulin dependent diabetes mellitus. N Engl J Med 329:977–986, 1993.

MISCELLANEOUS RENAL DISORDERS

123. What are the risk factors associated with aminoglycoside nephrotoxicity?
1. Dose and duration of drug therapy
2. Recent aminoglycoside therapy
3. Preexistent renal or liver failure
4. Elderly age
5. Volume depletion
6. Concurrent nephrotoxin administration
7. Potassium and/or magnesium depletion

Fumes D: Aminoglycoside nephrotoxicity. Kidney Int 33:900–911, 1988.

124. Which antibacterial agents should be avoided completely in renal failure?
Tetracyclines, nitrofurantoin, nalidixic acid, and bacitracin.

125. How should antibiotic doses be adjusted in patients with renal failure?
Several antibiotics need dosage modification in the presence of renal failure, notably aminoglycosides, most cephalosporins, many penicillins, and vancomycin. The adjustments can be made by maintaining the usual dose and varying the dosing interval, maintaining the dosing interval and varying the dose, or a combination of the two. The objective is to obtain a therapeutic drug concentration–time profile that is therapeutic and not toxic. For most commonly used antibiotics, dosing guidelines have been established and are readily accessible. No adjustment is needed for erythromycin, doxycycline, rifampin, and oral vancomycin.

Benett WM: Drug Prescribing in Renal Failure. Philadelphia, American College of Physicians, pp 15–35, 1993.

126. What are some of the commonly encountered drug-drug interactions seen in renal failure?
Drug interactions are fairly common in patients with renal failure.
- Concomitant use of **metoclopramide** with **digoxin** decreases the absorption of the digoxin due to decreased gastric motility. The digoxin dose may have to be increased. On the other hand, **quinidine** impairs renal excretion of digoxin, and hence the digoxin dose may have to be decreased.
- **Antacids** impair the gastric absorption of **β-blockers** and **ferrous sulfate**. It is recommended to allow 1–2 hours between the two agents.
- An important interaction occurs between **Scholl's solution**, an alkali that contains sodium citrate, and **aluminum hydroxide**. Citrate increases aluminum absorption so that aluminum toxicity may result. The combination has to be avoided.
- **Azathioprine** levels in the blood are elevated when used in conjunction with **allopurinol** due to decreased xanthine oxidase metabolism of azathioprine. The azathioprine dose therefore has to be decreased and leukocyte counts followed.
- Finally, many drugs alter the **cyclosporine** levels in the plasma. **Phenytoin, phenobarbital**, and **rifampin** increase cyclosporine clearance by the liver, and higher doses may be needed. On the other hand, **erythromycin, amphotericin B**, and **ketoconazole** decrease cyclosporine clearance by the liver, and hence the dose may have to be decreased.

127. How does pregnancy affect renal function?

Due to increased blood volume and hyperdynamic circulation in pregnancy, renal hemodynamics are altered. Most importantly, clearances of urea, creatinine, and uric acid are increased, leading to a decrease in the serum concentrations of these compounds. Urine protein excretion rates are increased. There is some dilation of the collecting system, including the ureters, partially due to the pressure from the gravid uterus but mainly due to the effect of progestational hormones on the muscular tone of the ureters. All of these changes revert to normalcy once the patient delivers.

128. What is the impact of pregnancy on renal disease?

Most renal diseases with proteinuria demonstrate increases in proteinuria during pregnancy. In diabetics with no renal disease, pregnancy does not adversely affect the renal function. However, there are no data about effects of pregnancy on renal function in patients with advanced diabetic nephropathy. Lupus nephritis is associated with an increased rate of spontaneous abortion and increased fetal loss. However, there is no evidence that pregnancy affects the long term prognosis of lupus nephritis.

129. What is a simple renal cyst? How is it distinguished from a malignant cyst?

Simple cysts represent 60–70% of renal masses. They are common after age 50, most often asymptomatic, and usually detected as incidental findings in radiologic procedures done for other reasons. On sonography, a simple cyst has smooth, sharply delineated margins, no echoes within the mass, and a strong posterior wall echo indicating good transmission through the cyst. These features generally exclude the possibility of malignancy. However, if there is any further suspicion, a CT scan should be done. CT findings consistent with a simple cyst include fluid that is homogeneous with a density of 0–20 Hounsfield units and no enhancement of the cyst fluid following the administration of radiocontrast media.

Characteristics of Renal Cystic Disorders

FEATURE	SIMPLE CYSTS	ADPKD	ARPKD	ACKD	MCD	MSK
Inheritance pattern	None	Autosomal dominant	Autosomal recessive	None	Often present, variable pattern	None
Incidence or prevalence	Common, increasing with age	1/200 to 1/1000	Rare	40% in dialysis patients	Rare	Common
Age of onset	Adult	Usually adults	Neonates, children	Older adults	Adolescents, young adults	Adults
Presenting symptom	Incidental finding, hematuria	Pain, hematuria, infection, family screening	Abdominal mass, renal failure, failure to thrive	Hematuria	Polyuria, polydipsia, enuresis, renal failure, failure to thrive	Incidental, UTIs, hematuria, renal calculi
Hematuria	Occurs	Common	Occurs	Occurs	Rare	Common
Recurrent infections	Rare	Common	Occurs	No	Rare	Common
Renal calculi	No	Common	No	No	No	Common
Hypertension	Rare	Common	Common	Present from underlying disease	Rare	No
Diagnosis	Ultrasound	Ultrasound, gene linkage analysis	Ultrasound	CT scan	None reliable	Excretory urogram
Renal size	Normal	Normal to very large	Large initially	Small to normal, occ. large	Small	Normal

ADPKD = autosomal dominant polycystic kidney disease; ARPKD = autosomal recessive polycystic kidney disease; ACKD = acquired cystic kidney disease; MCD = medullary cystic disease; MSK = medullary sponge kidney. Adapted from Grantham JJ: Cystic diseases of kidney. In Goldman L, Bennett JC, et al (eds): Cecil Textbook of Medicine, 21st ed. Philadelphia, W.B. Saunders, 2000.

130. You are asked to examine a 53-year-old male admitted to the hospital with fever, chills, right flank pain, and dysuria. Two years ago when he was being evaluated for newly detected hypertension, he was noted to have polycystic kidney disease. Urinalysis showed 15–20 RBC, plenty of WBC, and 3+ bacteria. An abdominal ultrasound read as unremarkable except for bilateral polycystic kidneys showing one of the renal cysts in the right kidney filled with highly echogenic material. At this point, your next step in management is to:
1. Order a urine culture
2. Start intravenous ampicillin
3. Start intravenous ciprofloxacin
4. Begin surgical drainage of the cyst.

The correct response is 3. The urinalysis is clearly indicative of an active urinary infection and hence although urine culture would be ordered it would not affect the immediate management. The ultrasound is suggestive of an infected cyst. Since ampicillin does not penetrate the cyst wall and reach adequate concentrations to clear the infection, ciprofloxacin is the appropriate antibiotic of choice. Surgical drainage is needed only in cases resistant to intravenous antibiotics.

131. List the renal manifestations of sickle cell disease.
1. Hematuria
2. Renal infarction and papillary necrosis, which may predispose to UTI
3. Abnormal tubular function:
   a. Reduced concentrating ability
   b. Reduced acid and potassium secretion
   c. Increased uric acid and creatinine secretion
   d. Increased phosphate reabsorption
4. Nephrotic syndrome, which may progress to renal failure

132. What are the causes of papillary necrosis?
Renal papillary necrosis is one of the most common renal complications of sickle cell anemia. The other common conditions in which this renal complication is observed include analgesic nephropathy and diabetes mellitus.

133. What are the renal manifestations of infective endocarditis? What is the pathogenesis of these lesions?
Renal manifestations in infective endocarditis include incidental microscopic or gross hematuria and proteinuria. Renal failure is usually mild or absent. The histologic exam in these cases reveals focal proliferative glomerulonephritis. Rarely, a rapidly progressive renal failure with extensive crescent formation is reported. Nephrotic syndrome is rare. Serum IgG and C3 levels are often decreased, and immunofluorescence often demonstrates IgG, IgM, and in subendothelial and subepithelial deposits, suggesting an immune-complex etiology.

134. What is the "internist's tumor"?
Renal cell carcinoma, because the condition is often diagnosed by its systemic, rather than urologic, manifestations. These systemic effects include fever, anemia, hypercalcemia, galactorrhea, feminization or masculinization, and Cushing's.

135. Describe the major differences between fibromuscular dysplasia and atherosclerotic renal artery stenosis.

	FIBROMUSCULAR DYSPLASIA	ATHEROSCLEROSIS
Age at onset	< 40 years	> 45 years
Gender	80% female	Primarily males
Distribution of lesion	Distal main renal artery and intrarenal branches	Aortic orifice and proximal main renal artery
Progression	Uncommon	Common, may progress to complete occlusion

136. What history or physical findings suggest renovascular hypertension (HTN)?

Renovascular HTN comprises about 0.2–5% of all cases of HTN. Clues to the presence of renal artery stenosis may be derived from the history and physical exam. Onset of HTN before age 20 or after age 50 should suggest the possibility of renovascular HTN. Similarly, the development of a refractory phase in a previously stable hypertensive patient, the presence of spontaneous hypokalemia, and the presence of an abdominal bruit makes renovascular HTN very probable. Fibromuscular disease is common in young white females, while atheromatous disease is more likely in middle-aged men, especially when there is evidence of atheromatous vascular disease elsewhere. Family history is not helpful in suspecting renovascular HTN.

137. How do you confirm renovascular HTN? What laboratory tests or imaging techniques are useful in screening for renovascular HTN?

A high plasma renin profile is seen in approximately 80% of patients with renovascular HTN, as opposed to 15% in essential HTN. Another screening test often used is the **captopril test**. The administration of oral captopril causes a reactive rise of renin which is greater in patients with renovascular as opposed to essential HTN. The overall sensitivity is 74% and specificity 89%.

Ultrasound determination of renal size (a difference of > 1.5 cm between the two kidneys) is very important in suggesting renal artery stenosis. **Captopril renography** has now replaced isotope renography as the screening procedure of choice, since the sensitivity is 92% and specificity 93%. The rationale for this test is that the GFR and renal blood flow of an ischemic kidney are dependent on the effects of angiotensin on the efferent glomerular arterioles and hence fall markedly with ACE inhibition. Thus, captopril causes decreased isotope uptake by the ischemic kidney.

Mann SJ, Pickering TG: Detection of renovascular hypertension. Ann Intern Med 117:845–853, 1992.

138. And how is the diagnosis confirmed?

The confirmation of renal artery stenosis is by renal angiography.

139. You are following a 47-year-old diabetic male with chronic renal failure. He suffered a stroke a year ago and 3 years ago he had triple vessel coronary bypass surgery. His blood pressure has gone out of control despite multiple antihypertensive medications. His laboratory studies show a blood urea nitrogen of 35 mg/dl, serum creatinine 4.6 mg/dl, sodium 138 mEq/L, potassium 3.3 mEq/L, cholesterol 368 mg/dl, and triglycerides 320 mg/dl. What tests would you employ to confirm the cause of his resistant hypertension?

Renovascular hypertension is a strong possibility in this patient. Because of advanced azotemia, a routine isotope renal flow scan is not useful since visualization of the kidneys is poor at this level of renal function. Magnetic resonance angiography (MRA) or a spiral computed tomography (CT) is very useful in this context. In centers where there is local expertise, a color flow Doppler ultrasonography can be used. However, angiography is necessary for confirmation. If the degree of suspicion is very strong, one may proceed to angiography directly. Keep in mind that there is a risk of contrast induced renal failure in this setting.

140. How do you diagnose ARF secondary to rhabdomyolysis? Are there clues to this form of ARF?

Rhabdomyolysis can cause ARF due to acute tubular necrosis (ATN). It occurs in various clinical conditions, including trauma, ischemic tissue damage following a drug overdose, alcoholism, seizures, and heat stroke (especially in untrained subjects or those with sickle cell trait). Hypokalemia and severe hypophosphatemia can also precipitate rhabdomyolysis. It is the most common cause of ARF in patients abusing illicit IV drugs.

Typically, these patients have pigmented granular casts in urine sediment, a positive orthotolidine test in the urine supernatant (indicating the presence of heme), and markedly elevated plasma creatine kinase and other muscle enzymes, owing to their release from damaged muscle tissue. Other characteristics of ARF due to rhabdomyolysis include hyperphosphatemia, hyperkalemia, and a disproportionate increase in plasma creatinine (all of these being due to release of cellular constituents). A high anion-gap metabolic acidosis and severe hyperuricemia are also characteristic, and oliguria or anuria is common.

The mechanism of renal failure is not completely understood. Although myoglobin is not directly nephrotoxic, concurrent vasoconstriction or volume depletion decreases the renal perfusion and rate of urine flow in tubules, thereby promoting the precipitation of these pigment casts.

BIBLIOGRAPHY

1. Bennett JC, et al (eds): Cecil Textbook of Medicine, 20th ed. Philadelphia, W.B. Saunders, 2000.
2. Brenner EM, Rector FC (eds): The Kidney, 6th ed. Philadelphia, W.B. Saunders, 2000.
3. Greenberg A: Primer on Kidney Diseases—National Kidney Foundation, 2nd ed. San Diego, Academic Press, 1998.
4. Rose BF: Pathophysiology of Renal Disease, 2nd ed. New York, McGraw-Hill, 1987.
5. Schrier RW (ed): Diseases of the Kidney, 6th ed. Boston, Little, Brown, 1997.
6. Schrier RW (ed): Renal and Electrolyte Disorders, 5th ed. Boston, Lippincoot-Raven, 1997.

8. ACID/BASE AND ELECTROLYTES

Sharma S. Prabhakar, M.D.

In all things you shall find everywhere the Acid and the Alcaly.
Otto Tachenius (1670)
Hyppocrates Chymacus, Ch. 21.

Hence if too much salt is used in food, the pulse hardens.
Huang Ti (The Yellow Emperor) (2697–2597 B.C.)
Nei Chung Su Wen, Bk. 3, Sect. 10, tr. by Ilza Veith,
in The Yellow Emperor's Classic of Internal Medicine.

REGULATION OF SODIUM, WATER, AND VOLUME STATUS

1. List the osmolality and electrolyte concentrations of serum and commonly used intravenous (IV) solutions.

Osmolality and Electrolyte Concentrations of Commonly Used IV Solutions

SERUM AND SOLUTIONS*	OSMOLALITY (mOsm/kg)	GLUCOSE (g/l)	SODIUM (mEq/L)	CHLORIDE (mEq/L)
Serum	285–295	65–110	135–145	97–110
5% D/W	252	50	0	0
10% D/W	505	100	0	0
50% D/W	2520	500	0	0
1/2 NS (0.45% NaCl)	154	0	77	77
NS (0.9% NaCl)	308	0	154	154
3% NS	1026	0	513	513
Ringer's lactate	272	0	130	109

*D/W = dextrose in water; NS = normal saline. Ringer's lactate also contains 28 mEq/L lactate, 4 mEq/L K^+, and 4.5 mEq/L Ca^{2+}.

2. How do you estimate a patient's serum osmolality?

A close estimate can be derived from measurements of the serum sodium (Na^+), glucose, and blood urea nitrogen (BUN), using the following equation:

$$\text{Osmolality} = 1.86 \times [Na^+] + \frac{\text{Glucose}}{18} + \frac{\text{BUN}}{2.8} + 9$$

3. What percentage of the adult human body consists of water? What percentage of the water content is intracellular versus extracellular?

Approximately 60% of the adult man and 50% of the adult woman are water. About two-thirds of this volume is intracellular, and one-third is extracellular. About 20% of the extracellular fluid volume is plasma water.

4. What are the sources and daily amounts of water gain and loss?

The average adult male gains and loses 2600 ml of water each day. The gains occur from direct fluid ingestion (1400 ml/day), from the fluid content of ingested food (850 ml/day), and as a product of water produced by oxidation reactions (350 ml/day). Water losses occur through urine (1500 ml/day), perspiration (500 ml/day), respiration (400 ml/day), and feces (200 ml/day).

5. Discuss the necessary factors that allow the kidney to adequately excrete free water.

The required factors are:

1. There must be a filtrate formed to allow for renal excretion of free water. The lower the glomerular filtration rate (GFR), the lower the kidney's ability to respond rapidly to a free-water challenge with excretion of free water.

2. Glomerular filtrate must escape reabsorption in the proximal tubule to get to the diluting segment (ascending loop of Henle), where free water is created. Pathologic states involving vigorous fluid reabsorption in the proximal tubule are associated with a compromised ability to excrete free water. Examples include true volume depletion and states of decreased effective arterial blood volume, such as congestive heart failure, cirrhosis, and nephrotic syndrome.

3. An adequately functioning diluting segment must be present. Intrinsic disorders of function of this segment are unusual. Endogenous prostaglandin E_2 and loop diuretics inhibit NaCl transport in this segment and can thereby limit formation of free water.

4. The free water formed by the diluting segment must leave the nephron without being reabsorbed by the collecting tubule. This nephron segment is intrinsically impermeable to water but is made permeable by antidiuretic hormone (ADH).

6. Explain the meaning of serum sodium concentration with respect to sodium balance and water balance.

Serum Na^+ concentration $[Na^+]$, (in mEq/L) reflects the concentration of this cation in extracellular fluid (ECF). Because its units are measured as mass per unit volume, $[Na^+]$ indicates the relative relationship between Na^+ and water in the body. It is not indicative of total body Na^+ content but is more an indication of the water status (hydration) of the body. $[Na^+]$ may be low, normal, or increased with any given perturbation of total body Na^+ content.

Alterations of the $[Na^+]$ reflect alterations in free-water balance. Therefore, a true low $[Na^+]$ indicates a free-water excess compared to Na^+ content, and a high $[Na^+]$ indicates a relative free-water deficit.

7. What happens to the serum Na^+ concentration in response to loss of isotonic fluid, as in hemorrhage?

Isotonic fluid losses in and of themselves cause a decrease in ECF volume with no change in $[Na^+]$. If, however, these losses are replaced with hypotonic fluids, dilutional hyponatremia results.

8. What is meant by a state of "decreased effective arterial blood volume"?

The extracellular space is dynamic, with an ongoing balance between its capacity and its actual volume. Both of these parameters are biologically monitored and normally coordinated to maintain optimal tissue perfusion. A state of decreased effective arterial blood volume occurs when there is a large capacity combined with a smaller volume. This is seen most commonly with congestive heart failure, cirrhosis, and nephrotic syndrome.

9. Why does Na^+ have an effective distribution in total body water despite being confined largely to the extracellular space?

Na^+ is the major determinant of serum osmolality, and changes in its concentration lead to water shifts between the extracellular and intracellular compartments. This osmotic shift of water gives Na^+ an effective distribution greater than its chemical distribution and equivalent to that for total body water.

10. What is the diluting segment of the nephron?

The diluting segment is the thick ascending limb of the loop of Henle. This segment actively reabsorbs NaCl without water. This process leads to urine that is hyposmotic compared to plasma, creating free water for excretion.

11. What is the initial step in evaluating a patient with hyponatremia?

Determining the serum osmolality (either measured or calculated).

- **Hyperosmolar** hyponatremia (serum osmolarity > 295 mOsm/kg H_2O) usually results from administration of hypertonic solutions of dextrose or mannitol.

- **Isotonic** hyponatremia (serum osmolality 280–295 mOsm/kg H_2O) is seen with administration of isotonic solutions of dextrose and mannitol.
- **Hyposmolar** hyponatremia (serum osmolality < 280 mOsm/kg H_2O) can be associated with low, normal, or increased volume status and is seen with diuretic administration, salt-losing renal conditions, SIADH, chronic renal failure, and a wide range of other causes.
- **Pseudohyponatremia** is artifactual depression of serum Na^+ that results from excessive amounts of lipids and proteins leading to reduction of the plasma fraction of water.

12. How can patients with hyposmolar hyponatremia be categorized according to their history and physical findings?

Patients with hyposmolar hyponatremia can be categorized according to their volume status as estimated from the physical exam and history.

1. **Low volume status:** Supported by a history of volume loss or decreased intake and orthostatic blood pressure changes on examination. These patients need to have the lost volume replaced to turn off the factors that limit the kidney's ability to excrete free water.

2. **Expanded volume:** Supported by a history of a condition with decreased effective arterial blood volume and an examination showing edema. Patients must have therapeutic attention directed to their underlying disorder. If the hyponatremia is mild and symptomatic, free-water restriction, in addition to specific treatment of the underlying disorder, would be the suggested

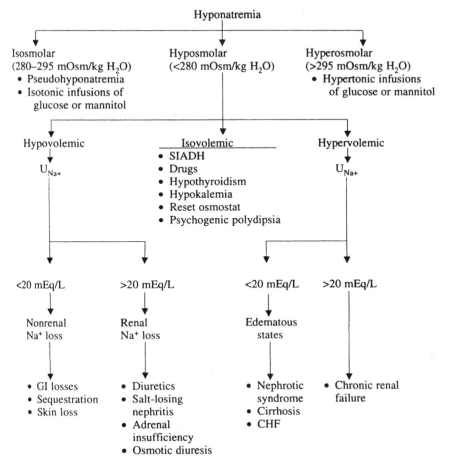

initial therapeutic approach. If the hyponatremia is severe and symptomatic, more aggressive treatment with hypertonic saline and furosemide may be required.

3. **Apparently normal volume status (euvolemia):** A wide variety of pathologic processes must be considered in the diagnostic evaluation, including SIADH and drugs that can limit free-water excretion (e.g., chlorpropamide).

13. How do pseudo-hyponatremia and spurious hyponatremia differ?

Pseudo-hyponatremia occurs when a quantitative serum Na^+ measurement is performed on a given volume of plasma that contains a greater-than-normal amount of water-excluding particles, such as lipid or protein. In this setting, plasma water (which contains the Na^+) comprises a smaller fraction of the plasma volume, leading to a factitiously low serum Na^+ concentration (when expressed in mEq/L). The Na^+ concentration in plasma water is normal, and therefore patients are asymptomatic. Attention should be directed to hyperlipidemia or hyperproteinemia.

Spurious hyponatremia results from hyperosmolality of the serum (i.e., from hyperglycemia), resulting in movement of intracellular water to the extracellular space and subsequent dilution of the Na^+ in the ECF. These patients are not symptomatic from hyposmolality (as are patients with true hyponatremia). If they are symptomatic at all, it is due to their hyperosmolar state. Attention should be directed to correcting the hyperosmolar state.

It is important to distinguish these two categories of hyponatremia from true hyponatremia associated with hyposmolality because the diagnostic workup and therapeutic management are different.

14. How do you correct the serum Na^+ for a given level of hyperglycemia?

Hyperglycemia, one of the causes of spurious hyponatremia, causes a decrease in the measured serum Na^+ concentration. For each increase in serum glucose of 100 mg/dl up to 600 mg/dl (an increase of 500, or 5×100 mg/dl), the serum Na^+ decreases by 8.0 mEq/L (5×1.6 mEq/L).

15. What is essential hyponatremia?

Essential hyponatremia, or "sick cell syndrome," denotes hyponatremia in the absence of a water diuresis defect. One hypothesis is that the osmoreceptor cells in the hypothalamus are reset so that they maintain a lower plasma osmolality. This is seen in several conditions, such as congestive heart failure, cirrhosis, and pulmonary tuberculosis, and is diagnosed by demonstrating normal urinary Na^+ concentration and dilution in the face of hyponatremia. Generally, this entity does not require treatment.

16. What are the signs and symptoms of hyponatremia?

The manifestations are mainly attributable to CNS edema, which is usually not seen until the serum Na^+ falls to 120 mEq/L or less. Symptoms range from mild lethargy to seizure, coma, and death. The signs and symptoms of hyponatremia are more a function of the rapidity of the drop in serum Na^+ than the absolute level. In patients with chronic hyponatremia, there has been time for solute equilibration, resulting in less CNS edema and less severe manifestations. In acute hyponatremia, there is no time for equilibration, and so smaller changes in serum Na^+ are accompanied by larger degrees of CNS edema and more severe manifestations.

17. Why is hyponatremia often seen after transurethral resection of the prostate (TURP)?

Often during the TURP procedure, large volumes of solutions containing mannitol, glycerol, or sorbitol are used to irrigate the prostate. A variable fraction of these fluids is absorbed into the systemic circulation, producing hyponatremia.

18. How do you manage hyponatremia in edematous states?

Treatment depends on the underlying etiology, any symptoms, and the rapidity of the drop in serum Na^+. In general, patients with edematous states such as the nephrotic syndrome, who have ECF expansion, have some degree of hyponatremia if they are not water-restricted. Generally, this condition is asymptomatic and requires no treatment. Treatment is required only if the hyponatremia is severe (< 125 mEq/L), and especially if there are symptoms such as lethargy, confusion, stupor, and coma.

19. A 41-year-old black man is hospitalized with acute bacterial meningitis. His chemistry profile shows a BUN and creatinine of 11 and 1.2 mg/dl, respectively, but his serum Na^+ is 127 mEq/L. How do you evaluate his hyponatremia and correct it?

Hyponatremia in the setting of bacterial meningitis (or any pathologic CNS process) is usually due to the syndrome of inappropriate ADH secretion (SIADH). SIADH is a form of hyponatremia involving sustained or spiking levels of ADH that are inappropriate for the osmotic or volume stimuli that normally affect ADH secretion. The essential points in the diagnosis of SIADH are:

    1. Presence of hypotonic hyponatremia

    2. Inappropriate antidiuresis (urine osmolality higher than expected for the degree of hyponatremia)

    3. Significant Na^+ excretion when the patient is normovolemic

    4. Normal renal, thyroid, and adrenal function

    5. Absence of other causes of hyponatremia, volume depletion, or edema

Thus, the workup includes measurement of serum and urine Na^+ concentration and osmolality. In most cases, urinary osmolality exceeds plasma osmolality, often by > 100 mOsm/l. Urinary Na^+ excretion exceeds 20 mEq/L unless the patient is wasting, and it improves with fluid restriction. In most cases, restriction of fluids to 1000–1200 ml/day is all that is needed. Occasionally, patients with symptomatic and marked hyponatremia may require demeclocycline therapy and/or hypertonic saline.

20. Which conditions are associated with SIADH?

Differential Diagnosis of SIADH

Malignant neoplasia	Pulmonary disorders
Carcinoma (bronchogenic, duodenum, pancreatic, urethral, prostatic, bladder)	Tuberculosis
	Pneumonia
Lymphoma, leukemia	Mechanical ventilators with positive pressure
Thymoma, mesothelioma, Ewing's sarcoma	Pneumonia (bacterial, viral, mycobacterial, fungal)
	Asthma, cystic fibrosis
CNS disorders	Pneumothorax
Trauma, subarachnoid hemorrhage, subdural hematoma, Rocky Mountain spotted fever	Lung abscess
Infection (encephalitis, meningitis, brain abscess)	**Drugs**
Tumors	Chlorpropamide
Porphyria	Thiazide diuretics
Guillain-Barré syndrome	Oxytocin
Psychosis, delirium tremens	Vincristine
Stroke	Haloperidol
Multiple sclerosis	Nicotine
	Phenothiazines
	Tricyclic antidepressants
	Others
	Other Conditions
	"Idiopathic" SIADH
	Hypothyroidism

21. What is cerebral salt-wasting?

Due to impaired renal water excretion, this condition is associated with hyposmolar hyponatremia in patients with cerebral trauma or disease. It mimics SIADH in all aspects including hypouricemia except that in this syndrome patients are volume-depleted, while in SIADH, patients are euvolemic. The high urinary Na^+ despite hypovolemia reflects renal salt-wasting. The etiology of this salt-wasting is unknown, although increased secretion of cerebral natriuretic factors is one likely explanation. A circulating factor that impairs renal tubular Na^+ reabsorption is another likely possibility.

Al-Mufti H, Arieff AI: Cerebral salt wasting syndrome: Combined cerebral and distal tubular lesion. Am J Med 77:740, 1984.

22. How do you estimate the free-water deficit in a patient with hypernatremia?

It can be assumed that the patient has lost free water without salt, and thus the patient has reduced total body water (TBW) but maintains the same total body Na^+ content. This change results in an increase in the serum Na^+ concentration that is proportional to the decrease in TBW. In other words, the ratio of the initial serum Na^+ (which is assumed to be normal) to the current serum Na^+ (which is higher than normal) is equal to the ratio of the present TBW (which is less than normal) to the initial TBW (which is assumed to have been normal).

$$\text{Current TBW} \div \text{Initial TBW} = \text{Initial } \{Na^+\} \div \text{Current } \{Na^+\}$$

This relationship can be used to calculate the current TBW. Subtracting this value from the initial (normal) TBW yields the estimated free-water deficit. This calculated free-water deficit must be replaced with fluids.

23. What are the manifestations of hypernatremia?

The manifestations of hypernatremia are basically those of hyperosmolality and are similar to the symptoms manifested by other causes of hyperosmolality, such as hyperglycemia. These are produced mainly by fluid shifts from the CNS and increased CNS osmolality, resulting in "shrinking" of the brain. The symptoms range from lethargy to seizures, coma, and death. The severity of the symptoms depends on the severity of the hyperosmolality and the speed with which it develops.

24. What are some common causes of hypernatremia?

Diabetes insipidus

Severe dehydration due to extrarenal fluid losses (e.g., burns, excessive sweating, etc.)

Hypothalamic disorders (e.g., tumors, granulomas, cerebrovascular accidents) leading to defective thirst and vasopressin regulation

25. How do you correct hypernatremia?

Once the free-water deficit is calculated, hypernatremia is usually corrected by replacement of the water. In mild cases, this can be accomplished by simply having the patient drink or, if IV fluids are used, dextrose in water can be given. If salt-containing fluids are deemed necessary, the equivalent free-water volume must be given. For example, if half-normal saline is used (1 liter of which contains 500 ml of NS and 500 ml of free water), then twice the amount of the estimated free-water deficit is needed to correct the free-water deficit.

This volume deficit should be replaced slowly. The first half is given over 24 hours. If the patient is hemodynamically unstable, with signs of severe ECF volume depletion, therapy with 0.9% normal saline is warranted before dextrose infusion is started.

POTASSIUM BALANCE

26. How is potassium distributed between the intracellular fluid (ICF) and extracellular fluid (ECF) compartments?

A 70-kg man contains approximately 3500 mEq of K^+ (approximately 50 mEq/kg body weight). The vast majority of this (98%) is in the ICF space. Therefore, the amount in the ECF compartment (the portion that we routinely measure) represents only a small percentage of the total body K^+.

27. How is the large chemical gradient between intracellular and extracellular K^+ concentration maintained?

The Na^+, K^+-ATPase pump actively extrudes Na^+ from the cell and pumps K^+ into the cell. This pump is present in all cells of the body. In addition, the cell is electrically negative compared to the exterior, which serves to keep K^+ inside the cell.

28. Given the relatively small extracellular compared to intracellular concentration of K^+, why are some electrical processes (cardiac conduction, skeletal and smooth muscle contraction) sensitive to changes in the ECF K^+ concentration?

It is the ratio of the ECF to ICF K^+ concentration more than the absolute level of either that determines the sensitivity of these electrical processes. Because the ECF concentration of K^+ is small compared to the ICF concentration, a small absolute change in ECF K^+ concentration results in a large change in the ECF:ICF K^+ ratio.

29. What are some common factors that influence the movement of K^+ between the intracellular and extracellular compartments?

1. **Acid-base changes:** Acidemia (increased concentration of H^+ in serum) leads to intracellular buffering of H^+, with subsequent extrusion of K^+ into the ECF, increasing the concentration of K^+ in this compartment.

2. **Hormones:** Insulin, epinephrine ($\beta2$-mediated), growth hormone, and androgens all promote net movement of K^+ into cells.

3. **Cellular metabolism:** Synthesis of protein and glycogen is associated with intracellular K^+ binding.

4. **Extracellular concentration:** All other things being equal, K^+ tends to enter the cell when its extracellular concentration is high and vice versa.

30. How is K^+ handled by the kidney?

Most of the filtered K^+ is reabsorbed in the proximal tubule, and there is net secretion or net resorption in the distal nephron, depending on the body's K^+ needs. Under most conditions, we are in K^+ excess, and the kidney must excrete K^+ to maintain whole-body K^+ balance. K^+ restriction leads to renal K^+ conservation, but this process is neither as rapid nor as efficient as the process for Na^+.

31. How does aldosterone influence K^+ metabolism?

Aldosterone is the main regulatory hormone for K^+ metabolism. It promotes Na^+ resorption and K^+ secretion in the distal nephron, gut, and sweat glands. Quantitatively, its greatest effect is in the kidney. Its secretion is increased by an increasing K^+ concentration in the ECF and is decreased by low K^+ concentrations.

32. What is meant by transtubular K^+ gradient (TTKG)? How does it help in evaluating a patient with hyperkalemia?

Asymptomatic hyperkalemia is a common presentation of patients with mineralocorticoid deficiency. Na^+ deficiency and volume depletion are not seen unless there is concomitant glucocorticoid deficiency. Na^+ balance is maintained by other factors, such as angiotensin II and catecholamines, although the ability to conserve Na^+ maximally is generally lost. Thus, urine $Na^+ <$ 10 mEq/L is unusual in primary hypoaldosteronism.

To diagnose hypoaldosteronism, the first step is to exclude drug-induced hyperkalemia (such as ACE inhibitors, β-blockers, NSAIDs, heparin, or K^+-sparing diuretics). The next step is to obtain morning samples of plasma for renin, aldosterone, and cortisol measurements. Administration of furosemide (20–40 mg) at 6 PM and 6 AM before samples are drawn enhances the utility of the test by stimulating plasma renin activity in normal persons but not in those with hypoaldosteronism.

TTKG is an indirect method of evaluating the effect of aldosterone on the kidney. The principle is to measure K^+ at the end of the cortical collecting tube, after all the distal K^+ secretion has taken place:

$$TTKG = \frac{U_{K^+}/(U_{osm}/P_{osm})}{P_{K^+}}$$

It is assumed that urine osmolality (U_{osm}) at the end of the cortical collecting tube is the same as that of plasma (P_{osm}) because the interstitium here is iso-osmotic, and that there is no further K^+ secretion or resorption. But, since ADH-mediated water permeability continues in the medullary collecting tubule, the K^+ concentration in this duct rises.

The above formula is applicable as long as the urine Na^+ concentration is 0.25 mEq/L, since Na^+ delivery should not be a limiting factor. The TTKG in normal subjects is 8–10 on a normal diet. On a high K^+ diet, TTKG is > 11 because of increased K^+ secretion. Thus, in a hyperkalemic subject, a TTKG < 5 mEq/L indicates impaired tubular K^+ secretion and is highly suggestive of hypoaldosteronism.

Ethier JH, et al: The trans-tubular potassium gradient in patients with hypokalemia and hyperkalemia. Am J Kidney Dis 15:309, 1990.

33. Name some conditions that can lead to increased renal K^+ excretion.

1. Increased dietary K^+ intake
2. Increased aldosterone secretion (as in volume depletion)
3. Alkalosis
4. Increased flow rate in the distal tubule
5. Increased Na^+ delivery to the distal nephron. This promotes Na^+ resorption in exchange for K^+ secretion in the distal nephron. The process is accelerated in the presence of aldosterone.
6. Decreased chloride concentration in tubular fluid in the distal nephron. This allows for Na^+ to be resorbed with a less-permeable ion (e.g., bicarbonate or sulfate) that increases the negativity of the tubular lumen in the distal nephron. The increased negativity of the tubular lumen promotes K^+ secretion.
7. Natriuretic agents. Drugs, such as the loop diuretics, thiazides, and acetazolamide, lead to increased Na^+ delivery to the distal nephron, volume depletion with increased aldosterone secretion, and subsequent increased renal K^+ excretion.

34. How do the potassium-sparing diuretics work?

Some natriuretic agents are K^+-sparing in that they inhibit K^+ secretion in the distal nephron. These agents include spironolactone, triamterene, and amiloride.

35. In addition to the kidney, what is the other major route of K^+ loss?

The GI tract. Fluids in the lower GI tract, particularly those of the small bowel, are high in K^+. Therefore, diarrhea can result in significant losses of K^+. However, upper GI losses, such as vomiting or nasogastric suction, cause renal K^+ loss. This renal K^+ loss is multifactorial and includes the following:
  • Alkalosis
  • Volume depletion, which leads to increased aldosterone secretion
  • Chloride depletion from the loss of HCl in gastric fluid. This leads to a high tubular concentration of HCO_3^-, which is a relatively nonresorbable anion.

36. What can cause a spuriously elevated serum K^+ determination?

1. **Hemolysis**, with the release of intraerythrocytic K^+.
2. **Pseudohyperkalemia**, seen in marked thrombocytosis or leukocytosis. It is due to the disproportionately increased amounts of the normally released K^+ that occurs with clotting. This can be corrected by inhibiting clotting and measuring the plasma K^+ concentration.

37. List the common causes of hyperkalemia.

Causes of Hyperkalemia

1. Inadequate excretion	**3. Shift of K+ from tissues**
Renal disorders	Tissue damage (muscle crush, hemolysis,
Acute renal failure	internal bleeding)
Severe chronic renal failure	Drugs (succinylcholine, arginine, digitalis
Tubular disorders	poisoning, β-blockers)
Hypoaldosteronism	Acidosis
Adrenal disorders	Hyperosmolality
Hyporeninemic (as in tubulointerstitial	Insulin deficiency
diseases, drugs such as NSAIDs, ACE	Hyperkalemic periodic paralysis
inhibitors, β-blockers)	
Diuretics that inhibit K+ secretion	**4. Pseudohyperkalemia**
(spironolactone, triamterene, amiloride)	Thrombocytosis
	Leukocytosis
2. Excessive intake	Poor venipuncture technique
	In vitro hemolysis

Singer GG, Brenner BM: Fluids and electrolytes. In Fauci A, et al (eds): Harrison's Principles of Internal Medicine, 14th ed. New York, McGraw-Hill, 1998, with permission.

38. Describe the general diagnostic approach to patients who have disturbances in serum K+ concentration.

In the initial approach, it is important to determine whether the disturbance results from:
1. Abnormal K+ intake or metabolism (excessive catabolism or anabolism)
2. Intra- and extracellular compartmental shifts
3. Disturbances in renal excretion or extrarenal loss

After the patient is placed in one of these three categories, it is possible to narrow the differential diagnosis, order appropriate diagnostic tests, and decide on the appropriate management. Disturbances of intake can be investigated by history and physical examination. The possibility of cellular shifts can be investigated by looking for any of the disturbances that result in compartmental movement of this cation. Determination of the urinary K+ concentration can help in distinguishing renal from nonrenal causes. High urinary K+ excretion in the setting of hypokalemia is compatible with a renal cause for K+ deficiency. In contrast, an appropriately low urinary K+ excretion in the setting of hypokalemia suggests extrarenal (possibly GI) losses.

39. How does hypokalemia present clinically?

The major manifestations are seen in the neuromuscular system. When K+ falls to 2.0–2.5 mEq/L, muscular weakness and lethargy are seen. With further decreases, the patient manifests paralysis with eventual respiratory muscle involvement and death. Hypokalemia also can cause rhabdomyolysis, myoglobinuria, and paralytic ileus. Prolonged hypokalemia can lead to renal tubular damage (called hypokalemic nephropathy).

40. How do you manage a patient with hypokalemia?

Management must be directed at the disturbance causing the abnormal K+ concentration. If hypokalemia is associated with alkalosis, then the alkalosis should be corrected in addition to providing K+ supplements.

In general, patients with K+ depletion should be given supplements slowly to replace the deficit. The oral route is preferred because of its safety as well as efficacy. Some instances require more rapid repletion with IV supplements, but this should not exceed 20 mEq/hr. Cardiac monitoring should accompany infusions of > 10 mEq/hr.

41. What are the manifestations of hyperkalemia besides ECG changes?

The most important manifestation is the increased excitability of cardiac muscle. With severe elevations in K^+, a patient can suffer diastolic cardiac arrest. Skeletal muscle paralysis also can be seen. Again, the symptoms produced by hyperkalemia are dependent on the rapidity of the change. Patients with chronically elevated serum K^+ levels can tolerate higher levels with fewer symptoms than patients with acute hyperkalemia.

42. How is hyperkalemia managed?

Treatment depends on the extent of the hyperkalemia and the clinical setting. Mild levels of hyperkalemia (5.0–5.5 mEq/L) associated with the hyporenin–hypoaldosterone syndrome are tolerated well and usually require no treatment. Higher levels not associated with ECG changes may require treatment with a synthetic mineralocorticoid.

Hyperkalemia occasionally presents as a medical emergency with very high levels (> 7.0 mEq/L) and cardiac conduction system abnormalities as determined by the ECG changes (see Chapter 3). In this emergent setting, management includes:

1. IV calcium must be administered to immediately counteract the effect of hyperkalemia on the conduction system.

2. This must be followed by maneuvers to shift K^+ into cells, thereby decreasing the ratio of extra- to intracellular K^+. This can be accomplished by administering glucose with insulin and/or bicarbonate to increase serum pH.

3. Finally, a maneuver to remove K^+ from the body must be instituted, such as a cation-exchange resin (Kayexalate) and/or hemodialysis or peritoneal dialysis.

43. A 61-year-old woman with end-stage renal disease (ESRD) missed her dialysis twice and presents to the emergency department with a serum K^+ of 6.4 mEq/L. How would you manage this patient?

The severity of hyperkalemia is assessed by both the serum K^+ level and ECG changes. If the ECG shows only tall T waves and the serum K^+ is < 6.5 mEq/L, the hyperkalemia is mild, whereas K^+ levels of 6.5–8.0 mEq/L are associated with more severe ECG changes, including absent P waves and wide QRS complexes. At higher K^+ levels, ventricular arrhythmias tend to appear, and the prognosis is grave unless proper treatment is given.

The first step is to obtain an ECG or observe the cardiac monitor. If it shows only tall T waves (as is likely in this situation), the patient can be treated with:

1. **Hypertonic glucose infusion**, along with 10 units of insulin (e.g., 10 units of insulin with 200–500 ml of 10% glucose in 30 min followed by 1 L of the same in the next 4–6 hours).

2. **Sodium bicarbonate**, 50–150 mEq given by IV (if the patient is not in fluid overload).

Both of these maneuvers shift K^+ into cells and start acting within an hour. Total body K^+ can be decreased by using cation-exchange resins, such as sodium polysterone sulfonate; usually, 20 gm with 20 ml of 70% sorbitol solution is started every 4–6 hours.

If the ECG shows the more severe changes, the patient should first receive 10% calcium gluconate (10–30 ml IV) while being monitored. Arrangements must be made to dialyze the patient as soon as possible to correct the hyperkalemia.

44. A 71-year-old diabetic with a nonhealing foot ulcer is on tobramycin and piperacillin. This patient has a resistant hypokalemia. How do you approach this problem?

Aminoglycosides and penicillins are both known to deplete serum K^+. The former do this by defective proximal tubular K^+ resorption and the latter by increased renal K^+ excretion induced by the poorly resorbable anion (penicillin). With aminoglycosides, magnesium-wasting is another complication. Hence, in addition to K^+ repletion, correction of hypomagnesemia is important, since hypokalemia is often resistant to correction unless the magnesium deficit is also corrected.

45. A 67-year-old white man with congestive heart failure treated with furosemide has a serum K⁺ of 2.4 mEq/L. How would you correct his K⁺ deficit?

Hypokalemia is an important complication of diuretic therapy (except with K⁺-sparing diuretics). It is important to monitor serum K⁺ periodically in these patients, especially those with cardiac illnesses who are likely to be on digoxin because hypokalemia can exacerbate digitalis toxicity. The K⁺ deficit requires replacement (except in patients who are on minimal doses of diuretics), particularly if serum K⁺ is < 3 mEq/L. The serum K⁺ level is not an exact indicator of the total body deficit, but severe hypokalemia with serum K⁺ of < 3 mEq/L is usually associated with a deficit of approximately 300 mEq. KCl elixir or tablets are the treatment of choice. Enteric-coated K⁺ supplements are known to cause gastric ulceration.

46. What is Bartter's syndrome?

Bartter's syndrome is a rare disorder characterized by hyperreninemic hyperaldosteronism, hyperplasia of juxtaglomerular apparatus, and hypokalemic alkalosis. There is also hypersecretion of vasodilatory prostaglandins, which help to maintain normal blood pressure despite hyper-reninemia. The primary defect seems to be impaired NaCl reabsorption in the thick ascending loop of Henle or distal tubule. Recent genetic studies indicate the defect involves a mutation of Na⁺-K⁺-2Cl cotransporter or K⁺ channel in the thick ascending limb of Henle. The diagnosis is often made by exclusion. Surreptitious use of diuretics and vomiting (urine Cl⁻ is often low!) can mimic most of the findings of this syndrome. Treatment consists of a K⁺-sparing diuretic (such as amiloride in higher doses of 10–40 mg) and NSAIDs to raise the plasma K⁺ by reversing the physiologic abnormalities.

Stein JH: The pathogenetic spectrum of Bartter's syndrome. Kidney Int 28:85, 1985.

Wingo C: Disorders of potassium balance. In Brenner B, Rector CR (eds): The Kidney, 6th ed. Philadelphia, W.B. Saunders, 2000.

47. A 55-year-old man with a history of congestive heart failure and chronic obstructive pulmonary disease (COPD) presents with extreme weakness and fatigue. His medications include digoxin 0.25 mg a day, hydrochlorothiazide 50 mg a day, and albuterol inhalations for his asthma. The patient reports a few days of exacerbation of COPD symptoms, forcing him to use the inhaler more frequently. What is the likely cause of his weakness?

The most likely cause of weakness in this patient is severe hypokalemia resulting from overuse of beta-agonists such as albuterol especially in the presence of potassium losing diuretics, since both effects could be additive. The hypokalemic effects of inhaled beta agonists are often so potent that they are used to treat patients with hyperkalemia acutely.

ACID-BASE REGULATION

48. What is the Henderson-Hasselbalch equation? What is its significance?

An acid-base disorder is suspected on clinical grounds and confirmed by arterial blood gas (ABG) analysis of the pH, PaCO2, or bicarbonate concentration. The Henderson-Hasselbalch equation is used to confirm that a given set of these parameters is mutually compatible:

$$pH = pKa + \log \frac{\{HCO_3^-\}}{\alpha CO_2 \times PaCO_2} = 6.1 + \log \frac{\{HCO_3^-\}}{0.03 \times PaCO_2}$$

The value of pK_a, the negative log of the equilibrium constant K, and the CO_2 solubility coefficient (αCO_2) are constant at any given set of temperature and osmolality. In plasma, at 37°C, the $pK_a = 6.1$ and $\alpha CO_2 = 0.03$.

The Henderson-Hasselbalch equation shows that pH is dependent on the ratio of $[HCO_3^-]$ to $PaCO_2$ and not on the absolute individual values alone. A primary change in one of the values usually leads to a compensatory change in the other value. This serves to limit the degree of the resulting acidosis or alkalosis.

49. The integrated action of which three organs is involved in acid-base homeostasis?

The **liver**, **lungs**, and **kidneys** cooperate to maintain acid-base balance. The liver metabolizes proteins contained in the standard American diet such that net acid (protons) is produced. Hepatic metabolism of organic acids (lactate) can consume acid, which is the equivalent of producing bicarbonate. Acid released into the ECF titrates HCO_3^- to H_2O and CO_2. This CO_2 and the CO_2 produced from cellular metabolism are excreted by the lungs. The kidney reclaims the filtered HCO_3^- and excretes the accumulated net acid.

50. What is the fate of a load of nonvolatile acid administered to the body?

The acid load is initially buffered by extracellular (40%) and intracellular (60%) buffers. These buffers minimize the decrease in pH that otherwise would occur. The major ECF buffer is the HCO_3^- system, and most intracellular buffering is provided by histidine-containing proteins. The administered acid reduces ECF HCO_3^-, and new HCO_3^- is then regenerated by the kidney during the process of proton (acid) secretion. Therefore, the administered acid is initially buffered and eventually excreted by the kidney.

51. Name the two major roles of the kidney in monitoring acid-base balance.

The kidney must **reclaim** the filtered HCO_3^- and **regenerate** the HCO_3^- lost by acid titration. This latter process is equivalent to acid excretion. Reclamation of HCO_3^- is quantitatively a more important process than regeneration (4500 mEq/day versus 70 mEq/day). Nevertheless, without regeneration of new HCO_3^- (excretion of acid), the plasma HCO_3^- concentration could not be maintained, and net acid retention would result.

52. Which two principal urinary buffers allow for net acid excretion (new HCO_3^- regeneration)?

Dibasic phosphate and ammonia. By accepting a proton, they become monobasic phosphate and ammonium ions, respectively, and are excreted in the urine. The phosphate is measured as titratable acid, and the ammonium is measured directly. Urinary excretion of these two substances minus urinary HCO_3^- excretion constitutes net acid excretion.

53. What are the four primary acid-base disturbances? How are they characterized?

Metabolic acidosis, **metabolic alkalosis**, **respiratory acidosis**, and **respiratory alkalosis**.

In the steady-state maintenance of normal acid-base balance, the addition of H^+ to the body fluids is balanced by their excretion, such that the H^+ concentration of the ECF remains relatively constant at 40 nM (40×10^{-9} M, or pH = 7.40). An imbalance in this process that leads to a net increase in $[H^+]$ is called acidosis. Alkalosis refers to an imbalance that leads to a net decrease in $[H^+]$.

54. What is meant by *metabolic* and *respiratory* when referring to these acid-base disturbances?

Metabolic and **respiratory** are terms used to describe how the imbalance occurred. Describing a disorder as **metabolic** infers that the imbalance leading to the change in H^+ occurred either because of addition of nonvolatile acid or base or because of a gain or loss of available buffer (HCO_3^-). HCO_3^- as a buffer reduces the concentration of free H^+ in solution. Referring to an acid-base disorder as **respiratory** infers that the net change in $[H^+]$ occurred secondary to a disturbance in ventilation that resulted in either a net increase or decrease in CO_2 gas in the ECF.

- **Metabolic acidosis** means there has been a net increase in $[H^+]$ as a result of a net gain in nonvolatile acid or from a net loss of HCO_3^- buffer.
- **Respiratory acidosis** means that there has been a net increase in $[H^+]$ as a result of decreased ventilation, leading to CO_2 retention.
- **Metabolic alkalosis** denotes a net decrease in $[H^+]$ that occurs as a result of gain of HCO_3^- or loss of acid.
- **Respiratory alkalosis** means that there has been a net decrease in $[H^+]$ because of increased ventilation leading to decreased CO_2.

Note that these disorders refer to the imbalance that leads to the directional change in $[H^+]$ and do not denote what the final $[H^+]$, PCO_2, and $[HCO_3^-]$ will be. Two important facts should be kept in mind:

1. There are compensatory changes that occur in response to these disorders
2. More than one acid-base disturbance may occur simultaneously; the final parameters measured depend not only on the algebraic sum of the different disorders but also on their respective compensatory responses.

55. How are the four primary acid-base disorders diagnosed?

Relationships Between HCO_3^- and $PaCO_2$ in Simple Acid-Base Disorders

CONDITION	PRIMARY DISTURBANCE	PREDICTED RESPONSE
Metabolic acidosis	$\downarrow HCO_3^-$	$\Delta PaCO_2$ ($\downarrow$) = 1–1.4 ΔHCO_3^-*
Metabolic alkalosis	$\uparrow HCO_3^-$	$\Delta PaCO_2$ ($\uparrow$) = 0.4–0.9 ΔHCO_3^-*
Respiratory acidosis	$\uparrow PaCO_2$	Acute: ΔHCO_3^- ($\uparrow$) = 0.1 $\Delta PaCO_2$
		Chronic: ΔHCO_3^- ($\uparrow$) = 0.25–0.55 $\Delta PaCO_2$
Respiratory alkalosis	$\downarrow PaCO_2$	Acute: ΔHCO_3^- ($\downarrow$) = 0.2–0.25 $\Delta PaCO_2$
		Chronic: ΔHCO_3^- ($\downarrow$) = 0.4–0.5 $\Delta PaCO_2$

* After at least 12 to 24 hours.
Hamm L: Mixed acid-base disorders. In Kokko JP, Tannen KL (eds): Fluids and Electrolytes, 3rd ed. Philadelphia, W.B. Saunders, 1996, p 487, with permission.

56. What are secondary acid-base disturbances?

The phrase *secondary acid-base disturbance* is actually a misnomer. More correctly stated, these are compensatory physiologic responses to the cardinal acid-base disturbances. They usually alleviate the change in H^+ concentration and therefore the pH that otherwise would occur. This can be seen more clearly by examining the mass-action equation defining the relationship of H^+, HCO_3^-, and the $PaCO_2$:

$$[H^+] = \frac{PaCO_2}{\{HCO_3^-\}} \times 24$$

This equation is derived from the more familiar Henderson-Hasselbalch equation. One can see that in the setting of metabolic acidosis, in which there is a primary decrease in $[HCO_3^-]$, the $[H^+]$ increases. It is also evident that the increase in $[H^+]$ in this setting can be alleviated by concomitantly decreasing the $PaCO_2$, which is exactly what occurs as a result of a ***physiologic*** increase in ventilation. This situation is properly described as metabolic acidosis with a directionally appropriate respiratory response. It is incorrect to describe the condition as primary metabolic acidosis with secondary respiratory alkalosis; to say that a patient has respiratory alkalosis is to say that a patient has ***pathologic*** hypoventilation, which is not the case in this situation. There are tables and formulas that can be used to calculate the expected respiratory response to a given degree of metabolic acidosis.

If the decrease in $PaCO_2$ in response to the degree of metabolic acidosis is exactly what we would have predicted from the formulas, then the patient is said to have one acid-base disorder: metabolic acidosis. In contrast, if the measured decrease in $PaCO_2$ is more than that predicted for the degree of metabolic acidosis, then the patient has an ***additional*** (not secondary) acid-base disorder: respiratory alkalosis in addition to metabolic acidosis. In other words, the patient has a mixed disorder, which is actually very common. If the measured $PaCO_2$ is higher than predicted, then the patient has an additional respiratory acidosis.

57. What is a respiratory acidosis?

Respiratory acidosis is a drop in the pH (acidosis) caused by alveolar hypoventilation. The alveolar hypoventilation leads to a rate of excretion of CO_2 that is less than its metabolic production. This net gain in CO_2 causes a rise in the $PaCO_2$. The lungs may be subject to diffuse hypoventilation (global alveolar hypoventilation), or only parts of the lungs may be involved (regional alveolar hypoventilation). As can be seen in the Henderson-Hasselbalch equation, any increase in the $PaCO_2$, if not accompanied by an increase in $[HCO_3^-]$, leads to a measurable drop in the pH.

58. How do you treat respiratory acidosis?

Treatment is aimed at the correction of the cause of the hypoventilation. This may involve the treatment of airway obstruction or, in respiratory failure, even mechanical ventilation.

59. What is a respiratory alkalosis?

Respiratory alkalosis, the opposite of respiratory acidosis, is a rise in pH (alkalosis). It is due to alveolar hyperventilation, which in turn leads to an increase in the excretion of CO_2 and a drop in the $PaCO_2$.

60. What are the causes of respiratory alkalosis?

Causes of Respiratory Alkalosis

1. CNS stimulation of ventilation:
   a. Physiologic (voluntary, anxiety, fear, fever, pregnancy)
   b. Pathologic (intracranial hemorrhage, stroke, tumors, brainstem lesions, salicylates)
2. Peripheral stimulation of ventilation:
   a. Reflex hyperventilation due to abnormal lung or chest wall mechanics (pulmonary emboli, myopathies, interstitial lung diseases)
   b. Arterial hypoxemia, high altitudes
   c. Pain
   d. Congestive heart failure, shock of any etiology
   e. Hypothermia
3. Hyperventilation with mechanical ventilation
4. Others:
   a. Severe liver disease
   b. Uremia

61. Are the plasma electrolytes alone (Na^+, K^+, Cl^-, and HCO_3^-) sufficient to determine a patient's acid-base status?

No. Remember that the regulatory systems of the body work to maintain the pH (or $[H^+]$), and that pH is a function of the ratio of $PaCO_2$ and $[HCO_3^-]$. The pH is not determined by the absolute value of $PaCO_2$ or $[HCO_3^-]$ alone.

Thus, a set of plasma electrolytes demonstrating a normal $[HCO_3^-]$ does not necessarily indicate a normal acid-base status. Furthermore, a low $[HCO_3^-]$ and high $[Cl^-]$ could represent either a metabolic acidosis (probably a nonanion gap acidosis) or a chronic respiratory alkalosis with an appropriate metabolic response (renal lowering of $[HCO_3^-]$ as a response to the chronically low $PaCO_2$). This is an attempt to maintain a more normal pH.

Likewise, a high $[HCO_3^-]$ with low $[Cl^-]$ may represent a metabolic alkalosis or a chronic respiratory acidosis with an appropriate metabolic response (renal increase in $[HCO_3^-]$ in response to chronically high $PaCO_2$) in an attempt to maintain a more normal pH. Note that without an accompanying pH and $PaCO_2$, one cannot tell if an abnormal $[HCO_3^-]$ is due to a metabolic cause (a metabolic acidosis or alkalosis) or to a metabolic response to a primary respiratory disorder. This illustrates the importance of obtaining ABGs (with a pH and $PaCO_2$) in addition to a $[HCO_3^-]$ to properly assess a patient's acid-base status.

62. What is meant by the anion gap?

The anion gap represents the difference between the routinely measured cations and anions in the plasma. It is usually calculated as follows:

$$\text{Anion gap} = [Na^+][Cl^-] + [HCO_3^-]$$

Since electroneutrality is always maintained in solution, there is no actual anion "gap." This gap is composed predominantly of negatively charged proteins in plasma and averages 12 ± 3

mEq/L. An increase is most commonly caused by addition of an acid salt (H^+A^-), which reduces plasma HCO_3^- concentration by titration. Electroneutrality is maintained in the face of the reduced plasma HCO_3^- concentration by the accompanying anion. Since the anion is not measured routinely in the electrolyte profile, the routine measurement would reveal only decreased HCO_3^- concentration. With plasma Na^+ and Cl^- remaining unchanged, this reduced HCO_3^- concentration leads to an increased anion gap. Note that the anion gap would not change if the added acid were HCl. Other circumstances that can increase the anion gap include increased protein concentration and alkalemia, which increase the net negative charge on plasma proteins. The presence of a large quantity of cationic (positively charged) proteins, as with multiple myeloma, can reduce the anion gap.

63. What is the conceptual difference between an anion-gap and a non-anion-gap metabolic acidosis?

An anion gap acidosis is caused by the addition of a nonvolatile acid to the ECF. Examples include diabetic ketoacidosis, lactic acidosis, and uremic acidosis. A non-anion-gap acidosis commonly (but not exclusively) represents a loss of HCO_3^-. Examples include lower GI losses from diarrhea and urinary losses due to renal tubular acidosis. Therefore, when approaching a patient with an anion-gap acidosis, one should look for the source and identity of the acid gained. By contrast, when evaluating a patient with a non-anion-gap acidosis, one should begin by looking for the source of the HCO_3^- loss.

64. What are the causes of anion-gap metabolic acidosis?

The mnemonic KUSMAL can be used to remember the differential diagnosis of anion-gap metabolic acidosis.

K — Ketones (diabetic, alcohol, starvation)
U — Uremia
S — Salicylates
M — Methyl alcohol
A — Acid poisoning (ethylene glycol, paraldehyde)
L — Lactate (circulatory/respiratory failure, sepsis, liver disease, tumors, toxins)

Morganroth ML: An analytical approach in the diagnosis of acid-base disorders. J Crit Illness 5:138–150, 1990.

65. What is the significance of plasma osmolal gap? How does it help in the evaluation of a patient with metabolic acidosis?

The plasma osmolal gap is the difference between the measured and calculated plasma osmolality. Plasma osmolal gap of .25 mOsm/kg suggests, in a patient with anion-gap metabolic acidosis, the possibility of ingestion of methanol or ethylene glycol. Isopropyl alcohol and ethanol increase the osmolal gap but not the anion gap, since acetone is not an anion.

66. What are the common causes of a non-anion-gap metabolic acidosis?

Causes of a Non-anion-Gap Metabolic Acidosis

Associated with K^+ loss	Drugs
Diarrhea	Acetazolamide
Renal tubular acidosis (proximal or distal)	Amphotericin B
Interstitial nephritis	Amiloride
Early renal failure	Spironolactone
Urinary tract obstruction	Toluene ingestion
Post-hypocapnia	**Urethral diversions**
Infusions of HCl (HCl, arginine HCl, lysine HCl)	Ureterosigmoidostomy
	Dual bladder
	Ileal ureter

Toto RD: Metabolic acid-base disorders. In Kokko JP, Tannen RL (eds): Fluids and Electrolytes, 3rd ed. Philadelphia, W.B. Saunders, 1996.

67. How does the serum albumin level affect the interpretation of anion gap?

The anion gap is significantly influenced by serum albumin level. If the concentration of serum albumin falls to 2 gm/dl (which is approximately half the normal), the expected normal anion gap should be reduced to half.

68. Why is the anion gap lower in patients with multiple myeloma?

The paraproteins that accumulate in multiple myeloma are usually positively charged since they are rich in lysine and arginine. If there is a significant accumulation of these positively charged particles, the measured cations remain in the normal range. But, since these "unmeasured" cations are associated with Cl^- (which is measured), the calculated anion gap will be reduced proportionately and may even become negative.

69. Why is ammoniagenesis reduced in renal failure?

Renal ammoniagenesis is an important mechanism for removal of acid and H^+ from the body. Ammonia then combines with H^+ to form ammonium, which is then excreted in the urine. In renal failure, with reduction in the renal mass, there is a decrease in the ATP stores. Consequently, less ATP can be used to oxidize glutamine to ammonia. This is an important mechanism for defective acidification in chronic renal failure.

70. How is the urine anion gap useful in the evaluation of metabolic acidosis?

Measuring urine electrolytes and calculating the urine anion gap are useful diagnostically in the evaluation of some cases of hyperchloremic metabolic acidosis.

$$\text{Urine anion gap} = \text{Unmeasured cations} - \text{unmeasured anions} = (Na^+ + K^+) - Cl^-$$

In normal subjects excreting 20–40 mEq of NH_4^+/L, the urine anion gap is positive or near zero. On the other hand, in metabolic acidosis, the NH_4^+ excretion increases if the renal acidification mechanisms are intact. Consequently, urinary Cl^- excretion also increases to maintain electroneutrality. Urinary Cl^- therefore exceeds cation $(K^+ + Na^+)$ excretion, and the urine anion gap is negative (often –20 to > –50 mEq/L. On the other hand, in acidosis where the renal acidification mechanisms are impaired (as in renal failure and renal tubular acidosis), the urine anion gap remains positive, as in normal subjects.

Battle DC, et al: The use of the urine anion gap in the diagnosis of hyperchloremic metabolic acidosis. N Engl J Med 318:594, 1988.

71. In which two situations should the urine anion gap not be used?

1. In **ketoacidosis**, the excretion of ketoacids neutralize the increased excretion of NH_4^+ cations, decreasing the negativity of anion gap.

2. In **hypovolemia**, the avid proximal Na^+ reabsorption causes decreased distal Na^+ delivery resulting in a defect in acidification. The Cl^- reabsorption that accompanies Na^+ prevents NH_4Cl excretion, and the urine anion gap remains positive.

72. What causes a decreased anion gap?

Certain disorders are associated with an anion gap that is lower than normal. This can be due to an increase in **unmeasured cations** like (K^+, Ca^{++}, or Mg^{++}), the addition of **abnormal** cations (lithium), or an increase in **cationic immunoglobulins** (plasma cell dyscrasias). It also can be decreased by loss of unmeasured anions such as albumin (serum hypoalbuminemia) or if the effective negative charge (on albumin) is decreased by severe acidosis.

73. What is renal tubular acidosis (RTA)?

This term refers to a disorder of tubular function in which the kidney has a compromised ability to excrete acid and/or recover filtered HCO_3^- in the setting of higher than normal [H^+] in the ECF. The laboratory presentation is that of a non-anion-gap metabolic acidosis.

74. Describe the four types of RTA.

Type I RTA (distal or classic RTA) is characterized by reduced net proton secretion by the distal nephron in the setting of systemic acidemia. Since the distal nephron is largely responsible for net acid excretion, patients with this disorder have continuous net acid retention (less net acid excretion than net acid production) and are therefore not in net acid balance. The diagnosis is made by demonstrating an inappropriately alkaline urine (pH > 5.5) in the setting of an acidemic serum (pH < 7.36) and by excluding the presence of drugs that alkalinize the urine (acetazolamide) or urea-splitting bacteria in the urine that can increase the urinary pH.

Type II RTA (proximal RTA) is characterized by a reduced capacity for HCO_3^- recovery by the proximal tubule but intact distal nephron function. These patients waste HCO_3^- in the urine until the ECF concentration of HCO_3^- is reduced to a level such that the reduced filtered load of HCO_3^- (GFR × plasma HCO_3^-) can now be more completely resorbed and the urine becomes nearly bicarbonate free. The reduction in plasma HCO_3^- concentration results in an increase in $[H^+]$. However, in the steady-state condition of low plasma HCO_3^-, these patients can excrete an appropriately acid urine (pH < 5.5) because distal nephron function is intact, and they are thus in acid balance (amount of acid excreted equals amount of acid produced), unlike the situation described for type I.

Type III RTA represents a variant of Type I, and the term is rarely used.

Type IV RTA is characterized by reduced aldosterone effect on the renal tubules, which may result in insufficient secretion of acid necessary to maintain normal acid-base status. These patients nevertheless can excrete an appropriately acid urine in the face of acidemic stress. Unlike the other types of RTA, type IV RTA is commonly associated with hyperkalemia due to a coexisting reduction in K^+ secretion. This disorder is commonly seen in patients with hyporenin-hypoaldosteronism but also is seen in isolated aldosterone deficiency and resistance.

75. How are the common types of renal tubular acidosis managed?

Type I (distal) RTA: Alkali is given in amounts necessary (usually 1–2 mEq/kg/day) to correct the acidosis and to buffer the acid being retained. K^+ supplements are commonly required at the initiation of treatment but usually not in the steady-state treatment once the acidosis has been corrected.

Type II (proximal) RTA: Alkali is not usually required in adults because they do not have net acid retention and have only mild acidemia. But because the chronic acidemia inhibits bone growth in children, they must be treated with large amounts of alkali (10–20 mEq/kg/day) as well as large K^+ supplements (the increased urinary HCO_3^- losses are accompanied by accelerated urinary K^+ losses).

Type IV RTA: The clinically mild degrees of acidemia rarely require alkali treatment. Hyperkalemia is more commonly a clinical concern and dictates whether mineralocorticoid replacements with synthetic steroids are required.

76. What is lactic acidosis?

Lactic acidosis is due to the accumulation of lactic acid, the end product of glycolysis. This accumulation leads to a depletion of the body's buffers and a drop in pH. Lactate, being an unmeasured anion, is one of the causes of an increased anion-gap acidosis.

77. What are the causes of lactic acidosis?

1. **Cellular hypoxia:** Oxygen is required for the oxidative phosphorylation of the lactic acid produced by glycolysis. Anything interfering with the available cellular supply of O_2 or its utilization will lead to the accumulation of lactic acid. This category includes respiratory failure, circulatory failure, and CO poisoning. This also can be seen in thiamine deficiency and has been reported in patients on long-term total parenteral nutrition (TPN) without supplementation with thiamine.

2. **Decreased hepatic utilization of lactic acid:** Seen in advanced hepatocellular insufficiency of any cause.

3. **Cyanide poisoning:** CN causes increased lactic acid production because it blocks oxidative phosphorylation, leading to increased glycolysis, decreased utilization of lactic acid, and therefore lactic acid accumulation.

4. **Alcohol consumption:** Alcohol causes a modest increase in lactic acid production. In association with caloric depletion, the lactic acidosis can be severe.

5. **Neoplasms with a large tumor burden:** Neoplasms can lead to increased production of lactic acid, even with sufficient O_2, since the tumor cells can have higher rates of glycolysis than normal cells.

6. **Diabetic ketoacidosis (DKA):** DKA is associated with increased lactic acid levels even in the absence of shock or other etiologies.

7. **Lactic acidosis X:** This is a condition in which severe lactic acidosis occurs without obvious cause.

8. **Factitious lactic acidosis:** When blood is stored for prolonged periods of time, the red and white cells generate lactic acid in the tube as it is stored. It is most commonly seen in patients with high WBC counts.

78. What is metabolic alkalosis?

Metabolic alkalosis is a disorder characterized by a directional decrease in [H^+] from metabolic causes. It results from addition of excess HCO_3^- or alkali or loss of acid. Note that a low Cl^- and a high HCO_3^- concentration can result from both metabolic alkalosis as well as from a metabolic response to a respiratory acidosis. However, the pH and $PaCO_2$ help to differentiate these two disorders.

79. What are the common causes of metabolic alkalosis?

Chloride-Responsive (Urine $Cl^- < 10$ mEq/L)	Chloride-Resistant (Urine $Cl^- > 20$ mEq/L)
Gastric fluid loss	Primary aldosteronism
Postdiuretic therapy	Primary reninism
Posthypercapnia	Hyperglucocorticoidism
Congenital chloride diarrhea	Hypercalcemia
	Potassium depletion
	Liddle's syndrome
	Bartter's syndrome
	Chloruretic diuretics

Toto RD: Metabolic acid-base disorders. In Kokko JP, Tannen RL (eds): Fluids and Electrolytes, 2nd ed. Philadelphia, W.B. Saunders, 1990, p 356.

Those forms of alkalosis responsive to chloride salt administration are generally associated with ECF fluid volume depletion and low urinary Cl^- concentration in spot urine tests, whereas the Cl^- unresponsive alkaloses are associated with ECF volume expansion and urine $Cl^- > 20$ mEq/L.

80. Which is the most common acid-base disturbance seen in cirrhosis?

Primary respiratory alkalosis due to centrally mediated hyperventilation is the most common acid-base disturbance in patients with severe hepatic disease, especially with superimposed encephalopathy. The exact etiology is unclear but may be related to the hormonal imbalance associated with liver failure. Estrogens and progesterone have been implicated, a situation somewhat similar to that seen in pregnancy.

81. How do you diagnose a mixed acid-base disorder?

Sometimes two or more primary acid-base disturbances are seen in the same patient, usually in critical care units. The steps in diagnosis are as follows:

1. Define the primary disturbance and the compensatory process involved. The primary disturbance is identified by the direction of the changes in pH, HCO_3^-, and $PaCO_2$ levels.

2. Determine if the pulmonary or renal compensation is appropriate (see Question 55). Two facts must be kept in mind while making these interpretations. First, adequate compensation takes 12–24 hrs to occur, and second, "overcompensation" never occurs in primary acid-base disturbances.

3. Consider the patient's history and clinical presentation to formulate a differential diagnosis.

- In combined **metabolic and respiratory acidosis**, even though the HCO_3^- and $PaCO_2$ may not be changed, pH is distinctly lower.
- In **combined metabolic acidosis and metabolic alkalosis**, the pH and HCO_3^- can be lower, normal, or higher, but an elevated anion gap with a high or normal HCO_3^- suggests the diagnosis.
- **A combined metabolic alkalosis and respiratory acidosis** (which can be seen in patients with ARDS or COPD who are vomiting) causes higher HCO_3^- levels than predicted compensation for a given high $PaCO_2$.

In general, the underlying clinical condition gives clues to the possible mixed acid-base disturbance, which can then be defined using the nomograms of expected compensation.

Narins R, Emmett M: Simple and mixed acid-base disorders: A practical approach. Medicine 59:161–187, 1980.

82. A 34-year-old woman is admitted to the hospital because of nausea and vomiting for the last 2 days. She admits to taking several aspirin pills to alleviate her joint pains before she noticed epigastric pain and vomiting. Her arterial blood gas analysis reveals the following: pH 7.64, P_{CO_2} 32, and plasma bicarbonate 33 mEq/L. What kind of acid-base disorder is present in this patient?

The patient has an alkalotic state since the pH is higher than normal range. Since the patient presented with significant emesis, it is logical to think that the primary disturbance is metabolic alkalosis, which is supported by the fact that plasma bicarbonate is significantly elevated. The expected respiratory compensatory response is to increase P_{CO_2} by 6–7 mmHg for every 10 mEq/L increase in plasma bicarbonate. However, in this patient the P_{CO_2} is actually lower than normal indicating a primary respiratory alkalosis. Thus, this patient has a mixed acid-base disorder. The combined metabolic and respiratory alkalosis explains why the pH is so disproportionately high.

83. In what situations are potentially fatal mixed acid-base disorders commonly encountered?

In general, combined respiratory and metabolic acidosis or metabolic and respiratory alkalosis can result in pH changes that are fatal. Some of the common examples are:

1. An alcoholic with ketoacidosis (metabolic acidosis) may have superimposed vomiting from gastritis (metabolic alkalosis) and hyperventilation associated with withdrawal (respiratory alkalosis).

2. A combination of metabolic acidosis and respiratory alkalosis is seen typically in patients with sepsis, salicylate intoxication, and severe liver disease.

3. Metabolic acidosis can coexist with metabolic alkalosis in patients with renal failure or with alcoholic or diabetic ketoacidosis (acidosis) who are vomiting or having gastric suction (alkalosis).

4. Vomiting in a pregnant female or a patient with liver failure causes a mixture of respiratory and metabolic alkalosis.

CALCIUM, PHOSPHATE, AND MAGNESIUM METABOLISM

84. How is calcium distributed in the body and in the serum?

A 70-kg man has approximately 1000 gm of calcium in his body. Of this, bone contains 99%, whereas the ECF and ICF contain only 1%. Furthermore, only about 1% of skeletal calcium is freely exchangeable with ECF calcium.

The routine measurement for serum calcium (normal = 9–10 mg/ml = 4.5–5.0 mEq/L = 2.25–2.5 mM/L) measures total calcium. Approximately 40% of this is protein-bound, 5–10% is complexed to other substances (e.g., phosphate, sulfate), and 50% is ionized.

85. Why is it important to recognize the differences between ionized and protein-bound calcium?

It is the ionized fraction of calcium that determines the activity of this electrolyte in cellular and membrane function. It is possible to vary the concentration of total calcium without changing the ionized fraction by changing the protein concentration. By contrast, it is also possible to vary the ionized fraction without changing the total concentration by changing serum pH. Increasing serum pH decreases the ionized fraction of calcium and vice versa.

86. What are the major sites of calcium resorption in the nephron?

About 50% of the filtered calcium is reabsorbed in the proximal tubule, and most of the remainder (about 40% of the total) is reabsorbed in the loop of Henle, primarily the ascending limb of the loop of Henle. A small amount of calcium is reabsorbed in the distal convoluted tubule and an even smaller amount in the collecting tubule.

87. What are the major hormones involved in calcium metabolism?

Parathyroid hormone (PTH), vitamin D, and calcitonin.

PTH is secreted in response to a decrease in serum calcium and promotes calcium resorption from bone because it enhances renal resorption of calcium and excretion of phosphate. Low serum calcium concentration stimulates 1-hydroxylation of 25-hydroxyvitamin D by the kidney to form 1,25-dihydroxyvitamin D (the active form of vitamin D). This hormone promotes calcium resorption from the gut and mineralization of bone. Increases in serum calcium lead to increased secretion of calcitonin. This hormone inhibits bone reabsorption and 1-hydroxylation of 25-hydroxyvitamin D and thereby ameliorates hypercalcemia.

88. Name some factors that affect renal calcium excretion.

With some exceptions, renal calcium handling varies directly with renal Na^+ handling. Therefore, renal calcium excretion is increased by saline diuresis, loop diuretics, and volume expansion. In contrast, renal calcium excretion is decreased in volume depletion and other states associated with renal salt retention. One notable exception to this general rule is that the natriuresis associated with thiazide diuretics is accompanied by decreased, rather than increased, urinary calcium excretion.

89. What are pseudohypocalcemia and pseudohypercalcemia?

These terms refer to an alteration of the total calcium concentration in the setting of a normal ionized fraction. Since the ionized fraction is normal, these patients are asymptomatic. Abnormalities in the concentration of serum proteins are a common cause of these disorders.

90. How do you correct the total serum calcium level for changes in the serum albumin?

Hypoalbuminemia causes a decrease in the total serum calcium level without a change in the level of ionized calcium. For each decrease of 1.0 g/dl in serum albumin, one should expect a drop in the total serum calcium of approximately 0.8 mg/dl.

91. What are some common causes of true hypocalcemia?

Hypoparathyroidism (usually following thyroid or parathyroid surgery)
Vitamin D deficiency
Magnesium depletion (usually at levels < 0.8 mEq/L)
Liver disease (decreased synthesis of 25-hydroxyvitamin D)
Renal disease (hyperphosphatemia and decreased synthesis of 1,25-dihydroxyvitamin D)
Acute pancreatitis
Tumor lysis syndrome
Rhabdomyolysis

92. What are some common causes of true hypercalcemia?

Primary hyperparathyroidism (approximately 50% of cases), malignancy, use of thiazide diuretics, vitamin D excess, hyper- and hypothyroidism, granulomatous disorders, immobilization, and milk-alkali syndrome.

93. What are the signs and symptoms of hypocalcemia?

The symptoms are dependent on the magnitude of the decrease in serum calcium, the rate of the drop, and its duration. The symptoms of hypocalcemia are due to the resultant decrease in the excitation threshold of neural tissue. This causes an increase in excitability, repetitive responses to a single stimulus, reduced accommodation, or even continuous activity of neural tissue. The varied symptoms and signs include:

Signs and Symptoms of Hypocalcemia

Tetany and paresthesia	QT interval prolongation on the ECG
Altered mental status (lethargy to coma)	Increased intracranial pressure
Seizures	Lenticular cataracts

94. What are Trousseau's and Chvostek's signs?

Both are indications of the latent tetany caused by hypocalcemia. Of the two signs, Trousseau's is more specific and reliable.

1. **Trousseau's sign:** A sphygmomanometer is placed on the arm and inflated to greater than systolic blood pressure and left in place for at least 2 minutes. A positive response is carpal spasm of the ipsilateral arm. Relaxation takes 5–10 seconds after the pressure is released.

2. **Chvostek's sign:** Tapping the facial nerve between the corner of the mouth and the zygomatic arch produces twitching of the ipsilateral facial muscle, especially the angle of the mouth. This sign may be seen in 10–25% of normal adult patients.

95. What are the symptoms and signs of hypercalcemia?

Symptoms include weakness, constipation, nausea, anorexia, polyuria, polydipsia, and pruritus. Severe hypercalcemia may present with progressive CNS symptoms of lethargy, depression, obtundation, coma, and seizures. Rapid onset is more likely to be symptomatic than a slowly progressive level, regardless of the ultimate level at presentation.

96. Describe the appropriate treatment for hypercalcemia.

Treatment depends on the calcium level and symptoms of the patient. Acute, symptomatic hypercalcemia should be treated aggressively, first with saline infusion to expedite calcium excretion. Most patients with hypercalcemia are significantly volume-depleted as a result of the osmotic diuresis related to the hypercalciuria.

1. **Normal saline** should be given at a rapid rate, 300 ml/hr or more, with KCl and possibly magnesium added to the solution depending on measured blood values. After the patient is volume-repleted, furosemide may be given to promote calciuresis. Care must be taken to keep input equal to or greater than output, to avoid making the patient hypovolemic again.

2. **Mithramycin** is effective when the patient cannot tolerate large fluid loads due to congestive heart failure or third-space losses or if there is an inadequate response to IV volume replacement. It should be given at a dose of 15 mg/kg (i.e., 1–2 mg) IVSS for one dose. The dose can be repeated if necessary, but doses more frequent than every 3–7 days have been associated with renal and hepatic toxicity. Mithramycin also can cause a coagulopathy, which can lead to serious bleeding complications.

3. **Calcitonin** is useful for decreasing serum calcium and has the added advantage of rapid onset of action. It may be given in the presence of renal insufficiency, thrombocytopenia, or when mithramycin is contraindicated. Its disadvantage is that rapid resistance often develops, probably related to the development of antibodies. This resistance can sometimes be delayed by concomitant administration of prednisone.

4. **Bisphosphonates** inhibit osteoclast activity and are effective with those cancers in which this mechanism is present. They are given as IV infusion over 5 days or as oral tablets.

Less significant levels of hypercalcemia can be treated with other agents, such as glucocorticoids (prednisone, 20–40 mg/day), phosphates (1–6 g/day), prostaglandin inhibitors (aspirin and NSAIDs), or oral bisphosphonates. All of these agents are less effective but may suffice for chronic maintenance.

Bilizekian JP: Management of acute hypercalcemia. N Engl J Med 326:1196–1203, 1992.

97. What are the major sites of phosphate resorption in the nephron?

Phosphate is resorbed predominantly in the proximal tubule, with small amounts being absorbed in the distal tubule.

98. What factors increase excretion of urinary phosphate?

PTH
Alkalosis
Saline diuresis
Ketoacidosis
Increased dietary phosphate intake

99. What factors can lower serum phosphate by shifting this ion into cells?

Insulin, glucose (by stimulating insulin secretion), and alkalosis.

100. In which clinical situations can hypophosphatemia develop?

1. **Decreased dietary intake**
   a. Decreased intestinal absorption due to vitamin D deficiency, malabsorption, steatorrhea, secretory diarrhea, vomiting, or phosphate binders
   b. Alcoholism
2. **Shifts from serum into cells**
   a. Respiratory alkalosis as seen in sepsis, heat stroke, hepatic coma, salicylate poisoning, gout, etc.
   b. Recovery from hypothermia
   c. Hormonal effects of insulin, glucagon, androgens, etc. (recovery from diabetic ketoacidosis)
   d. Carbohydrate administration (hyperalimentation, fructose or glucose infusions)
3. **Increased excretion into urine**
   a. Hyperparathyroidism
   b. Renal tubule defects as in aldosteronism, SIADH, mineralocorticoid administration, diuretics, corticosteroids
   c. Hypomagnesemia
4. **Spurious**
   a. Mannitol infusion

101. What are the main disturbances thought to be responsible for the abnormalities of calcium and phosphate metabolism seen with progressive renal disease?

Patients with progressive renal disease develop hyperphosphatemia, hypocalcemia, and secondary hyperparathyroidism. They are also at risk of developing at least two kinds of bone disease. The main disturbances that contribute to these abnormalities are:

1. A rise in inorganic phosphate concentration in the serum due to poor renal excretion. This leads to a decrease in serum calcium concentration and stimulation of PTH secretion. The increased PTH secretion leads to increased bone resorption and osteitis fibrosa cystica.

2. Resistance to the action of vitamin D. One function of this hormone is to promote calcium resorption from the gut. Decreased gut resorption of calcium exacerbates the hypocalcemia and reduces available calcium for bone mineralization.

3. Defective synthesis of 1,25-dihydroxyvitamin D (the active form of this hormone). Reduced levels of 1,25-dihydroxyvitamin D result in defective bone mineralization (osteomalacia in adults, rickets in children).

102. How does magnesium depletion affect calcium and phosphate metabolism?

Magnesium depletion results in decreased secretion and end-organ responsiveness of PTH. This leads to functional hypoparathyroidism and the resultant effects on the serum level and urinary excretion of calcium and phosphate. This disorder can be corrected with magnesium repletion.

103. What are the major nephron sites for magnesium resorption?

Magnesium is resorbed predominantly in the thick ascending limb of the loop of Henle, with a smaller amount being resorbed in the proximal tubule.

104. What are some common causes of magnesium deficiency?

- Dietary insufficiency (decreased intake, protein-calorie malnutrition, prolonged IV feeding)
- Intestinal malabsorption
- Chronic loss of GI fluids
- Diuretics
- Other drugs (gentamicin, cisplatin, pentamidine, cyclosporine)
- Alcoholism
- Hyperparathyroidism
- Lactation

105. What is the milk-alkali syndrome?

The presence of hypercalcemia, increased BUN and creatinine, increased serum phosphate, and metabolic alkalosis in a patient ingesting large quantities of milk and calcium carbonate-containing antacids. The patient usually presents with nausea, vomiting, anorexia, weakness, polydipsia, and polyuria. If it continues, metastatic calcification can occur, leading to mental status changes, nephrocalcinosis, band keratopathy, pruritus, and myalgias. The treatment is withdrawal of the milk and antacid.

106. What electrolyte abnormalities are seen in HIV infection?

Apart from the main proteinuric syndrome caused by focal sclerosis (so-called HIV nephropathy), a variety of electrolyte disorders are commonly seen in patients with HIV. Asymptomatic **hyperkalemia** is a common manifestation. The hyperkalemia may be due to many possible causes, including hyporenin-hypoaldosteronism, adrenal insufficiency, drugs such as pentamidine and trimethoprim-sulfamethoxazole, and even isolated hypoaldosteronism. **Hyponatremia** is frequently caused by hypovolemia, adrenal insufficiency, and SIADH due to associated pulmonary or cerebral diseases. Other electrolyte abnormalities include hypocalcemia, hypomagnesemia, and hypouricemia. Hypercalcemia has been seen in association with lymphomas and cytomegalovirus infection.

Glassock RJ, Cohen AH, Danovitch G: Human immunodeficiency virus (HIV) infection and the kidney. Ann Intern Med 112:35, 1990.

Klotman PE : AIDS and the Kidney: Semin Nephrol 18:4, 1998.

107. What are the common electrolyte abnormalities seen in alcoholics?

Hypokalemia is seen in one-half of hospitalized, withdrawing alcoholics. This does not necessarily mean a total body K^+ deficit. Respiratory alkalosis, inadequate dietary intake, and GI losses (vomiting, diarrhea) are the common etiologic factors for hypokalemia. Withdrawal as well as severe liver disease can cause respiratory alkalosis in alcoholics.

Hypophosphatemia (< 2.5 mg/dl) is a common finding in hospitalized severe alcoholics, noted in more than half (50%) of patients in some series. The common predisposing factors are respiratory alkalosis, decreased dietary intake, transcellular shifts due to glucose administration, and, rarely, associated proximal tubular injury leading to phosphate wasting.

Chronic alcoholism is the most common cause of **hypomagnesemia** in the U.S. It is seen in alcoholics who are withdrawing and more commonly in those who had withdrawal seizures. GI losses, cellular uptake, dietary deficiencies, and possibly lipolysis leading to fatty acid-magnesium precipitation are the possible causes.

Hyponatremia sometimes is seen in beer-drinkers who ingest large quantities of beer, which is virtually solute-free. When this free-water volume exceeds the excretory capacity of the kidney, hyponatremia results.

BIBLIOGRAPHY

1. Brenner BM, Rector FC (eds): The Kidney, 6th ed. Philadelphia, W.B. Saunders, 2000.
2. Rose BD: Clinical Physiology of Acid-Base and Fluid and Electrolyte Disorders, 4th ed. New York, McGraw-Hill, 1994.
3. Schrier RW (ed): Renal and Electrolyte Disorders, 5th ed. Boston, Lippincott-Raven, 1997.
4. Seldin DW, Giebisch G (eds): The Regulation of Acid-Base Balance. New York, Raven Press, 1992.
5. Bennett JC, et al (eds): Cecil Textbook of Medicine, 20th ed. Philadelphia, W.B. Saunders, 2000.

9. HEMATOLOGY

Mark M. Udden, M.D.

> *Blood is the originating cause of all men's diseases.*
> The Talmud, *Baba Nathra, III.58a*

> *The blood is the life.*
> The Bible, *Deuteronomy 12:23*

HYPOPROLIFERATIVE ANEMIAS

1. What are the two most helpful laboratory tests in the initial evaluation of anemia?

Reticulocyte count and peripheral blood film. The peripheral blood film demonstrates important abnormalities of red blood cell (RBC) shape, size, or hemoglobinization. In addition, an impression of the white blood cell (WBC) count and platelet count can be obtained. RBCs also must be examined for the presence of inclusions (such as Howell-Jolly bodies).

2. What are reticulocytes? Why count them?

Reticulocytes are young RBCs newly released from the marrow. They can be detected by their lacy network of RNA. If the reticulocyte count is high, blood loss or hemolysis is likely to be the cause of anemia. If the reticulocyte count is low, a primary marrow disorder (hypoproliferative anemia) should be considered.

Physiologic Classification of Anemia

LOW RETICULOCYTE COUNT	HIGH RETICULOCYTE COUNT
Hypoproliferative anemia	Blood loss
	Response to treatment of iron, folate, or vitamin B12 deficiency
	Hemolysis

From Cavill I: The rejected reticulocyte. Br J Haematol 84:563–565, 1992.

The old method of determining the reticulocyte count relied on a manual count of 1000 cells stained with new methylene blue. Currently reticulocyte count usually is determined by flow cytometric analysis of thiazole orange-stained cells or other automated analysis, which leads to greater reproducibility and allows discrimination between mature and immature reticulocytes. The release of immature reticulocytes is often a sign of early marrow recovery after bone marrow transplantation or response to treatment in deficiency states.

3. How are mean cell volume (MCV) and red cell distribution width (RDW) used in the evaluation of anemias?

The complete blood count (CBC) now includes the MCV, and many clinical laboratories also determine an index of the heterogeneity of cell size (RDW). In iron-deficiency anemia, for example, RBCs have been produced during periods of iron sufficiency and varying degrees of deficiency. Thus, cell size in iron-deficiency anemia is more heterogeneous than in thalassemia minor, in which all of the cells are small. This difference results in a larger RDW for iron-deficiency anemia and a normal RDW for thalassemia. Current automated devices for determining the CBC can also determine the mean cellular hemoglobin content of reticulocytes. A decrease in reticulocyte cellular hemoglobin content is an early indicator of iron deficient erythropoiesis.

Classification of Anemias Based on MCV and RDW

MCV LOW		MCV NORMAL		MCV HIGH	
RDW NORMAL	RDW HIGH	RDW NORMAL	RDW HIGH	RDW NORMAL	RDW HIGH
Chronic disease	Iron deficiency	Normal	Early or mixed	Aplastic	Folate or
Nonanemic	HbS-α or β	Chronic disease	nutritional	anemia	vitamin B12
heterozygous	thalassemia	Nonanemic	deficiency		deficiency
thalassemia	Hb H	or enzyme	Anemic abnor-		Sickle cell
Children		abnormality	mal hemoglobin		anemia ($\frac{1}{3}$
		Splenectomy	Myelofibrosis		of cases)
		CLL (except	Sideroblastic		Immune
		extreme high	anemia		hemolytic
		lymphocyte	Myelodysplasia		anemia
		number)			Cold agglu-
		Acute blood loss			tinins
					Preleukemia
					Newborn

Note: Chronic liver disease, chronic myelogenous leukemia, and cytotoxic chemotherapy may be associated with high or normal MCV and high or normal RDW. CLL = chronic lymphocytic leukemia.
From Bessman JD: Automated Blood Counts and Differentials: A Practical Guide. Baltimore, Johns Hopkins University Press, 1986, p 11, with permission.

4. What are the causes of hypochromic microcytic anemias? How are iron studies used in their differentiation?

Hypochromic microcytic anemias are the most frequently encountered anemias in hospitalized and ambulatory patients. A working knowledge of these anemias and their laboratory diagnosis is essential to avoid wasting time and resources.

Causes of Hypochromic Microcytic Anemias

	NORMAL	IDA	ANEMIA OF CHRONIC DISEASE	SIDERO-BLASTIC ANEMIA	THALASSEMIA
Serum iron (μg/dl)	115 (70–180)	< 70	30 (15–65)	> 180	Normal or elevated
TIBC (μg/ml)	340	> 400	200	250	250
Transferrin saturation (%)	35 (25–50)	< 16	15 (10–40)	80 (60–100)	Normal or elevated
Marrow hemosiderin	2+	0	3+	4+	2+ to 4+
Serum ferritin	Normal	Decreased	Slightly elevated	Elevated	Normal or elevated

IDA = iron-deficiency anemia; TIBC = total iron-binding capacity.

Note that a bone marrow examination in sideroblastic anemia shows increased iron stores and abnormal iron distribution in ringed sideroblasts. Both iron-deficiency anemia and anemia of chronic disease have a low transferrin saturation. In iron-deficiency anemia, the TIBC is often increased, whereas anemia of chronic disease is marked by an unusually low TIBC. Iron stores are usually normal in thalassemia-minor, although β-thalassemia major may be complicated by iron overload.

Measurement of the serum soluble transferrin receptor protein (sTfR) may help to distinguish iron deficiency (sTfR is high) from anemia of chronic disease (sTfR is in the normal range) when the ferritin is elevated due to tissue damage.

Cook JD: The measurement of serum transferrin receptor. Am J Med Sci 318:269–276, 1999.
Massey AC: Microcytic anemia: Differential diagnosis and management of iron deficiency anemia. Med Clin North Am 76:549–566, 1992.

5. Summarize the symptoms and signs of iron deficiency.

Patients may have the symptoms of **anemia**: fatigue, dyspnea on exertion, and, in certain cases in which underlying cardiac disease exists, signs of congestive heart failure or angina. In many cases, however, the anemia develops insidiously and is well-tolerated. Iron deficiency is associated with **pica**. Adults may crave ice, starch, or even dirt. Iron-deficient children in older neighborhoods may eat lead-containing paint chips, leading to the association of iron deficiency and plumbism. Iron deficiency is also associated with **esophageal webs** (sometimes causing dysphagia), painless stomatitis, and spooning of the fingernails (**koilonychia**).

Moore DF Jr, Sears DA: Pica, iron deficiency, and the medical history. Am J Med 97:390–393, 1994.

6. In the treatment of iron-deficiency anemia, how much iron should be administered, in what form, and for how long?

Iron is best given as ferrous sulfate in a formulation that does not include enteric coating. Typically, patients take 325 mg orally 3 times/day until the anemia corrects and for several months thereafter. This regimen provides 60 mg of elemental iron per tablet, or 180 mg/day. Of this, 18–36 mg can be absorbed and utilized by an otherwise unimpaired marrow. Intravenous iron therapy (as iron dextran) has been used in patients undergoing renal dialysis to optimize the response to erythropoietin therapy. Certain patients with ongoing blood loss (e.g., inflammatory bowel disease or Osler-Weber-Rendu syndrome) who cannot tolerate iron orally or who cannot absorb enough iron from the gut also benefit from iron dextran replacement.

When a low serum ferritin value is used to make the diagnosis of iron deficiency, the ferritin can be checked to verify that iron stores have increased with therapy. In some instances, patients improve, but the anemia does not fully correct. If the ferritin has normalized, another cause of anemia (i.e., coexistent thalassemia minor) should be sought. A useful guide to success is the occurrence of reticulocytosis about 10 days after initiation of iron therapy.

Goodnough LT, Skikne B, and Brugnara C: Erythropoietin, iron and erythropoiesis. Blood 96:823–833, 2000.

7. What are common causes of iron deficiency?

Diet, malabsorption, chronic blood loss, and chronic intravascular hemolysis. The last-mentioned disorder is usually seen in paroxysmal nocturnal hemoglobinuria, a rare stem cell disorder, or in patients with malfunctioning cardiac valves. Examination of a urine sediment stained for iron discloses iron-laden tubular cells (hemosiderosis).

Common Causes of Iron Deficiency

1. Chronic blood loss
   - Gastrointestinal: gastritis, peptic ulcer disease, GI varices, GI malignancy, polyps, diverticulosis, telangiectasia (Osler-Weber-Rendu disease, scleroderma), angiodysplasia, long-distance running
   - Menstrual loss and pregnancy
2. Dietary deficiency (infants)
3. Malabsorption: sprue, postgastrectomy patients
4. Others: chronic intravascular hemolysis, idiopathic pulmonary hemosiderosis, repetitive phlebotomy

8. What are the causes and consequences of iron overload?

Iron overload results from chronic administration of iron to non–iron-deficient persons, chronic transfusion therapy, and disorders associated with increased absorption of dietary iron (hemochromatosis, thalassemia intermedia or major, and certain refractory anemias, such as sideroblastic anemia).

Although hereditary hemochromatosis, an autosomal recessive disorder, affects approximately 1 in 300 people, it is frequently missed. Many patients are diagnosed only after significant damage to the heart or liver has occurred. Iron overload has many effects, including:

1. Cardiomyopathy, arrhythmias
2. Hepatic dysfunction and cirrhosis
3. Hepatoma
4. Endocrine dysfunction (hypothyroidism, hypogonadotrophic hypogonadism, hyperpigmentation, diabetes mellitus)
5. Arthropathy (chondrocalcinosis, synovial fluid containing calcium pyrophosphate or hydroxyapatite crystals)
6. Osteopenia and subcortical cysts
7. Peripheral neuropathy

9. What are the appropriate screening tests for hemochromatosis?

The serum transferrin saturation (serum iron divided by the total iron-binding capacity) is frequently used to screen for hemochromatosis. Because of the diurnal variation in serum iron, a fasting morning sample is best. A serum transferrin saturation > 50 % for women and > 60 % for men suggests the possibility of iron overload. Mutations in the HFE gene may account for most white patients, who appear to have genetic hemochromatosis. Homozygosity for C282Y or the combination of C282Y and another mutation H63D in the HFE can be detected by the polymerase chain reaction assay. Use of this genetic method in population studies shows that not all patients who appear to have the hemochromatosis genotype develop clinical iron overloading. Similarly, some white patients and most black patients with clinical iron overloading have a normal HFE genotype. Measurement of serum ferritin and assessment of hepatic iron (usually on liver biopsy) and/or a PCR study of HFE should be considered next in the evaluation of suspected hemochromatosis. Elevated serum ferritin levels, however, can occur in a number of inflammatory conditions without iron overload. Treatment of hemochromatosis is simple: patients are recommended for phlebotomy with assessment of serum ferritin to determine success of therapy.

Andrews NC: Disorders of iron metabolism. N Engl J Med 341:1986–1995, 1999.

10. When is it appropriate to order hemoglobin electrophoresis to evaluate hypochromic microcytic anemia?

When iron stores are established as normal. The microcytic disorders that may be detected are β-thalassemia minor and the so-called thalassemic hemoglobinopathies (including hemoglobin [Hb] E in Asians). β-Thalassemia minor is marked by an increased Hb A_2 and sometimes increased fetal Hb. Iron deficiency results in a decreased pool of α-chains, for which the β chain of Hb A and the δ chain of Hb A_2 must compete. Beta chains are more successful, resulting in diminished Hb A_2 during iron deficiency. For this reason, a search for β-thalassemia may be thwarted when patients are also iron-deficient.

Beutler E: The common anemias. JAMA 259:2433–2437, 1988.

11. Which diseases are usually associated with the anemia of chronic disease (ACD)?

ACD is typified by a low serum iron, low TIBC, and low percent saturation but increased iron stores, as evidenced by an increased ferritin. Traditionally, ACD is associated with inflammatory states, including malignancy, rheumatologic disease, and infection. However, a study of hospitalized patients showed that the laboratory pattern of ACD occurs in a significant number of anemic patients who do not have inflammatory conditions. These patients were severely ill with complications of diabetes, renal failure, and hypertension.

Cash JM, Sears DA: The anemia of chronic disease: Spectrum of associated disease in a series of unselected hospitalized patients. Am J Med 87:638, 1989.

12. What are the causes of macrocytosis?

Macrocytosis, or a large MCV, is not always associated with folate or vitamin B12 deficiency. Anemia with macro-ovalocytic RBCs (megaloblastic) is much more specific for folate or vitamin B12 deficiency.

Causes of Macrocytosis

Megaloblastic anemia (macro-ovalocytosis)	Sideroblastic anemia*
Alcoholism	Chronic obstructive pulmonary disease
Malignancy	Artifacts and idiopathic
Hemolysis (usually poorly compensated)	Pregnancy
Aplastic anemia	Liver disease
Hypothyroidism	Drugs (AZT, azathioprine, anticonvulsants)
Refractory anemias (myelodysplasia)	

* Often marked by dual populations of RBCs—one hypochromic microcytic and the other macrocytic. From Colon-Otero G, et al: A practical approach to the differential diagnosis and evaluation of the adult patient with macrocytic anemia. Med Clin North Am 76:581–596, 1992; and Savage DG, et al: Etiology and diagnostic evaluation of macrocytosis. Am J Med Sci 319:343–352, 2000.

13. How are folate and vitamin B12 deficiency states recognized? How do they differ?

Common features of B12 and folate deficiency are those of megaloblastic anemia:

1. **Marrow:** hyperplastic marrow demonstrating a markedly ineffective erythropoiesis; megaloblastic RBCs with open, granular nuclei, and mature cytoplasm or nuclear-cytoplasmic asynchrony; giant metamyelocytes.

2. **Peripheral blood:** macro-ovalocytosis with occasional Howell-Jolly bodies and basophilic stippling; hypersegmented neutrophils; variable degree of neutropenia and thrombocytopenia.

3. **Megaloblastic changes:** affect rapidly proliferative cells of mouth, gut, small intestine, and cervix, showing immature-looking nuclei (indeed, some cervical Pap smears are mistakenly read as atypical or malignant).

Distinguishing Features of Folate vs. Vitamin B12 Deficiency

FEATURE	VITAMIN B12	FOLATE
Neurologic disease	Subacute, combined systems	None, or associated with alcohol
Diet	Normal	Alcoholism, junk food, "tea and toast," no green leafy vegetables
Serum folate level	Normal	Low
RBC folate level	Low or normal	Low
Response to physiologic dose of folate (200 mg/day)	Absent*	Present
Urine formiminoglutamic acid	Absent	Increased
Serum methylmalonic acid	Increased	Normal
Homocysteine levels	Increased	Increased

* Pharmacologic dose of folate (1 mg/day) can correct anemia but may exacerbate neurologic symptoms. From Babior BM: The megaloblastic anemias. In Williams WJ, et al (eds): Hematology, 5th ed. New York, McGraw-Hill, 1995.

14. What processes may interrupt B12 absorption?

1. Pernicious anemia associated with gastric atrophy and loss of intrinsic factor due to an autoimmune-mediated attack on the gastric mucosa.

2. Postgastrectomy: After total gastrectomy, megaloblastic anemia develops 5–6 years later.

3. Disorders of the small intestine: ileal resection, Crohn's disease, sprue.

4. Competition with intestinal flora: blind-loop syndrome, fish tapeworm (*Diphyllobothrium latum*).

5. Pancreatic disease: deficiency of R-binders with chronic pancreatitis.

6. Dietary: strict vegetarians (no meat or eggs or milk), breastfed infants of strict vegetarians.
Pruthi RK, Tefferi A: Pernicious anemia revisited. Mayo Clin Proc: 69:144–150, 1994.

15. Describe the pattern of neurologic disease associated with B12 deficiency. Is the severity of anemia a good predictor of neurologic involvement?

B12 deficiency is associated with the findings of combined systems disease:
- Posterior column: paresthesia, disturbed vibratory sense, loss of proprioception
- Pyramidal: spastic weakness, hyperactive reflexes
- Cerebral: dementia, psychosis (megaloblastic madness), optic atrophy

Folate deficiency may be associated with peripheral neuropathy in alcoholics. Of interest is the lack of correlation between severity of anemia and neurologic manifestations of B12 deficiency. A recent study suggests that a significant minority of patients with peripheral neuropathy or other neurologic manifestations of B12 deficiency have a normal hematocrit and MCV, but low or low-normal B12 levels. It is possible that serum methylmalonic acidemia and homocystinemia are better indicators.

Lindebaum J, et al: Neuropsychiatric disorders caused by cobalamin deficiency in the absence of anemia or macrocytosis. N Engl J Med 318:1720, 1988.

16. Who should receive folate supplementation?
- Elderly, poor, and alcoholic patients
- Patients receiving hyperalimentation or hemodialysis
- Premature infants, infants on synthetic diets, and children fed on goat's milk
- Patients with sprue or other small intestinal disease
- Patients with hemolysis or exfoliative dermatitis
- Pregnant women and women in the periconceptual period
- Homocystinemia (usually in conjunction with B6 and B12)

17. How much folate is required in pregnant women? Why?

Developmental anomalies of the fetal neural tube have been associated with poor folate intake early in pregnancy. For this reason, it has been recommended that women of child-bearing age consume 400 mg/day of folate. This recommendation is controversial because folate supplementation may mask symptoms of vitamin B12 deficiency.

Cziezel AE, Dudas I: Prevention of the first occurrence of neural-tube defects by periconceptional vitamin supplementation. N Engl J Med 327:1832–1835, 1992.

18. When are bone marrow biopsy and aspiration indicated?

Bone marrow biopsy and aspiration are safe, easily performed, and particularly helpful in evaluating pancytopenia, thrombocytopenia, neutropenia, and hypoproliferative anemia. Because of the high prevalence of iron-deficiency anemia and anemia of chronic disease, a hypoproliferative (low reticulocyte count) anemia does not always require bone marrow biopsy if iron studies are consistent. The diagnosis of a sideroblastic anemia requires a bone marrow study to demonstrate the presence of ringed sideroblasts.

Indications for Bone Marrow Biopsy and Aspirate

1. Pancytopenia: myelodysplasia, aplastic anemia, myelophthisic states, hypersplenism, megaloblastic anemia
2. Anemia: sideroblastic anemia, refractory anemia, pure red cell aplasia
3. Staging of malignancy: Hodgkin's disease, leukemias, non-Hodgkin's lymphoma, small cell carcinoma of the lung, multiple myeloma
4. Thrombocytopenia: evaluation of idiopathic thrombocytopenic purpura
5. Neutropenia
6. Infectious diseases: typhoid, tuberculosis, pancytopenia seen in AIDS, brucellosis
7. Lipid-storage diseases

19. What are the diagnostic criteria for severe aplastic anemia?

Aplastic anemia is marked by peripheral pancytopenia and a hypocellular bone marrow aspirate. Commonly used criteria for severe aplastic anemia are as follows:

- Marrow biopsy cellularity < 25%
- Neutrophil counts < $0.5 \times 10^9/l$
- Platelet counts < $20 \times 10^9/l$
- Corrected reticulocyte count < 1%

Patients meeting these criteria have a median survival of < 6 months; only 20% survive 1 year.

20. What is the best therapy for aplastic anemia in a young person?

For patients who are under age 40, bone marrow transplantation (BMT) from an HLA-identical sibling is the current standard of care. HLA-identical but nonrelated donors may be used for such patients. For nontransfused patients, 80% long-term survival rates have been achieved with BMT, although survival may be accompanied by disabling graft-vs.-host disease in 10–20%.

Patients who do not have donors or who are otherwise unsuitable candidates for BMT have been successfully treated with immunosuppressive regimens. The most effective has been antithymocyte globulin (ATG), which produces remission rates of 40–60%. ATG or antilymphocyte globulin is administered via a central line in daily doses of 15–40 mg/kg for 4–10 days. Severe serum sickness and thrombocytopenia are consequences.

Patients frequently have partial responses, freeing them from infections or the need for transfusions. Unfortunately, relapses occur in 10%, and some patients, although clinically improved at first, develop myelodysplastic syndromes later. Recently, cyclosporine has been employed in the treatment of aplastic anemia with good results.

Young NS, Barrett AJ: The treatment of severe acquired aplastic anemia. Blood 85:3367–3377, 1995.

21. Who should receive erythropoietin (EPO) therapy for anemia?

EPO deficiency regularly accompanies end-stage renal disease, and the resultant anemia is the principal indication for use of EPO. Recent studies suggest a role for EPO in patients with AIDS-related anemia, particularly when they receive zidovudine. The anemia of chronic disease is associated with inappropriately low EPO levels in some people with rheumatoid arthritis or malignancy. EPO has also been used with success to improve the ability of patients to undergo autologous blood donation before surgery. It also has been beneficial in the treatment of anemia of prematurity and myelodysplasia.

Erslev AJ: Erythropoietin. N Engl J Med 324:1939–1944, 1991.

22. Alcoholics admitted to the hospital are frequently anemic. List the causes.

Primary bone marrow toxicity of alcohol
Vacuolated marrow erythroid cells
Megaloblastic erythropoiesis due to folate deficiency
Hypophosphatemia
Sideroblastic anemia

Hemolytic anemia
Hypersplenism
Spur cell anemia
Iron-deficiency due to hemorrhage

23. How should you evaluate anemia in the alcoholic?

Savage and Lindenbaum found that megaloblastic changes in the marrow usually were not associated with disorderly iron accumulation in the macrophages, as in anemia of chronic disorders. They emphasize the multifactorial nature of anemia. See algorithm on the following page for their guide to the work-up of anemia in alcoholics.

HEMOLYTIC ANEMIAS

24. Patients with hemolytic anemia have shortened RBC survival. What are the laboratory features of hemolysis?

During hemolysis, the bone marrow responds to the premature destruction of RBCs by increasing its production of RBCs 7–8-fold. This expansion is marked by reticulocytosis. Other clues to accelerated RBC destruction are:

1. Indirect hyperbilirubinemia-acholuric jaundice (unconjugated bilirubin is not secreted in urine)
2. Hemoglobinuria
3. Fall of hemoglobin > 1 gm/7 days in the absence of bleeding or massive hematoma

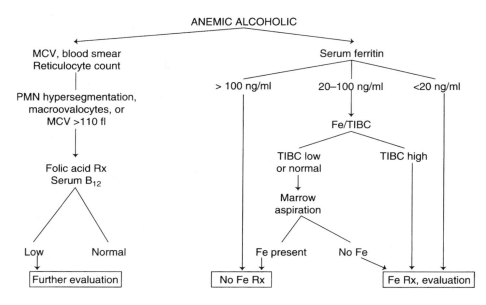

Diagnostic and therapeutic approach to anemia in alcoholics. (Adapted from Savage D, et al: Anemia in alcoholics. Medicine 65:322, 1986, with permission.)

25. How is intravascular hemolysis distinguished from extravascular?

Laboratory Studies in Hemolysis

INTRAVASCULAR	EXTRA- AND INTRAVASCULAR
Hemoglobinemia	Increased reticulocyte count
Hemoglobinuria	Increased indirect, unconjugated bilirubin
Hemosiderinuria	Increased urobilinogen
Low serum haptoglobin	
Methemalbumin	
Low serum hemopexin	
Increased lactate dehydrogenase	

From Udden MM: Hemolytic anemias: Intravascular. In Goldman L, Bennett JC (eds): Cecil Textbook of Medicine. Philadelphia, W.B. Saunders, 2000, pp 882–884.

Examples of intravascular hemolytic disorders include hemolytic transfusion reactions, paroxysmal nocturnal hemoglobinuria, march hemoglobinuria, and RBC fragmentation syndromes.

26. Name the three basic types of RBC defects that lead to hemolysis in the hereditary hemolytic anemias. Give examples of each.

MEMBRANE DISORDERS	HEMOGLOBIN ABNORMALITIES	ENZYMATIC DEFECTS
Spherocytosis	Sickle cell anemia	G6PD deficiency
Elliptocytosis	Unstable hemoglobins	Pyruvate kinase
Stomatocytosis	Thalassemia	5'-nucleotidase
Xerocytosis		

The RBC is extraordinarily adapted to a circulatory system that requires resistance to shear stresses in the arterioles and suppleness to negotiate small orifices in the spleen and capillaries.

27. Name the major acquired hemolytic disorders.
Whereas hereditary disorders are examples of intracorpuscular defects, acquired hemolytic disorders typically result from extracorpuscular defects. Examples include autoimmune hemolytic anemia, fragmentation syndromes, malaria, hypersplenism, and physical agents such as heat, copper, and certain oxidants.

28. What are the complications of hereditary spherocytosis?

Aplastic crises (associated with parvovirus B19)	Pigment gallstones
Hemolytic crises	Splenomegaly
Megaloblastic crises (increased demand for folate)	Stasis ulcers

29. A patient presenting with life-long anemia and spherocytosis on the peripheral blood film probably has hereditary spherocytosis (HS). How do you confirm the diagnosis?
Patients with HS, usually an autosomal dominant disorder, may have affected siblings as well as an affected parent. But, as in other autosomal dominant disorders, the spontaneous mutation rate is significant (10%). Paternity need not be questioned when neither parent is affected.

A confirmatory test frequently obtained is the **osmotic fragility test**. The patient's blood is incubated in a series of tubes containing decreasing concentrations of saline. In increasing hypotonic media, RBCs swell until a critical hemolytic volume is reached, beyond which the RBC membrane ruptures. Because the RBC in HS is already a sphere, lysis occurs in media of relatively high osmotic strength. Osmotic fragility, therefore, is increased. Normal RBCs are underfilled spheres and can accommodate a lot of water before reaching their critical hemolytic volume.

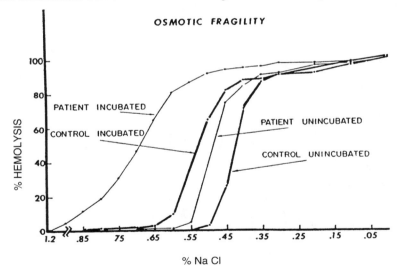

Osmotic fragility of unincubated and incubated RBCs from a normal person and from a patient with hereditary spherocytosis. (From Rappaport S: Introduction to Hematology, 2nd ed. Philadelphia, J.B. Lippincott, 1987, p 135, with permission.)

30. What therapeutic interventions can be made in HS?
  1. **Diet:** Patients should receive dietary supplementation with folate.
  2. **Splenectomy:** Older children and adults who have symptomatic anemia with ordinary viral illness or who have troublesome splenomegaly usually undergo splenectomy. Splenectomy

prevents aplastic crises and gallstone formation, and many people who have adapted to mild anemia feel better. After splenectomy, the risk for overwhelming pneumococcal bacteremia is increased, and greater morbidity and mortality rates result from this and other encapsulated organisms. Risks are lessened by administration of pneumococcal, *Haemophilus influenzae* B, and meningococcal vaccines. Decisions about attempts to cure HS by splenectomy should be individualized.

31. Describe the underlying membrane structural defects associated with HS.

HS is marked by decreased amounts of spectrin, the principal membrane protein found in erythrocytes. Spectrin has self-associative properties and forms a lattice with other RBC membrane proteins and actin. This supportive lattice on the inner aspect of the lipid bilayer gives the RBC its unique properties of strength and suppleness. Deficiency of spectrin correlates with the degree of hemolysis, changes in osmotic fragility, and response to splenectomy. The molecular mechanisms underlying HS include structural changes in spectrin itself, loss of ankyrin (a protein that links spectrin to the transmembrane protein band 3), and structural abnormalities of band 3. Most of these defects occur in what investigators call the "vertical interaction" in the red blood cell membrane cytoskeleton between band 3, ankyrin, and spectrin. Two mutations are associated with additional morphologic changes. A spectrin beta-chain mutation is associated with acanthocytic spherocytes that are accentuated by splenectomy. A truncated band-3 protein is associated with so-called pincered red blood cells. A deficiency of spectrin, for whatever reason, accounts for the decreased membrane surface area and spherocytosis.

Tse WT, Lux SE: Red blood cell membrane disorders. Br J Haematol 104:2–13, 1999.

32. What is hereditary elliptocytosis (HE)? What are its most important subsets?

HE includes a broad spectrum of disorders that result in an elliptical RBC shape and hemolysis. In general, HE results from genetic defects that arise in the horizontal interaction of the red blood cell membrane cytoskeleton that depends on alpha spectrin–beta spectrin association and interaction of spectrin with band 4.1 protein to form a high-molecular-weight oligomeric structure.

1. Some families have a normal hematocrit and a mild reticulocytosis (**mild common HE**).

2. Others have a more striking degree of hemolysis and anemia and more bizarre RBC morphology, which is **common HE with chronic hemolysis**.

3. Infants who have hemolytic HE at birth may later have striking hemolysis with bizarre RBCs and jaundice (**infantile poikilocytosis**).

4. Severe anemia accompanies the rare cases of **homozygous HE**.

5. **Hereditary pyropoikilocytosis** is another rare variant of HE in which the spectrin is abnormally sensitive to heat. The peripheral blood picture resembles that seen in hemolysis associated with severe burns. Most patients with HE and its variants have a structural abnormality of the spectrin protein that results in failure of the protein to self-associate into higher order tetramers and oligomers.

6. **Spherocytic elliptocytosis** is an unusual autosomal dominant disorder in which the elliptocytes are rounded. Spherocytes and increased osmotic fragility are also found.

7. Resistance to malarial infection accompanies **Southeast Asian ovalocytosis**. The central pallor in these cells is separated by a transverse ridge. This disorder is associated with an abnormal band-3 protein that leads to membrane rigidity but only mild hemolysis.

33. What is the most common enzymatic defect in RBCs leading to hemolysis? How is it diagnosed?

Glucose-6-phosphate dehydrogenase (G6PD) deficiency. Hundreds of variants of this X-linked enzyme have been characterized. Because this is the first enzyme in the hexose monophosphate pathway, G6PD deficiency compromises the RBC's ability to regenerate NADPH from NADP+. NADPH is necessary for the reduction of glutathione-containing disulfides (GSSG to GSH). The RBC as a carrier of oxygen is highly vulnerable to oxidative attack when GSH is depleted. Oxidation results in precipitation of hemoglobin, which can be detected as Heinz bodies by supravital staining with crystal violet. The diagnosis is established by measuring the enzymatic activity of G6PD.

34. How do patients with G6PD deficiency present?

Most patients are well until they come into contact with an oxidant drug. Some experience hemolysis with infections. Hepatitis in G6PD-deficient persons can result in spectacular jaundice. In the Mediterranean region, ingestion of fava beans can result in a severe hemolytic episode. It is important to identify potentially oxidant drugs (e.g., nitrofurantoin, phenazopyridine [pyridium], primaquine, sulfacetamide, sulfamethoxazole, sulfanilamide, sulfapyridine).

African-Americans have an increased prevalence (about 10% of men) of type A2, which is unstable, losing G6PD activity as the RBC ages. During a hemolytic episode, the G6PD activity is normal because the young RBCs survive and the older, deficient RBCs are lost. The deficiency, therefore, is not recognized until months later when the patients no longer have reticulocytosis.

Beutler E: Glucose-6-phosphate dehydrogenase deficiency. N Engl J Med 324:169–174, 1991.

35. Many abnormal hemoglobins with single amino acid changes are known. Of these, which sickle or participate in the sickling process during deoxygenation?

Sickle hemoglobin coexists with other β-chain variants to produce a spectrum of disorders from clinically insignificant conditions such as sickle trait to severe disease represented by homozygous SS.

Sickle Syndromes

SICKLE CELL DISEASE	SICKLE CELL TRAIT
SS (homozygous)	AS
Sβ-thalassemia	S-hereditary persistence of fetal hemoglobin
SC	
SD Los Angeles	
SO Arab	

36. What is the incidence of sickle hemoglobinopathies in births among African-Americans?

AS	8.0% (1 of 12)	AC	3.00%	SBo	0.03%
SS	0.16%	SC	0.12%		

Note that the incidence of SBo and SC is approximately that of SS. In adults, as many patients with sickle β-thalassemia or SC will be seen as homozygous S patients. Although SBo is clinically similar to SS disease, SB+ and SC patients are more likely to have palpable spleens and may experience splenic sequestration/infarctive crises as adults rather than in early childhood, as is the case with SS disease. SC patients also tend to have higher hematocrits. They may present with blindness due to retinopathy or aseptic necrosis of the hip. The hemoglobin S gene also can be found in Sicily, Northern Greece, Turkey, the eastern province of Saudi Arabia, and central India.

Serjeant GR: Sickle Cell Disease, 2nd ed. New York, Oxford University Press, 1992, pp 16–28.

37. What are the predictors for adverse outcomes in children with sickle cell disease?

Analysis of outcomes of infants entered into the Cooperative Study of Sickle Cell Disease showed that adverse outcomes later in life were associated with the appearance of the following three manifestations of sickle cell disease during the first 2 years of life:

1. Dactylitis (hand/foot syndrome)   3. Leukocytosis
2. Severe anemia (hemoglobin < 7.0 gm/dl)

Miller ST, et al: Prediction of adverse outcomes in children with sickle cell disease. N Engl J Med 342:83–89, 2000.

38. What are the main clinical manifestations of sickle hemoglobinopathies?

Hemolytic anemia
  Gallstones
  Increased folate needs
  Aplastic crises
  Indirect hyperbilirubinemia
  Increased lactate dehydrogenase

Chronic end-organ damage
  Retinopathy
  Aseptic necrosis of the hip
  Osteomyelitis
  Isosthenuria, hematuria, chronic renal failure
  Nephrotic syndrome

Periodic vaso-occlusive disease ("crises")	Hyposplenism
Pain crises	Pneumococcal septicemia
Chest syndrome	Increased morbidity with other encapsu-
Abdominal pain	lated organisms
Stroke	**Reproductive**
Splenic infarct	High-risk pregnancy
Splenic sequestration syndrome	Impotence
Multiorgan failure syndrome	
Priapism	

Serjeant GR: Sickle cell disease. Lancet 350:725–730, 1997.

39. Is any morbidity truly associated with sickle trait?

Because 8% of African-Americans are heterozygous for sickle trait, this is an important question. The following abnormalities have been associated with sickle trait:

Splenic infarction at high altitude	Pulmonary embolism
Hyposthenuria	Glaucoma, anterior chamber bleeds
Hematuria	Sudden death following exertion
Bacteriuria and pyelonephritis in pregnancy	Bacteremia in women

Sears DA: Sickle cell trait. In Embury SH, et al (eds): Sickle Cell Disease: Basic Principles and Clinical Practice. New York, Raven Press, 1994.

40. What are sickle crises?

Patients with sickle cell disease are susceptible to sudden, unheralded vaso-occlusive events that are called crises. The most common event is a simple pain crisis affecting the limbs, low back, chest, or abdomen. Sometimes specific organs are affected by definite infarcts, including the bone and spleen (if splenic tissue has been preserved). The chest syndrome is marked by episodes of dyspnea, fever, pain, and sudden appearance of an infiltrate on chest x-ray consistent with pneumonia. As often as not, no infection exists; instead, there is probably a sickle vaso-occlusion. Recent studies of chest syndrome have emphasized the role of fat embolism from bone marrow infarcts and rib infarcts. Splinting while the patient is suffering a rib infarct may lead to hypoventilation and pulmonary vaso-occlusion. Incentive spirometry has been advocated to reduce the risk of chest syndrome in patients hospitalized with sickle crises and chest pain.

In a recent multicenter study, acute chest syndrome often occurred as a complication in patients admitted for other reasons. Thirteen percent of patients who developed chest syndrome required mechanical ventilation, and 3% died. Half of the deaths involved infections. Thus, antibiotics, along with transfusion therapy, have an important place in management.

Vichinsky EP, et al: Causes and outcomes of the acute chest syndrome in sickle cell disease. N Engl J Med 342:1855–1865, 2000.

41. How are patients in a sickle crisis managed? How often do crises occur?

Patients with chest syndrome often receive antibiotics and require oxygen. When hypoxemia continues despite oxygen therapy, exchange transfusions are helpful. The pathophysiology of the pain crisis is not well understood. Of note, most patients experience pain relatively infrequently—once every year or two. About 20% of patients, however, are troubled by more frequent crises and may visit the emergency department or hospital monthly. Why some homozygotes do poorly while others do relatively well is one of the mysteries of sickle cell disease. Similarly, it is not known what initiates crises or what mechanisms of spontaneous recovery terminate crises while patients are receiving only supportive care. The severity and duration of crises are variable. Stays for patients requiring hospitalization vary from 3–10 days.

Platt OS, et al: Pain in sickle cell disease: Rates and risk factors. N Engl J Med 325:11–16, 1991.

42. What routine health maintenance measures are used in patients with sickle cell anemia?

Now that many states routinely screen all births for hemoglobin S, practice guidelines for follow-up of parents and identified infants have been developed. Parents are taught to bring in their child when he or she is febrile and to examine the child for splenic enlargement. Penicillin prophylaxis is emphasized. Children should receive the polyvalent pneumococcal vaccine at age 2 years, *Haemophilus influenzae* type B vaccine, and hepatitis B immunization.

For adults, routine health maintenance includes genetic counseling about the risk of sickle cell disease in relatives or children. Patients are given folate supplementation and periodic oph-thalmoscopic exams. All adults should receive pneumococcal vaccine if they have not already been vaccinated. As patients get older, periodic review of renal function seems prudent.

43. Is pregnancy safe for women with sickle cell anemia?

With modern obstetric care, the risks of pregnancy have been greatly reduced. However, most obstetricians consider such pregnancies to be high risk and advocate close follow-up. The maternal mortality rate is < 2%, and the incidence of stillbirths and neonatal deaths is < 15%.

There is some controversy over the appropriate use of blood transfusions during prenancy. A recent study suggests that patients who receive prophylactic transfusions during pregnancy do no better than those who are transfused only when symptomatic. Many women with sickle cell disease are successful mothers. However, women who are often ill and require frequent hospi-talizations for control of pain may require a great deal of support from other family members if they are to have children. Women who do not wish to become pregnant can be placed on oral contraceptives.

Koshy M, et al: Prophylactic red cell transfusions in pregnant patients with sickle cell disease. N Engl J Med 319:1447, 1988.

44. Under what circumstances should RBC transfusion be considered in the treatment of sickle cell disease?

Strong indications	Relative indications	Not indicated
Aplastic crises	Before general anesthesia	Management of typical
Hypoxemia and chest syndrome	During pregnancy	pain crises
CNS events, stroke	Priapism	
Sequestration crises	Before arteriography	

A national cooperative study found that simple transfusions to an arbitrary level of hemoglo-bin seemed to enable patients to undergo general anesthesia with no worse outcome than patients who had exchange transfusions. Because less blood was used, the conservative transfusion proto-col was complicated less often by alloimmunization.

Vichinsky EP, et al: A comparison of conservative and aggressive transfusion regimens in the periopera-tive management of sickle cell disease. N Engl J Med 333:206–213, 1995.

45. What are the hazards of RBC transfusions in patients with sickle cell disease?

Hazards include transmission of hepatitis, iron overload, and sensitization (which can be a significant problem). Delayed transfusion reactions occur in patients with a history of transfu-sions but with a negative crossmatch. After a few days, an anamnestic response occurs that re-sults in hemolysis due to the sudden appearance of an IgG antibody. Delayed transfusion reactions usually involve Rh, Kidd, Kell, or Duffy antigens. Delayed transfusion reactions can mimic a crisis and may result in death. Alloimmunization occurred in 30% of patients with sickle cell disease compared with 5% of a control group. Half of those alloimmunized had a recogniz-able delayed transfusion reaction.

46. A patient with sickle cell disease presents with a history of a viral syndrome, followed by dramatic worsening of the anemia. What entity needs to be strongly considered?

Aplastic crisis. Typically, patients have a flu-like illness, with or without an evanescent rash, fever, and myalgias, followed 5–10 days later by weakness and dyspnea. The patient presents with a sharply reduced hematocrit. A key finding is the nearly absolute absence of reticulocytes. This disorder is in fact a transient pure red cell aplasia. The platelet and WBC counts are usually unaffected. Bone marrow shows the absence of erythroid progenitors, except for a few "giant pronormoblasts."

This syndrome is caused most often by **parvovirus B19**, which seems to have a unique tropism for erythroid progenitors. In patients with hemolysis, parvovirus-induced aplasia is significant, because the duration of aplasia (5–10 days) coincides with the half-life of RBCs. Thus, cessation of RBC production for 10 days in a patient with a hematocrit of 22% and RBC lifespan of 9 days spells trouble. Transfusions of packed RBCs are life-saving. The 10-day cessation of erythropoiesis caused by the parvovirus goes unnoticed in a normal person with a hematocrit of 40% and an RBC lifespan of 120 days. The parvovirus may be the cause of fifth disease, arthritis, and spontaneous abortions.

Saarinen UM, et al: Human parvovirus B19-induced epidemic acute red cell aplasia in patients with hereditary hemolytic anemia. Blood 67:1411, 1986.

47. What treatment options are available for the patient with severe (> 3 crises/year) sickle cell anemia?

Perhaps the greatest therapeutic advance in sickle hemoglobinopathy was the recognition that certain chemotherapeutic agents can reverse the developmental "switch" from fetal to adult hemoglobin (Hb) synthesis. The rise in Hb F in each RBC suppresses sickling and offers the promise of reduced hemolysis and vaso-occlusive phenomena. A double-blinded trial of hydroxyurea was halted early when it was shown to reduce the rate of crises by about 40% and also to reduce the incidence of chest syndrome and frequency of transfusions. Issues related to compliance with daily medications, frequent follow-up, and the potential for leukemogenesis have spurred the search for alternative agents that increase Hb F production.

Bone marrow transplantation (BMT) also has been used in the treatment of severe sickle cell disease with good results. It is controversial because of the morbidity and mortality associated with allogeneic BMT and graft-vs.-host disease. The longevity enjoyed by most patients and the promise of regimens such as hydroxyurea cast doubt on the usefulness of BMT except for the sickest patients.

Charache S, et al: Effect of hydroxyurea on the frequency of painful crises in sickle cell anemia. N Engl J Med 332:317–322, 1995.

Steinberg MH: Management of sickle cell disease. N Engl J Med 340:1021–1030, 1999.

48. Which disorders result in decreased α-chain production? Why are they less severe than disorders of β-chain production?

Thalassemia minor is a frequent cause of microcytic hypochromic anemia. It is due to an imbalance of α- and β-chain production. The genetic information for the α-chain of hemoglobin is organized as two adjacent genes on chromosome 16. Thus, normal people have four copies of the gene for α hemoglobin. In α-thalassemias, deletions of one or more of these genes result in a deficiency of α-chains and an excess of β-chains. A study of Chinese patients with Hb H disease found that adult patients had significant disability due to iron overload despite the absence of a need for chronic transfusion therapy.

Deletion of a single gene is silent, but deletion of two genes is noticed as a microcytic mild anemia, with a normal hemoglobin electrophoresis. About 30% of African-Americans are heterozygous for a single-gene deletion; thus, α-thalassemia is found in about 2.0%. Asians have a much higher incidence of a chromosome 16 with two deleted α-genes and therefore are at risk for bearing children with only one or no functional α genes. People with only one functional α-gene have a mild hemolytic anemia (Hb H disease). Hemolysis results from oxidative attack by the β_4 tetramers present in the RBCs of affected people.

Hydrops fetalis in association with a tetramer of γ-chains (hemoglobin Bart's) is the cause of death at birth of a fetus with four α-gene deletions.

In **beta-thalassemia major**, the absence of β-chains results in the presence of α_4, a tetrameric α-chain protein that is highly toxic to the RBC membrane. Developing RBCs perish in the marrow or limp out to live a short, withered existence in the circulation. Erythropoiesis is highly ineffective. Patients have tremendous expansion of the bone marrow and extramedullary hematopoiesis. Affected children are transfusion-dependent; if not transfused aggressively, they develop pathologic fractures and significant growth retardation.

Oliveri N: The β-thalassemias. N Engl J Med 341:99–109, 1999.

49. Is there an effective treatment for children with beta-thalassemia major?

Aggressive transfusion therapy has greatly improved the outlook for these children. Iron overload is the price for this therapy. Chelation with deferoxamine by continuous subcutaneous infusion with a pump has been effective in reducing iron burden and prevents the onset of cardiomyopathy. However, the expense and inconvenience of chelation therapy are burdensome to patients when they reach young adulthood. Noncompliance with subcutaneus chelation has led to the pursuit of an effective oral agent.

Children with thalassemia major have been successfully treated with BMT. In the very young, graft-vs.-host disease is less frequent, and mortality and morbidity rates seem to be acceptable. After restoration of normal hematopoiesis, iron overload can be aggressively treated by phlebotomy.

Lucarelli G, et al: Marrow transplantation in patients with thalassemia responsive to iron chelation therapy. N Engl J Med 329:840, 1993.

50. A 20-year-old woman with a history of two previous laparotomies for abdominal pain presents with confusion, fever, tachycardia, abdominal pain, and peripheral neuropathy. Her mother had a similar history and died at a young age. What disorder do you suspect? How do you make a diagnosis?

The history is strongly suggestive of porphyria, acute intermittent type (AIP), which results from a deficiency of porphobilinogen deaminase. Physicians must be aware of two unfortunate facts about porphyria: (1) many people carry a diagnosis that is not based on adequate testing, amd (2) many others with the disease are unrecognized. Hence, before embarking on specific therapy, laboratory studies must be obtained to confirm the diagnosis.

Clinical Features of AIP

Autosomal dominant inheritance
Urine: δ-aminolevulinic acid, porphobilinogen, uroporphyrin
Symptoms and signs:
Abdominal pain: fever, leukocytosis, vomiting, constipation
Neurologic manifestations: peripheral neuropathy, paraplegia, Guillian-Barré, respiratory arrest,
cranial nerve findings, psychosis, seizure, coma
Other: hyponatremia, hypertension, tachycardia

Treatment includes carbohydrate infusions, hematin, beta blockers, and observation for respiratory compromise while appropriate lab studies are obtained to confirm the diagnosis. The patient should avoid barbiturates, anticonvulsants, estrogens, oral contraceptives, and alcohol.

Tefferi A, et al: Acute porphyrias: Diagnosis and management. Mayo Clin Proc 69:991–995, 1994.

51. A young man presents with symptomatic cyanosis. What are the most likely hematologic causes?

1. **Congenital methemoglobinemia** due to abnormal hemoglobin (M-hemoglobinopathy). Congenital cyanosis is transmitted as an autosomal dominant disorder. The M-hemoglobins are among the 400 or more human hemoglobin variants that have been reported in various parts of the world and are generally known by place names of first discovery, such as M-Boston, Saskatoon, Milwaukee, and Kochikuro. M-hemoglobins have been identified only rarely in blacks. These hemoglobins stabilize iron in its oxidized (Fe^{+3}) state and have a muddy brown appearance.

2. **Methemoglobin reductase** (cytochrome b_5 reductase) deficiency, which is an autosomal recessive disorder. Cyanosis caused by hypoxemia requires at least 5 gm/dl of deoxyhemoglobin to be noticeable, whereas only 1.5 gm/dl of methemoglobin will be recognized.

Differential Diagnosis of Cyanosis

1. Hypoxemia
   - Pulmonary disease
   - Cardiac right-to-left shunting
   - Shock, congestive heart failure
   - Low oxygen affinity hemoglobin

Table continued on following page

Differential Diagnosis of Cyanosis (Continued)

2. Methemoglobinemia	
• Congenital	• Acquired
M-hemoglobin	Drugs (dapsone, certain topical anesthetics)
Cytochrome b$_5$ reductase	Chemicals (well-water nitrates)
3. Sulfhemoglobinemia	

From Jaffe E: Methemoglobinemia in the differential diagnosis of cyanosis. Hosp Pract 20(12):92–110, 1985; and Dinneen SF, Mohr DN, Fairbanks VF: Methemoglobinemia from topically applied anesthetic spray. Mayo Clin Proc 69:886–888, 1994.

52. What disorder is associated with chronic intravascular hemolysis, anemia, iron-deficiency, and dark urine after waking from sleep?

Paroxysmal nocturnal hemoglobinuria (PNH), an acquired clonal or oligoclonal disorder that results in increased sensitivity to complement. Most patients have chronic hemolysis, hemoglobinuria, and hemosiderinuria without the paroxysmal nocturnal component. The sucrose hemolysis test is a useful screen. An old but favorite pimp question is to ask for the two disorders that result in a low leukocyte alkaline phosphatase score—chromic myelogenous leukemia and PNH.

PNH also has a close relationship to aplastic anemia. Some patients with aplastic anemia have a typical PNH defect but produce few cells. PNH may arise after a hypoplastic event. The hemolytic disorder is complicated by unusual thrombi, including Budd-Chiari syndrome.

53. What is the cause of PNH on the molecular level?

The biochemical defect leading to increased complement lysis has been a hot topic for decades. New research has focused on abnormalities of the many proteins that are linked to the cellular membrane by a glycosylphosphatidylinositol anchor. These proteins usually are reduced or absent in PNH. Japanese investigators have identified abnormalities in an X-linked gene PIG-A (phosphatidylinositol glycan class A) that apparently are responsible for PNH in the patients studied to date.

Hillmen P, et al: Natural history of paroxysmal nocturnal hemoglobinuria. N Engl J Med 333:1253–1258, 1995.

54. Compare the laboratory and clinical features of warm and cold antibody-mediated immune hemolytic anemias.

	WARM	COLD
Antibody	IgG	IgM
Complement	±	+
Spontaneous agglutination	-	+++
Active temperature	37°C	4°C
Antigen	Rh(pan)	I,i
Response to therapy with:		
Steroids	Good	Poor
Splenectomy	Good	Poor
Gloves, warmth	None	Good

Cold agglutinin disease may be a self-limited disorder brought on by mycoplasmal infection (usually anti-I) or infectious mononucleosis (usually anti-i). Chronic cold agglutination disease may be an idiopathic syndrome or associated with a lymphoproliferative disorder. In contrast, warm autoimmune hemolytic anemia is associated with lupus, chronic lymphocytic leukemia, Hodgkin's disease, non-Hodgkin's lymphomas, and certain drugs.

55. How is the Coombs' test used to evaluate autoimmune hemolytic anemia?

The Coombs' test is used to detect antibodies on RBCs (direct Coombs' or direct antiglobulin test positive) or in plasma. In the **direct test**, the RBCs are washed and incubated with an antiglobulin serum (rabbit or other species) and then examined for agglutination. In the **indirect test**, the serum is reacted with a panel of RBCs bearing antigens of interest. Antibodies, if present in the sera, bind to the RBCs bearing the relevant antigen. The panel cells are washed to reduce nonspecific binding, then incubated with an antiglobulin serum to detect agglutination. The antiglobulin reagent is necessary because antibodies attached to RBCs are usually IgG in low numbers and cannot ordinarily cross-link to agglutinate. The antiglobulin serum bridges these antibodies, favoring agglutination.

In autoimmune hemolytic anemia, the direct test is usually positive, indicating the presence of an autoantibody on the RBCs. The indirect test, indicating the presence of the same antibody in serum, also may be positive. Persons who have been exposed to blood or have had a miscarriage or abortion may develop antibodies to certain antigens on the transfused RBCs that do not exist on native RBCs. Later they have a positive indirect Coombs' test and negative direct Coombs' test.

56. What are the possible causes of fragmented RBCs on a peripheral smear from a patient with a hemolytic anemia?

Fragmentation hemolysis is characterized by the appearance of schistocytes, helmet cells, burr cells (echinocytes), and spherocytes. The hemolysis is intravascular and can be associated with a wide variety of conditions:

Macroangiopathic

Valve hemolysis	Extracorporeal circulation
Endocardial cushion defect repair	

Microangiopathic (thrombocytopenia often present)

Cavernous hemangiomas	Malignant hypertension
Thrombotic thrombocytopenic purpura (TTP)	Scleroderma
Hemolytic uremic syndrome	Disseminated carcinomatosis
Eclampsia/preeclampsia	Disseminated intravascular coagulation (DIC)

57. What important syndrome is characterized by the triad of thrombocytopenia, fragmentation hemolysis, and fluctuating neurologic signs?

TTP, which is perhaps the most spectacular of the fragmentation syndromes. Patients may present with seizures, coma, paresis, or more subtle neurologic signs and thrombocytopenia. The classic triad may be complemented by fever and renal abnormalities to give a pentad of findings. The mainstay of treatment is plasmapheresis/plasma exchange. Corticosteroids also may be of benefit. About 20 % of patients have a subsequent relapse. During remission, unusually large, multimeric von Willebrand factor (vWF) has been identified in the cirulation. New evidence points to the role of an acquired metalloprotease inhibitor in the pathogenesis of TTP. The metalloprotease appears to degrade multimeric vWF to a smaller, less thrombogenic protein. Treatment with plasmapheresis may remove such an inhibitor, which has the characteristics of an immunoglobulin, whereas plasma exchange should act to replace the missing metalloprotease. The pathogenesis of ticlopidine-induced TTP may be similar.

Moake JL: Moschowitz, multimers, and metalloprotease. N Engl J Med 339:1629-1631, 1998.

58. How does hemolytic uremic syndrome (HUS) differ from TTP?

In HUS, renal failure is the predominant organ syndrome associated with thrombocytopenia and fragmentation hemolysis. Metalloprotease activity, absent in TTP, is present in HUS, indicating a different pathogenesis. Recently, HUS has been observed after infection with *Escherichia coli* O157:H7, a newly arising contaminant of undercooked meat. This *E. coli* serotype elaborates a shiga-like toxin that may participate in the genesis of HUS.

LEUKOCYTES

59. What is the lower limit for the absolute neutrophil count?

For adults, the level below which neutropenia is a consideration is 1.8×10^9/L (1800/mm^3). African-Americans have a lower mean neutrophil count, which may be encountered during routine exams. However, they do not have an increased incidence of infections, nor do they have increased severity of infectious diseases. When the neutrophil count is $< 0.5 \times 10^9/L$ (500/mm^3), neutropenia is severe, and there is a greater propensity for compromised response to infection.

60. What causes neutropenia?
Decreased production
Drug-induced: alkylating agents, antimetabolites, antibiotics, phenothiazines, tranquilizers, certain diuretics, anti-inflammatory agents, antithyroid drugs, others
Hematologic diseases: idiopathic, cyclic neutropenia, Chèdiak-Higashi syndrome, aplastic anemia, infantile genetic disorders
Tumor invasion, myelofibrosis
Nutritional deficiency: vitamin B12, folate (especially in alcoholics)
Infection: tuberculosis, typhoid fever, brucellosis, tularemia, measles, dengue, mononucleosis, malaria, viral hepatitis, leishmaniasis, AIDS
Peripheral destruction
Antineutrophil antibodies and/or splenic or lung (alveolar macrophage) trapping
Autoimmune disorders: Felty's syndrome, rheumatoid arthritis, systemic lupus erythematosus
Drugs as haptens: aminopyrine, α-methyl dopa, phenylbutazone, mercurial diuretics, some phenothiazines
Wegener's granulomatosis
Peripheral pooling (transient neutropenia)
Overwhelming bacterial infection (gram-negative septicemia)
Hemodialysis
Cardiopulmonary bypass
Stock W, Hoffman R: White blood cells. 1: Non-malignant disorders. Lancet 355:1351–1357, 2000.

61. Which drugs commonly cause neutropenia?
The cytotoxic chemotherapeutic agents (including alkylating agents and antimetabolites) as well as immunosuppressive drugs are obvious choices, but other drugs such as phenothiazines, antithyroid drugs, or chloramphenicol may cause neutropenia in a dose-dependent fashion by inhibiting cell replication. Immune-related neutropenia may be seen with penicillins, cephalosporins, and other agents. The more common agents associated with idiosyncratic neutropenia are listed below:

Analgesics/anti-inflammatory agents	Antibiotics	Others
Indomethacin	Chloramphenicol	Phenytoin
Para-aminophenol derivatives	Penicillins	Cimetidine
Acetaminophen	Sulfonamides	Captopril
Phenacetin	Cephalosporins	Chlorpropamide
Pyrazolone derivatives	Phenothiazines	
Aminopyrine	Antithyroid drugs	
Dipyrone		
Oxyphenbutazone		
Phenylbutazone		

International Agranulocytosis and Aplastic Anemia Study: Risks of agranulocytosis and aplastic anemia. JAMA 256:1749, 1986.

62. What is the significance of finding myelocytes, metamyelocytes, and nucleated RBCs in the peripheral blood?
Leukoerythroblastosis, or the presence of immature WBCs and nucleated RBCs, often is associated with a malignancy that has metastasized to the bone marrow. Numerous other, less serious conditions also affect leukoerythroblastosis, sometimes transiently:

Malignancies	Nonmalignant conditions
Solid tumors	Hemolysis, including sickle cell disease
Prostate	Thrombocytopenic purpura
Breast	Infancy
GI	GI bleeding

Lymphoma   Renal transplants
Myelofibrosis   Septicemia
Leukemia   Chronic lung disease
Preleukemia   Myocardial infarction
                            Liver disease

63. Describe the features of lymphocytosis caused by infections.

When infections (usually viral) cause lymphocytosis, the lymphocyte morphology is unusual or atypical. Thus, infection with Epstein-Barr virus (EBV) or cytomegalovirus (CMV) can cause an infectious mononucleosis syndrome of fever, sore throat, lymphadenopathy, hepatosplenomegaly, and, in the case of EBV, an increased titer of the heterophile antibody. An acute lymphocytosis may be associated with primary infection with HIV-1.

In EBV infection, B cells are penetrated by the virus, eliciting a polyclonal T-cell response manifested in the peripheral blood as atypical lymphocytosis. Cold agglutinin disease also may occur in EBV disease. The IgM antibodies are usually directed against the i antigen. These disorders are usually self-limited. CMV, toxoplasmosis, and, less commonly, EBV infection during the first trimester of pregnancy have been associated with serious developmental defects in the newborn.

Causes of Heterophile-Negative Mononucleosis

Cytomegalovirus	Adenovirus	Toxoplasma
HIV-1	Herpes simplex II	Rubella

MYELOPROLIFERATIVE DISORDERS

64. Polycythemia is frequently encountered by internists. Before you embark on a long and expensive work-up, what two steps are necessary?

There is no point in pursuing a work-up of polycythemia without demonstrating that (1) the RBC mass is increased and (2) hypoxemia is not present as a cause of secondary erythrocytosis. Many patients who take diuretics have an increased hematocrit, but typically they also have decreased plasma volume and normal RBC mass. Some patients who are not taking diuretics (usually smokers) have so-called "stress erythrocytosis," with normal RBC mass and reduced plasma volume. Patients with chronic lung disease or congenital heart disease resulting in significant left-to-right shunts are also polycythemic.

Djulbegovic B, et al: A new algorithm for the diagnosis of polycythemia. Am Fam Physician 44:113–120, 1991.

65. List the major and minor criteria widely used to diagnose polycythemia vera (PCV).

The Polycythemia Study Group has developed the following guidelines to establish a diagnosis of PCV:

Category A (major criteria)
1. Increased red cell mass
    Males: > 36 ml/kg
    Females: > 32 ml/kg
2. Normal SaO_2 (> 90%)
3. Splenomegaly

Category B (minor criteria)
1. Thrombocytosis: platelets > 400 x 109/l
2. Leukocytosis: WBC > 12×10^9/L
3. Elevated leukocyte alkaline phosphatase (LAP)
4. Elevated B12 level (> 900 pg/ml) or unbound B12-binding capacity (> 2200 pg/ml)

A diagnosis of PCV is supported by finding either (1) all three criteria of category A or (2) increased RBC mass, normal SaO_2, and two of the criteria in category B. Although these criteria are useful, important causes of secondary polycythemia need to be considered. Carboxyhemoglobin should be measured if the patient is a heavy smoker, and in certain families a high-affinity hemoglobin may be identified by determining the P_{50} (oxygen half-saturation pressure). Several kindreds have alterations in the gene for the erythropoietin receptor, resulting in familial erythrocytosis. A neoplasm-producing ectopic erythropoietin also may result in erythrocytosis. Typically, these are obvious, but CT scans or liver scans may be necessary to evaluate the possibility of an occult neoplasm of the kidney or liver. In PCV the erythropoietin level is usually low or normal, whereas in secondary conditions, erythropoietin levels are increased.

Berlin NI: Diagnosis and classification of the polycythemias. Semin Hematol 12:339–351, 1975.

66. Once the diagnosis of PCV is established, how are patients treated? What are the expected complications of therapy?

Treatment of PCV is important, because untreated patients are uncomfortable and at risk for life-threatening thrombotic events. Initially, phlebotomy of 500 ml of blood every other day as tolerated is undertaken until the hematocrit is reduced to a normal range. Some patients are not well-controlled and require myelosuppressive therapy with hydroxyurea. As phlebotomy proceeds, patients develop iron deficiency, which reduces the rate at which phlebotomy is necessary for control of the disease.

An important study by the Polycythemia Vera Study Group compared treatment with phlebotomy, 32P, or chlorambucil. Phlebotomy alone was associated with an increased incidence of stroke and other thrombotic events, whereas treatment with chlorambucil or 32P was associated with a high incidence of transformation into acute leukemia. Therefore, patients who are over age 70 or those who have had previous thrombotic events may do better with hydroxyurea and occasional phlebotomy. Phlebotomy alone usually suffices for younger patients.

Tefferi A, Solberg LA, Silverstein MN: A clinical update in polycythemia vera and essential thrombocythemia. Am J Med 109:141–149, 2000.

67. What is the typical cytogenetic abnormality found in chronic myelogenous leukemia (CML)? Do any other hematologic malignancies share this finding?

The cytogenetic marker of CML is the **9:22 translocation**, in which portions of the long arms of chromosomes 9 and 22 are exchanged, resulting in a shortened 22 or **Philadelphia chromosome** (Ph[1]). This balanced translocation results in the juxtaposition of an oncogene c-abl originating on chromosome 9 with genes in the breakpoint cluster region (bcr) of chromosome 22. Cell lines established from CML cells express a new mRNA, which reflects the chimeric gene produced by the fusion of the bcr and c-abl genes. From this mRNA, a unique tyrosine phosphoprotein kinase, P210 bcr-abl, is translated, which may act to phosphorylate tyrosine residues in important cellular proteins. A small minority of patients with CML have normal cytogenetics, but the c-abl/bcr translocation is found by studies at the molecular level.

Some patients with acute lymphoblastic leukemia (ALL) also have 9:22 translocations. Although some of these may have been lymphoblastic transformations of CML, most are thought to be de novo leukemias with subtle differences in the location of the c-abl translocation into the bcr region of 22.

Sawyers C: Chronic myeloid leukemia. N Engl J Med 340:1330–1340, 1999.

68. How is CML differentiated from a leukemoid reaction?

Occasionally patients who have an inflammatory disease, infection, or cancer have a leukocytosis up to, but usually not over, 50×10^9/L. In some instances, the cause may not be apparent, and CML is a consideration. The two entities may be differentiated by the characteristics outlined below:

	CML	LEUKEMOID REACTION
Juvenile neutrophils (e.g., metamyelocytes, myelocytes)	+	
Basophilia	+	–
Eosinophilia	+	–
Marrow fibrosis	±	–
Splenomegaly	±	–
Leukocyte alkaline phosphatase	Low	Increased
Philadelphia chromosome	+	–

+ = present; – = absent.

69. What is the prognosis of CML?

Despite control of symptoms with agents such as hydroxyurea, CML uniformly transforms into an acute leukemia that is typically poorly responsive to chemotherapy. The median survival of patients ranges from 39–47 months. After the first year, the risk of transformation into blast phase is about 20% per year. Thus, a minority of patients have long survival timess of 10–25 years with CML.

70. Describe the clinical and laboratory features of acceleration of CML into blast phase.

Certain clinical events herald the transformation of CML from chronic to blast phase, including an enlarging spleen (with splenic infarcts), increased basophilia and eosinophilia, fever, fibrosis in the marrow, and resistance to hydroxyurea. In many instances, an accelerated phase (marked by an increased percentage of blasts and promyelocytes) occurs before frank leukemia.

In about two-thirds of cases of transformation into acute leukemia, a new cytogenetic abnormality appears in addition to the Philadelphia chromosome. These new cytogenetic abnormalities suggest that the Ph^1 clone evolves into a more malignant cell. Four typical chromosomal changes are seen in the setting of transformation: (1) a second Ph^1 chromosome, (2) trisomy 8, (3) isochromosome 17, and (4) trisomy 19. Of interest, the phenotype of a leukemic cell in the blast crisis of CML is variable. Although most patients have blasts with the characteristics of myeloid cells, about one-third have cells that are lymphoid in character. Less often, the cells have features of erythroblastic leukemia or megakaryocytic leukemia.

71. Compare the roles of interferon and BMT in the treatment of CML.

Recent studies have shown the usefulness of α-interferon in the treatment of CML in the chronic phase, particularly for patients who have thrombocytosis as a manifestation of CML. Treatment with α-interferon can result in loss of the cytogenetic abnormality; in a significant number of patients, no Ph^1 chromosome was detected in mitotic figures obtained from bone marrow aspirate after treatment. Whether this form of therapy delays the onset of blast crises is unknown.

BMT is the only current therapy that offers a hope of cure for CML. Although the peritransplant mortality rate is significant, the long-term outlook is better for young patients who have CML and an HLA-identical sibling. Patients should undergo BMT during the chronic phase, because once patients reach blast crises, the outlook is poorer.

An exciting development in the therapy of CML is the design of a synthetic inhibitor of the ABL tyrosine kinase, STI-571. This drug acts as an active signal transduction inhibitor (STI) and causes apoptosis of CML cells. In clinical trials it has few side effects and is highly active in the chronic phase of CML, demonstrating the usefulness of targeting the specific molecular pathology of a leukemic disorder.

Deininger, MWN, Goldman JM, Melo JV: The molecular biology of chronic myeloid leukemia. Blood 96: 3343–3356, 2000.

72. Patients presenting with large spleens, fibrotic marrows, and teardrop-shaped erythrocytes on the peripheral blood film have what myeloproliferative disorder?

Myelofibrosis, or agnogenic myeloid metaplasia. This myeloproliferative disease is marked by splenomegaly, tear-drop RBCs, fibrotic marrow, and immature erythroid and myeloid cells in peripheral blood (leukoerythroblastic blood picture). Extramedullary hematopoiesis is usually present in the liver and spleen. Patients may have neutrophilia, thrombocytosis, and anemia, but other patients, typically with massively enlarged spleens, may be cytopenic instead. Patients with enlarged spleens and neutrophilia resemble patients with CML. Determination of the presence of Ph^1 chromosome may distinguish the two.

The fibroblast proliferation that is typically present in the marrows of such patients is polyclonal and appears to be fostered by fibroblast growth factors released by abnormal megakaryocytes. Patients may be troubled by bone pain and often have radiographic evidence of osteosclerosis. Massive splenomegaly may lead to portal hypertension and varices. Treatment is largely supportive and ineffective. As in other myeloproliferative diseases, transformation into acute leukemia has been observed in some patients.

Tefferi A: Myelofibrosis with myeloid metaplasia. N Eng J Med 342:1255–1265, 2000.

73. Patients without massive splenomegaly may have platelet counts above 1,000,000/ml ("platelet millionaires"). What myeloproliferative disease do they have?

Patients may become platelet millionaires for various reasons. Occasionally patients with severe **iron deficiency** and concurrent hemorrhage or inflammatory disease have platelet counts > 1,000,000/ml. Once iron deficiency is corrected or the inflammatory disorder resolves, platelet counts return to normal levels.

Another myeloproliferative disorder, **essential thrombocythemia**, should be considered when the platelet count rises above 600,000/ml, although a count > 1,000,000/ml is the rule. Patients also have evidence of clonal proliferation. Physical exam may show modest splenic enlargement and purpura. Patients often are troubled by hemorrhage due to poorly functioning platelets. Purpura, epistaxis, and gingival bleeding are typical manifestations and may be exacerbated by aspirin. Erythromelalgia, characterized by a localized burning pain and warmth of the distal extremities, is commonly seen. Dramatic relief is obtained with small doses of aspirin. Also seen are neurologic manifestations such as dizziness, seizures, and transient ischemic attacks.

Tefferi A, et al: Issues in the diagnosis and management of essential thrombocythemia. Mayo Clin Proc 69:651–655, 1994.

74. List the causes of thrombocytosis.

Reactive	Myeloproliferative disorders
Malignancy	Essential thrombocythemia
Iron deficiency	Polycythemia vera (PCV)
Splenectomy	CML (Ph[1]+)
Inflammatory bowel disease	Myelofibrosis
Infection	Myelodysplastic syndromes
Collagen-vascular diseases	

Iron studies, collagen vascular screen, and cytogenetic studies of the bone marrow aspirate are helpful in differentiating these disorders. PCV may present as essential thrombocythemia and iron deficiency with chronic GI blood loss. When the iron deficiency is corrected, the erythrocytosis of PCV becomes evident.

Buss DH, et al: Occurrence, etiology, and clinical significance of extreme thrombocytosis: A study of 280 cases. Am J Med 96:247–253, 1994.

75. What is the most likely complication in a patient with a myeloproliferative disease who presents with a swollen, hot ankle?

Patients with myeloproliferative syndromes (PCV, CML, myelofibrosis, essential thrombocythemia) may develop hyperuricemia and gout. Thus, arthritis in such patients should be investigated thoroughly, including arthrocentesis and examination for intracellular, negatively birefringent crystals under polarized light.

ACUTE MYELOGENOUS LEUKEMIA (AML)

76. Which cytogenetic abnormalities have been described in AML?

At least 90% of patients with AML have cytogenetic abnormalities. Some of these, when detected, indicate a relatively good prognosis, and others bode ill. Specific morphologic variants of AML have been linked to characteristic cytogenetic abnormalities, as shown in the table below.

CYTOGENETIC ABNORMALITY	LEUKEMIA TYPE	PROGNOSIS
Trisomy 8	M2	Average
t(8;21)	M2 with splenomegaly, chloromas, Auer rods	Good
t(15;17)	M3, many promyelocytes, DIC	Good
inv 16	M4 with abnormal eosinophils	Good
t(9;11)	M5, monocytic leukemia	Average

Table continued on following page

CYTOGENETIC ABNORMALITY	LEUKEMIA TYPE	PROGNOSIS
t(6;9)	M2 with increased basophils	Average
t(4;11)	Biphenotypic leukemia lymphoid and monocytic phenotype	Poor
5q-, 7-, 5-, 7-	Therapy-related leukemia	Poor

From Löwenberg B, Downing JR, Burnett A: Acute myeloid leukemia. N Eng J Med 341:1051–1062, 1999.

77. How is AML classified? How do the subtypes differ in natural history and complications?

The diagnosis of AML M1–M5 requires a cellular bone marrow aspirate with blasts representing > 30% of all nucleated WBCs. If erythroblasts comprise > 50% of the nucleated bone marrow cells, erythroleukemia (M6) is present. If the marrow is cellular but blasts account for < 30% of the nucleated RBCs, myelodysplasia is present. Peroxidase stain is important in the definition of AML; in practice, the blasts are peroxidase (or Sudan black)-positive in AML and peroxidase-negative in acute lymphoblastic leukemia (ALL).

French-American-British (FAB) Classification of AML

TYPE	DESCRIPTION	CRITERIA
M1	Myeloblastic leukemia without maturation	> 3% of blasts are peroxidase-positive. A few granules, Auer rods, or both; one or more distinct nucleoli; no further maturation
M2	Myeloblastic leukemia with maturation	> 50% of marrow cells are myeloblasts and promyelocytes. Myelocytes, metamyelocytes, and mature granulocytes are seen; eosinophilia may predominate in some cases
M3	Hypergranular promyelocytic leukemia	Majority of cells are abnormal promyelocytes, reniform (kidney-shaped) nuclei, bundles of Auer rods; also some have closely packed bright pink or purple granules
M4	Myelomonocytic leukemia	> 20% of bone marrow, peripheral blood nucleated cells, or both are promonocytes and monocytes; an eosinophilic variant is also recognized
M5	Monocytic leukemia (M5a = poorly differentiated) (M5b = differentiated)	Granulocyte component, 10% of marrow cells, monocytoid cells have a fluoride-sensitive esterase reaction cytochemically
M6	Erythroleukemia	> 50% of cells are erythroblasts; myeloblasts represent >30% of nonerythroid nucleated cells
M7	Megakaryoblastic	> 30% of marrow cells are blasts; platelets peroxidase-positive on electron microscopy, or blasts react with antiplatelet monoclonal antibodies; marrow fibrosis is prominent; cytoplasmic budding is also a feature

From Bennett JM, et al: Proposal for the classificiation of the acute leukemias. Br J Hematol 33:451, 1976.

78. How does the presentation and treatment of acute promyelocytic leukemia (APL) differ from other AML subtypes?

Patients with APL present with lower WBC counts and may have a normal count when first examined. Careful attention to the morphology of the circulating WBCs discloses the presence of the hypergranular blasts or blasts with multiple Auer rods. Less frequently the blasts are hypogranular.

A significant hemorrhagic diathesis may complicate either the presentation or the treatment of APL with standard AML chemotherapy. A picture resembling disseminated intravascular coagulation (DIC) is characteristic and may be accompanied by CNS bleeding, which is sometimes fatal. Patients may require intensive support with platelets, fresh frozen plasma, and cryoprecipitate. In the past, heparin has been used to abrogate the consumptive coagulopathy.

79. What gene rearrangement defines APL?

The 15:17 translocation, which involves a rearrangement of a receptor for retinoic acid (retinoic acid receptor-α, or RAR-α). Administration of all-trans retinoic acid (ATRA) results in maturation of the promyelocyte to a granulocyte, so that complete morphologic and cytogenetic remission can be attained without the hemorrhagic diathesis. Although these remissions are short-lived, the combination of ATRA and chemotherapy seems to be the best way to treat patients with APL. ATRA does have side effects, the most important of which is the retinoic-acid syndrome of capillary leak, pulmonary infiltrates, and hypoxemia. Complete remissions of APL also have been achieved in patients treated with arsenic trioxide. This compound causes incomplete differentiation and apoptosis of the leukemic cells.

The reverse transcriptase polymerase chain reactions (rt-PCR) now allow the detection of minimal disease at the level of the gene rearrangement—a much more sensitive way to assess the presence of leukemic cells than counting blasts in the marrow or screening the karyotypes of marrow cells for the 15:17 translocation. The presence of the PML-RAR-α gene rearrangement detected by rt-PCR may predict relapse.

Tallman MS, et al: Acute promyelocytic leukemia: A paradigm for differentiation therapy with retinoic acid. Blood Rev 8:70–78, 1994.

80. What are the main causes of death in AML?

Infection, hemorrhage from thrombocytopenia, or resistant disease. Refractoriness to platelet transfusions is a significant problem in patients who become sensitized to donor platelets. The use of filters to remove contaminating lymphocytes appears to reduce this complication of transfusion support. Resistance to chemotherapy may be related to changes in the leukemic cells that affect the ability of drugs to enter the cell. The multidrug resistance phenotype is conferred by enhanced expression of a membrane protein, p-glycoprotein, which actively pumps a wide variety of chemotherapeutic agents out of the cell. Expression of this protein at diagnosis may confer a worse prognosis.

Ross DD, et al: Enhancement of daunorubicin accumulation, retention, and cytotoxicity by verapamil or cyclosporin A in blast cells from patients with previously untreated acute myeloid leukemia. Blood 82:1288–1299, 1993.

81. Which organisms most frequently cause infection during induction chemotherapy-induced bone marrow aplasia?

Patients receiving induction chemotherapy usually endure a period of absolute granulocytopenia (leukocyte nadir) at a time when there have been breakdowns of important barriers to infection. These breakdowns include mucositis throughout the GI tract and the presence of chronic indwelling venous catheters.

Organisms Causing Infection in AML

BACTERIA	FUNGI
Pseudomonas aeruginosa	Candida spp.
Escherichia coli	Aspergillus spp.
Staphylococcus aureus	Phycomycetes spp.
Klebsiella aerobacter	
Proteus vulgaris	
Bacteroides spp.	
α-Hemolytic streptococci	
Staphylococcus epidermidis	

Antibiotic therapy usually is designed to cover the bacterial pathogens on this list. If after a period of adequate treatment the patient remains febrile, amphotericin is usually begun. Controversy still rages over the need for reverse isolation, enteric sterilization with antibiotics, or other prophylactic measures that may be taken to reduce infection.

82. What proportion of patients with AML attain complete remission? How many survive for 5 years or more?

In the Toronto Leukemia Study, the complete remission (CR) rate among 272 patients with AML ranged from 43.8–85.3%, depending on the exclusion criteria used. The lower remission rate occurred in patients who were elderly (> age 70), had an antecedent myelodysplastic syndrome, or had partial treatment. A younger patient with no previous hematologic disorder had a 70–85% chance of attaining CR, which may last for 11–16 months on average. Of those who attain CR, 20% survive for > 5 years.

Recently the Cancer and Leukemia Group B found that younger patients (< 40 years) had a 75% CR rate and a 4-year disease-free survival rate of 32%, whereas older patients had CR and disease-free rates of 47% and 14%, respectively. During induction chemotherapy, the younger patients died because they had disease resistant to two courses of therapy, but the older patients died more often during treatment-induced hypoplasia. Growth factors such as G-CSF and GM-CSF have been used to stimulate granulopoiesis after chemotherapy with mixed results.

Mayer RJ, et al: Intensive postremission chemotherapy in adults with acute myeloid leukemia. N Engl J Med 331:896–903, 1994.

83. Young patients with AML in first remission are usually evaluated or considered for BMT. Do syngeneic (identical twin) transplants or allogeneic (HLA-identical) transplants fare better after BMT?

Patients in remission who are age 40 or younger and have HLA-identical siblings are usually evaluated for BMT. In comparisons of BMT vs. maintenance or other forms of postinduction chemotherapy, patients receiving transplants seem to have an advantage. This advantage may be due to the intensity of the preoperative regimen for BMT, which includes lethal doses of chemotherapy, often in conjunction with total body irradiation. However, studies of identical-twin donor-recipient pairs indicate that the recipients have a higher relapse rate than HLA-identical sibling transplants. These studies indicate an important "graft-vs.-leukemia" effect of allogeneic BMT. The relatively recent recognition of cytogenetic abnormalities with "good prognosis" has led some centers to treat patients having 8:21, 15:17 translocations or inv (16) with intensive chemotherapy alone. In such patients, BMT is reserved for relapse.

Appelbaum FR, et al: Chemotherapy vs marrow transplantation for adults with acute nonlymphocytic leukemia: A five-year follow-up. Blood 72:179–184, 1988.

84. What are the most important causes of death in patients undergoing BMT?

BMT is a challenging mode of therapy. After conditioning, patients become pancytopenic during the 3 weeks or so that is required for engraftment. During that time, they are prone to **infectious complications** similar to those experienced by patients undergoing remission-induction chemotherapy for AML. These patients are treated prophylactically with antibiotics and transfusions of RBCs and platelets. Blood products must be irradiated to prevent **graft-vs.-host disease** from lymphocytes in the donor units. After engraftment, **interstitial pneumonitis** is a frequent complication, with a high mortality rate. Some of these deaths are due to infectious agents such as CMV. Recently, a severe form of **veno-occlusive disease** of the liver has emerged as a cause of morbidity and mortality after BMT.

85. Describe the clinical findings in graft-vs.-host disease (GvHD).

One consequence of engraftment is the potential for GvHD, which is caused by T cells from the donor. GvHD may be either acute or chronic. **Acute GvHD** arises during the first 100 days after transplant, with donor T lymphocytes targeting the host's skin, liver, and GI tract. Patients may have mild skin rashes or more severe disease resulting in toxic epidermal necrolysis.

Diarrhea and transient elevation of liver enzymes may occur and, in some patients, are more severe, resulting in massive diarrhea and liver failure. Immunologic competence is also delayed by GvHD, so that patients are susceptible to new infections, including those mediated by encapsulated organisms such as pneumococci.

Chronic GvHD results in the same organ involvement, with additional features of a scleroderma-like illness. Dry eyes, dry mouth, myasthenia, bronchiolitis, and infections are also observed.

ACUTE LYMPHOBLASTIC LEUKEMIA (ALL)

86. Can ALL be reliably differentiated from AML (M1) by examination of the peripheral blood smear only?
No. Although hematologists can sometimes distinguish between the two entities by looking at the morphology of the blasts, there is a high rate of discordance with the results of special studies. Flow cytometry is frequently used to show typical lymphoid markers in ALL and myeloid markers in AML. Some patients with leukemia show evidence of both types of markers and are called biphenotypic. AML can be differentiated from ALL by using sensitive markers such as CD19 and CD7 for B- and T-cell lineages, respectively, and CD 13 or CD33 for AML.

Distinguishing Cytologic Features of ALL and AML

WRIGHT'S STAIN MORPHOLOGY	AML	ALL
Cytoplasm	More abundant	Scanty
Granules	Sometimes present	Absent
Nucleoli	3–5 distinct	1–3, often indistinct
Auer rods	May be present	Absent
STAINING CHARACTERISTICS		
Peroxidase or Sudan black	+	–
Periodic acid–Schiff	+/-	+

From Pui C-H, Evans WE: Acute lymphoblastic leukemia. N Engl J Med 339:605–615, 1998.

87. What are the indicators of a poor prognosis in adults with ALL?
ALL has an 80% cure rate in young children with good prognostic features, but in adults the outlook is much worse. Certain features at presentation of ALL in adults confer a poorer prognosis and may suggest the need for highly aggressive therapy. Adults are more likely than children to show:
 • Unfavorable chromosomal abnormalities, such as Ph[1] and 8:14 translocation
 • Biphenotypic disease and other than early pre-B immunophenotype
 • Leukocytosis at presentation
 • Multidrug resistance
 • Mediastinal mass
Copelan EA, McGuire EA: The biology and treatment of acute lymphoblastic leukemia in adults. Blood 85:1151–1168, 1995.

LYMPHOPROLIFERATIVE DISEASE

88. What is the most common leukemia of adults?
Chronic lymphocytic leukemia (CLL), which is a neoplastic growth of lymphocytes, most often B lymphocytes. Patients are often elderly, and CLL is detected during examination for other problems. Lymphadenopathy and splenomegaly are also relatively common. Some patients present only with an elevated WBC count, composed of lymphocytes with a normal morphology.

89. List the diagnostic criteria for CLL.
 1. Sustained lymphocyte count > 10×10^9/liter. Morphology should be "typical."
 2. Bone marrow involvement (> 30% lymphocytes)

3. B-cell immunophenotypes (typically weak expression of membrane immunoglobulin, CD 20, expression of the T-cell antigen CD5).

To make a diagnosis of CLL, criterion 1 should be satisfied along with either criterion 2 or 3. If criterion 1 is not satisfied (lymphocyte count < 10×10^9/L), criteria 2 and 3 must be present.

International Workshop on Chronic Lymphocytic Leukemia: Chronic lymphocytic leukemia: Recommendations for diagnosis, staging, and response criteria. Ann Intern Med 110:236–238, 1989.

90. Patients with CLL are typically staged to determine prognosis and therapy. What are the current staging systems?

Many patients with CLL present with limited disease and live without problems from leukemia. Because most are elderly, death from other causes is most likely. Patients with more advanced disease, however, do less well; unfortunately, chemotherapy has not improved survival. Treatment is usually given to patients who have anemia, thrombocytopenia, or bulky lymphadenopathy. Two staging systems have been in use for CLL:

Rai Staging System for CLL

STAGE	CLINICAL FEATURES	SURVIVAL (MO)*
0	Lymphocytosis in blood and bone marrow only	> 120
I	Lymphocytosis and enlarged lymph nodes	95
II	Lymphocytosis plus hepatomegaly, splenomegaly, or both	72
III	Lymphocytosis and anemia (hemoglobin < 110 gm/L)	30
IV	Lymphocytosis and thrombocytopenia (platelets <100×10^9/L)	30

* Weighted median survival was derived from 8 series that involved a total of 952 patients.

Binet Staging System for Chronic Lymphocytic Leukemia

STAGE	CLINICAL FEATURES	SURVIVAL (MO)*
A	Hemoglobin > 100 gm/L; platelets > 100×10^9/L and < 3 areas involved[†]	> 120
B	Hemoglobin > 100 gm/L; platelets > 100×10^9/L and > 3 areas involved	61
C	Hemoglobin < 100 gm/L or platelets < 100×10^9/L or both (independent of the areas involved)	32

* Weighted median survival was derived from 8 series that involved a total of 1117 patients.
† Cervical, axillary, and inguinal lymph nodes (whether unilateral or bilateral); spleen; and liver.
From International Workshop on Chronic Lymphocytic Leukemia: Chronic lymphocytic leukemia: Recommendations for diagnosis, staging, and response criteria. Ann Intern Med 110:236–238, 1989.

91. What are the complications of CLL?

- Autoimmune phenomena (warm antibody autoimmune hemolytic anemia, immune thrombocytopenia, neutropenia)
- Pure red cell aplasia
- Hypogammaglobulinemia
- Transformation into a large cell lymphoma with poor prognosis (Richter's syndrome)

Rozman C, Montserrat E: Chronic lymphocytic leukemia. N Engl J Med 333:1052–1057, 1995.

92. Which lymphoproliferative disorder is associated with pancytopenia, splenomegaly, absence of lymphadenopathy, and circulating lymphoid cells with multiple projections?

Hairy cell leukemia (HCL). Although an uncommon malignancy (2% of all leukemias), HCL receives a great deal of attention because of advances in treatment and the unusual infections observed in the course of the disease. HCL is an important consideration in the work-up of patients who present with pancytopenia. Although the bone marrow aspirate is often scanty, characteristic "hairy" lymphs may be observed. The biopsy may show a diffusely involved marrow with mononuclear cells situated in a network of fibrosis. Some patients have presented with aplastic anemia.

Although hairy cells may be present in the marrow, the biopsy picture is one of profound hypocellularity. The hairy cell is a B lymphocyte with an immunophenotype consistent with a cell between a CLL-lymphocyte and a plasma cell. Hairy cells also possess the Tac antigen (CD25), a receptor for interleukin-2, usually seen on activated T cells. The distinctive cytochemical feature of the hairy cell is a tartrate-resistant acid phosphatase activity. In the past many patients improved after splenectomy. Interferon has been used successfully in alleviating this disorder, but recent trials show that the most effective agent is the purine analog 2-chlorodeoxyadenosine.

The differential diagnosis of a patient with splenomegaly and circulating abnormal but relatively mature lymphocytes includes HCL, CLL, leukemic phase of non-Hodgkin's lymphoma, and splenic lymphoma with villous lymphocytes (SLVL). SLVL shows many features of HCL, including lymphocytes with projections or villi. However, the lymphocyte in SLVL has usually just one or two polar projections. SLVL is considered to be the leukemic counterpart of marginal zone lymphoma.

Catovsky D: Chronic lymphoproliferative disorders. Curr Opin Oncol 7:3–11, 1995.

93. What infectious complications are seen in HCL?

The course of HCL is marked by an increased incidence of infections with atypical mycobacteria or fungi, such as *Histoplasma* and *Cryptococcus* spp. There also may be an increased incidence of bacterial infections and perhaps legionellosis. Factors contributing to the occurrence of atypical mycobacterial and fungal infections may include decreased neutrophils, absolute monocytopenia, and inability to form granuloma normally.

Westbrook CA, Golde DW: Clinical problems in hairy cell leukemia: Diagnosis and management. Semin Oncol 11:514, 1984.

HODGKIN'S AND NON-HODGKIN'S LYMPHOMAS

94. What are the common presentations of Hodgkin's disease?

Most patients often present with lymphadenopathy in the neck or axilla; lymph nodes are nontender, rubbery, and discrete. Sometimes the nodes wax and wane in size until attention is sought. Important symptoms in the staging of Hodgkin's disease are fever, weight loss (> 10% of body weight), and night sweats. Some patients are troubled by pruritus. Hodgkin's disease tends to originate in central lymph nodes, so that some patients present with mediastinal lymphadenopathy.

95. How does Hodgkin's disease spread? How does this pattern affect staging?

Hodgkin's disease is thought to spread from a unifocal site to contiguous lymph nodes. There may be early hematogenous dissemination to the spleen, with subsequent spread to the splenic hilar and retroperitoneal nodes as well as the liver. If large tumor masses develop, there may be extension into adjacent organs. Often the spleen is significantly involved in the absence of palpable splenomegaly. Hence, some centers recommend staging laparotomy to avoid missing splenic and hepatic disease. The importance of staging in Hodgkin's disease is to determine the extent of disease and thereby decide on therapy.

Ann Arbor Staging of Hodgkin's Disease

STAGE	SUBSTAGE	INVOLVEMENT
I	I	Single lymph node
	IE	Single extralymphatic organ
II	II	≥ Lymph nodes on same side of diaphragm
	IIE	With localized extralymphatic site
III	III	Lymph nodes above and below diaphragm
	IIIE	With localized extralymphatic site
	IIIS	With isolated splenic site
	IIISE	With both extralymphatic and splenic sites
IV	IV	Disseminated or diffuse involvement of one or more extralymphatic sites
	IVA	Asymptomatic
	IVB	Fever, sweats, weight loss > 10% body weight

Aisenberg A: The staging and treatment of Hodgkin's disease. N Engl J Med 299:1228, 1978.

96. What are the histologic subtypes of Hodgkin's disease? Which carry the worst prognosis?

Nodular sclerosis	35%
Mixed cellularity	33%
Lymphocyte predominant	16%
Lymphocyte depletion	16%

Nodular sclerosis more frequently affects women, whereas the other three types more often affect men. Although staging generally determines the outlook, histologic subtype is also important. Nodular-sclerosing and lymphocyte-predominant subtypes tend to present with limited disease. Lymphocyte depletion is associated with more advanced disease, retroperitoneal involvement, and presentation in older adults.

97. What is the classic cell seen in the lymph nodes of patients with Hodgkin's disease?

The Reed-Sternberg (RS) cell, a large cell with two nuclei, each possessing a distinct nucleolus. RS cells are plentiful in mixed-cellularity and lymphocyte-depletion Hodgkin's disease, but in nodular-sclerosis and lymphocyte-predominant disease they are overwhelmed by reactive lymphocytes, PMNs, and eosinophils. In nodular sclerosis, retraction of the cells surrounding the RS cell during fixation produces the lacunar cell. Also present are bands of fibrosis. The pathology of Hodgkin's disease is not straightforward; diagnostic confusion surrounds the newly recognized entities, T-cell–rich B-cell lymphoma and peripheral T-cell lymphomas.

Banks PM: The pathology of Hodgkin's disease. Semin Oncol 17:683–695, 1990.

98. When should patients with Hodgkin's disease undergo staging laparotomy?

Patients first must undergo a comprehensive clinical staging evaluation before surgical staging is contemplated. The key elements in the clinical staging are as follows:

• Detailed history
• Detailed physical exam, with attention to lymph node areas, spleen, and liver
• Laboratory: complete blood count, erythrocyte sedimentation rate, alkaline phosphatase, renal and liver function tests
• Radiology: posteroanterior and lateral views of chest, abdominal and chest CT scans, bilateral lower-extremity lymphangiogram
• Bone marrow aspirate and biopsy

Once this evaluation is complete, surgical staging with laparotomy can be considered. There is no need for staging laparotomy if disseminated or diffuse extralymphatic involvement is found, unless the results would change therapy. In centers where treatment includes chemotherapy for limited disease, the need for laparotomy is less apparent. Unfortunately, staging laparotomy carries a high morbidity due to pulmonary emboli, subphrenic abscesses, stress ulcers, and wound infections.

Urba WJ, Longo DL: Hodgkin's disease. N Engl J Med 326:678–687, 1992.

99. In patients cured of Hodgkin's disease, what are the late sequelae of therapy?

The most important of the late sequelae are myelodysplasia, leukemia, and non-Hodgkin's lymphoma (3–10 years after therapy). Certain complications of the high-dose irradiation are also evident: acute radiation pneumonitis with fever, cough, and shortness of breath. Cardiac effects of irradiation include pericarditis, pericardial effusions, and pericardial fibrosis. Coronary artery disease may be accelerated. Neurologic effects of irradiation include Lhermitte's syndrome (paresthesia produced by flexion of the neck). Hypothyroidism is also a frequent sequelae of radiation therapy.

Bookman MA, Longo DI: Concomitant illness in patients treated for Hodgkin's disease. Cancer Treat Rev 13:77, 1986.

100. How does the pattern of lymph node involvement in non-Hodgkin's lymphoma (diffuse vs. nodular) correlate with the pace of disease progression?

In nodular lymphomas, the neoplastic lymphocytes congregate into aggregates that superficially resemble germinal centers. Lymphomas of this type generally pursue an indolent course. Diffuse lymphomas tend to behave in a more aggressive manner. Other adverse prognostic factors include older age, elevated lactate dehydrogenase, two or more extranodal sites, T-cell phenotype, and masses > 10 cm.

101. How often do patients with lymphoma have bone marrow involvement?

Bone marrow involvement is extremely common in non-Hodgkin's lymphoma, whereas it is relatively uncommon in Hodgkin's disease. Diffuse well-differentiated lymphocytic lymphoma is associated with bone marrow involvement in 100% of cases. Small, cleaved-cell lymphomas, follicular and diffuse types, are associated with bone marrow involvement in 40–50% of cases. Large-cell lymphomas are less likely to spread to the marrow (15% incidence). When bone marrow involvement occurs in large cell lymphoma, there is a greater risk for CNS disease.

102. In Africa, Denis P. Burkitt described an aggressive neoplasm that bears his name. What are the salient clinical features of this lymphoma?

Burkitt's lymphoma results from a proliferation of B lymphocytes with a striking appearance. They present as round or oval cells with abundant basophilic cytoplasm-containing vacuoles that stain positively for fat. The tissue is replaced with a monotonous infiltrate of cells with interspersed macrophages, giving a "starry sky" appearance. When it presents as a leukemia, it is classified as L3 in the FAB scheme. These cells proliferate rapidly and have a potential doubling time of 24 hours. In African Burkitt's lymphoma, patients present with large extranodal tumors of the jaws, abdominal viscera (including kidney), and ovaries and retroperitoneum. In the American form of Burkitt's lymphoma, patients present with intra-abdominal tumors arising from the ileocecal region or mesenteric lymph nodes. In Africa, the disease is associated with Epstein-Barr virus, but this association is less common in American cases.

103. What characteristic cytogenetic abnormalities are seen in Burkitt's lymphoma?

A t(8:14) translocation is recognized in most cases. The proto-oncogene *c-myc* is located on chromosome 8 and usually becomes translocated to the locus of the heavy-chain immunoglobulin gene. This results in the activation of *c-myc*. Burkitt's is now classified as a subset of small non-cleaved cell lymphoma (SNCL). SNCL is a frequent neoplasm diagnosed in association with HIV infection and has a predilection for CNS and bone marrow involvement.

Mashal RD, Canellos GP: Small non-cleaved cell lymphoma in adults. Am J Hematol 38:40–47, 1991.

104. When should patients with non-Hodgkin's lymphoma receive chemo- or radiotherapy?

In an evaluation of patients with favorable histology and stage III or IV disease, it was found that deferral of treatment until patients became symptomatic did not adversely affect survival. In fact, during the course of nontreatment, spontaneous regression was frequently observed. The median time to treatment was 31 months. Thus, in the absence of curative chemotherapy for indolent lymphomas, deferral of treatment is a reasonable course, provided patients are followed closely.

PLASMA CELL DYSCRASIAS

105. Which disorders are associated with the presence of a serum monoclonal immunoglobulin paraprotein?

Monoclonal immunoglobulins are detected frequently as a result of the routine availability of serum protein determinations and electrophoresis. Secondary monoclonal gammopathy must be distinguished from the monoclonal gammopathy associated with multiple myeloma, benign monoclonal gammopathy of uncertain significance, solitary plasmacytoma, amyloidosis, lymphoma, and Waldenström's macroglobulinemia.

Disorders Associated with Monoclonal Gammopathy

Collagen vascular diseases (SLE, scleroderma, Sjögren's disease, rheumatoid arthritis)	Infectious disease (tuberculosis, subacute bacterial endocarditis, AIDS, purpura fulminans)
Crohn's disease	Hepatitis, cirrhosis
Skin disease (pyoderma gangrenosum, psoriasis, scleromyxedema, urticaria)	Myeloproliferative diseases
	Post-BMT
Gaucher's disease	Cryoglobulinemia

From Foerster J: Plasma cell dyscrasias: General considerations. In Wintrobe's Clinical Hematology, 10th ed. Baltimore, Williams & Wilkins, 1999, p 2620.

106. How do you differentiate multiple myeloma (MM) from benign monoclonal gammopathy (BMG)?

	MM	BMG
M-protein	> 3.5 gm/dl	< 3.5 gm/dl
IgG IgA	> 2.0 gm/dl	< 2.0 gm/dl
Anemia or other cytopenia	Usually present	Absent
Urine protein	> 500 mg/24 hr	< 500 mg/24 hr
Bones	Lytic lesions or osteoporosis	Normal
Marrow plasma cells	> 10%	< 10%
Serum β_2-microglobulin	> 3.0 mg/L	<3.0 mg/L
Calcium	Elevated in 30%	Normal
Creatinine	± Elevation	Normal
Change in monoclonal protein with time	Increases	No change

The discovery of a monoclonal protein on serum protein electrophoresis should be followed by a careful work-up for MM. Patients who have a small serum spike, normal CBC, no proteinuria, and no lytic lesions, hypercalcemia, or renal dysfunction usually are followed with periodic serum protein electrophoresis. Patients meeting some of the criteria for MM but showing no progression with follow-up are described as having indolent MM. Such patients generally do not have anemia or lytic bone lesions.

107. What are the common complications of multiple myeloma?

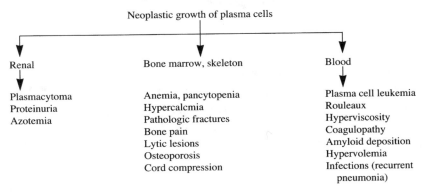

Neoplastic growth of plasma cells

Renal	Bone marrow, skeleton	Blood
Plasmacytoma	Anemia, pancytopenia	Plasma cell leukemia
Proteinuria	Hypercalcmia	Rouleaux
Azotemia	Pathologic fractures	Hyperviscosity
	Bone pain	Coagulopathy
	Lytic lesions	Amyloid deposition
	Osteoporosis	Hypervolemia
	Cord compression	Infections (recurrent pneumonia)

108. What are the renal manifestations of multiple myeloma?

Myeloma kidney
    Dense tubular casts and progressive azotemia
    Hyperviscosity
Renal tubular dysfunction
    Isosthenuria
    Renal tubular acidosis
    Adult Fanconi syndrome

Glomerulonephritis
Urate nephropathy
Pyelonephritis
Dye-nephropathy
Hypercalcemia renal damage
Plasma cell infiltration
Amyloid kidney
Nephrotic syndrome

109. Describe the clinical manifestations of Waldenström's macroglobulinemia.

Waldenström's macroglobulinemia is a B-cell disorder of proliferating plasmacytoid lymphs that produce an IgM monoclonal protein. Patients frequently have hepatosplenomegaly, lymphadenopathy, and bone marrow involvement. The elderly are affected most often. Neurologic disease, including peripheral neuropathy and cerebellar dysfunction, is also seen. A prominent feature is retinopathy with large sausage-shaped, dilated retinal veins. Bleeding and purpura are also common. Of particular importance is the recognition of hyperviscosity syndrome, which also may occur in MM. This syndrome can respond dramatically to plasmapheresis, because IgM does not have a large extravascular distribution.

Dimopoulos MA, Alexanian R: Waldenstrom's macroglobulinemia. Blood 83: 1452–1459, 1994.

110. Outline the manifestations of the hyperviscosity syndrome.

Global CNS dysfunction and stupor	Hypervolemia, congestive heart failure
Retinopathy	Headache, vertigo, ataxia
Retinal hemorrhages	Stroke
Papilledema	Coagulopathy

111. Patients with the λ-light-chain type of MM are prone to develop amyloidosis. What are the clinical and laboratory clues to the presence of this systemic disorder?

Amyloid is a lardaceous substance that accumulates in the tissues of patients with various disorders, including MM. The amyloid in MM is composed of light chains, most often of the λ type, arranged in a β-pleated sheet. When stained with Congo red and viewed under polarized light, amyloid shows an apple-green birefringence. Patients may develop purpura from skin involvement, hepatosplenomegaly, macroglossia, orthostatic hypotension, congestive heart failure, malabsorption, nephrotic syndrome, peripheral neuropathy, and carpal tunnel syndrome. Of interest, the consequences of amyloid include an acquired factor X deficiency, resulting in a prolonged PT and PTT and functional hyposplenism. The latter results in the presence of Howell-Jolly bodies, even though the spleen is present.

Gertz MA, Kyle RA: Primary systemic amyloidosis—a diagnostic primer. Mayo Clin Proc 64:1505–1519, 1989.

HEMOSTASIS

112. Define the primary and secondary phases of hemostasis.

Hemostasis is a complicated process with several components, all of which must work well for normal hemostasis to occur. The two overlapping phases of the formation of a clot or hemostatic plug are (1) **primary hemostasis**, in which the ruptured vessel wall interacts with platelets that must adhere and aggregate to form the basis of the clot, and (2) **secondary hemostasis**, in which clotting factors circulating in the blood activate each other in a cascade that results in the activation of thrombin and the deposition of fibrin around the platelet plug.

113. How do disorders of primary and secondary hemostasis differ in clinical presentations?

	PRIMARY	SECONDARY
Onset	Immediate	Delayed, hours after trauma
Sites, type of lesion	Mucosa, GI, GU, skin (purpura, petechiae)	Joints, retroperitoneum, muscles, hematuria, hematomas
Components involved	Vessel wall, platelet adhesion	Generation of fibrin from fibrinogen
Typical disorder	von Willebrand disease	Hemophilia A (factor VIII deficiency)

From Schafer AI: Approach to bleeding. In Loscalzo J, Schafer AI (eds): Thrombosis and Hemorrhage, 2nd ed. Boston, Blackwell, 1998, p 461.

114. What conditions are associated with immune thrombocytopenias?

1. Collagen-vascular diseases (systemic lupus erythematosus)
2. Impaired immunity (Bruton's agammaglobulinemia, IV drug users, HIV-1 infection)
3. Lymphoid neoplasias (Hodgkin's disease, non-Hodgkin's lymphoma, CLL)
4. Drug-induced (quinine, quinidine, hydrochlorothiazide, gold, heparin)

5. Others (thyrotoxicosis, sarcoidosis, antithymocyte globulin, solid tumors, anaphylaxis)
6. Isoimmune (post-transfusion purpura, fetal-maternal isoimmunization)

115. Describe idiopathic thrombocytopenic purpura (ITP).

In ITP, an autoantibody arises (usually IgG) that interacts with the patient's own platelets. Sometimes these antibodies interact with specific antigens related to functional proteins; platelets coated with the auto-IgG are then sequestered and removed by macrophages in the spleen, liver, and bone marrow. Production of megakaryocytes, as judged by a bone marrow aspirate, appears to be normal. However, recent studies indicate that megakaryocytopoiesis is, in fact, suboptimal for the degree of peripheral destruction. Thus, megakaryocytes may be affected by the autoantibody of ITP. ITP implies no known cause and is a diagnosis of exclusion. ITP occurs early in HIV infection, often before typical AIDS-defining illness.

Diagnosis does not always require a bone marrow aspirate and biopsy. Treatment remains empiric. Patients typically respond to prednisone. Refractory ITP or relapsed ITP may require splenectomy and/or additional immunosuppressive therapy. Treatment with intravenous IgG often produces a significant, though transient increase in the platelet count.

George JN, et al: Idiopathic thrombocytopenic purpura: A practice guideline developed by explicit methods for the American Society of Hematology. Blood 88:3–40, 1996.

116. What disorders are associated with nonimmune destruction of platelets?

Thrombocytopenia occurs with a wide variety of disorders of hematopoiesis. Of most concern are situations that result in the increased peripheral destruction of platelets. Some of these conditions may have immune components. The following disorders are associated with increased platelet destruction:

Infections
  Sepsis, gram-negative or gram-positive
  Viral, rickettsial
  Histoplasmosis
  Malaria
  Typhoid, brucellosis
Hypersplenism
Extracorporeal circulation, hypothermia

Microangiopathic disease
  Disseminated intravascular coagulation
  Thrombotic thrombocytopenic purpura
  Eclampsia, preeclampsia
  Burns
Cavernous hemangiomas
  Kasabach-Merritt syndrome
Massive transfusion

117. Name the most common hereditary disorder resulting in a prolonged bleeding time.

Von Willebrand's disease, an autosomal dominant disorder, results from several abnormalities in the production of a large, multimeric adhesive protein, von Willebrand factor (VWF). Classic VWF (type 1) disease results from decreased release of vWF from the endothelial cell. VWF is also synthesized by megakaryocytes and is a constituent of the α-granules of platelets. Decreased presence of VWF at the site of endothelial damage results in impairment of platelet adhesion and consequently poor primary hemostasis.

Patients with von Willebrand's disease have problems with epistaxis, hematuria, menorrhagia, GI bleeding, and bleeding after trauma. In classic type I disease, the platelet count is normal, but the bleeding time is prolonged. Factor VIII activity is also reduced in the plasma of patients with type 1 disease. The reduction of VWF seems to shorten the circulating life of factor VIII. Understanding of the pathophysiology of von Willebrand's disease has advanced rapidly so that now multiple types are recognized.

Phillips M, Santhouse A: von Willebrand disease: Recent advances in pathophysiology and treatment. Am J Med Sci 316: 77–86, 1998.

118. What are the hereditary disorders of platelet function?

Because von Willebrand disease is associated with platelet dysfunction, it is often considered with disorders resulting from congenital structural abnormalities of the platelet. These bleeding disorders are identified by a prolonged bleeding time and abnormal functional behavior in platelet aggregation tests. Three of these disorders are described below:

Hereditary Disorders Resulting in Platelet Dysfunction

	VON WILLEBRAND'S DISEASE	BERNARD-SOULIER SYNDROME	GLANZMANN'S THROMBASTHENIA
Defect	Reduced or abnormal factor VIII:VWF	Absence of platelet gp Ib, a receptor for VWF	Absence of platelet gp IIb, IIIa, a receptor for VWF and fibrinogen
Inheritance	Autosomal dominant	Autosomal recessive	Autosomal recessive
Platelet appearance	Normal	Macrothrombocytes	Normal
Aggregometry			
Ristocetin	Decreased	Decreased	Normal
ADP	Normal	Normal	Decreased
Collagen	Normal	Normal	Decreased

gp = glycoprotein, VWF = von Willebrand factor, ADP = adenosine diphosphate.

119. What conditions result in an acquired platelet defect?

The biggest offender in this category is aspirin. Platelet cyclooxygenase is irreversibly inhibited by low doses of aspirin. As a result, the platelet has lifelong impaired function. Aspirin exacerbates the bleeding tendencies associated with von Willebrand's disease and other platelet disorders and by itself can produce prolongation of the bleeding time. It is important to note that the bleeding time does not predict the risk of hemorrhage in an individual patient. The potential benefit of this aspirin effect is to reduce platelet activity in critical areas, such as a stenosed coronary artery. The typical finding in platelet aggregometry with aspirin-treated platelets is the absence of the secondary wave of aggregation produced by ADP.

Another important acquired disorder of platelet function is that associated with uremia. Although the pathogenesis of this mild hemostatic defect is poorly understood, it appears that the administration of the vasopressin analog desmopressin increases VWF and shortens the bleeding time.

George JN, Shattil SJ: The clinical importance of acquired abnormalities of platelet function. N Engl J Med 324:27–39, 1991.

120. What two factor deficiencies result in hemophilia? What is their pattern of inheritance?

Hemophilia results from a deficiency of factor VIII (hemophilia A) or factor IX (hemophilia B). These are X-linked disorders, and the family history of an affected boy reveals affected maternal uncles and cousins. Patients may have mild or severe disease. Severe disease requires frequent administration of factor VIII or IX concentrates. In the past, hemophilia was a crippling disorder because of the frequency of hemarthroses and arthritis. Prophylactic administration of factor VIII concentrate after trauma has reduced the incidence of complications dramatically.

Hoyer LW: Hemophilia A. N Engl J Med 330:38–47, 1994.

121. How necessary is a preoperative measurement of prothrombin time (PT) and partial thromboplastin time (PTT) in patients without a history of bleeding?

Although physicians routinely order a preoperative or prebiopsy PT and PTT, the value of these tests as screens for coagulation defects has been disputed. In recent studies, no advantage was seen in performing either test in asymptomatic patients. The low prevalence of clinically important, yet unsuspected bleeding disorders results in more false-positive than true-positive results. However, both tests are indicated in symptomatic patients and for monitoring of warfarin (via PT) or heparin (via PTT) administration.

Suchman AL, Griner PA: Diagnostic uses of the activated partial thromboplastin time and prothrombin time. Ann Intern Med 104:810–816, 1986.

122. What questions about bleeding problems need to be asked in the history?

The patient interview should include questions about personal or family history of bleeding problems, including prolonged bleeding after dental extraction, injury, or surgical procedure.

Patients should be asked about frequent nosebleeds, menorrhagia, melena, and bruising. A history of liver disease, obvious malnutrition, or malabsorption syndrome also should be sought. Although irrelevant to PT and PTT, a recent history of aspirin ingestion needs to be sought. The physical exam should include inspection of the skin and mucosa for purpura or petechiae, hematomas, and ecchymotic lesions.

123. What hereditary disorders result in a prolonged PTT without bleeding?

When routine preoperative screening PT and PTT tests are obtained, occasional patients have a dramatic, reproducible prolongation of the PTT but no historical or physical findings to suggest a hemostatic disorder. Familial disorders causing this phenomenon are (1) hereditary deficiency of factor XII (Hageman factor) and (2) deficiency of factors in the contact activation system that activates XII, including Fletcher factor (prekallikrein) and Fitzgerald factor (high-MW kininogen). These disorders produce an interesting in-vitro phenomenon that does not seem to result in any hemorrhagic tendency. In fact, Mr. Hageman, the first person recognized to be deficient in factor XII, died of pulmonary embolism.

124. What is the lupus anticoagulant (LA)? What is its relationship to the antiphospholipid syndrome?

LA is an autoantibody that binds to the phospholipid component required in the formation of the prothrombin activation complex. Its presence on the phospholipid disrupts the association between factor Xa, prothrombin, factor V, and calcium, leading to an abnormally long PTT (and sometimes PT). The name is truly a misnomer because in vivo it is not an anticoagulant, nor does it occur only in patients with lupus. There is a high but incomplete level of concordance with other known phospholipid antibodies, such as anticardiolipin antibodies.

The term **antiphospholipid antibody syndrome** (APS) refers to patients with antiphospholipid antibodies that react with cardiolipin or with β_2-glycoprotein I. Some of these patients also may have typical LAs. APS and LA are associated with thrombosis (arterial and venous), recurrent pregnancy loss, and thrombocytopenia.

Greaves M: Antiphospholipid antibodies and thrrombosis. Lancet 353: 1348–1353, 1999.

125. What are the causes of disseminated intravascular coagulation (DIC)?

Infections
  Viral (epidemic hemorrhagic fevers, herpes, rubella)
  Rickettsial (Rocky Mountain spotted fever)
  Bacterial (gram-negative sepsis, meningococcemia)
  Fungal (histoplasmosis)
  Protozoan (malaria)
Neoplasms
  Carcinomas (prostate, pancreas, breast, lung, ovary)
  Acute promyelocytic leukemia
Vascular disease
  Cavernous hemangiomas (Kasabach-Merritt syndrome)
  Aneurysms
Collagen-vascular disease
  Vasculitis
  Polyarteritis
  Systemic lupus erythematosus
Obstetric complications
  Abruptio placentae
  Septic abortion
  Amniotic fluid embolism
  Intrauterine fetal death
  Saline-, urea-induced abortions
  Eclampsia
Hemolytic transfusion reactions
Hypothermia-rewarming
Shock
Cocaine-induced rhabdomyolysis
Use of factor IX concentrates

Colman RW, et al: Disseminated intravascular coagulation. Annu Rev Med 30:359, 1979.

126. When DIC is present, which coagulation tests are abnormal?

DIC occurs in patients with inappropriate activation of thrombin and disseminated clotting, which in turn is associated with increased fibrinolysis. During this process, multiple coagulation factors are consumed. Byproducts of thrombin and plasmin activity circulate as well. As endothelial cell damage occurs, there is consumption of platelets and, in some instances, fragmentation of RBCs, resulting in significant intravascular hemolysis. Although DIC is often a hemorrhagic condition, certain patients present with thrombotic complications: digital ischemia, decreased mentation, migrating thrombophlebitis, and renal involvement.

Laboratory Findings in DIC

Peripheral blood smear	
Platelets	↓
Red cell fragmentation	Present
PT, PTT	Both ↑
Fibrinogen	↓
Fibrin degradation products	↑
D-dimers	↑
Platelet count	↓

From Levi M, Ten Cate H: Disseminated intravascular coagulation. N Engl J Med 341: 586–592, 1999.

127. How does the bleeding diathesis associated with liver disease resemble DIC?

The liver may not be the seat of the soul, but it is definitely the site of production of all clotting factors (except von Willebrand factor). Severe liver disease compromises hemostasis in a number of ways. Most readily detected is a decrease in the activity of the vitamin K-dependent factors II, VII, IX, and X. Patients with severe liver disease have a prolonged PT and PTT that does not improve after the administration of vitamin K.

Low fibrinogen levels also elaborate a poorly functioning fibrinogen. Dysfibrinogenemia produces prolongation of the PT, PTT, and thrombin time. With the onset of cirrhosis and portal hypertension, splenomegaly and a reduced platelet count occur. Because the liver is also an important organ of clearance of plasminogen activators, increased fibrin degradation products may be measured. Thus, the laboratory abnormalities in severe liver disease may mimic DIC.

128. Patients receiving certain antibiotics develop prolongation of the PT and PTT. Which antibiotics, and why?

Certain β-lactam antibiotics reduce the prothrombin level. This characteristic is associated with a methylthiotetrazole substitution that appears to inhibit microsomal carboxylase activity, which in turn results in decreased γ-carboxylation of the vitamin K-dependent factors. Antibiotics in general may reduce vitamin K levels by destroying the bacterial flora of the gut, which also provide vitamin K. Thus, the combination of prolonged reduced feeding and antibiotic administration is associated with vitamin K deficiency and bleeding diathesis. When β-lactam antibiotics with the methylthiotetrazole substitution are administered, the inhibition of the vitamin K-dependent carboxylase results in the more rapid onset of a bleeding diathesis.

Platelet function can be impaired by several antibiotics, such as carbenicillin or ticarcillin. Platelet function also may be affected by some of the β-lactam antibiotics (e.g., moxalactam), prolonging the bleeding time. Presumably, antibiotics interact with the platelet membrane to block receptor-mediated aggregation. Unfortunately, some patients who receive β-lactam antibiotics experience a "double whammy" of hypoprothrombinemia and platelet dysfunction. Bleeding may be avoided by concomitant administration of vitamin K and using the lowest antibiotic dose possible. Patients may benefit from platelet transfusions.

129. Which congenital disorders are associated with an increased incidence of deep venous thromboembolism (DVT)?

The occurrence of DVT in a young person, a family history of thrombosis, thrombosis at unusual sites (such as the mesenteric vein), or recurrent thrombosis without precipitating factors suggests a hypercoagulable state. Activated protein C inhibits coagulation by inactivating factors Va and VIIIa. A mutation in factor V (V_{Leiden}), arg506 to gly, results in resistance of factor Va to activated protein C (APC). APC resistance has a remarkably high prevalence in certain populations and may account for 30% of patients thought to have a congenital or hereditary susceptibility to thrombosis ("thrombophilia"). Patients with these disorders need careful evaluation and family screening. Symptomatic pastients are cautiously managed with warfrain anticoagulation.

Primary Hereditary Factors Associated with Hypercoagulability

FACTOR	PREVALENCE OF PATIENTS WITH DVT (%)
Factor V Leiden	20
Prothrombin G20210A	6
Protein C deficiency	3
Protein S deficiency	2
Antithrombin III deficiency	1
Homocystinemia	10

From Rosendaal FR: Venous thrombosis: A multicausal disease. Lancet 353:1167–1173, 1999.

130. What serious complication can occur with anticoagulation therapy in patients with congenital hypercoagulable states?

Proteins C and S are vitamin K-dependent anticoagulants. When patients are placed on warfarin for treatment of DVT, the goal of therapy is to reduce the activity of procoagulant factors (VII included). This effect is monitored by following the PT, which detects early changes in the activity of factor VII. When warfarin therapy is initiated, particularly at high doses or in patients with a congenital deficiency, the levels of protein C may drop precipitously before the onset of anticoagulation because of decreased factor VII activity. One consequence of this drop is a serious disorder, known as warfarin skin necrosis.

131. What are the acquired causes of hypercoagulability?

Secondary Hypercoagulable States

Abnormalities of coagulation and fibrinolysis	Abnormalities of blood vessels and rheology
Malignancy	Conditions promoting venous stasis (immobilization, obesity, advanced age, postoperative state)
Pregnancy	
Use of oral contraceptives	Artificial surfaces
Infusion of prothrombin complex concentrates	Vasculitis and chronic occlusive arterial disease
Nephrotic syndrome	Homocystinuria
Disseminated intravascular coagulation	Hyperviscosity (polycythemia, leukemia, sickle cell disease, leukoagglutination, increased serum viscosity)
Antiphospholipid antibody syndrome,	
Lupus anticoagulant	
Abnormalities of platelets	Thrombotic thrombocytopenic purpura
Myeloproliferative disorders	
Paroxysmal nocturnal hemoglobinuria	
Hyperlipidemia	
Diabetes mellitus	
Heparin-induced thrombocytopenia	

Adapted from Schafer AI: The hypercoagulable states. Ann Intern Med 102:818, 1985, with permission.

132. What is thrombopoietin?

Thrombopoietin acts in concert with other growth factors, such as IL-3, IL-6, and IL-11, to increase the number of megakaryocytic precursors. Thrombopoietin appears to be the predominant factor in megakaryocyte maturation. Thrombopoietin levels vary inversely with platelet counts in bone marrow failure syndromes. Mature platelets remove thrombopoietin from plasma so that levels are low when the platelet count is high. However, patients with clonal disorders associated with thrombocytosis, such as essential thrombocytosis, may have elevated thrombopoietin levels because of the decreased binding of thrombopoietin to presumably abnormal megakaryocytes and platelets.

Kaushansky K: Thrombopoietin. N Engl J Med 339:746–754, 1999.

133. Why does the platelet count need to be monitored in patients receiving heparin?

Heparin-induced thrombocytopenia (HIT) occurs in 1–3 % of patients who receive heparin as prophylaxis or treatment for thrombosis or when heparin is used to flush catheters. Heparin-naive patients may develop thrombocytopenia 7–10 days after initiation of the drug. Unlike other causes of drug-induced thrombocytopenia, HIT is associated with thrombosis—venous and arterial. Heparin should be discontinued, and another form of anticoagulation (heparan, argatroban or hirudin) should be substituted.

Warkentin TE, Kelton JG: A 14-year study of heparin-induced thrombocytopenia. Am J Med 101:502–507, 1996.

BIBLIOGRAPHY

1. Hoffbrand AV, Fantini B (eds): A Century of Hematology. Semin Hematol 36(Suppl 7), 1999.
2. Lee GR, et al (eds): Wintrobe's Clinical Hematology, 10th ed, Baltimore, Williams & Wilkins, 1999.
3. Loscalzo J, Schafer AI (eds): Thrombosis and Hemorrhage, 2nd ed. Boston, Blackwell, 1998.
Useful websites
www.hematology.org
www.bloodline.net

10. PULMONARY MEDICINE

Sheila Goodnight-White, M.D.

If a man will begin with certainties, he shall end in doubts; but if he will be content to begin with doubts, he shall end in certainties.
Francis Bacon (1561–1626)
Advancement of Learning (1605)

DIAPHRAGM, n. A muscular partition separating disorders of the chest from disorders of the bowels.
Ambrose Bierce (1842–1914)
The Devil's Dictionary

PHYSIOLOGY

1. Define hypoxemia.
Hypoxemia usually is defined as a partial arterial oxygen tension (PaO_2) < 60 mmHg.

2. List and explain the five basic pathophysiologic mechanisms that can cause hypoxemia.
1. **Decreased inspired oxygen (PIO_2).** Any condition that leads to a decrease in the oxygen content of inspired gas can lead to hypoxemia. This form of hypoxemia can be expressed as a decrease in the FIO_2 (fraction of inspired gas composed of oxygen) or significant changes in barometric pressure (P_{atm}). Situations leading to this problem include high altitude, flying in a nonpressurized airplane cabin, or rebreathing expired gases (as in a paper bag or closed space).
2. **Hypoventilation.** Any condition that interferes with the normal movement of gas in and out of the alveoli (decreased minute ventilation), resulting in the inability to maintain normal arterial carbon dioxide (CO_2), leads to hypoxemia. Examples include CNS impairment, respiratory muscle fatigue, or neuromuscular disease. In patients with normal lungs, the rise in the partial pressure of CO_2 in arterial blood ($PaCO_2$) is associated with a fall in PaO_2, as defined by the alveolar gas equation. The result is a normal alveolar-arterial oxygen difference.
3. **Diffusion abnormality.** Any condition that interferes with the normal diffusion of oxygen from the alveolar space into the capillaries can lead to hypoxemia. For example, all causes of diffuse interstitial pulmonary fibrosis may result in hypoxemia.
4. **Ventilation-perfusion (V/Q) abnormalities.** Any condition that leads to a mismatching of ventilation and perfusion can cause hypoxemia. Most pulmonary disorders are associated with some degree of V/Q mismatching. This is the most common cause of hypoxemia and is responsive to oxygen therapy.
5. **Shunt.** Any condition that leads to perfusion of nonventilated lung can lead to hypoxemia. A shunt is an absolute mismatching of ventilation and perfusion in which there is perfusion of alveoli with absolutely no ventilation. Examples include pulmonary arteriovenous (AV) fistulae, intracardiac shunts, and conditions characterized by perfusion of alveoli that are filled with pus, fluid, or other substances (pneumonia, pulmonary edema, intrapulmonary hemorrhage). Hypoxemia secondary to shunting is refractory to oxygen therapy.

3. How can the five basic mechanisms of hypoxemia be differentiated?
The values of PaO_2, $PaCO_2$, alveolar–arterial oxygen (A–aO_2) difference, and response to breathing 100% oxygen can be used to separate the basic causes of hypoxemia.

Differentiation of the Causes of Hypoxemia

MECHANISM	PaO_2	$PaCO_2$	A–aO_2 GRADIENT	RESPONSE TO 100% O_2
PIO_2	↓	↔ or ↓	↔	N/A
Hypoventilation	↓	↑	↔	N/A
Diffusion abnormality	↓	↔ or ↓	↑	Yes
V/Q mismatch	↓	↔ or ↓	↑	Yes
Shunt	↓	↔ or ↓	↑	No

↓ = decreased, ↔ = normal, ↑ = increased, N/A = not applicable.

4. What is the alveolar-arterial oxygen difference (PA-aO_2)?

The alveolar-arterial oxygen difference aids in evaluating the effectiveness of gas exchange. The PA-aO_2 is the difference in the partial pressure of oxygen between alveolar air (PAO_2) and arterial blood (PaO_2):

$$PA\text{-}aO_2 = PAO_2 - PaO_2$$

A normal PA-aO_2 is usually < 10 mmHg in a patient breathing room air. In conditions that interfere with gas exchange between the alveoli and pulmonary capillaries, the PA-aO_2 increases. In pure hypoventilation, when lung function is not impaired, the PA-aO_2 is normal.

5. How do you calculate the PA-aO_2?

The PA-aO_2 can be calculated by estimating the alveolar PO_2 (PAO_2) using a simplified form of the alveolar gas equation and then subtracting this estimate from the arterial PO_2 (PaO_2), as measured by arterial blood gas analysis:

$$PAO_2 = PIO_2 - (PaCO_2/RQ)$$

PIO_2 (partial pressure of oxygen in inspired gas) is calculated as follows:

$$PIO_2 = FIO_2 (P_{atm} - PH_2O)$$

The RQ is the respiratory quotient (usually assumed to be 0.8), FIO_2 is the fraction of the inspired gas that is oxygen (21% in room air), P_{atm} is the atmospheric pressure (760 mmHg at sea level), and PH_2O is the vapor pressure of water (assumed to be 47 mmHg). Therefore, in a patient breathing room air with a PAO_2 of 94 mmHg and $PaCO_2$ of 40 mmHg, the PAO_2 is calculated as follows:

$$PAO_2 = 0.21 (760 - 47) - 40/0.8 = 150 - 50 = 100 \text{ mmHg}$$

Therefore, the PA-aO_2 is within normal limits:

$$PA\text{-}aO_2 = PAO_2 - PaO_2 = 100 - 94 = 6 \text{ mmHg}$$

6. Does the PA-aO_2 increase with age?

Yes. Oxygenation normally decreases slightly with increasing age. An age-adjusted normal PA-aO_2 can be estimated as follows: 2.5 + 0.21(age). Thus, a healthy 70-year-old is expected to have a PA-aO_2 of approximately 17 mmHg. Of course, this equation yields only an approximation; there may be a great deal of individual variation.

7. How is the RQ used in the alveolar air equation? What factors affect its value?

The RQ is the ratio of CO_2 produced per unit of O_2 consumed at the cellular level. It ranges from 0.7 when fatty acids are the substrate to 1.0 when carbohydrates are the substrate. Usually, a value of 0.8 can be used, which reflects the normal mixture of substrates.

8. What is the oxyhemoglobin equilibrium curve? What does it demonstrate?

The oxyhemoglobin equilibrium curve (or dissociation curve) is a plot of the hemoglobin percent saturation (SaO_2) against the PaO_2. It demonstrates the binding reaction of hemoglobin and oxygen.

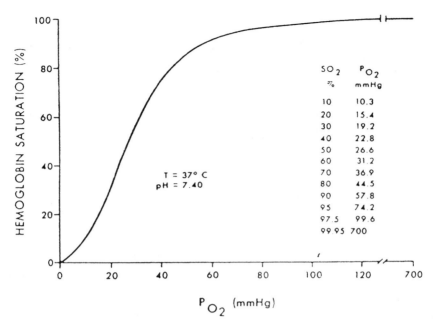

SO$_2$ %	PO$_2$ mmHg
10	10.3
20	15.4
30	19.2
40	22.8
50	26.6
60	31.2
70	36.9
80	44.5
90	57.8
95	74.2
97.5	99.6
99.95	700

Normal oxyhemoglobin dissociation curve for humans. (From Murray JF: The Normal Lung, 2nd ed. Philadelphia, W.B. Saunders, 1986, p 174, with permission.)

The sigmoid-shaped curve shows that the binding (or releasing) of oxygen and hemoglobin is not a linear relationship (as is the case with dissolved oxygen). Oxygen is readily released at the lower range of PaO$_2$ values but very tightly held at the upper range of PaO$_2$ values—i.e., the affinity of hemoglobin for oxygen increases as more oxygen molecules bind to it. This enables the oxygen content of blood to remain high at high PaO$_2$ levels but still allows hemoglobin to release oxygen readily as the PaO$_2$ drops below 60 mmHg (the "steep" part of the curve).

9. How do you calculate the oxygen content of blood (CaO$_2$)?

CaO$_2$ includes the oxygen bound to hemoglobin, represented by hemoglobin (Hb) and percent saturation (SaO$_2$), and the oxygen dissolved in solution in the plasma, represented by PaO$_2$. It can be calculated as follows:

$$CaO_2 = O_2 \text{ bound to Hb} + O_2 \text{ dissolved in plasma}$$
$$= (1.34 \times Hb \times SaO_2) + (PaO_2 \times 0.003)$$

The normal value is 16–20 ml/100 ml of blood. Over 99% of the oxygen content of blood is bound to hemoglobin. Only a very minor part of the total is dissolved oxygen (that which is measured by PaO$_2$). The obvious clinical importance of this fact is that any therapy that raises the PaO$_2$ while allowing the patient to remain anemic will have minimal effect on the oxygen-carrying capacity of the blood.

10. What is the P$_{50}$?

P$_{50}$ is the PaO$_2$ that corresponds to a hemoglobin saturation (SaO$_2$) of 50% under conditions of standard temperature (37°C) and pH (7.40). Normally it is 26.6 mmHg. P$_{50}$ is a measure of the affinity of hemoglobin for oxygen. A higher P$_{50}$ represents less hemoglobin affinity for oxygen, whereas a lower P$_{50}$ represents increased hemoglobin affinity for oxygen. The P$_{50}$ varies with conditions that shift the oxyhemoglobin equilibrium curve.

11. Clinicians refer to a shift of the oxyhemoglobin equilibrium curve to the left or right. What does this mean?

Because the curve represents the affinity of hemoglobin for oxygen over the range of PaO_2, a shift in the curve in either direction represents a change in that affinity. A shift of the curve to the left represents an increase in the affinity of hemoglobin for oxygen; i.e., oxygen is taken up more readily and released less readily for any given PaO_2. Conversely, a shift to the right represents a decrease in affinity; i.e., oxygen is taken up less readily and released more readily.

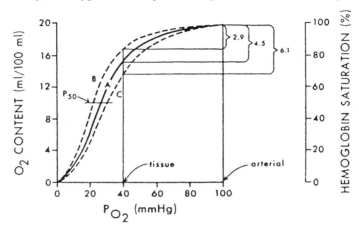

Effects of increases and decreases in O_2 affinity on the amount of O_2 available at the PO_2 values prevailing in arterial blood and tissues. Curve A = normal blood, curve B = blood with increased affinity (decreased P_{50}); and curve C = blood with decreased affinity (increased P_{50}). (From Murray JF: The Normal Lung, 2nd ed. Philadelphia, W.B. Saunders, 1986, p 175, with permission.)

12. What factors can shift the oxyhemoglobin equilibrium curve?

SHIFT TO THE LEFT (↑ Hb/O_2 AFFINITY)	SHIFT TO THE RIGHT (↓ Hb/O_2 AFFINITY)
Hypothermia	Hyperthermia/fever
Alkalosis	Acidosis
Hypocapnia	Hypercapnia
↓ 2,3DPG	↑ 2,3DPG
↑ Carboxyhemoglobin	↓ Carboxyhemoglobin
Hemoglobin F (Chesapeake, Yakima, Ranier)	Hemoglobin E (Seattle, Kansas)

DGP = diphosphoglycerate.

13. If the dissolved oxygen content of blood, measured by the PaO_2, is so small compared with the oxygen bound to hemoglobin, why do we measure and follow the PaO_2 as we treat patients?

The oxyhemoglobin equilibrium curve answers this question. The PaO_2, although directly measuring only a tiny fraction of the total oxygen content of blood, is related to the total oxygen content through the dissociation curve. As the PaO_2 drops below 60 mmHg, the curve is very steep, whereas at a PaO_2 over 60 mmHg, the curve is flat. A drop of PaO_2 from 100 to 60 mmHg (drop of 40 mmHg) represents a drop of SaO_2 from 99% to 90%, a loss of only 9% of the blood's total oxygen content. However, a further drop of 40 mmHg (from a PaO_2 of 60 to 20 mmHg) represents a drop in SaO_2 from 90% to about 30%, or a loss of 60% of the blood's total oxygen content. Therapeutic guidelines call for maintaining the PaO_2 above 60 mmHg. Below this level, small decreases in PaO_2 are accompanied by very large drops in the SaO_2 and therefore very large drops in the total oxygen content of blood.

14. When is oxygen toxic?

Oxygen toxicity is an iatrogenic disease caused by prolonged administration of high concentrations of supplemental oxygen, usually an FiO_2 greater than 60% for longer than 72 hours. Toxicity can occur earlier with higher concentrations of oxygen. Initially, it is manifested by an acute exudative phase, consisting of a decrease in vital capacity, interstitial and alveolar edema, decreased lung compliance, decreased diffusion capacity, and an increased $A–aO_2$ gradient. The chronic proliferative phase also has been seen in humans and animals on prolonged oxygen therapy. Oxygen toxicity is thought to result from the effect of oxygen free radicals on the lung interstitium.

15. What is the goal of oxygen therapy?

The goal of oxygen therapy is to provide adequate supplemental oxygen to maintain tissue oxygenation, usually at a PaO_2 just over 60 mmHg. Attempts to increase the PaO_2 further do not result in significant increases in the oxygen content of blood but may increase the risk of oxygen toxicity. Because of oxygen toxicity, use of high concentrations of therapeutic oxygen (> 60%) should be limited to as short a duration as possible.

DIAGNOSTIC TECHNIQUES

16. What are the indications for bronchoscopy?

Diagnostic uses
- Evaluation of indeterminate lung lesions (abnormal chest film)
- Assessment of airway patency, including problems associated with endotracheal tubes, wheeze, and stridor
- Investigation of unexplained symptoms (e.g., cough, hemoptysis, stridor) or unexplained findings (recurrent laryngeal nerve paralysis, recent diaphragmatic paralysis)
- Evaluation of suspicious or malignant sputum cytology
- Preoperative staging of cancer
- Bronchoalveolar lavage for interstitial lung disease
- Specimen collection for selective cultures/suspected infection
- Determination of the extent of injury secondary to burns, inhalation, and other mishaps

Therapeutic uses
- Removal of mucous plugs/secretions, foreign bodies
- Assistance with difficult endotracheal intubations
- Treatment of endobronchial neoplasms

Prakash UBS, et al: Bronchoscopy in North America: The ACCP survey. Chest 100:1668–1675, 1991.

17. What are the contraindications and complications of fiberoptic bronchoscopy?

Although there are no *absolute* contraindications to bronchoscopy, sound clinical judgment should guide any decision concerning an invasive procedure with potential risk for morbidity and mortality. Well-trained and experienced bronchoscopists, careful supervision, and consideration of potentially high-risk conditions (e.g., uremia, thrombocytopenia, pulmonary hypertension, bleeding diathesis) reduce morbidity and mortality risks.

In a large series of over 24,000 cases, the mortality rate was 0.01% and the complication rate was 0.08%. In 4,273 consecutive flexible bronchoscopies reviewed in another large study, the rate of major complications (e.g., significant hemorrhage, pneumothorax, respiratory failure) was 0.5%, and the rate of minor complications (e.g., syncope, epistaxis, bronchospasm) was 0.8%. Complications resulting from fiberoptic bronchoscopy include reaction to topical anesthetic, trauma, laryngospasm, bronchospasm, hypoventilation, pneumothorax, hemorrhage, cardiac arrhythmia, myocardial infarction, hypoxemia, ruptured lung abscess with flooding of airways, and post-bronchoscopy fever/infection.

Pue CA, Pacht ER: Complications of fiberoptic bronchoscopy at a university hospital. Chest 107:430–432, 1995.

18. Which conditions place patients at increased risk during bronchoscopy?

Bleeding diathesis	Inability to cooperate with the exam
Hypoxia	Cardiac arrhythmias
Unstable asthma	Recent myocardial infarction
Acute hypercapnia	Partial tracheal obstruction
Hepatitis	Uremia
Lung abscess	Immunosuppression
Superior vena cava syndrome	Respiratory failure requiring mechanical ventilation

19. What is the most common clinical use of pulmonary function tests (PFTs)?

PFTs help to identify and quantify abnormalities of the pulmonary system, which usually are categorized as obstructive or restrictive. By far the most common use of PFTs is the evaluation of obstructive airway disease. Causes of an obstructive ventilatory defect include emphysema, bronchitis, asthma, bronchiolitis, and upper airway obstruction (tumors, foreign bodies, stenosis, and edema). Obstruction is defined as a decrease in forced expiratory flow rates. The FEV_1 (forced expiratory volume in 1 second) and FEV_1/FVC (forced vital capacity) are both reduced. Other supporting data include increased residual volume and increased airway resistance.

20. What lung volumes and capacities are measured with PFTs?

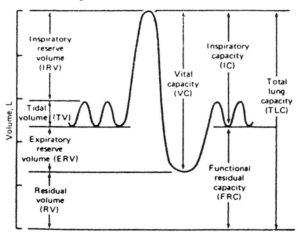

Summary of lung volumes and capacities measured with PFTs. (From Fishman AP: Pulmonary Diseases and Disorders. New York, McGraw-Hill, 1998, p 150, with permission.)

Functional residual capacity (FRC) is the volume of air that remains in the lungs at the end of a normal respiration.

Tidal volume (TV) is the volume of air that is drawn into the lungs during inspiration from the end-expiratory position (it also leaves the lungs passively during expiration in the course of quiet breathing).

Expiratory reserve volume (ERV) is the maximal volume of air that can be forcibly exhaled after a quiet expiration has been completed (i.e., from the end-expiratory position).

Residual volume (RV) is the volume of air that remains in the lungs after a maximal expiratory effort.

Inspiratory capacity (IC) is the maximal volume of air that can be inhaled from the end-expiratory position. It consists of two subdivisions: tidal volume and inspiratory reserve volume (IRV).

Total lung capacity (TLC) is the total volume of air contained in the lungs at the end of a maximal inspiration.

Vital capacity (VC) is the volume of air that is exhaled by a maximal expiration after a maximal inspiration.

21. What are the common causes of restrictive pulmonary disease?
- Interstitial lung disease (fibrosis, pneumoconiosis, edema)
- Chest wall disease (kyphoscoliosis, neuromuscular disease)
- Space-occupying lesions (tumors, cysts)
- Pleural disease (effusion, pneumothorax)
- Extrathoracic conditions (obesity, ascites, pregnancy)

22. What are the PFT findings suggestive of a restrictive ventilatory defect?
A restrictive defect implies that lung volumes are decreased with normal expiratory flow rates (decreased vital capacity, normal expiratory flow rates, and normal maximal voluntary ventilation). Certain diagnosis of a restrictive process rests on a decreased total lung capacity (TLC). Other supporting data for a restrictive defect may include decreased lung compliance and decreased diffusion of carbon monoxide (DL_{CO}).

23. Which test helps to differentiate between emphysema and chronic bronchitis as the cause of an obstructive ventilatory defect?
The finding of an obstructive pattern associated with a normal single-breath DL_{CO} argues against emphysema, whereas an obstructive defect with a decreased DL_{CO} suggests the presence of anatomic emphysema with a concomitant loss of alveolar capillary bed.

American Thoracic Society: Standards for the diagnosis and care of patients with chronic obstructive pulmonary disease. Am J Respir Crit Care Med 152(Pt 2):S77–S120, 1995.

24. What causes a reduced DL_{CO}?
The diffusing capacity of carbon monoxide (DL_{CO}) estimates the transfer of oxygen from the alveolus to the red blood cell. The diffusion is determined by the thickness of the alveolar-capillary membrane, the "driving pressure" or oxygen tension difference between the alveolus and capillary, and the area of the alveolar-capillary membrane.

Causes of Decreased Diffusing Capacity

DECREASED AREA FOR DIFFUSION	INCREASED THICKNESS OF ALVEOLAR-CAPILLARY MEMBRANE
Emphysema	Idiopathic pulmonary fibrosis
Lung/lobe resection	Pulmonary sarcoidosis
Bronchial obstruction, as by tumor	Asbestosis
Multiple pulmonary emboli	Alveolar proteinosis
Anemia	Hypersensitivity pneumonitis, including farmer's lung
Miscellaneous	Histiocytosis X
High CO back pressure from smoking	Congestive heart failure
Pregnancy	Collagen vascular disease
Ventilation-perfusion mismatch	Drug-induced alveolitis or fibrosis

From Hyatt RE, Scanlon PD, Nakamura M: Interpretation of Pulmonary Function Tests: A Practical Guide. Philadelphia, Lippincott-Raven, 1997, p 45 with permission.)

25. What are the indications for preoperative PFTs? How do they help to assess postoperative risk?
Patient factors

Known pulmonary dysfunction	Advanced age
Current smoking, especially	Obesity
if > 1 pack/day	Thoracic cage deformity (e.g., kyphoscoliosis)
Chronic productive cough	Neuromuscular disease (e.g., amyotrophic lateral
Recent respiratory infection	sclerosis, myasthenia gravis)

Procedural factors
Thoracic or upper abdominal operation
Pulmonary resection
Prolonged anesthesia

Guidelines for Estimating Postoperative Risks

TEST	INCREASED RISK	HIGH RISK
FVC	< 50% predicted	< 1.5 L
FEV_1	< 2.0L or < 50% predicted	< 1 .0 L
MVV		< 50 % predicted
$PaCO_2$		> 45 mmHg

FVC = forced vital capacity, FEV_1 = forced expiratory volume in 1 second, MVV = maximal voluntary ventilation, $PaCO_2$ = arterial tension of carbon dioxide.
From Hyatt RE, Scanlon PD, Nakamura M: Interpretation of Pulmonary Function Tests: A Practical Guide. Philadelphia, Lippincott-Raven, 1997, p 95, with permission.

PLEURAL EFFUSION

26. What are the two basic types of pleural effusion?
    A pleural effusion represents an increase in fluid in the pleural space, which may be due to increased hydrostatic pressure, decreased oncotic pressure, decreased pleural space pressure (lung collapse), obstruction of lymphatic drainage, or increased permeability. A **transudative** effusion classically is associated with volume overload states, such as congestive heart failure, nephrotic syndrome, and cirrhosis. An **exudative** effusion is a protein-rich effusion secondary to inflammation of the pleura or failure of lymphatic protein removal. Exudates occur in neoplasms, infection, and various collagen vascular diseases.

27. What findings on physical examination are suggestive of a pleural effusion?
    Small effusions (< 500 ml) frequently have minimal findings. Larger effusions demonstrate dullness to percussion, diminished breath sounds, and reduced tactile and vocal fremitus over the involved hemithorax. Large effusions (> 1500 ml), with concomitant atelectasis, demonstrate bronchial breath sounds, egophony (a sound on auscultation like the bleating of a goat), and inspiratory lag. Pleural friction rubs may be noted in the early stages or as the effusion resolves.

28. Which diagnostic tests are used to distinguish transudative from exudative pleural effusions? What are Light's criteria?
    Thoracentesis (percutaneous removal of pleural fluid) is used to obtain pleural fluid for analysis. An exudative pleural effusion meets one or more of the following criteria (Light's criteria), whereas a transudative meets none:
    1. Pleural fluid protein/serum protein ratio > 0.5
    2. Pleural fluid lactate dehydrogenase (LDH)/serum LDH ratio > 0.6
    3. Pleural fluid LDH > two-thirds the upper limit of normal for serum
    Other tests that may be helpful include pleural fluid glucose, pH, cell count and WBC differential, amylase, Gram stain, special stains as clinically indicated, and culture. Pleural glucose < 60% of the serum value suggests infection, rheumatoid arthritis, or neoplasm. A pH < 7.30 suggests empyema/infection. An elevated amylase in a left-sided pleural effusion may be secondary to pancreatitis. Pleural fluid WBC counts and differentials are usually of limited value, but lymphocyte predominance may suggest tuberculosis or malignancy. Cytologic examination is indicated if a neoplasm is suspected.

29. Which radiologic test should be performed in patients with suspected pleural effusion?
    A small amount of pleural fluid can be detected as the obliteration of the posterior part of the diaphragm on lateral chest x-ray (CXR). When a larger amount of fluid is present, the lateral

costophrenic angle on the posteroanterior radiograph is blunted. When pleural fluid is suspected, lateral decubitus films should be obtained to detect free fluid gravitating to the dependent side and accumulating between the chest wall and lung. The amount of fluid present can be roughly quantified by measuring the distance between the inner border of the chest wall and the outer border of the lung. When this distance is < 10 mm, the amount of fluid present is small, and usually a diagnostic thoracentesis should be performed under ultrasonographic guidance.

30. What is an empyema?

Empyema describes the presence of infected liquid or frank pus in the pleural space. It may result from infection of a contiguous structure, instrumentation of the pleural space, or hematogenous spread of infection. The diagnosis is made by examination of the pleural fluid obtained from thoracentesis. A Gram stain and culture of the pleural fluid may reveal the causative organism.

31. What is the significance of a parapneumonic effusion?

A parapneumonic effusion is any effusion associated with pneumonia. As many as 40% of all pneumonias may be associated with a pleural effusion. Morbidity and mortality rates are higher in pneumonias with effusion than in pneumonia alone. Most effusions resolve without specific intervention. However, the effusion may be complicated and require tube thoracotomy (chest tube) or surgical decortication. In addition to protein and LDH analysis, pleural fluid pH, Gram stain/culture, and glucose may help to classify parapneumonic effusions and determine an appropriate treatment plan.

Classification and Treatment Scheme for Parapneumonic Effusions and Empyema

CLASS/DESCRIPTION	TREATMENT
Class 1: nonsignificant pleural effusion Small < 10 mm thick on decubitus film	No thoracentesis indicated
Class 2: typical parapneumonic pleural effusion > 10 mm thick Glucose > 40 mg/dl, pH >7.20 Gram stain and culture negative	Antibiotics alone
Class 3: borderline complicated pleural effusion 7.00 < pH > 7.20 and/or LDH >1000 and Glucose > 40 mg/dl Gram stain and culture negative	Antibiotics plus serial thoracentesis
Class 4: simple complicated pleural effusion pH < 7.00 and/or glucose < 40 mg/dl and/or Gram stain or culture positive Not loculated, no frank pus	Tube thoracostomy plus antibiotics
Class 5: complex complicated pleural effusion pH < 7.00 and/or glucose < 40 mg/dl and/or Gram stain or culture positive Multiloculated	Tube thoracostomy plus thrombolytics (rarely requires thoracoscopy or decortication)
Class 6: simple empyema Frank pus present Single locule or free flowing	Tube thoracostomy ± decortication
Class 7: complex empyema Frank pus present Multiple locules	Tube thoracostomy plus thrombolytics Often requires thoracoscopy or decortication

From Light RW: Pleural Diseases. Baltimore, Williams & Wilkins, 1995, p 142, with permission.

32. What other procedures are available if routine pleural fluid analysis fails to diagnose an exudative effusion?

A definitive diagnosis cannot be made in approximately 20% of patients with an exudative effusion. In patients with a suspected neoplasm or tuberculous pleural effusion, a closed-needle biopsy of the parietal pleura may establish the diagnosis. Although the overall yield from pleural fluid cytology is slightly higher, needle biopsy of the pleura is positive in 40% of patients with malignant pleural disease. When tuberculous pleuritis is suspected, a portion of the biopsy should be sent for culture. The initial biopsy is positive for granuloma in 50–80% of patients. The combined results of pleural fluid culture and biopsy have a diagnostic sensitivity of 90% for tuberculosis. Other procedures to be considered are bronchoscopy, if the patient has a parenchymal abnormality on CXR or CT scan; thoracoscopy, which allows direct visualization of the pleural surface; and guided or open pleural biopsy.

HEMOPTYSIS

33. What is hemoptysis? What is its differential diagnosis?

Hemoptysis is defined as blood in the sputum and includes the full range of bloody sputum, from blood streaks to frank blood. In addition to history and physical examination, all patients should have a CXR. Further diagnostic procedures should be guided by the findings of these studies.

Most Common Causes of Hemoptysis

Neoplasm	**Bronchiectasis/infections**
Bronchial carcinoma	Mycobacteria, especially tuberculosis
Metastatic lung cancer	Fungal infections
Adenoma	Lung abscess
Vascular disorders	Necrotizing pneumonia
Pulmonary infarct/embolism	Paragonimiasis
Mitral stenosis	Hydatid cyst
Iatrogenic rupture of pulmonary artery	
by balloon-tipped catheter	**Miscellaneous**
Bronchial-arterial fistula	Anticoagulant therapy
Ruptured thoracic aneurysm	Coagulopathies
Arteriovenous malformation	Goodpasture's syndrome
Vasculitis	Trauma
Behçet's disease	Lymphangioleiomyomatosis
Wegener's granulomatosis	

From Jean-Baptiste E: Clinical assessment and management of massive hemoptysis. Crit Care Med 28:1642–1647, 2000, with permission.

34. What is massive hemoptysis?

Massive hemoptysis implies copious bleeding and has been defined as the expectoration of > 600 ml of blood in a 24-hour period. The prognosis depends on the etiology and magnitude of the bleeding. This potentially lethal and alarming clinical situation requires expeditious evaluation, close observation, and possible surgical intervention.

PNEUMOTHORAX

35. Which population of patients is most likely to experience a primary spontaneous pneumothorax? In which patients is a secondary spontaneous pneumothorax most often seen?

Primary spontaneous pneumothorax, occurring in patients with no history of pulmonary disease, is believed to result from spontaneous rupture of a subpleural emphysematous bleb. Primary spontaneous pneumothorax has a peak incidence at 20–30 years of age, is more common in smokers and exsmokers, has a 4:1 male-to-female ratio, and is seen most often in tall, thin people. **Secondary spontaneous pneumothorax**, occurring in patients with underlying pulmonary disease, is most often seen with chronic obstructive pulmonary disease (COPD).

36. What is the likelihood that spontaneous pneumothorax will recur?

Recurrence rates for both primary and secondary spontaneous pneumothorax range from 10–50%, and approximately 60% of those patients have a third recurrence. After three episodes, the recurrence rate exceeds 85%. Therefore, repeated spontaneous pneumothorax should be treated by pleurodesis or surgical intervention (including parietal pleurectomy).

37. What causes pneumothorax?

Spontaneous pneumothorax, although not common, should be considered in any patient with a history of underlying lung disease and unexplained clinical decompensation. Causes of pneumothorax secondary to underlying lung disease include COPD, asthma, lung abscess, adult respiratory distress syndrome (ARDS), AIDS/*Pneumocystis carinii* pneumonia, neoplasm, Marfan's syndrome, sarcoidosis, cystic fibrosis, tuberculosis, and eosinophilic granuloma. Pneumothorax may be iatrogenic (after thoracentesis or transbronchial biopsy or secondary to barotrauma) or traumatic. Catamenial pneumothorax is rare and occurs in women at the time of menstruation. IV drug abuse (attempting to inject the subclavian or internal jugular vein) also may cause pneumothorax.

38. How does pneumothorax present clinically?

Spontaneous pneumothorax usually occurs at rest. Pleuritic chest pain and dyspnea of acute onset are the most common complaints. The acute pleuritic pain, which is localized to the side of the pneumothorax, may become more of a dull ache with time. Symptoms, especially dyspnea, are more pronounced in patients with underlying pulmonary disease. Findings on physical exam include sinus tachycardia, reduced breath sounds, reduced tactile fremitus, hyperresonance, and reduced chest wall excursion on the ipsilateral side. Findings may be subtle with small pneumothoraces.

39. What is a tension pneumothorax?

Tension pneumothorax is due to unidirectional flow of air into the pleural space from which it cannot escape. Tension pneumothorax develops when intrapleural pressure exceeds atmospheric pressure during expiration, causing collapse of the involved lung, shift of the mediastinum, and potentially acute deterioration in cardiopulmonary status.

40. When should the diagnosis of tension pneumothorax be suspected?

Tension pneumothorax is a medical emergency and requires prompt relief of the positive pleural pressure. It usually is heralded by sudden deterioration in cardiopulmonary status. It should be suspected:

1. In any patient with a history of pneumothorax
2. After a procedure known to cause pneumothorax
3. In patients receiving mechanical ventilation
4. During cardiopulmonary resuscitation, if it is difficult to ventilate the patient or if electromechanical dissociation is present

On physical exam, tension pneumothorax should be suspected if the patient has signs of a significant pneumothorax (no tactile fremitus, markedly decreased or absent breath sounds, and hyperresonance on percussion), cardiopulmonary compromise (rapid pulse, hypotension, cyanosis, electromechanical dissociation), and possibly a shift of the trachea away from the involved side.

41. What is Hamman's sign?

Mediastinal emphysema or pneumomediastinum can be detected on auscultation by the presence of a mediastinal "crunch" coinciding with cardiac systole and diastole. It is named after the American physician, Louis Hamman (1877–1946).

Collins RK: Hamman's crunch: an adventitious sound. J Fam Pract 38:284–286, 1994.

INFECTIONS

42. What is the most common cause of community-acquired pneumonia (CAP)?

CAP is defined as pneumonia contracted in the community rather than in the hospital setting. The most common cause of CAP is *Pneumococcus* spp., which account for up to 55% of cases requiring hospitalization. Other causes include *Mycoplasma* and *Legionella* spp., *Haemophilus influenzae*, atypical organisms, and viruses. However, the cause and incidence of CAP vary depending on the community, patient age, and comorbidities.

43. Which CAPs are seen more commonly in alcoholic patients?

As in nonalcoholic patients, pneumococcal pneumonia is the most frequent cause of CAP. Although at risk for the usual pathogens, alcoholics have a higher incidence of pneumonia due to gram-negative organisms (including *Klebsiella pneumoniae* and *Haemophilus influenzae*), anaerobic pneumonia secondary to aspiration, and *Staphylococcus aureus*.

44. What clinical manifestations and laboratory tests may help to diagnose pneumonia?

1. **History**

Fever	Cough (productive vs. nonproductive)
Dyspnea	Pleuritic pain
Abdominal pain	Malaise

2. **Physical examination**

Fever	Tachycardia
Cyanosis (with severe pneumonia)	Tachypnea

3. **Auscultation**

Crackles	Pectoriloquy
Egophony	Dullness to percussion (with pleural effusion)

4. **Laboratory tests**

Sputum Gram stain and culture	WBC count (elevated, normal, low)

5. **Chest x-ray** showing consolidation/infiltrate (bilateral?) and/or pleural effusion
6. **Other evaluations**

Oxygen saturation	Arterial blood gas

45. What factors predispose to the development of pneumococcal pneumonia?

- Severe underlying illness such as multiple myeloma, lymphoma, and leukemia
- Cirrhosis and renal failure
- Poorly controlled diabetes mellitus
- Sickle cell anemia
- Splenectomy
- Advanced age

46. Which factors determine the prognosis of pneumococcal pneumonia?

The mortality rate associated with pneumococcal pneumonia ranges from 6% to 19% in hospitalized patients without complications. Prognosis is worsened by the presence of the following:

Underlying illnesses

Alcoholism	Bronchiectasis
COPD	Hemoglobin SS and SC disease
Congestive heart failure	Bronchogenic carcinoma
Diabetes mellitus	Multiple myeloma

Other factors

Hypogammaglobulinemia	Bacteremia
Age > 60 yr	Delay in onset of therapy
Multilobar involvement	Pneumococcal serotype 3
Leukopenia	Extrapulmonary involvement

Munson MA: Pneumococcal infections. JAMA 246:1942, 1981.

47. What are the common risk factors for the development of anaerobic pneumonia? Which bronchopulmonary segments are most commonly involved?

Approximately 25% of patients with anaerobic pneumonia report a history of transient loss of consciousness, especially seizures or alcohol-related loss of consciousness. Other predisposing factors include poor oral hygiene, dysphagia, endobronchial obstruction, and any risk factor for aspiration. The posterior segment of the right upper lobe and superior segment of the right lower lobe are most commonly involved, followed by the posterior segment of the left upper lobe and superior segment of the left lower lobes. Patients usually aspirate in the supine position, in which these segments are dependent. The right lung is involved more frequently than the left, because the right mainstem bronchus comes off at a less acute angle than the left.

48. Which risk factors predispose to the development of nosocomial pneumonia?

- Increased severity of underlying illness
- Previous hospitalization
- Indwelling urethral catheters
- Presence of intravascular catheters
- Intubation (especially prolonged intubation)
- Recent thoracic or upper abdominal surgery
- Use of broad-spectrum antibiotics (increased risk of superinfection).

49. Which organisms most commonly cause nosocomial pneumonia?

Hospital-acquired pneumonia is the number one cause of nosocomial mortality. Nosocomial pneumonia, a pneumonia occurring > 48 hours after admission, is caused most commonly by gram-negative organisms, including *Pseudomonas aeruginosa, Klebsiella pneumoniae, Escherichia coli, Enterobacter* spp., and extended-spectrum, beta lactamase-producing gram-negative bacilli. *Staphylococcus aureus*, including methicillin-resistant organisms, *Streptococcus pneumoniae*, anaerobes, *Candida* spp., enterococci, and polymicrobial infections are also common. There is an increasing incidence of infections caused by resistant organisms. The mortality rate of nosocomial pneumonia remains high (30–50%) despite antimicrobial therapy.

50. What radiographic patterns are commonly observed in HIV-infected patients?

PATTERN	DISEASE
Diffuse reticulonodular infiltration	*Pneumocystis carinii* pneumonia
	Disseminated tuberculosis
	Disseminated histoplasmosis
	Disseminated coccidioidomycosis
	Lymphocytic interstitial pneumonitis
Focal airspace consolidation	Bacterial pneumonia
	Kaposi's sarcoma
	Cryptococcal pneumonia
Normal	*Pneumocystis carinii* pneumonia
	Disseminated *Mycobacterium avium* complex
	Disseminated histoplasmosis
Adenopathy	Tuberculosis
	Kaposi's sarcoma
	Disseminated *Mycobacterium avium* complex
Pleural effusion	Kaposi's sarcoma
	Tuberculosis
	Non-Hodgkin's lymphoma
	Pyogenic empyema

Modified from Zurlo JJ: Respiratory infections and the acquired immunodeficiency syndrome. In Bone RC (ed): Pulmonary and Critical Care Medicine. St. Louis, Mosby, 1997, with permission.

51. Which pathogens cause lower respiratory tract infections in HIV-infected patients?

PATHOGEN	WELL-RECOGNIZED	UNUSUAL
Bacteria	*Streptococcus pneumoniae* *Haemophilus influenzae*	Many species
Mycobacteria	*Mycobacterium tuberculosis* *M. avium* *M. kansasii*	Many species
Fungi	*Pneumocystis carinii** *Cryptococcus neoformans* *Histoplasma capsulatum* *Coccidioides immitis*	*Aspergillus* spp. *Candida* spp.
Protozoa	None *Cryptosporidium* spp.	*Toxoplasma gondii*
Viruses	None Varicella-zoster Herpes simplex Epstein-Barr virus	Cytomegalovirus

* *P. carinii* has been reclassified as a fungus.
Modified from Zurlo JJ: Respiratory infections and the acquired immunodeficiency syndrome. In Bone RC (ed): Pulmonary and Critical Care Medicine. St. Louis, Mosby, 1997, with permission.

52. Describe the characteristic clinical features of *P. carinii* pneumonia (PCP).
PCP is the most common AIDS-defining illness and should be suspected in the appropriate clinical setting. Features of PCP include fever, dyspnea, nonproductive cough, and progression of symptoms over several weeks. The chest x-ray typically shows bilateral infiltrate, but may be relatively normal-appearing. Laboratory findings usually include hypoxemia, lymphopenia, and a CD4 count < 200 ml.
Bartlett JG, et.al: Community-acquired pneumonia in adults: Guidelines for management. Clin Infect Dis 26: 811–838, 1998.

TUBERCULOSIS

53. What symptoms are associated with tuberculosis (TB)?
The symptoms associated with TB are often nonspecific. Common complaints include productive cough, weight loss, weakness, anorexia, night sweats, and generalized malaise. These nonspecific symptoms are most often subacute or chronic (> 8 wk) in duration. Both fever, present in one-third to one-half of the patients, and hemoptysis correlate with cavitary disease and positive sputum smears.

54. Describe the common anatomic distribution of CXR changes in postprimary (reactivation) TB. What is the differential diagnosis?
In postprimary TB, CXR abnormalities are located predominantly in the apical and posterior segments of the upper lobes (85%). Although the anterior segment of the upper lobes may be affected, a lesion found only in the anterior segment suggests a diagnosis other than TB (e.g., malignancy). The superior segments of the lower lobe account for approximately 10% and the remainder of the lower lobe for < 7%. The right lung is more often affected than the left.

55. Which diseases may be associated with infiltrates in the upper lobes?
The differential diagnosis of upper lobe infiltrates with or without cavitation includes atypical mycobacterial infections, silicosis, pneumonia, malignancy, pulmonary infarct, ankylosing spondylitis, actinomycosis, fungal infections, and nocardial infection.

56. What specific factors are associated with an increased risk for developing TB?

Medical high risk (increased susceptibility)

Silicosis	Diabetes mellitus
Chronic renal failure	HIV infection
Alcoholism	Steroids
Weight loss	Weight loss $\geq$ 10% ideal body weight
Malignancy	Immunosuppressive therapy
Gastrectomy	

High risk of exposure

Foreign birth	Elderly patients in nursing home
Low socioeconomic status	Physicians
Prisoners	Hospital employees
IV drug users	

Joint Statement of the American Thoracic Society and the Centers for Disease Control and Prevention: Targeted tuberculin testing and treatment of latent tuberculosis infection. Am J Respir Crit Care Med 161(4 Pt 2):S221–S247, 2000.

57. How is active M. tuberculosis infection diagnosed?

Because many months of medical therapy are required for adequate treatment of TB, a definitive diagnosis by culture is recommended. A negative tuberculin (purified protein derivative [PPD]) skin test in patients with no underlying disease (patients who are not anergic) or overwhelming TB infection makes the diagnosis of TB unlikely. A positive PPD without CXR changes also makes the diagnosis of active pulmonary TB unlikely and reflects previous exposure. A positive PPD and typical CXR findings or response to antituberculous medications may provide a presumptive diagnosis of TB, which should be verified by culture.

58. What clinical problems are associated with the treatment of TB?

1. **Drug resistance.** Primary resistance (resistant organisms in the initial infection) is increasing in the U.S. and is most common for isoniazid (INH). Resistance to both INH and rifampin may be seen. Primary drug resistance can vary with location and ethnic background and is higher in foreign-born patients. Secondary drug resistance develops during treatment.

2. **Noncompliance.** Multiple drug regimens given over an extended period (6 months or more) may lead to failure to complete therapy. Supervised biweekly home therapy helps to ensure compliance and is now highly recommended.

3. **Medication side effects.** Hepatotoxicity, the most important side effect, is seen in 2–5% of patients. It occurs most frequently with INH therapy, less frequently with rifampin, and rarely with pyrazinamide (PZA). Other side effects include retrobulbar optic neuritis, hyperuricemia, thrombocytopenia (ethambutol), hyperglycemia (rifampin), and peripheral neuropathy (INH).

O'Brien RJ: Drug-resistant tuberculosis: Etiology, management, and prevention. Semin Respir Infect 9:104–112, 1994.

59. How do you monitor for adverse drug reactions during TB therapy?

Before therapy is started, baseline liver function tests (INH, rifampin, PZA); CBC with platelets, blood urea nitrogen, creatinine, and calcium (INH, rifampin); uric acid (PZA, ethambutol); and visual acuity (ethambutol) should be performed. For persons with liver disease/alcoholism or age > 35 years, liver function tests should be performed periodically and symptoms monitored. Patients receiving INH should be questioned monthly about potential symptoms. All patients should be fully informed of potential complications of therapy.

60. Why is multidrug therapy used in the treatment of TB?

Work by Canetti over 30 years ago established the large numbers of organisms found in tuberculous cavities. Spontaneous resistance develops in 1 in 100,000–1,000,000 organisms. Therefore, single-drug therapy may lead to the selection of resistant organisms and treatment failure.

61. What is the major role of identifying latent tuberculosis infection (LTBI)?

The identification and treatment of LTBI is an essential part of the strategy to eliminate TB in the U.S. The American Thoracic Society (ATS) and the Centers for Disease Control and Prevention (CDC) use the term LBTI treatment rather "preventive therapy" or "chemoprophylaxis," both of which are misleading and confusing. INH and other antimicrobial agents have little effect on an infection in which microbial multiplication is minimal or absent. What is actually taking place is treatment of a potentially subclinical but active infection.

Joint Statement of the American Thoracic Society and the Centers for Disease Control and Prevention: Targeted tuberculin testing and treatment of latent tuberculosis infection. Am J Respir Crit Care Med 16(4 Pt 2):S221–S247, 2000.

62. What are the guidelines for determining a positive tuberculin skin test reaction?

INDURATION ≥ 5MM	INDURATION ≥ 10 MM	INDURATION ≥ 15 MM
HIV-positive status	Recent arrivals (< 5 yr) from high-	No risk factor for TB
Recent contact with TB case	prevalence countries	
CXR changes consistent with	Injection drug users	
old TB	Residents and employees of high-risk	
Patients with organ transplant or	congregate settings (e.g., prisons, jails,	
immunosuppression (receiving >	nursing homes, homeless shelters)	
15 mg prednisone or equivalent	Mycobacteriology lab personnel	
for > 1 month)	High-risk clinical conditions: silicosis,	
	diabetes, chronic renal failure, some	
	hematologic malignancies (leukemia,	
	lymphoma), specific malignancies	
	(lung, head and neck), weight loss >	
	10% ideal weight	

From American Thoracic Society: Diagnostic standards and classification of tuberculosis in adults and children. Am J Respir Crit Care Med 161:1376–1395, 2000, with permission.

63. Which infectious agents can mimic TB?

Fungal infections, especially histoplasmosis and coccidioidomycosis, can mimic pulmonary TB. Histoplasmosis has similar presenting symptoms and CXR findings and should be considered in any differential diagnosis when TB is considered. Lymph node involvement is more common with histoplasmosis than TB. Complications secondary to lymph node and mediastinal involvement include fibrosing mediastinitis (rare), pericarditis (rare), esophageal encroachment, superior vena cava syndrome, and tracheal/airway encroachment.

Nocardia spp. (gram-positive, aerobic, partially acid-fast organisms) can mimic pulmonary TB. Symptoms include fever, night sweats, and productive cough. CXR findings with cavitation are frequent. Previously, nocardiosis was viewed as infection by a primary pulmonary pathogen. It is now recognized more frequently as an opportunistic infection in patients with underlying disease, such as pulmonary alveolar proteinosis. Most strains are susceptible to sulfonamides.

64. What are the mechanisms of hemorrhage from the site of previous pulmonary TB?

- Reactivation of TB
- Bronchiectasis
- "Scar carcinoma" (adenocarcinoma)
- Erosion of a vessel by a broncholith (calcified lymph node)
- Fungal infection (usually aspergillosis) in the cavity
- Rasmussen's aneurysm (terminal pulmonary artery)

NEOPLASTIC DISEASE

65. How does lung cancer rank in cancer-related deaths?

Lung cancer is the leading cause of cancer deaths for both men and women in the United States, with over 170,00 deaths per year. Fewer than 15% of patients survive for 5 years, and over 85%

present with advanced disease. Cigarette smoking accounts for over 80% of risk, with environmental exposures and genetic factors contributing to the rest. Approximately 50 tumor suppressor genes (p53, p16) and over 100 oncogenes (K-*ras* mutation, c-*myc* oncogene) have been described.

Rom WN, et al: State of the art: Molecular and genetic aspects of lung cancer. Am J Respir Crit Care Med 161:1255–1367, 2000.

66. Which CXR and clinical criteria can help distinguish between a benign and malignant pulmonary nodule?

A pulmonary nodule can be described as a rounded lesion measuring < 3 cm at maximal diameter on a CXR. Although no single characteristic or group of characteristics definitely predicts the nature of a solitary pulmonary nodule, the following chart may be useful.

Differentiation of Benign and Malignant Solitary Pulmonary Nodules

FACTOR	BENIGN	MALIGNANT
Clinical		
Age	< 40 yr (except hamartoma)	> 45 yr
Sex	Female	Male
Symptoms	Absent	Present
History	Lives in area of high granuloma incidence, exposure to TB, mineral oil medication	Diagnosis of primary lesion elsewhere
Skin tests	Positive, usually with specific infectious organisms	Negative or positive
Roentgenographic		
Size	Small (< 2 cm in diameter)	Large (> 2 cm in diameter)
Location	No predilection (except for TB [upper lobes])	Predominantly upper lobes (except for lung metastases)
Definition and contour	Margins well-defined and smooth	Margins ill-defined, lobulated, umbilicated
Calcification	Almost pathognomonic of benign lesion, particularly if of a laminated, multiple punctuate, or "popcorn" variety	Very rare, may be eccentric (scar carcinoma)
Satellite lesions	More common	Less common
Serial studies with no change over 2 years	Almost diagnostic of benign lesion	Most unlikely
Doubling time	< 30 or > 490 days	30–490 days

From Frazer RG, et al: Diagnosis of Diseases of the Chest, 3rd ed. Philadelphia, W.B. Saunders, 1989, p 1390, with permission.

67. How should you follow up an abnormal CXR?

Evaluation is directed by the patient's symptoms. If there is evidence of infection, treatment should begin before further evaluation. If the CXR is still abnormal after treatment or reveals an obvious mass, tissue diagnosis is imperative. Tissue diagnosis may be obtained by expectorated sputum, bronchoscopy with biopsy, or percutaneous fine-needle aspiration and cytology. Once the tissue diagnosis is established, treatment plans can be made. If the abnormality is a solitary pulmonary nodule, the algorithm on the following page may be used.

68. What are the most common histologic types of lung cancer?

Squamous cell carcinoma, adenocarcinoma, small cell carcinoma, bronchoalveolar cell, and large cell undifferentiated carcinoma. Lung cancer is slightly more frequent in the right lung, in the upper lobes, and in the anterior segment. Both squamous and small cell carcinomas occur more commonly in a central location, whereas adenocarcinoma usually develops more peripherally. All major cell types have been associated with cigarette smoking.

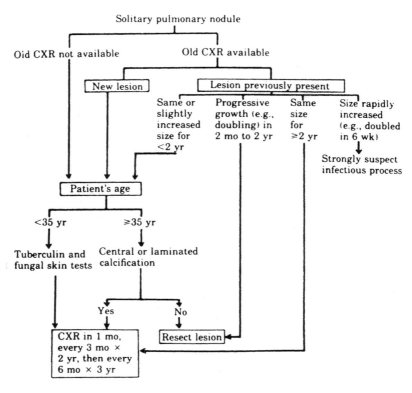

Algorithm for evaluation of solitary pulmonary nodule. (From Casciato DA, Lowitz BB: Manual of Clinical Oncology, 2nd ed. Boston, Little Brown, 1988, p 120, with permission.)

Lung Malignancies and Associated Clinical Syndromes

TYPE	RELATIVE INCIDENCE (%)	MAJOR CXR LOCATION	ASSOCIATED CLINICAL SYNDROMES
Non-small lung cancer	70		
Adenocarcinoma	30–35	Peripheral	Hypertrophic osteoarthropathy
Bronchioloalveolar cell carcinoma	10-15%	Peripheral	Voluminous watery sputum
Squamous cell	25–30	Central	Hypercalcemia
Large cell	10–15	Peripheral	Gynecomastia, galactorrhea
Small cell lung cancer	20–25%	Central	Paraneoplastic syndromes

69. What complications are associated with lung cancer?

COMPLICATION	COMMON CELL TYPE	PREVALENCE (%)	ASSOCIATED ABNORMALITIES
Pancoast's tumor	Squamous cell	2–5	Horner's syndrome
Superior vena cava syndrome	Non-small cell		Facial swelling, dilated neck and chest wall veins, confusion
Central airway obstruction	Squamous cell		Flattened inspiratory or expiratory limbs of flow-volume loop on PFT

Table continued on following page

COMPLICATION	COMMON CELL TYPE	PREVALENCE (%)	ASSOCIATED ABNORMALITIES
Paraneoplastic syndromes			
SIADH	Small cell	5–10	Hyponatremia
Hypercalcemia	Squamous cell		Lethargy, confusion
Eaton-Lambert syndrome	Small cell		Fatigability
Increased ACTH	Small cell	25	Cushing's syndrome
Digital clubbing	Non-small cell		Pain, swelling

SIADH = syndrome of inappropriate antidiuretic hormone, ACTH = adrenocorticotropic hormone.
Modified from Kukafka DS, Travaline JM: Lung cancer. In Criner GJ, D'Alonzo (eds): Pulmonary Pathophysiology. Madison, CT, Fence Creek Publishing, 1999, p 308, with permission.

70. Describe the symptoms and location of a Pancoast tumor.

First described in 1932 by Henry Khunrath Pancoast, a Philadelphia radiologist, this tumor is located in the extreme apex of the upper lobe of the lung and represents approximately 4% of all lung cancers. Although the tumor may be of various cell types, the most common is squamous cell carcinoma. Pancoast's original criteria included the following characteristics: arm/shoulder pain, Horner's syndrome, destruction of bone, and atrophy of the hand muscles.

71. List the most common pulmonary complications of lung cancer.

Atelectasis, postobstructive pneumonia secondary to endobronchial obstruction, hemoptysis, pleural effusion, and respiratory failure. Symptoms also may include cough, wheezing, stridor, chest pain, and hemoptysis.

72. What is Eaton-Lambert syndrome (ELS)?

ELS is a paraneoplastic myopathy; that is, it is associated with malignancy but not secondary to the direct effects of the tumor or its metastases. ELS is most often seen with small cell carcinoma. Clinically, it resembles myasthenia gravis (MG), but careful neurologic and electromyographic (EMG) examination can distinguish between the two. Unlike MG, ELS involves proximal muscle groups, has little response to neostigmine challenge, and demonstrates increased muscular response/strength to repetitive stimulation on EMG tracings.

73. What symptoms and x-ray changes are associated with hypertrophic pulmonary osteoarthropathy (HPO)?

HPO is one of the many varied paraneoplastic syndromes and more often is associated with squamous cell carcinoma. The patient complains of a deep burning pain, usually in the distal extremity. There is usually clubbing of the fingers and/or toes, periostitis of the long bones, and occasionally polyarthritis. The most commonly involved bones are the tibia, fibula, humerus, radius, and ulna. The x-ray of the extremity reveals subperiosteal new bone formation. The cause is unknown, and the abnormalities resolve with treatment of the primary tumor. HPO is seen more often in squamous cell and adenocarcinoma, less frequently with small cell lung cancer.

74. Which tumors commonly metastasize to the lung?

Lung cancer	Genitourinary (renal, prostate, bladder)
Colorectal carcinoma	Breast cancer
Thyroid cancer	Testicular cancer
Ovarian cancer	Melanoma
Pancreatic/hepatic	Gastric
Head and neck	Sarcoma

Endobronchial metastases occur most commonly in renal cell carcinoma, melanoma, and breast carcinoma.

PULMONARY THROMBOEMBOLISM

75. What are the predisposing factors for the development of pulmonary emboli (PE)?

- Injury or surgery of the pelvis and lower extremities
- Previous history of deep venous thrombosis (DVT)
- Prolonged general anesthesia
- Burns
- Pregnancy and postpartum period
- Right ventricular failure
- Immobility

- Age
- Obesity
- Cancer
- Estrogen-containing medications (high-dose)
- Coagulation disorders (including deficiency of protein C, antithrombin III, protein S, factor V Leiden mutation)
- Activated protein C resistance, dysfibrinogenemia
- Antiphospholid antibodies/lupus anticoagulant

Goldber SZ: Pulmonary embolism. N Engl J Med 339:93–104, 1999.

76. What is the mortality rate for PE?

PEs occur in over 600,000 people per year, resulting in over 50,000 deaths. The mortality rate is slightly over 10%, and 30% are diagnosed antemortem.

77. What CXR findings are associated with PE?

Often the interpretation of the CXR of patients with acute PE is "normal," although subtle non-specific abnormalities are generally found. Examples include differences in diameters of vessels that should be similar in size, abrupt cut-off of a vessel followed distally, increased radiolucency in some areas, regional oligemia (Westermark's sign), a peripheral wedge-shaped density over the diaphragm (Hampton's hump), or an enlarged right descending pulmonary artery (Palla's sign).

78. What findings are associated with pulmonary infarction?

Approximately 1 in 10 PEs results in pulmonary infarction. Pleuritic chest pain, hemoptysis, and low-grade fever are present when infarction has occurred. Pulmonary infarction is classically described as a wedge-shaped infiltrate that abuts the pleura (Hampton's hump). It often is associated with a small pleural effusion that is usually exudative and may be hemorrhagic.

79. How is the diagnosis of PE established?

It is impossible to diagnose PE on clinical grounds alone; therefore, further testing is needed. The V/Q scan is usually the starting point of the evaluation. Although highly sensitive, it is non-specific, and interpretation may be difficult in patients with underlying pulmonary disease. Angiography is often reserved for unstable patients, when thrombolysis is considered, or when less invasive tests (guided by the clinical situation) are nondiagnostic.

80. What major complications may be associated with pulmonary angiography?

Pulmonary angiography is still the gold standard to demonstrate PE, but the procedure is not without risk. Complications may include death (< 0.5%), cardiac perforation, arrhythmias, contrast reaction, renal insufficiency secondary to dye, and bleeding. Overall, the risk of major complications is 4% and appears to be the highest in the most critically ill patients.

American Thoracic Society: The diagnostic approach to acute venous thromboembolism. Am J Respir Crit Care Med 160:1043–1066, 1999.

81. What is the role of D-dimers in the evaluation of suspected PE?

The enzyme-linked immunosorbent assay (ELISA) has a high negative predictive value. Recent data for the use of rapid D-dimer assays are encouraging; however, this test is not recommended as a standard part of the PE diagnostic evaluation.

American Thoracic Society: The diagnostic approach to acute venous thromboembolism. Am J Respir Crit Care Med 160:1043–1066, 1999.

82. Name two types of nonthrombotic PE.

Fat emboli and amniotic fluid emboli. The pulmonary vasculature filters the venous circulation and is exposed to nonthrombotic emboli. Fat embolism usually follows bone trauma or fracture, and symptoms begin 12–36 hours after the event. Clinical manifestations include altered mental status, respiratory decompensation, anemia, thrombocytopenia, and petechiae. Amniotic fluid embolism results from entrance of amniotic fluid into the venous circulation, with consequent shock and disseminated intravascular coagulation (DIC).

OBSTRUCTIVE AIRWAY DISEASE

83. What causes chronic obstructive pulmonary disease (COPD)?

Cigarette smoking has a primary role in most cases of COPD, but the disease does not have a single cause. Pulmonary function declines normally with aging, and patients who experience a rate of loss that significantly exceeds the norm are classified as having COPD. Contributing factors include:

1. **Cigarette smoking.** Cigarette/tobacco smoking is associated with a dose-related risk (usually expressed in pack-years) of developing COPD, although there is great individual variation. Not all smokers develop COPD, even those with a high-dose history.

2. **Air pollution.** Although it is difficult to measure, there is an association between COPD and air pollution, especially sulfur dioxide and particulate matter.

3. **Mucosal hypersecretion and bronchial infection.** Both have been associated with COPD, but the causal relation is uncertain.

4. **Sex and race.** The higher prevalence of COPD in men is due to sex-related differences in cigarette smoking. Some studies have suggested that white men may be more susceptible than black men.

5. **Allergic factors.** Patients with a history of allergic disorders may be at higher risk, but the role is probably minor.

6. **Hereditary factors.** Hereditary deficiency of alpha$_1$-antitrypsin is associated with diffuse emphysema, and there may be other contributing genetic factors.

7. **Sociologic factors.** The association of COPD with lower socioeconomic groups is probably due to differences in cigarette smoking, occupational factors, and air pollution.

8. **Occupational factors.** Occupations at increased risk include coal mining, fire fighting, grain handling, and copper smelting (sulfur dioxide exposure). Occupational exposures that increase risk include poison gas (mustard gas), granite dust, carbon black, cotton (byssinosis), hemp, and toluene diisocyanate.

Niewoehner DE: Clinical aspects of chronic airflow obstruction. In Baum GL, Wolinsky E (eds): Textbook of Pulmonary Diseases, 4th ed. Boston, Little, Brown, 1989.

84. Define chronic bronchitis.

Chronic bronchitis is defined by its symptoms, which include a productive cough on most mornings for 3 or more consecutive months for 2 or more consecutive years.

85. Define emphysema.

Unlike chronic bronchitis, which is described in terms of symptoms, emphysema is an anatomic/structural term. Emphysema is an abnormal enlargement of air-containing space distal to the terminal bronchioles accompanied by destruction of alveolar tissue.

86. What are the key aspects in the clinical evaluation of patients with COPD?

History
- Smoking: age at initiation, quantity smoked per day, still smoking (if not, date of cessation)
- Environmental factors: may disclose important risk factors
- Cough (chronic, productive): frequency and duration, productive (especially on awakening), presence of blood
- Wheezing
- Dyspnea
- Acute chest illnesses: frequency, productive cough, wheezing, dyspnea, fever

Physical examination
- Chest

 Airflow obstruction evidenced by wheezing during auscultation on slow or forced breathing, prolonged forced expiratory phase

 Severe emphysema indicated by overdistention of lungs in stable state, low diaphragmatic position, decreased intensity of breath and heart sounds

 Severe disease suggested by pursed-lip breathing, use of accessory respiratory muscles, indrawing of lower interspaces
- Other: unusual positions to relieve dyspnea at rest, digital clubbing (suggests lung cancer or bronchiectasis), mild dependent edema (may be seen in absence of right heart failure)

Laboratory tests
- CXR: diagnostic only of severe emphysema but essential to exclude other lung disease
- Spirometry (before and after bronchodilator use): essential to confirm presence or reversibility of airflow obstruction and to quantify maximal level of ventilatory function
- Lung volumes: FVC only, except in special instances (e.g., presence of giant bullae)
- DL_{CO}: unnecessary except in special instances (e.g., dyspnea out of proportion to severity of airflow limitation)
- Arterial blood gases: not needed in stage I airflow obstruction (FEV_1 > 50% predicted); essential in stages II and III (FEV_1 < 50% predicted) and in very severe airflow obstruction (major monitoring tool)

American Thoracic Society: Standards for the diagnosis and care of patients with chronic obstructive pulmonary disease. Am J Respir Crit Care Med 152:S77–S120, 1995.

87. What radiographic changes are associated with COPD?

The CXR findings are secondary to overdistention of the lungs. Examples include a low, flat diaphragm; increased retrosternal airspace (on lateral x-ray); and an elongated, narrow heart shadow. Bullae, which appear as rounded radiolucent areas, are occasionally seen and reflect emphysematous changes.

88. Describe the findings of PFTs in patients with COPD.

The early signs, symptoms, and radiographic changes of COPD are variable and nonspecific; therefore, PFTs are important in the diagnosis of COPD. Patients show evidence of airway obstruction, such as decreased vital capacity and expiratory flow rates (i.e., FEV_1 or $FEF_{25-75\%}$). There is also evidence of lung hyperinflation and air trapping, manifested by increases in RV, FRC, and TLC. Most patients respond to bronchodilators, although the response is variable and usually improves by only 15–20% above prebronchodilator values.

89. Pink puffers and blue bloaters—what are they?

They are the two distinct clinical patterns of gas exchange abnormalities seen in patients with advanced COPD. In most patients, however, there is significant overlap of features. Both patterns usually result from long-term cigarette smoking. The reason for the two different presentations is not clearly defined.

Pink puffers tend to be thin and dyspneic but maintain relatively normal PaO_2 and $PaCO_2$ levels. They breathe with hyperinflated lungs and fast, shallow respirations. They remain relatively free of cor pulmonale. The pathophysiology seems to be that of severe emphysema, and their symptoms result primarily from the loss of lung elastic recoil, with relatively little intrinsic airway disease.

Blue bloaters tend to be overweight, with minimal dyspnea but significant coughing and sputum production. They suffer from cor pulmonale, respiratory infections, and chronic CO_2 retention. Although they usually have some degree of emphysema, the pathophysiology is significant small and large airway inflammation. Symptoms are largely due to intrinsic airway disease.

90. What complications are associated with COPD?

Frequent exacerbations and respiratory decompensation characterize COPD. Upper respiratory tract infections, pneumonia, medical noncompliance, and environmental changes (e.g., temperature, allergens, irritants) can induce exacerbations. Complications include sleep disturbances due to nocturnal desaturation, acute and chronic respiratory failure, chronic cor pulmonale, spontaneous pneumothorax, and impairment of pulmonary function secondary to large bullae.

91. What is cor pulmonale?

Cor pulmonale, or pulmonary heart disease, is right-sided congestive heart failure caused by an increase in pulmonary vascular resistance (pulmonary hypertension) due to intrinsic lung disease. Examples include pulmonary parenchymal diseases (e.g., COPD, sarcoidosis, pneumoconiosis, restrictive lung disease) and pulmonary vascular diseases, (e.g., primary pulmonary hypertension, recurrent pulmonary embolism, scleroderma). Cor pulmonale is a major cause of morbidity and mortality in COPD.

92. What is the prognosis of severe COPD? How is the severity staged?

Prognosis is based on age, severity of hypoxemia, presence of hypercapnia, and severity of airflow obstruction (FEV_1). Of these, the most relevant is the FEV_1. The severity of COPD is staged on the basis of airflow obstruction:

Stage I	$FEV_1 > 50\%$ predicted
Stage II	FEV_1 35–49 % predicted
Stage III	$FEV_1 < 35\%$ predicted

93. How is COPD treated?

1. **Removal of risk factors.** The most important component is the cessation of smoking and removal of other risk factors (i.e., environmental and occupational).

2. **Bronchodilators.** Although the airway obstruction is largely fixed, with only a small reversible component, most patients experience a small improvement in symptoms with the use of bronchodilator therapy.

3. **Corticosteroids.** Patients who are most likely to respond include those with recurrent attacks of wheezing and a relatively significant response to inhaled bronchodilators (FEV_1 increase > 20%). Because of the risk of side effects, the lowest possible dose should be used, preferably inhaled steroids (if needed chronically) or an alternate-day oral regimen.

4. **Diuretics.** Diuresis is indicated for relief of the symptoms of cor pulmonale.

5. **Antibiotic therapy.** If indicated for acute bacterial exacerbation, "targeted" (i.e., aimed at the most common pathogens) agents should be used (preferably the least expensive).

6. **Continuous oxygen therapy.** In patients for whom it is indicated, long-term oxygen therapy decreases the morbidity and mortality rates of COPD.

7. **Phlebotomy.** In the past, this procedure was commonly performed in patients with COPD and secondary erythrocytosis. At present, with the appropriate use of long-term oxygen therapy, phlebotomy is rarely necessary.

94. Which classes of bronchodilator drugs are available for treatment of obstructive airway diseases?

1. **Anticholinergic agents** compete with acetylcholine at its receptors. The current congener, ipratropium bromide (Atrovent), is available for inhalational use and causes far fewer systemic side effects than atropine. It also has an extended duration of action compared with atropine.

2. **Beta-adrenergic agonists**, which are available for oral, parenteral, or inhalational use, produce bronchodilation by directly stimulating the β_2 receptors on the bronchial smooth muscle cell. Currently available agents offer increased duration of action and increased β_2 selectivity. Oral agents should be reserved for patients unable to use inhaled agents.

3. **Methylxanthines**, which are available for oral or parenteral use, include aminophylline, theophylline, and related compounds. To achieve maximal benefit from theophylline and to minimize toxic effects, the serum level must be maintained within the therapeutic range of 10–20 gm/ml.

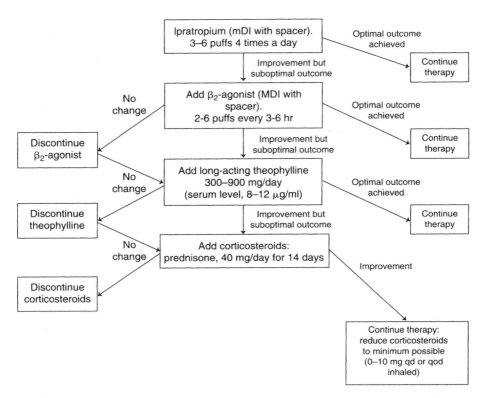

Typical regimen for treatment of COPD. (Adapted from Ferguson CT, Cherniack RM: Management of chronic obstructive pulmonary disease. N Engl J Med 328:1017–1022, 1993.)

95. Why is theophylline beneficial in patients with COPD?

Theophylline is classified as a bronchodilator. However, because in most patients COPD has a small reversible component, the significance of theophylline's bronchodilatory effects in COPD is questionable. Various other possible beneficial actions have been attributed to theophylline:

- Increased mucociliary clearance
- Increased respiratory drive
- Improved cardiovascular function
- Increased diaphragmatic contractility
- Decreased dyspnea
- Improved exercise capacity

96. Discuss the toxic effects of theophylline.

The toxic effects of theophylline occur with increasing frequency as the serum level exceeds 20 mg/ml. They can be seen even within the therapeutic range of 10–20 mg/ml. The serious toxicities (especially seizures and cardiac arrhythmias) usually are not seen until the serum levels rise above 30 mg/ml, but they can occur at lower serum levels and often are not preceded by less severe signs of toxicity. The common toxic effects are as follows:

1. **Gastrointestinal:** nausea, vomiting, diarrhea, and abdominal pain

2. **Cardiac:** various arrhythmias (including sinus tachycardia, multifocal atrial tachycardia, and extrasystoles)

3. **Neurologic:** headache, nervousness, insomnia, tremor, and seizures

97. What factors affect the clearance of theophylline?

Theophylline is cleared mainly through hepatic oxidation and demethylation; hepatic metabolites and unmetabolized theophylline are excreted in the urine. Any increase or decrease in theophylline clearance necessitates increasing or decreasing the maintenance dose to maintain therapeutic serum levels and avoid toxicity.

Factors Affecting Theophylline Clearance and Dosage Requirements

INCREASED CLEARANCE (LARGER DOSAGE REQUIRED)*	DECREASED CLEARANCE (SMALLER DOSAGE REQUIRED)
Major change (26–50%)	
Cigarette smoking	Hepatic insufficiency
Phenytoin	Heart failure
Rifampin	Cor pulmonale
Isoproterenol IV	Viral pneumonia
Phenobarbital	Cimetidine
Carbamazepine	Mexiletine
Aminoglutethimide	Ciprofloxacin, other quinolones
	Allopurinol
	Erythromycin
	Influenza vaccination
	Triacetyloleandomycin (TAO)
	Propranolol
	Oral contraceptives
Smaller change (10–25%)[†]	
Low-carbohydrate, high-protein diet	Verapamil
	Nifedipine
Charcoal-cooked food	Tetracycline
Isoniazid	Hydrocortisone
Ketoconazole	Aluminum hydroxide
	Magnesium hydroxide
	Thiabendazole

* Serum levels must be used for guidance in increasing dosage.
† Data supporting these changes are less well documented.
From American Thoracic Society: Standards for diagnosis and care of patients with chronic obstructive pulmonary disease. Am J Respir Crit Care Med 152(5):S87, 1995, with permission.

98. When should antibiotics be given to patients with an acute exacerbation of COPD?

Antibiotics are recommended if two or three of the following are present:
- Increasing dyspnea
- Increased sputum production
- Purulent sputum

Anthonisen NR, et at: Antibiotic therapy in exacerbations of COPD. Ann Intern Med 106:196–204, 1987.

99. What are the criteria for continuous low-flow oxygen therapy?

The role of oxygen therapy was largely established in the early 1980s by the Nocturnal Oxygen Therapy trial in the U.S. and by the Medical Research Council trial in Great Britain. Oxygen therapy is indicated for any one of the following conditions:

1. $PaO_2 < 55$ mmHg in patients at rest and taking an optimal medical regimen.

2. PaO_2 is > 55 mmHg in patients at rest and taking an optimal medical regimen, if evidence of hypoxic end-organ dysfunction is indicated by one or more of the following:

- Cor pulmonale
- Secondary pulmonary hypertension
- Secondary erythrocytosis
- Impaired mentation

3. Patients whose PaO_2 drops below 55 mmHg with exercise and who have evidence of significant improvement in either or both of the following with oxygen therapy:

- Exercise duration
- Exercise performance or capacity

4. Patients whose PaO_2 drops below 55 mmHg during sleep and who have evidence of one or more of the following:

- Hypoxic organ dysfunction   • Significant cardiac dysrhythmia
- Disturbed sleep pattern

100. Does cessation of smoking have a beneficial effect on patients with COPD?
   Yes. The morbidity and mortality associated with COPD are reduced, and there is small but significant improvement in objective tests of pulmonary function and subjective symptom severity. These benefits are more dramatic in patients with mild COPD than in those with more advanced disease. Smoking is the leading cause of preventable morbidity and mortality, contributing to 20% of all deaths in the U.S. and over 80% of lung cancers and COPD. Smoking cessation should be continually encouraged.

101. What are the poor prognostic signs in an acute exacerbation of asthma?
- Pulse rate > 100/min   • Retraction of sternocleidomastoid muscles
- Pulsus paradoxus > 10 mmHg   • FEV_1 < 600 ml before treatment
- PEFR < 16% of predicted   • FEV_1 < 1600 ml after treatment
- $PaCO_2$ > 45 mmHg

102. What is Samter's syndrome?
   Approximately 4–20% of asthmatics are sensitive to aspirin. Of aspirin-sensitive patients, 90% have associated nasal polyposis and rhinosinusitis. This triad is known as Samter's syndrome.

103. What is bronchiectasis?
   It is a fixed dilatation of bronchi due to destructive changes in the elastic and muscular layers of the bronchial wall. The hallmark of bronchiectasis is overproduction of sputum. It was a more common disease before the advent of appropriate antibiotic therapy for pulmonary infection. Conditions predisposing to bronchiectasis include severe inflammation (including infections), congenital syndromes (e.g., cystic fibrosis, Kartagener's syndrome, Young's syndrome), airway obstruction, traction of the airways (e.g., fibrosis, TB, radiation), and anatomic malformations. Patients usually present with a chronic cough productive of large quantities of foul, often blood-tinged sputum. High-resolution CT scan has replaced bronchography as the gold standard for diagnosis.
   Mysliwiec,V, Pina JS: Bronchiectasis: The other obstructive lung disease. Postgrad Med 106:123–131, 1999.

INTERSTITIAL LUNG DISEASE

104. How are the interstitial lung diseases (ILDs) classified?
   ILD refers to a heterogeneous group of diseases with similar clinical and x-ray abnormalities. The CXR shows varying degrees of fibrotic changes (usually widespread). The most common symptoms include dyspnea and dry cough. PFTs reveal a restrictive defect. There are over 100 causes of ILD, and they often are classified according to known vs. unknown etiology.

Idiopathic fibrotic diseases
   Idiopathic pulmonary fibrosis   Lymphocytic interstitial pneumonitis
   Acute interstitial pneumonitis   Bronchiolitis obliterans organizing pneumonia (BOOP)
Connective tissue diseases
   Systemic lupus erythematosus   Rheumatoid arthritis
   Scleroderma   Ankylosing spondylitis
   Sjögren's syndrome   Others (less common)
Primary diseases
   Sarcoidosis   Acute respiratory distress syndrome
   Lymphangitic carcinoma   Eosinophilic granulomatosis
   Systemic vasculitides   Alveolar microlithiasis
   Lymphangioleiomyomatosis   Neurofibromatosis
   Eosinophilic pneumonia   Other rare diseases

Drug- and treatment-related causes

Oxygen	Radiation
Chemotherapy	Antiarrhythmic agents (amiodarone, others)
Antibiotics (macrodantin, others)	Anti-inflammatory agents (aspirin, gold, others)
Narcotics (morphine, cocaine, others)	

Occupational diseases

Pneumoconiosis	Hypersensitivity pneumonitis

Modified from Schwartz MI, King TE: Interstitial Lung Disease, 2nd ed. St. Louis, Mosby, 1993, with permission.

105. How are the ILDs classified according to clinical findings?

Spontaneous pneumothorax

Eosinophilic granuloma	Neurofibromatosis
Lymphangioleiomyomatosis	Tuberous sclerosis

Increased lung volumes

Eosinophilic granuloma	Neurofibromatosis
Tuberous sclerosis	Chronic hypersensitivity pneumonitis
Sarcoidosis	Lymphangioleiomyomatosis

Upper lobe predominance

Ankylosing spondylitis	Berylliosis
Eosinophilic granuloma	Neurofibromatosis
Silicosis	Chronic sarcoidosis

Pleural involvement

Asbestosis	Lymphangioleiomyomatosis (chylous effusion)
Sarcoidosis	Radiation pneumonitis
Collagen vascular disease	Drug-induced (nitrofurantoin)
Lymphangitic carcinoma	

Subcutaneous calcinosis

Scleroderma	Polymyositis-dermatomyositis

Hilar nodal eggshell calcification

Silicosis	Sarcoidosis

Kerley's B lines

Lymphoma	Lymphangitic carcinoma
Lymphangioleiomyomatosis	Pulmonary veno-occlusive disease
Chronic left ventricular failure	

Lando Y, O'Brien G: Interstitial lung disease. In Criner GJ, D'Alonzo (eds): Pulmonary Pathophysiology. Madison, CT, Fence Creek Publishing, 1999, p 263, with permission.

106. What is Hamman-Rich syndrome (HRS)?

In 1944, Hamman and Rich first described rapidly progressive and fatal pulmonary fibrosis for which no cause could be identified. HRS refers to rapidly progressive ILD of unknown etiology.

Hamman L, Rich AR: Acute diffuse interstitial fibrosis of the lungs. Bull Johns Hopkins Hosp 74:177–212, 1944.

107. Which pulmonary syndromes are associated with rheumatoid arthritis (RA)?

RA may be associated with ILD. The condition is more common in men, rarely precedes joint disease, and may be associated with cutaneous nodules. The most common pulmonary complication is pleural effusion. Other conditions include pulmonary vasculitis, parenchymal nodules, and bronchiolitis obliterans. In addition, Caplan's syndrome (rheumatoid pneumoconiosis) refers to the association of rheumatoid arthritis and nodules on CXR in patients with coalworker's pneumoconiosis. This syndrome has been associated with the risk for pneumothorax.

108. How prevalent is sarcoidosis?

Sarcoidosis is a multisystem disorder of unknown etiology that has a prevalence of approximately 20 cases/100,000 population. Although it may occur at any age, patients are usually

20–40 years of age. Women have a slightly higher prevalence, and in the U.S. sarcoidosis is more common in blacks than whites (10:1 ratio). Many organs may be involved, but the lung is involved most frequently (> 90% of cases).

109. How is sarcoidosis staged by CXR?

About 90% of patients have an abnormality on CXR at some time during the course of the disease. The following categories represent CXR patterns and are not "stages" of the disease, as usually understood. However, patients with stage I disease are more likely to have reversible sarcoidosis.

STAGE	CXR FINDINGS
0	Clear (< 10%)
I	Bilateral hilar adenopathy (25–40%)
II	Bilateral hilar adenopathy with pulmonary infiltrate (25–50%)
III	Pulmonary infiltrate without adenopathy (< 15%)

110. What clinical and laboratory abnormalities are associated with sarcoidosis?

Because sarcoidosis is a multisystem disease, clinical manifestations can be nonspecific. Symptomatic patients complain of malaise, fever, weight loss, or symptoms referable to the specific organ involved. Laboratory abnormalities are also nonspecific and include increased erythrocyte sedimentation rate, hyperglobulinemia, increased angiotensin-converting enzyme activity, and occasionally hypercalcemia and/or hypercalciuria.

111. How is the diagnosis of sarcoidosis established?

Sarcoidosis is a diagnosis of exclusion. The diagnosis rests on the combination of history, radiographic, and histologic findings. The typical pathologic finding is noncaseating granuloma. This finding, in conjunction with the appropriate clinical picture and lack of infectious etiology (e.g., TB, fungal), establishes the diagnosis. Although any involved organ may be biopsied for pathologic changes, transbronchial lung biopsy is positive in about 90% of cases.

112. What other diseases may be associated with nonnecrotizing granulomas?

The presence of nonnecrotizing granulomas is suggestive of, but not pathognomonic for, sarcoidosis. Other diseases associated with nonnecrotizing granulomas include mycobacterial and fungal disease, extrinsic allergic alveolitis, celiac disease, Crohn's disease, Whipple's disease, pneumoconiosis, drug reaction, foreign body reaction, syphilis, and berylliosis.

113. Which organs, in addition to the lung, are most frequently involved in sarcoidosis?

The lymph nodes, skin (25%), eyes (25%), and musculoskeletal system (arthralgias). Although the bone marrow, spleen, and liver are often involved, findings usually are not clinically significant. Skin manifestations include erythema nodosum and plaques. Ocular manifestations include both anterior and posterior uveitis and can lead to blindness. CNS and cardiac involvement are present in approximately 5% of patients.

114. Which patients with sarcoidosis should be treated?

Sarcoidosis is usually a self-limited disease, with 30–50% of cases spontaneously remitting, 20–30% remaining stable, and 30% demonstrating progression. Because therapeutic intervention is not without side effects, close observation of patients who are asymptomatic and without organ dysfunction is warranted. Therapy should be initiated in patients with significant systemic organ impairment (lung, eyes, heart, CNS, or extensive skin lesions) or evidence of hypercalcemia or hypercalciuria. Corticosteroids are the first line of therapy.

115. What is Goodpasture's syndrome?

Goodpasture's syndrome usually refers to a combination of glomerulonephritis and diffuse pulmonary hemorrhage associated with development of antiglomerular basement membrane (anti-GBM) antibodies and, less frequently, antipulmonary basement membrane antibodies. Some use the eponym more broadly to refer to all diseases characterized by glomerulonephritis and pulmonary hemorrhage.

116. Which diagnostic tests help to differentiate Goodpasture's syndrome from other pulmonary-renal syndromes?

Anti-GBM antibodies can be demonstrated in serum, renal tissue, and, less frequently, pulmonary tissue. Immunofluorescent staining of tissue reveals a linear pattern of deposition of IgG. Goodpasture's syndrome is predominantly a disease of young adults (mean age = 21 years) and is more common in males. The typical initial presentation is hemoptysis, but in rare cases renal involvement is the first symptom. The differential diagnosis includes other pulmonary-renal syndromes, including vasculitis, Wegener's granulomatosis, polyarteritis nodosa, uremia with pulmonary edema, and immune complex disease (e.g., systemic lupus erythematosus).

ACUTE RESPIRATORY DISTRESS SYNDROME

117. What are the hallmarks of acute respiratory distress syndrome (ARDS)?

The term ARDS is applied to diverse causes of lung injury characterized by an initial noxious event, followed by an interval of normal lung function, and then progressive and rapid hypoxemia and diffuse pulmonary infiltrates. The incidence of ARDS is estimated to be approximately 150,000 cases/year. The overall mortality rate remains at 40–60%; mortality is highest in cases associated with sepsis and aspiration.

118. Can cardiogenic pulmonary edema be distinguished from noncardiogenic pulmonary edema based on clinical and radiographic findings?

No. The two conditions can be differentiated by measurement of the pulmonary capillary wedge pressure (PCWP), which reflects left ventricular (LV) filling pressures (normally 6–12 mmHg). The PCWP is elevated in cardiogenic pulmonary edema, reflecting the elevated LV filling pressures, but it is normal in ARDS, because LV filling pressures are normal (the defect resulting in increased interstitial fluid is at the alveolocapillary membrane).

119. List the major clinical disorders associated with ARDS.

DIRECT LUNG INJURY	INDIRECT LUNG INJURY
Common causes	
Pneumonia	Sepsis
Aspiration of gastric contents	Severe trauma (with shock and multiple transfusions)
Less common causes	
Pulmonary contusion	Cardiopulmonary bypass
Fat emboli	Drug overdose
Near-drowning	Acute pancreatitis
Inhalation injury	Transfusions of blood products
Reperfusion pulmonary	

From Ware LB, Matthay MA: The acute respiratory distress syndrome. N Engl J Med 342:1334–1346, 2000.

120. List the potential complications of ARDS.

LV failure, secondary bacterial infection, DIC, pulmonary oxygen toxicity, barotrauma secondary to mechanical ventilation (pneumothorax, pneumomediastinum), and multisystem organ failure.

121. What is the prognosis of ARDS? How is it managed?

Despite increased understanding of the pathophysiology of ARDS, the mortality rate remains high (40–60%). The prognosis at the time of diagnosis depends on various factors: acute underlying diagnosis, etiology of ARDS, severity of illness, physiologic reserve, and comorbidity and preexisting conditions. Management involves ruling out treatable causes of respiratory failure, treatment of underlying disease processes, maintaining $PaO_2 > 5$ mmHg, hemodynamic and nutritional support, and avoidance of complications.

ENVIRONMENTAL LUNG DISEASE

122. What is pneumoconiosis?

The term is derived from the Greek words *pneumo* (lung) and *konis* (dust). It currently refers to an accumulation of inorganic dust in the lungs and the consequences of the tissue's response to the presence of the dust. The most common pneumoconioses are silicosis, asbestosis, and coalworker's pneumoconiosis (black lung).

123. What are the CXR abnormalities and clinical complications associated with silicosis?

Silicosis is a pulmonary disease secondary to the inhalation of quartz or silica dust. Occupations leading to potential exposure include mining, quarrying, sandblasting, pottery/stoneware production, and tunneling. The disease is characterized by focal pulmonary fibrosis that has a tendency to appear first in the upper lobes. Enlargement of the hilar lymph nodes and eggshell calcifications are suggestive of this process. Complications of silicosis include spontaneous pneumothorax, cor pulmonale, and infection with mycobacteria (TB and atypical mycobacteria) and fungi, increased frequency of connective tissue disorders, and possibly an increased risk of lung cancer (a cause-and-effect relationship cannot be established in most studies).

124. What clinical problems are associated with asbestos exposure?

Asbestosis (bibasilar-predominant pulmonary fibrosis), pleural plaques, pleural effusions, and malignancies are associated with a history of asbestos exposure. Asbestosis is a fibrotic disease of the lung and visceral pleura. The CXR shows interstitial fibrosis, beginning usually at the bases and progressing upward. Usually no hilar adenopathy is seen. Asbestos exposure increases the risk of malignancy, including lung cancer, GI cancer, and mesothelioma. There is no associated increase in infection or collagen vascular diseases.

125. Which tests are useful in diagnosing mesothelioma?

Because generous biopsy specimens are needed to diagnose mesothelioma, diagnosis is usually made after open thoracotomy. Periodic acid-Schiff (PAS) stain, immunoperoxidase staining for carcinoembryonic antigen (CEA) and keratin, and electron microscopy are useful in differentiating mesothelioma from adenocarcinoma. Mesothelioma lacks PAS-positive vacuoles and has weak staining with CEA antigen.

Antman KH, et al: Benign and malignant mesothelioma. Clin Chest Med 6:141–152, 1985.

MEDIASTINUM

126. Name the three major compartments of the mediastinum viewed on lateral CXR.

By convention, the mediastinum is divided into anterior, middle, and posterior compartments, according to its appearance on the lateral CXR (see figure at top of following page).

127. What are the components of the mediastinum?

Anterior mediastinum (includes everything forward of and superior to the heart shadow)
- Thymus gland
- Aortic arch and major branches
- Substernal extension of the thyroid or parathyroid glands
- Innominate veins
- Lymphatic vessels and lymph nodes

Middle mediastinum (extends from the anterior heart border to the anterior ventral border)
- Heart and pericardium
- Trachea and mainstem bronchi
- Pulmonary hila
- Lymph nodes
- Phrenic and vagus nerves

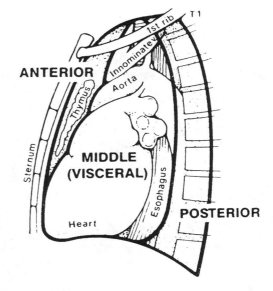

Three major compartments of the mediastinum. (From Shields TW: Chest wall, pleura, mediastinum, and diaphragm. In James EC, et al (eds): Basic Surgical Practice. Philadelphia, Hanley & Belfus, 1987, p 179, with permission.)

Posterior mediastinum (occupies space within the margins of the vertebrae on lateral film)
- Esophagus
- Descending aorta
- Azygous and hemiazygous veins
- Areolar connective tissue
- Thoracic duct and lymph nodes
- Vagus nerves and sympathetic chains

128. What is the most common mediastinal tumor in adults? In which compartment does it occur?

Thymic tumors, of which thymoma is the most common. The tumors usually are located in the anterior mediastinum and often are quite large. Most are benign, and, if the tumor is fully encapsulated, the prognosis is good. The mean age at presentation is 40–60 years. Symptoms may include cough, pain, and, in rare cases, fever.

129. What systemic syndromes may be associated with thymoma?

Forty to 70% of patients have at least laboratory evidence of a "parathymic syndrome." Approximately 35% of patients have myasthenia gravis (MG), although most patients with MG do not have thymoma. Other syndromes include erythrocyte aplasia, collagen vascular disease (lupus, rheumatoid arthritis, dermatomyositis), polycythemia/pancytopenia, and Cushing's syndrome.

130. What are the presenting signs and symptoms of superior vena cava obstruction?

Patients may complain of headache, chest pain, cough (sometimes associated with syncope or headache), lacrimation, and periorbital/facial edema. Symptoms are present in most patients for 2–4 weeks before hospitalization. Physical findings include neck vein distention; edema, plethora, and cyanosis of the face; tachypnea; edema of the upper extremities; paralysis of the vocal cords; and distention of retinal veins or veins beneath the tongue. Veins of the upper extremities do not empty when lifted above the level of the heart.

DIAPHRAGM

131. Name the three major diaphragmatic hernias.

Herniation of abdominal contents into the chest can occur through a region of congenital defect or weakness. Hiatal hernias (via the esophageal hiatus), with displacement of the stomach into the posterior mediastinum, are the most common. Herniation via the retrosternal foramen of Morgagni is often asymptomatic and appears as an abnormal shadow, frequently on the right heart border. Herniation via the posterolateral foramen of Bochdalek is more common in infancy.

132. What causes elevation of a hemidiaphragm on CXR?
Normally, the right hemidiaphragm is several centimeters higher than the left because of upward displacement by the liver. Elevation of a hemidiaphragm may be secondary to:
- Unilateral diaphragmatic paralysis
- Displacement secondary to intra-abdominal masses or ascites
- Loss of lung volume on the affected side
- Eventration of the diaphragm (a rare congenital disorder)
- Subpulmonic effusion

133. What are the most common causes of unilateral diaphragmatic paralysis?
Each diaphragm is innervated by a phrenic nerve originating from the third, fourth, and fifth cervical roots. Paralysis results from disruption of this nerve. The most common causes include invasion by bronchogenic carcinoma, thoracic trauma, surgical resection or disruption, and possibly postviral neuropathy. Slightly more than one-half of cases remain unexplained. Occasionally, recovery occurs. Unilateral diaphragmatic paralysis is usually asymptomatic.

134. How is the "sniff" test useful in evaluating unilateral diaphragmatic paralysis?
The diagnosis of unilateral diaphragmatic paralysis is suggested by elevation of one hemidiaphragm on CXR. Under fluoroscopy, this diagnosis can be confirmed by asking the patient to "sniff," which rapidly increases intra-abdominal pressure, lowers intrathoracic pressure, and causes an upward (paradoxical) movement of the affected diaphragm.

VENTILATORY SUPPORT

135. List the indications for initiation of mechanical ventilation.
Absolute indications

Apnea	Administration of paralyzing agents

Clinical examination alone

Ineffectual respiratory efforts	Inspiratory muscle fatigue

Arterial blood gas values plus clinical evaluation

Hypoxemia not corrected by other means	Progressive hypercarbia with acidosis

Johanson WG, et al: Critical care. In Murray JF, Nadel JA (eds): Textbook of Respiratory Medicine. Philadelphia, WB. Saunders, 1988, p 1994.

136. Which physiologic guidelines should be used to evaluate the need for ventilatory support in respiratory failure?
The need for ventilatory support should be based on a bedside assessment of impairment. Mechanical ventilation usually is indicated when one or more of the following five parameters of respiratory function are met:
1. Alveolar ventilation: increased $PaCO_2$ such that pH is < 7.20–7.25.
2. Work of breathing: minute ventilation to maintain $PaCO_2 > 15$–20 L/min or respiratory rate > 35 breaths/minute or dead space > 0.6 of tidal volume.
3. Lung expansion: maximal inspiratory force < 4–5 ml/kg or inspiratory vital capacity < 10–15 ml/kg.
4. Respiratory muscle strength: maximal inspiratory force < 25 cmH$_2$0 or inability to double resting minute ventilation.
5. Hypoxemia: $P(A\text{-}a)O_2 > 350$ on 100% or $PaO_2/FIO_2 < 200$ or right-to-left shunt > 20–25%.

137. What are the complications of endotracheal intubation?

IMMEDIATE	DELAYED	LATE
Difficult intubation	Self-extubation	Tracheomalacia
Local trauma	Infections (tracheobronchitis,	Tracheal perforation
Malposition of endotracheal	pneumonia)	Laryngeal dysfunction
tube	Mucosal edema, denudation	Subglottic/tracheal stenosis

From Johanson WG Jr, Peters JI: Critical care. In Murray JF, Nadel JA (eds): Textbook of Respiratory Medicine. Philadelphia, W.B. Saunders, 1988, p 1979.

APNEA SYNDROMES

138. How do you differentiate central apnea and obstructive sleep apnea?
Apnea refers to a pause in respiration for more than 10 sec. Both central sleep apnea (CSA) and obstructive sleep apnea (OSA) result in cessation of respirations. They are differentiated by a lack of respiratory effort in CSA vs. continued but ineffective respiratory effort in OSA. Hypopnea is defined as a reduction in airflow of at least 50% that results in a decrease in arterial saturation of 4% or more (due to partial airway obstruction). The number of apneas and hypopneas per hour is termed the respiratory distress index (RDI). This index is helps to determine the severity of OSA.

139. What are the clinical characteristics of a patient with OSA?

Obesity (common)	Sexual dysfunction
Daytime hypersomnia	Morning headache
Rarely awaken during sleep	Nocturnal enuresis
Loud snoring	Intellectual deterioration

140. How is the severity of OSA determined?
The severity of OSA is determined by many variables, including the RDI and oxygen saturation (SaO_2) as well as the severity of symptoms and potentially comorbid diseases.

CRITERION	MILD OSA	MODERATE OSA	SEVERE OSA
RDI	5–19	20–49	≥ 50
Minimal SaO_2 (%)	80–89	70–79	≤ 69

From Chervin R, Guilleminault C: Obstructive sleep apnea and related disorders. Neurol Clin 14:583–609, 1996.

BIBLIOGRAPHY

1. Baum GL, Wolinsky E (eds): Textbook of Pulmonary Diseases, 5th ed. Boston, Little, Brown, 1994.
2. Bone RC, et al (eds): Pulmonary and Critical Care Medicine, St. Louis, Mosby, 1997.
3. Fishman AP: Pulmonary Diseases and Disorders, 3rd ed. New York, McGraw-Hill, 1998.
4. Murray JF, Nadel JA (eds): Textbook of Respiratory Medicine, 2nd ed. Philadelphia, W.B. Saunders, 1999.
5. Parsons PE, Heffner JE (eds): Pulmonary/Respiratory Therapy Secrets. Philadelphia, Hanley & Belfus, 1997.

11. RHEUMATOLOGY

Richard A. Rubin, M.D.

The wolf, I'm afraid, is inside tearing up the place.
Flannery O'Connor (1925–1964)
Novelist, sufferer from lupus erythematosus (letter)

*Screw up the vise as tightly as possible—you have rheumatism; give it
another turn, and that is gout.*
Anonymous

1. Give an operational definition for rheumatic diseases.
Rheumatic diseases are syndromes of pain and/or inflammation in articular or periarticular tissues.

2. What is undifferentiated connective tissue disease (UCTD)? How is it different from mixed connective tissue disease (MCTD)?
An exact diagnosis of a rheumatic disease is not always possible at initial presentation. All of the clinical manifestations of a given rheumatic disease may not develop at once but may unfold over time, and many features are shared among different rheumatic diseases. Myositis, for example, can be found as a primary condition (polymyositis) or as part of other systemic diseases (dermatomyositis, systemic sclerosis, and even systemic lupus erythematosus [SLE]). In addition to shared clinical features, these illnesses may have shared serologic features. The most obvious example is antinuclear antibody (ANA), which may be found in various diseases, including SLE, systemic sclerosis, Sjögren's syndrome, inflammatory myopathies, Hashimoto's thyroiditis, and inflammatory bowel disease. When clinical and laboratory features suggest an autoimmune or inflammatory etiology but clinical and serologic heterogeneity make an exact diagnosis impossible, the designation **UCTD** has been used.

MCTD was first described as a separate entity in 1972 and is a more specific designation than UCTD. It is not the mixture or overlap of any rheumatic diseases; rather, MCTD is used specifically when features of SLE and systemic sclerosis are present with high titers of antibody to U_1RNP.

3. What is a "joint mouse"?
Osteocartilaginous bodies within a joint are often termed joint mice or loose bodies and occur commonly in osteoarthritis. They are believed to arise when bits of articular cartilage and subchondral bone break from the surface and enter the joint. There may be proliferation and deposition of new bone on these fragments.

4. What is chondromalacia patella?
Chondromalacia is a softening and degeneration of articular cartilage. In the patella, it is often associated with meniscal disease, knee laxity, or recurrent trauma. Typically, pain is associated with activity, often with descending stairs.

Moskowitz RW: Clinical and laboratory findings in osteoarthritis. In McCarty DJ, Koopman WJ (eds): Arthritis and Allied Conditions, 12th ed. Philadelphia, Lea & Febiger, 1993, pp 1735–1760.

5. How do bunions occur?
A bunion (hallux valgus) is a deviation of the proximal phalanx of the great toe toward the fibular side of the foot. It can be caused by biomechanical factors (tight and pointy-toed shoes that push the proximal phalanx across the other toes), inflammatory disease (gout or rheumatoid arthritis), or abnormal alignment (usually congenital) at the first metatarsal-cuneiform joint. If the cuneiform is abnormal, the first metatarsal may deviate excessively toward the midline (a primary

varus deformity), which leads to a valgus deformity (lateral deviation) of the great toe when the abnormal foot is placed into standard shoes.

6. What conditions are associated with avascular necrosis (AVN) of bone?

Trauma (femoral head fractures)
Hemoglobinopathies
Exogenous or endogenous overproduction
of glucocorticoids
Alcoholism
Human immunodeficiency virus (HIV)
Gaucher's disease
Pregnancy
Systemic lupus erythematosus (SLE)
Kidney transplantation
Lymphoproliferative diseases
Anticardiolipin antibody syndrome

7. What mechanisms contribute to bone loss with the use of glucocorticoids?

Use of glucocorticoids is a cornerstone of treatment of many rheumatic diseases, but one of its most concerning toxicities is accelerated bone loss. Corticosteroids have been shown to decrease intestinal absorption of calcium, increase urinary calcium excretion, and inhibit osteoblast function. Calcium loss from trabecular bone is greater than from cortical bone, although the mechanism for this difference is not known.

Sambrook PN, et al: Corticosteroid osteoporosis. Br J Rheum 34:8–12, 1995.

8. Describe the following eponymous disorders.

Behçet's syndrome: an inflammatory disease manifested principally by ocular inflammation and oral, nasal, and genital ulcerations. Other features include arthritis, thrombophlebitis, and vasculitis.

Buerger's disease (also called thromboangiitis obliterans): a vasculopathy in which acute inflammatory lesions produce occlusive thrombosis of arteries and veins. It has been associated overwhelmingly with tobacco use.

Caplan's syndrome: rheumatoid arthritis (RA) with pneumoconiosis.

Cogan's syndrome: an unusual vasculopathy associated with interstitial keratitis, sensorineural hearing loss, tinnitus, and vertigo. Systemic features such as fever, weight loss and fatigue are present in about one-half of patients.

DeQuervain's tenosynovitis: inflammation of the cellular lining and subsequent narrowing of the membrane (stenosing tenosynovitis) of the abductor pollicis longus and extensor pollicis brevis tendons at the radial styloid.

Dupuytren's contracture: nodular fibrosis of the palmar fascia and flexion contractures of the digits.

Ehlers-Danlos syndrome: a group of disorders characterized by hyperextensibility of skin and hypermobility of joints, predisposing to early development of osteoarthritis.

Kawasaki's disease (also called mucocutaneous lymph node syndrome): an acute febrile disease, usually in children under 5 years of age, associated with conjunctivitis, fissuring of the lips, strawberry tongue, painful lymphadenopathy, and vasculitis, especially of the coronary arteries.

Legg-Calvé-Perthes disease: idiopathic osteonecrosis of the femoral capital epiphysis usually in boys ages 3-8 that may result in a large flat femoral head.

Osgood-Schlatter disease (also called tibial tubercle apophysitis): inflammation at the site where the patellar tendon inserts onto the tibial tubercle. It is a probably a repetitive motion injury, usually occurring in adolescents, and presents as knee pain.

Saint Vitus' dance (also called Sydenham's chorea or chorea minor): a neurologic disorder consisting of abrupt, purposeless involuntary movements that disappear during sleep. It is found in patients with rheumatic fever.

Still's disease: a subset of juvenile rheumatoid arthritis that has systemic features (fever, lymphadenopathy, pleuropericarditis, hepatosplenomegaly, and leukocytosis) as major manifestations.

Sudek's atrophy (also called reflex sympathetic dystrophy): severe pain, edema, vasomotor abnormalities, and atrophy of bone, muscle and skin.

Tietze's syndrome (also called osteochondritis): painful enlargement of the upper costal cartilages.

9. Distinguish between Bouchard's nodes and Heberden's nodes.

Bouchard's nodes: one of the most common manifestations of osteoarthritis with bony enlargement of the proximal interphalangeal (PIP) joints.

Heberden's nodes: one of the most common manifestations of osteoarthritis with bony enlargement of the distal interphalangeal (DIP) joints. Women are affected more frequently than men (10:1 ratio). Heredity plays a particularly strong role in mothers, daughters, and sisters.

10. Distinguish between Charcot joint and Charcot-Leyden crystals.

Charcot joint: progressive degenerative arthropathy associated with a neuropathic joint; historically, it was associated most commonly with tabes dorsalis, but now it is seen most frequently with syrinx or diabetic neuropathy.

Charcot-Leyden crystals: crystals formed in the cytoplasm of disrupted eosinophils found in the sputum of asthmatics and in the synovial fluid of patients with eosinophilic synovitis.

11. Define the following disorders named after occupations or specific activities.

Housemaid's knee: prepatellar bursitis.

Little leaguer's shoulder: separation of the proximal humeral epiphysis probably secondary to the repetitive motion associated with pitching.

Tailor's seat (also called weaver's bottom): inflammation of the ischial bursa (the bursa that separates the gluteus maximus from the ischial tuberosity).

Tennis elbow: lateral epicondylitis.

Trigger finger: sticking or locking of a finger in flexion as a result of stenosing tenosynovitis. The finger can be extended manually, often with discomfort.

12. What are Milwaukee shoulder, slapped-cheek syndrome, and opera glass hands?

Milwaukee shoulder: degeneration of the glenohumeral joint with lysis of the rotator cuff (noted on x-ray by cephalad migration of the humeral head) associated with deposition of basic calcium phosphate and calcium pyrophosphate crystals.

Slapped-cheek syndrome: acute parvovirus infection in children.

Opera glass hands (also called arthritis mutilans): severe inflammatory destructive disease of the hands. Dissolution of bone causes a foreshortening of digits in the same way that opera glasses are foreshortened binoculars.

13. Define the following eponymous signs and tests.

Finkelstein's test: a maneuver to demonstrate de Quervain's tenosynovitis. A fist is made around the thumb, and ulnar motion of the wrist is produced. In patients with de Quervain's tenosynovitis, this maneuver reproduces the typical sharp, exquisite pain.

Phalen's sign: a test of diagnostic usefulness in carpal tunnel syndrome. By raising both arms, opposing the dorsum of the hands, and then slightly dropping the elbows (maximally flexing the wrist), one can reproduce the discomfort of carpal tunnel syndrome.

Shober test: a test for spinal flexion. Two points on the patient's lumbar spine (usually the lumbar sacral junction and a point 10 cm above) are marked while the patient is standing. The distance is remeasured after the patient bends to touch the toes (maximal forward flexion). An elongation < 5 cm suggests spine stiffness.

Tinel's sign: focal pain and electrical sensations elicited by tapping on a nerve at the site of entrapment.

14. What is POEMS syndrome?

A plasma cell dyscrasia characterized by **p**olyneuropathy, **o**rganomegaly, **e**ndocrinopathy, **m**onoclonal protein, and **s**kin changes, which may resemble scleroderma.

15. What are rice bodies?

Aggregates of fibrin frequently found in the synovial fluid of patients with RA.

16. Define RS3PE.

RS3PE is a remitting, symmetric, seronegative synovitis associated with pitting edema. It usually has an abrupt onset and affects primarily older men.

17. Which clinical syndromes are associated with complement deficiencies?

COMPLEMENT DEFICIENCY	DISEASE(S)
C1q	Glomerulonephritis and poikiloderma congenita
C1r	Glomerulonephritis, lupus-like syndrome
C1s	Lupus-like syndrome
C1INH	Discoid lupus, SLE, lupus-like syndrome
C4	SLE, Sjögren's syndrome
C2	SLE, discoid lupus, polymyositis, Henoch-Schönlein purpura, Hodgkin's disease, vasculitis, glomerulonephritis, common variable hypogammaglobulinemia
C3	Vasculitis, lupus-like syndrome, glomerulonephritis
C5	SLE, neisserial infection
C6	Neisserial infection
C7	SLE, rheumatoid arthritis, Raynaud's phenomenon and sclerodactyly, vasculitis, neisserial infection
C8	SLE, neisserial infection
C9	Neisserial infection

From Ruddy S: Complement deficiencies and rheumatic diseases. In Kelly WN, et al (eds): Textbook of Rheumatology, 4th ed. Philadelphia, W.B. Saunders, 1993, pp 1283–1289.

DIAGNOSIS

18. How much synovial fluid is present in the normal knee?

The knee normally has up to 4 ml of fluid. Detection of a joint effusion is important in the evaluation of patients with articular symptoms.

19. Which studies should generally be performed on synovial fluid after arthrocentesis?

Gram stain and bacterial culture may confirm the presence of an infective agent. In the right clinical setting, similar procedures for mycobacteria or fungi are important. A white blood cell (WBC) count with differential is one of the best indicators of the degree of inflammation. Evaluation for crystals by polarized light microscopy may confirm the diagnosis. Although a good deal has been written about various other tests (e.g., glucose, complement, rheumatoid factor, ANA, lactate dehydrogenase, protein), they add little diagnostic information.

20. What are the "string" and "mucin clot" tests?

The primary component of joint fluid is hyaluronic acid. It is quite viscous and makes a "string" when expressed from a syringe as a single drop. Dilute acetic acid causes hyaluronate and protein to clump and fall to the bottom of a test tube (producing the famous "mucin clot"). Inflammatory mediators cause fragmentation of the hyaluronate–protein complex, rendering it unable to form a good mucin clot.

Basically, these tests provide a crude bedside estimate of the level of synovial inflammation. Because the wet prep and total synovial fluid WBC count give more objective data, the mucin clot and string tests are primarily of historic interest. It is also probably true that when done in the traditional manner at the bedside, these tests violate regulations for the handling of body fluids established by the Occupational Safety and Health Administration and Clinical Laboratories Improvement Act.

Schumacher HR Jr: Synovial fluid analysis and synovial biopsy. In Kelly WN, et al (eds): Textbook of Rheumatology, 4th ed. Philadelphia, W.B. Saunders, 1993, pp 562–578.

21. Straight leg raising is a useful diagnostic maneuver in what common condition?

The straight leg-raising test is designed to reproduce back pain secondary to nerve root compression. The leg is lifted by the calcaneus with the knee remaining straight. Bringing the heel across the other leg (called cross-table straight leg raising) may increase the sensitivity of this maneuver.

22. What clinical features help to distinguish neurogenic from arterial claudication?

Progressive leg or back pain with walking (claudication) may result from either arterial insufficiency or nerve compression, but distinguishing between the two can be difficult. Absence of pedal pulses suggests arterial disease, although one study reported this sign in 9% of patients with spinal stenosis. Patients with arterial insufficiency often get relief of pain simply by pausing or slowing their pace. Patients with nerve compression rarely get relief unless they sit or lie down. Neurologic signs such as weakness, abnormal reflexes, and abnormal electromyographic/nerve conduction velocities are present in spinal stenosis but absent in arterial disease.

O'Duffy JD, Ebersold MJ: Spinal stenosis. In McCarty DJ, Koopman WJ (eds): Arthritis and Allied Conditions, 12th ed. Philadelphia, Lea & Febiger, 1993, pp 1601–1608.

23. What is onychodystrophy? With which diseases is it associated?

Separation of the nail plate, usually beginning at the free margin and progressing proximally, is called onychodystrophy. Both systemic and local processes are associated with this finding, including hypo- and hyperthyroidism, pregnancy, syphilis, trauma (particularly clawing), psoriasis, SLE, atopic dermatitis, eczema, use of solvents (including nail hardeners), and mycotic, pyogenic, or viral infections.

Domonkos AN, et al: Diseases of the skin appendages. In Andrews' Diseases of the Skin: Clinical Dermatology, 7th ed. Philadelphia, W.B. Saunders, 1982, pp 930–984.

24. Which rheumatic syndromes have been associated with uveitis?

Ankylosing spondylitis	Juvenile rheumatoid arthritis
Reactive arthritis	Sjögren's syndrome
Psoriasis	Sarcoidosis
Inflammatory bowel disease	Behçet's disease
Kawasaki disease	Relapsing polychondritis

Rosenbaum JT: Uveitis. In McCarty DJ (ed): Arthritis and Allied Conditions, 11th ed. Philadelphia, Lea & Febiger, 1989, pp 1563–1568.

25. Which diseases are associated with soft tissue calcification?

Soft tissue calcification detected by plain roentgenograms can be an important clue in the diagnosis of rheumatic conditions. A partial list includes:

Calcific tendinitis	Neuropathic arthropathy
Chondrocalcinosis	Parathyroid disease
Dermatomyositis	Renal osteodystrophy
Diabetes	Sarcoidosis
Ehlers-Danlos syndrome	Scleroderma
Neoplasia	Trauma

Resnick D, Niwayama G: Soft tissues. In Resnick D, Niwayama G (eds): Diagnosis of Bone and Joint Disorders, 2nd ed. Philadelphia, W.B. Saunders, 1988, pp 4171–4294.

26. Which conditions commonly mimic systemic vasculitis?

Bacterial endocarditis, atrial myxoma, and multiple cholesterol embolization syndrome have many of the same presenting signs and symptoms as systemic vasculitis. Thrombotic states, including hypercoagulability (as occurs with phospholipid antibodies), cryoglobulinemia, hemoglobinopathies, thrombotic thrombocytopenic purpura (TTP), or hemolytic uremic syndrome, may be confused with vasculitis. Drugs that induce vasospasm (cocaine, ergots, and other sympathomimetics) sometimes produce the arteriographic appearance of vasculitis. Finally, processes that produce vascular malformation, such as fibromuscular disease and moyamoya, may be included in the differential diagnosis of vasculitis.

Sack KE: Mimickers of vasculitis. In Koopman WJ (ed): Arthritis and Allied Conditions, 13th ed. Baltimore, Williams & Wilkins, 1997, pp 1525–1546.

27. What is the differential diagnosis of subcutaneous nodules?

Subcutaneous nodules are found in RA, rheumatic fever, and SLE. In addition, gouty tophi, synovial cysts, and xanthomas can sometimes appear as subcutaneous nodules.

28. What are Gottron's papules?

Patches of erythematous scaly plaques on knuckles in patients with dermatomyositis.

RHEUMATOID ARTHRITIS

29. Give an operational definition for RA.

RA is a systemic disease characterized clinically and pathologically by inflammation of diarthrodial joints. Although RA often is accompanied by a variety of extra-articular manifestations, arthritis is its major expression, and currently we must rely on the characteristics of this expression to recognize RA.

30. What are the American College of Rheumatology (ACR) criteria for RA?

Patients can be said to have RA if they satisfy at least four of the following seven criteria. Criteria 1–4 must be present for at least 6 weeks.

1. Morning stiffness around the joints, lasting at least 1 hour before maximal improvement.
2. Arthritis of 3 or more joints. A physician has observed simultaneous soft tissue swelling or fluid (not bony overgrowth alone) in at least 3 joint areas. The 14 possible joint areas include PIP, metacarpophalangeal (MCP), wrist, elbow, knee, ankle, and metatarsophalangeal (MTP) joints.
3. Arthritis of hand joints. At least one joint area is swollen, as above, in the wrist, MCP, or PIP joint.
4. Symmetric arthritis: simultaneous involvement of the same joint areas on both sides of the body.
5. Rheumatoid nodules: subcutaneous nodules over bony prominences or extensor surfaces or in juxta-articular regions, observed by a physician.
6. Serum rheumatoid factor (RF): demonstration of abnormal amounts of serum RF by any method that has been positive in < 5% of normal control subjects.
7. Radiographic changes typical of RA on posteroanterior hand and wrist x-rays, which must include erosions or unequivocal bony decalcification localized to or most marked adjacent to the involved joints (osteoarthritis changes alone do not qualify).

Arnett FC, et al: The American Rheumatism Association 1987 revised criteria for the classification of rheumatoid arthritis. Arthritis Rheum 31:315–324, 1988.

31. Discuss the HLA association with RA.

Upward of 90% of patients meeting the ACR criteria for RA have been found to have the HLA class II genes DR4 or DR1. Closer review shows that the specific alleles of these otherwise disparate genes have a common sequence at loci 67–74 of their DRB1 chains, which code for one side of the peptide-binding groove. The estimated prevalence of the susceptibility alleles in the general population (5–15%) makes it clear that most people with these alleles do not develop RA; therefore, genetic testing is not a useful tool in general clinical practice.

Nepom GT, Nepom B: Rheumatoid Arthritis: Genetics of the Major Histocompatibility Complex. In Klippel JH, Dieppe P (eds): Rheumatology CD ROM Version 2.0, 1998.

32. Does RA have a uniform onset?

Although some interesting patterns and observations of onset have been described, they are of little diagnostic usefulness. For example, patients have been documented to develop RA twice as commonly between October and March as between March and October. Most patients (50–70%) have an insidious onset of RA with gradual development of generalized achiness, fatigue, and stiffness. They notice actual joint swelling after weeks or months of nonspecific symptoms. Up to 15% of patients may have an abrupt onset of RA, with the explosive development of intense, symmetric, articular stiffness, pain, and swelling. Occasionally patients suffer intermittent attacks involving single or multiple joints that gradually quiet, leaving them asymptomatic for prolonged periods. Hench coined the term "palindromic rheumatism" for this presentation.

33. What is "gelling"?

Gelling describes the achiness and stiffness that occurs in patients with RA after a period of inactivity (such as getting up from the dinner table or rising from a seat after a movie). The stiffness that occurs on rising from bed in the morning is also a form of gelling.

34. Which joints are most commonly involved in RA?

RA is a symmetric polyarthropathy that can involve almost any diarthrodial joint. The hands and wrists are involved in over 90% of patients. About one-half of patients with RA develop x-ray evidence of hip involvement. Foot and ankle disease can have a major impact on function, although ankle involvement is rare in the absence of MTP involvement. Palpable swelling at the radiohumeral joint, along with incomplete extension, marks elbow involvement. Nodules and concomitant swelling of the olecranon bursae also may suggest elbow disease. Knee involvement is common. The thoracic and lumbar spine are rarely if ever involved with RA. The cervical spine is commonly involved and deserves special mention. Cervical spine involvement usually is heralded by pain with motion and occipital headache. Significant laxity at the alantoaxial joint with subluxation makes patients prone to slowly progressive, spastic quadriparesis. If this laxity is present, the hyperextension of the neck that occurs during intubation for general anesthesia can produce quadriplegia. Thus patients with neck pain or longstanding disease should undergo cervical spine evaluation before any surgical procedure. Other joints involved include the shoulders, temporomandibular joints, cricoarytenoid joints (sometimes explaining why patients commonly have "sore throats" without signs of pharyngitis), and ossicles of the ears (which may be in part responsible for some hearing loss).

35. What is Baker's cyst? How does it form? What is the major differential diagnosis?

Swelling of the knee capsule extending posteriorly to the popliteal fossa (hence the synonym popliteal cyst). Baker's cyst is thought to develop as the knee is flexed, producing a significant rise in intra-articular pressure and an outpouching of the synovium posteriorly. The cruciate ligaments may act as a one-way valve, making it hard for the fluid to resorb. Posterior rupture may lead to swelling of the leg below the knee. When rupture occurs, a crescentic hematoma may form beneath one of the malleoli. The major differential diagonsis is thrombophlebitis. Although a ruptured popliteal cyst may mimic thrombophlebitis, the increased pressure in the calf from the fluid may compress venous return and predispose to clot as well.

Kraag G, et al: The hemorrhagic crescent sign of acute synovial rupture [letter]. Ann Intern Med 85:477, 1976.

36. How does RA affect the synovium?

The synovium is a primary target for the inflammatory process in RA. Normal synovium is a thin, delicate structure (only one or two cells thick) and contains two types of synoviocytes: type A (macrophage-like cells derived from the bone marrow) and type B (fibroblast-like cells that probably are mesenchymal in origin). Early changes in the joints of patients with RA show both hypertrophy and hyperplasia of the synovial lining. Angiogenesis is a prominent and early change in RA synovium. Adhesion molecules appear, polymorphonuclear leukocytes (the predominant cell type in the articular fluid), and metalloproteinases are present in synovial fluid, and fibronectin is deposited on articular cartilage. White cells soon infiltrate the synovium, principally small lymphocytes, macrophages, and plasma cells. Although B cells are present, the majority of infiltrating cells are T lymphocytes with a phenotype characteristic of memory T cells.

37. What is pannus? Is it responsible for the articular destruction in RA?

Grossly, the synovium becomes boggy and edematous with villous projections. This congested proliferative synovium is called pannus. Histologically, there are two kinds of pannus: (1) a fibroblastic transitional pannus, which is more commonly found in large joints where progressive cartilage loss is characteristic, and (2) an intensely inflammatory type, which is more common in small joints and associated with juxta-articular erosive disease. New information has called into question the old hypothesis that pannus was solely responsible for articular destruction in RA. Normal articular surfaces do not support the adhesion of pannus. Electron micrographs suggest that damage to articular cartilage may precede the overgrowth of pannus. In addition, erosive disease has been seen in areas without pannus. Although the exact mechanism remains a mystery, it appears that articular damage in RA results from cartilage destruction that is a direct consequence of a relentless inflammatory attack that includes both pannus formation and soluble inflammatory mediators.

38. What mechanisms underlie the classic swan neck and boutonnière deformities?

The **swan neck deformity** describes flexion at the MCP and DIP joints with extension at the PIP joints. This deformity results from inflammation and subsequent contraction of interosseous and flexor muscles and tendons. Other contributing factors include tenosynovitis and destruction leading to MCP subluxation. Flexion at the MCP leads to exaggerated pull on the extensor tendon of the PIP. The flexion at the DIP is caused because the pull of the flexor tendon overcomes the pull of the extensor tendon.

Flexion contracture at the PIP with extension of the DIP is referred to as the **boutonnière deformity**. The pathogenesis of this deformity is thought to be related to injury of the extensor tendon. If it becomes lengthened or torn, the flexor tendons are unopposed. The altered mechanics and location of the joint lead to functional shortening of the lateral tendons and hyperextension of the DIP joint.

39. What is the mechanism for the development of cocked-up toes in RA?

Inflammation of the MTP joints in RA often leads to subluxation of the metatarsal heads and collapse of the arch of the foot. A claw-like or cocking up appearance of the toes follows.

McCarty DJ: Clinical picture of RA. In McCarty DJ, Koopman WJ (eds): Arthritis and Allied Conditions, 12th ed. Philadelphia, Lea & Febiger, 1993, pp 781–809.

40. What are rheumatoid factors (RFs)? Which conditions are associated with their presence in the circulation?

RFs are antibodies (usually IgM) directed at the Fc portion of the IgG molecule. RFs may be found in 1–5% of the normal population (a percentage that increases with age). The presence of RF is not specific for RA. Patients with other conditions that have rheumatic features, including sarcoidosis, interstitial lung disease, cryoglobulinemia, SLE, and Sjögren's syndrome, may have circulating RFs. Viral, parasitic, and other infectious diseases, including mononucleosis, hepatitis, malaria, tuberculosis, and bacterial endocarditis, may be associated with RFs. Up to 70% of patients with active hepatitis C infection have RFs in the circulation, probably because of the cross-reactivity between cryoglobulins (produced commonly in hepatitis C) and RF. Since chronic hepatitis can also produce achiness and occasionally a mild synovitis, careful attention should be paid to excluding hepatitis C (even if the patient has normal serum transaminase levels) before establishing a diagnosis of RA. Finally, human parvovirus B19 infection (fifth disease or slapped-cheek syndrome) may produce a symmetric polyarthropathy that can mimic RA, at times with modest titers of RFs in the circulation.

Fuchs HA, Sergent JS: Rheumatoid arthritis: The clinical picture. In Koopman WJ (ed): Arthritis and Allied Conditions: A Textbook of Rheumatology, 13th ed. Baltimore, Williams & Wilkins, 1997, pp 1041–1070.

41. How many RA patients have no circulating RF detectable?

Up to 25% of patients with clinical RA have no circulating RF. In addition, it may take as long as 2 years for the RF to become detectable. Thus, just when it would be most helpful diagnostically,

RF is least likely to be present. The titer has little prognostic value in an individual patient, and remeasurements provide little added information.

42. How many patients with RA test positive for ANAs?

Up to 25% of patients with established RA have circulating ANAs. Patients with RA and Sjögren's syndrome often have positive anti-Ro antibodies. ANA-positive patients with RA are often considered to have a poorer prognosis.

43. Does RA confer an increased mortality rate?

Yes. For many years, it was believed that although RA was a painful and destructive condition, it had no influence on mortality. Recent studies have shown that the average life expectancy is significantly shorter for patients with RA than for the general population (up to a twofold increase in mortality). Causes of death include factors attributable to RA itself or to drugs used to treat it (vasculitis, secondary amyloidosis, carditis, cervical myelopathy, rheumatoid lung disease, and drug toxicity), cardiovascular disease (the leading cause of death in RA patients), and malignancies. The risk for malignancy, taken as a whole, is not elevated in RA, although the incidence of lymphoma (especially non-Hodgkin's lymphoma), leukemia, and myeloma is higher in patients with RA than in the general population. Survival rates of patients with RA and malignancy are no different from those expected in the general population. Predictors of early mortality include older age, concomitant cardiovascular disease, high number of involved joints, high titer of RF, fewer years of formal education, and poor functional status.

Isomaki HA: Mortality in patients with rheumatoid arthritis. In Wolfe F, Pincus T (eds): Rheumatoid Arthritis: Pathogenesis, Assessment, Outcome and Treatment. New York, Marcel Dekker, 1994, pp 235–246.

44. How has the general approach to treatment of RA changed over the past decade? Why?

In the past, it was believed that not all cases of RA were severe; therefore, most patients did not warrant early treatment with potentially toxic medication. Treatment was instituted with the least toxic but also least effective medications, which were increased in a stepwise fashion as the disease flared or did not respond (the so-called pyramid approach). Unfortunately, it may take 6 months to learn whether the disease-modifying antirheumatic drug (DMARD) has failed, and considerable joint damage can be done in this period. This early articular damage leads to mechanical deformities that in turn produce disability and lack of function. In fact, more recent data have shown that most functional deterioration occurs early in the disease. One study revealed that patients treated in the traditional way suffered a moderate loss of function within 2 years, a severe loss of function within 6 years and a very severe loss by 10 years. If ability to maintain work status is used as a measure of function, statistics are even grimmer. Fifty percent of patients were disabled after 10 years and 60% after 15 years. An increased mortality rate (see previous question) has recently been recognized in patients treated in the traditional way. Therefore, in an attempt to improve outcome, most rheumatologists now recommend earlier initiation of DMARDs and a more aggressive approach to management.

Donnelly S, Scott DL: The morbidity of rheumatoid arthritis. In Wolfe F, Pincus T (eds): Rheumatoid Arthritis: Pathogenesis, Assessment, Outcome and Treatment. New York, Marcel Dekker, 1994, pp 207–234.

45. How is the functional capacity of RA patients classified? Why is it important?

Class I   No restrictions, able to perform normal activities
Class II   Moderate restriction, but able to perform normal activities
Class III   Marked restriction, inability to perform most duties of the patient's usual occupation or self-care
Class IV   Incapacitation or confinement to a wheelchair

Functional status may be one of the best predictors of premature mortality in patients with RA.

46. What classification scheme is available to describe the progression of RA?

Stage I: early
- No destructive changes on x-ray.
- X-ray evidence of osteoporosis is acceptable.

Stage II: moderate
- X-ray evidence of osteoporosis with or without slight subchondral bone destruction; slight cartilage destrution may be present.
- No joint deformities, although joint mobility may be limited.
- Adjacent muscle atrophy.
- Extra-articular soft tissue lesions such as nodules or tenosynovitis may be present.

Stage III: severe
- X-ray evidence of cartilage and bone destruction in addition to osteoporosis.
- Joint deformity, such as subluxation, ulnar deviation, or hyperextension, without fibrosis or bony ankylosis.
- Extra-articular soft tissue lesions such as nodules or tenosynovitis may be present.

Stage IV: terminal
- Criteria of stage III.
- Bony or fibrous ankylosis.

47. Which factors suggest an aggressive disease course in RA?

Explosive onset of disease with involvement of multiple joints, high titers of RF, positive ANA, nodules, lower socioeconomic status, and fewer years of formal education.

48. Do patients with RA develop gout with increased, decreased, or the same frequency as the general population?

There is a negative association between RA and gout.

49. How does pregnancy affect RA?

Signs and symptoms of RA subside in approximately 70% of women during pregnancy. No data suggest that RA has a detrimental effect on the fetus. However, arthritis should be assessed before pregnancy, if possible, because anesthesia and intubation can be problematic and even dangerous when cervical spine disease is present. Delivery also can be difficult if arthritis limits hip motion. Postpartum flares of disease occur in approximately 90% of women who experience improvement.

Griffin J: Rheumatoid arthritis: Biological effects and management. In Scott JS, Bird HA (eds): Pregnancy, Autoimmunity and Connective Tissue Disorders. Oxford, Oxford University Press, 1990, pp 140–162.

50. List the major extra-articular manifestations of RA.

- Nodules
- Pulmonary involvement
- Eye involvement
- Vasculitis
- Cardiac disease
- Felty's syndrome

51. What are rheumatoid nodules? Where are they found?

The classic rheumatoid nodule has a central area of necrosis surrounded by a rim of palisading fibroblasts that, in turn, is surrounded by a collagenous capsule with perivascular collections of chronic inflammatory cells. Rheumatoid nodules occur in 20–35% of patients with RA and can be found at the elbow, wrist, soles, Achilles tendon, head, or sacrum. RF is usually present. Accelerated nodule formation has been described in patients receiving methotrexate treatment for RA, even when methotrexate shows efficacy at calming the arthritis and the patient has had no previous nodule formation. Nodulosis goes away when methotrexate is discontinued.

52. What is the classic clinical setting for the development of vasculitis associated with RA?

The development of vasculitis classically occurs in patients with long-standing disease and severe joint disease with destruction, high titers of RF, and nodules. Men are affected more often than women. As with any systemic vasculopathy, constitutional features such as weight loss and fever are common findings, as are cutaneous manifestations (nail edge lesions, rashes, ulcers, and, less commonly, gangrene), neurologic manifestations (mononeuritis multiplex, CNS inflammation), ocular manifestations (scleritis, corneal melt and retinal vasculitis), and cardiopulmonary manifestations (alveolitis, pleurisy, pericarditis, aortitis, and arrhythmias).

Bacon PA, Moots RJ: Extra-articular manifestations of rheumatoid arthritis. In Koopman WJ (ed): Arthritis and Allied Conditions: A Textbook of Rheumatology, 13th ed. Baltimore, Williams & Wilkins, 1997, pp 1071–1088.

53. How does RA affect the heart?

Cardiac involvement in RA can take several forms. Although pericardial disease is present in nearly one-half of patients with RA at autopsy and up to one-third studied by echocardiography, the clinical impact of pericardial inflammation is usually minimal. Myocarditis also has been demonstrated and may be granulomatous with nodules. Conduction defects, coronary arteritis, and granulomatous aortitis also have been described.

54. How does RA affect the lungs?

Pulmonary disease is an extra-articular feature of RA that increases both morbidity and mortality. Pleural disease is a common postmortem finding, but it is usually not clinically relevant. Pneumonitis and interstitial fibrosis also occur in RA. Nodules may be present in the lung but precede articular disease only in rare cases; they may be present individually or in clusters and occasionally cavitate. Rarely, arteritis can be present; if present, it often leads to pulmonary hypertension. Finally, airway disease has been described, typically as reduced maximal mid-expiratory flow rate and maximal expiratory flow rate at 50% of functional capacity. In its most severe form, bronchiolitis obliterans can occur, with a uniformly unfavorable outcome.

In addition to the RA itself, the treating physician also should consider drug-induced lung disease. Methotrexate, d-penicillamine, gold salts, and even sulfasalazine have been associated with the development of pulmonary complications.

Anaya JM, et al: Pulmonary involvement in rheumatoid arthritis. Semin Arthritis Rheum 24:242–254, 1995.

55. What mechanism explains the low glucose level in pleural effusions of RA?

Low levels appear to result from a defect in the transport of glucose into the fluid.

56. What ocular abnormalities are seen in RA?

Episcleritis and scleritis.

57. Define Felty's syndrome.

Felty's syndrome describes the constellation of circulating neutropenia and splenomegaly in patients with established RA. Recurrent infections are common.

58. What is LGL syndrome?

Large granular lymphocyte (LGL) syndrome is a form of chronic lymphoproliferative disease. LGLs have azurophilic granules and normally compose about 10–15% of peripheral blood monocytes, a number that may rise as high as 90% in LGL syndrome. Up to one-third of reported patients with LGL syndrome have RA, making it the most frequently associated disease. Patients may have neutropenia and splenomegaly (pseudo-Felty's syndrome).

Bowman SJ, et al: The large granular lymphocyte syndrome with rheumatoid arthritis: immunogenetic evidence for a broader definition of Felty's syndrome. Arthritis Rheum 37:1326, 1994.

59. Does Still's disease occur in adults? How is it diagnosed?

Still's disease is the eponym assigned to systemic-onset juvenile arthritis. It has been reported in adults as a seronegative polyarthropathy associated with sudden-onset high fever and chills, with evanescent rash on the trunk and extremities. Bony erosions are uncommon, although fusion of the carpal bones may occur.

Reginato AJ: Adult onset Still's disease. In Schumacher HR Jr, et al (eds): Primer on the Rheumatic Diseases, 10th ed. Atlanta, Arthritis Foundation, 1993, pp 182–183.

60. What are the so-called COX₂ anti-inflammatory drugs? How do they differ from other NSAIDs?

All NSAIDs work by inhibiting cyclooxygenase (COX). This enzyme forms an important step in the production of many proinflammatory mediators, including prostaglandins. Without COX there are fewer circulating prostaglandins and therefore less inflammation and pain. As with most mediators in the body, prostaglandins do not have a unique function. They are important in regulating blood flow to the kidney, producing protective mucus in the stomach among many others. In fact, the toxicities of NSAIDs are related primarily to inhibition of all prostaglandins, whether they produce useful or harmful effects.

Recently two subtypes of COX have been described. The traditionally recognized enzyme, designated COX_1, seems to be most involved with normal cellular processes, often described as housekeeping functions. COX_2 seems to be involved more specifically in the synthesis of inflammatory mediators. It is normally not easily detectable in tissue and is thought to be "upregulated" under inflammatory conditions. Thus, a new group of NSAIDs designed for preferential inhibition of COX_2 have been developed. Because they do not inhibit the broader function of COX_1, there is less interference with housekeeping chores and therefore fewer side effects.

61. How do the effects of aspirin on platelets differ from those of other NSAIDs?

NSAIDs, including aspirin, decrease platelet aggregation by inhibiting the COX. Acetylated salicylates (such as aspirin) irreversibly destroy this enzyme, whereas other NSAIDs (including nonacetylated salicylates) allow the return of normal enzyme function once the drug level has dropped. Because COX_2 does not regulate platelet aggregation, newer COX_2 NSAIDs have little effect on platelet function.

62. What are the common side effects of methotrexate (MTX) in the treatment of RA?

Because of its effectiveness and its relatively quick onset of action (4–6 weeks compared with 4–6 months for hydroxychloroquine), MTX is widely used in the treatment of RA. Reported toxicities include stomatitis, alopecia, bone marrow suppression, macrocytosis, liver damage, and pulmonary disease. Pulmonary disease may be mild or potentially life-threatening (pneumonitis) and may begin as a benign but persistent cough. It appears that preexisting lung disease (especially interstitial disease) may predispose to MTX pulmonary toxicity.

Liver toxicity most commonly takes the form of transient elevation of serum transaminases. These episodes do not correlate with the more disturbing complication of hepatic fibrosis. Although the risk of fibrosis is unknown, long-term studies have produced waning concern about the need for liver biopsy after prolonged treatment. Because the drug is immunosuppressive, herpetic outbreaks as well as infections such as *Pneumocystis carinii*, *Nocardia asteroides*, and cytomegalovirus have been reported. MTX is teratogenic and should not be given to women who are or may become pregnant. It produces chromatin abnormalities in sperm and should not be given to men within 9–12 months of conception. MTX should not be used with trimethoprim/sulfamethoxazole because of increased toxicity. Modest doses (1 mg/day orally) of folic acid reduce some of the troubling toxicities of MTX without impairing its efficacy.

Golden MR, et al: The relationship of preexisting lung disease to the development of methotrexate pneumonitis in patients with rheumatoid arthritis. J Rheumatol 22:1043–1047, 1995.

Kremer JM, Phelps CT: Long-term prospective study of the use of methotrexate in the treatment of rheumatoid arthritis: Update after a mean of 90 months. Arthritis Rheum 35:138–145, 1995.

Weinblatt ME, et al: Long-term prospective study of methotrexate in the treatment of rheumatoid arthritis: 84-month update. Arthritis Rheum 35:129–137, 1995

63. What are some of the newer treatments for RA?

By and large, newer drugs have supplanted the older and more toxic DMARDs such as gold and D-penicillamine.

Leflunimide recently was approved by the FDA for treatment of RA. It is an inhibitor of pyrimidine synthesis, and thus seems to inhibit activated T and B lymphocytes. It is about as effective as MTX and has a rapid onset of action. Its toxicities are similar to those of MTX, although pulmonary interstitial disease has not been demonstrated. Its most common toxicity is diarrhea.

Tumor necrosis factor inhibitors are now available for treatment of RA. TNF-α is important in the production of inflammation in RA. Binding and inactivation of TNF-α produces significant reduction in inflammation. Two preparations are available: etanercept and infliximab. They have little toxicity, but some concern has been raised about allergy, irritation at the injection site (etanercept is available only for subcutaneous injection), and increased risk for serious infection. Because they are chimeric molecules, there is also a risk of developing blocking antibodies. The biggest drawback to their use is cost.

Cyclosporin A has been shown in double-blind placebo-controlled trials to be useful in the treatment of RA. Its toxicity, especially hypertension and potentially irreversible renal insufficiency (which probably is worsened by concomitant use of NSAIDs), make it difficult to use.

Minocycline also has been shown to be better than placebo in the treatment of RA. At best it is mildly effective and is rarely used except in the most limited disease. Its minimal success is probably due to its ability to inhibit metalloproteinases rather than to any antimicrobial effect.

SJÖGREN'S SYNDROME

64. What is Sjögren's syndrome?

Sjögren's syndrome is an inflammatory disease of exocrine glands manifested primarily by dryness of the eyes and mouth. It can occur as an isolated entity (primary Sjögren's syndrome) or in association with another rheumatic disease, commonly RA or SLE (secondary Sjögren's syndrome).

65. Which glands are most commonly involved in Sjögren's syndrome?

Major and minor salivary glands (including parotid and submandibular glands) as well as lacrimal glands are commonly involved.

66. How does one document keratoconjunctivitis sicca?

Many believe that Sjögren's syndrome is underdiagnosed. The first step is to ask the appropriate historical questions. Inquiries about eye grittiness or the ability to eat crackers without water have been suggested as nonleading ways to ask about dryness. Schirmer's test can document diminished output of the lacrimal glands. Likewise, biopsy of the salivary glands (usually in the lower lip), showing the presence of infiltrating lymphocytes, establishes the diagnosis.

Talal N: Sjögren's syndrome and connective tissue diseases association with other immunologic disorders. In McCarty DJ, Koopman WJ (eds): Arthritis and Allied Conditions, 12th ed. Philadelphia, Lea & Febiger, 1993, pp 1343–1356.

67. What percent of patients with primary Sjögren's syndrome subsequently develop a connective tissue syndrome?

If symptoms of an underlying connective tissue disease do not appear within 12 months of the keratoconjunctivitis sicca, the chances are approximately 10% that it will appear later in life.

68. Are patients with Sjögren's syndrome at increased risk for certain malignancies?

Yes—non-Hodgkin's lymphoma. The lymphomas are usually B cell-derived, and some patients also have serum protein spikes. The diagnosis of tumor may be difficult, given that the nonmalignant lymphoid infiltration of lymphocytes often simulates neoplasm (pseudolymphoma).

SYSTEMIC LUPUS ERYTHEMATOSUS

69. What are the most common clinical and laboratory features of SLE?

FEATURE	FREQUENCY (%)	FEATURE	FREQUENCY (%)
Positive ANA	97	Leukopenia	46
Arthritis/arthralgia	80	Anemia	42
Fever	48	Myalgia	60
Skin involvement	71	Nephritis	42
Low complement	51	Pleurisy	44
Elevated anti-dsDNA	46	CNS symptoms	32

From Wallace DJ: The clinical presentation in SLE. In Wallace DJ, et al (eds): Dubois' Lupus Erythematosus, 4th ed. Baltimore, Williams & Wilkins, 1993, pp 317–321.

70. What genes influence the development of SLE?

SLE is associated with MHC class II genes HLA DR2 and DR3. Inherited complement deficiencies, including the absence of C4A, C1Q, C1 R/S, and C2, have been associated with increased risk for the development of SLE. The receptor Fc gamma RIIa provides a protective effect in African Americans who otherwise would develop severe lupus. Sex chromosomes obviously play a role in the development of lupus given its profound female predominance.

71. Describe the common skin manifestations of SLE.

The skin is a frequent target organ in SLE. The classic lesion of **acute lupus** is the malar (butterfly) rash. which consists of an area of redness across the cheeks, usually involving the bridge of the nose, and often is exacerbated by ultraviolet light (artificial or sunlight). Atrophic dermal scarring does not develop with clearing of the rash.

Symmetric, superficial, nonscarring annular lesions of the shoulders, upper arms, and back are the classic lesions of **subacute cutaneous lupus**. Nonscarring alopecia often occurs concurrently. Patients may or may not have circulating anti-Ro antibodies. Lesions are highly photosensitive.

The skin lesions of **discoid lupus** (chronic cutaneous lupus erythematosus) most commonly occur over the face and neck. They eventually become hypopigmented and atrophic.

Less common skin lesions include urticaria, periungual erythema, bullae, livedo reticularis petechiae, purpura, and ecchymoses.

Sontheirmer RD: Clinical manifestations of cutaneous lupus erythematosus. In Wallace DJ, et al (eds): Dubois' Lupus Erythematosus, 4th ed. Philadelphia, Lea & Febiger, 1993, pp 285–301.

72. What is subacute cutaneous lupus (SCLE)?

Some consider this cutaneous eruption on a spectrum between chronic discoid lupus and acute cutaneous lupus. The lesions generally occur on the shoulders, upper chest, and neck and are symmetric and nonscarring. They can be annular and resemble psoriasis. Between 25–50% of patients have constitutional symptoms, and they may have circulating antibodies to Ro antigen. SCLE is associated with HLA-DRW3.

McCauliffe DP, Sontheimer RD: Subacute cutaneous lupus erythematosus. In Wallace DJ, et al (eds): Dubois' Lupus Erythematosus, 4th ed. Philadelphia, Lea & Febiger, 1993, pp 302–309.

73. Describe the relationship between discoid lupus and systemic lupus.

This area is somewhat controversial. Approximately 25% of patients with classic discoid lesions may have constitutional symptoms but do not meet the ARA criteria for SLE. Approximately 10% of patients with discoid lupus eventually develop SLE. These data are inexact, because early epidemiologic studies lumped SCLE and discoid lupus together in assessing risk for the development of systemic disease.

74. How commonly does SLE affect the GI tract?

GI manifestations may be present in up to 50% of patients with SLE. Anorexia, nausea, and vomiting are among the most common. Oral ulcerations (most commonly buccal erosions) were identified in 40% of one group of patients. Esophageal involvement, as esophagitis, esophageal ulceration, or esophageal dysmotility, seems to correlate with the presence of Raynaud's phenomenon. Intestinal involvement results in abdominal pain, diarrhea, and occasionally hemorrhage. Intestinal ischemia may be present and may progress to infarction and perforation. Pneumatosis intestinalis in SLE is usually benign and transient but may represent an irreversible necrotizing enterocolitis. In addition, pancreatitis and abdominal serositis are well-recognized. Abnormal liver functions also occur. A vasculitic process has been implicated in the pathogenesis of GI manifestations.

Wallace DJ: Gastrointestinal manifestations and related liver and biliary disorders. In Wallace DJ, et al (eds): Dubois' Lupus Erythematosus, 4th ed. Philadelphia, Lea & Febiger, 1993, pp 410–417.

75. What is the most common pathologic abnormality in patients with lupus CNS disease?

Small infarcts and hemorrhages are more commonly the source for the neuropsychiatric features of lupus than vasculitis. In fact, vasculitis, as suggested by such commonly used designations as "lupus cerebritis," occur in <15% of patients.

Johnson RT, Richardson EP. The neurological manifestations of systemic lupus erythematosus. Medicine 47:337–369, 1968.

76. What are the neuropsychiatric manifestations of SLE?

Because of the difficulty in establishing an unequivocal diagnosis, rates of CNS features cross a broad range. Neuropsychiatric manifestations of lupus may occur in around 70% of patients. Examples include psychosis (5%); cranial, autonomic, and peripheral neuropathies; migraine headaches; seizure; aseptic meningitis; pseudotumor cerebri; chorea; and cerebral infarction. Rarely transverse myelitis has been observed. Organic brain syndromes are easier to recognize in lupus when they are profound (delirium) but now are recognized more frequently as changes in mentation, such as mild memory loss and impaired concentration. The more subtle features of cognitive dysfunction may be the most common CNS syndrome in SLE. Abnormal SPECT or PET scanning and decreasing intellectual function, as measured by a standard battery of neurocognitive function tests, are present. The cause for this problem is not known, but cytokines are believed to play an important role.

Wallace DJ, Metzger AL: Systemic lupus erythematosus: Clinical aspects and treatment. In Koopman WJ (ed): Arthritis and Allied Conditions: A Textbook of Rheumatology, 13th ed. Baltimore, Williams & Wilkins, 1997, pp 1319–1345.

77. Describe the pulmonary manifestations of lupus.

Pulmonary involvement is fairly common in lupus and usually takes the form of pleurisy or pleural effusion. Up to 60% of patients may have pleuritic pain over the course of their illness. Effusions can be either transudative or exudative and in rare cases are the presenting feature. The so-called shrinking lung syndrome describes dyspnea associated with diaphragmatic dysfunction, probably secondary to chronic pleural scarring. Pulmonary parenchymal involvement or lupus pneumonitis has been described, as have pulmonary hemorrhage, pulmonary emboli, and pulmonary hypertension. Emboli and hypertension are more common when phospholipid antibodies are also present.

78. List some conditions associated with a positive ANA.

- Lupus
- Drug-induced lupus
- Rheumatoid arthritis
- Systemic sclerosis
- CREST syndrome
- Polymyositis
- Dermatomyositis
- Mixed connective tissue disease
- Chronic hepatitis
- Infectious mononucleosis

79. Is ANA one antibody?

No. The detection of the LE cell initiated the study of autoantibodies. With the development of immunofluorescent techniques, different staining patterns were discovered, and it became clear that many different nuclear antigens can elicit an antibody response. Thus, many antibodies can be classified as ANA. Detecting the specific antibody reaction requires more refined techniques.

Antinuclear Antibodies

ANTIGEN	ANTIBODY
Deoxyribose phosphate backbone of DNA	Anti-DNA (double-stranded or native)
Purine and pyrimidine bases	Anti-single-stranded DNA
H1, H2A, H2B, H3, H2A/H2B complex, H3/H4 complex	Antihistones
DNA topoisomerase I	Anti-SCL-70
Histidyl tRNA transferase	Anti-Jo-1
Kinetochore	Anticentromere
RNA polymerase I	Antinucleolar
Y1–Y5 RNA and protein	Anti-Ro
U1–6 RNA and protein	Anti-RNP (includes anti-Sm)

From von Mühlen CA, et al: Autoantibodies in the diagnosis of systemic rheumatic diseases. Semin Arthritis Rheum 24:323–358, 1995.

80. Do ANA staining patterns detect specific ANAs? What is their clinical relevance?

The fluorescence test for ANA is performed by incubating the patient's serum with a fixed monolayer of human larynx epithelioma cancer (HEp-2) cell lines. If ANAs are present in the serum, they bind to the nuclear component of the substrate. Next, fluorescent anti-Ig is added, which binds to antibodies (if present) in the test serum. With the fluorescent tag, the ANA can be directly visualized under fluorescent light. Different patterns of staining occur, and although they may provide some information, they do not identify the specific antibody present, nor are they specific for a disease entity. For example, the rim or peripheral pattern (usually associated with antibodies directed against nuclear membrane proteins) may be obscured if another autoantibody (staining a homogeneous pattern) is present.

81. Why is it helpful to know which specific ANA is present in a given patient?

Although no laboratory test is absolutely diagnostic for a rheumatic disease, the presence of certain autoantibodies in the appropriate clinical setting can be helpful. Some common disease associations include:

Ro/SSA	SLE, neonatal lupus syndrome, subacute lupus, Sjögren's syndrome, RA
DS DNA	SLE
Sm	SLE
Jo-1	Polymyositis with pulmonary involvement
Centromere	CREST syndrome
SCL-70	Systemic sclerosis

Craft J, et al: Antinuclear antibodies. In Kelly WN, et al (eds): Textbook of Rheumatology, 4th ed. Philadelphia, W.B. Saunders, 1993, pp 164–187.

82. Which drugs are commonly associated with the development of a clinical syndrome of lupus and a positive ANA?

Historically, a clinical syndrome of arthritis, fever, rash, and positive ANA was seen in some patients after initiating antihypertensive treatment with hydralazine. Since then, the development of circulating ANA or clinical symptoms has been demonstrated with many drugs, including procainamide, diphenylhydantoin, isoniazid, chlorpromazine, d-penicillamine, sulfasalazine, methyldopa, and quinidine. So-called slow acetylators more commonly develop clinical symptoms. The clinical features usually regress fairly promptly, although the laboratory abnormality may persist (sometimes indefinitely) when the drug is discontinued. The clinical features commonly present in drug-induced lupus rarely, if ever, include CNS disease or nephritis.

Fritzler MJ, Rubin RL: Drug-induced-lupus. In Wallace DJ, et al (eds): Dubois' Lupus Erythematosus, 4th ed. Philadelphia, Lea & Febiger, 1993, pp 442–453.

83. What antibody is often touted to be diagnostic for drug-induced lupus?

Although often touted to be diagnostic for drug-induced lupus, an antihistone antibody is not particularly helpful when a patient taking one of the above medications has features of lupus and a positive ANA. Although antihistone antibody is present in the syndrome of drug-induced lupus (perhaps as many as 90% of cases), it is also true that nearly 75% of patients with idiopathic disease may produce this antibody, making it of little diagnostic usefulness.

84. Does lupus nephritis recur in a transplanted kidney?

Disease activity in SLE often quiets with the onset of uremia and dialysis. Several studies note the ability to discontinue glucocorticoids without a return of extrarenal manifestations once dialysis has been initiated. Although there are reports of subsequent disease exacerbations, disease activity usually does not recur in transplanted kidneys.

85. Discuss the interaction of pregnancy and SLE.

1. Fertility is unaffected by the disease (i.e., patients become pregnant just as readily as women without lupus).

2. Although recent data suggest that pregnant patients with lupus do not have disease flares more frequently than nonpregnant patients, disease exacerbations during pregnancy do occur.

Because such flares can be severe, patients with SLE should be considered at high risk. Active disease during the antecedent 3–6 months may increase the risk of a flare.

3. Preeclampsia occurs more frequently in pregnant patients with lupus. There is also increased risk of miscarriage, abortion, intrauterine growth delay, and prematurity in patients with SLE compared with controls.

4. The Ro antibody crosses the placenta and is responsible for most of the neonatal lupus syndromes, including skin manifestations and congenital heart block.

Lochshin MD: Pregnancy does not cause systemic lupus erythematosus to worsen. Arthritis Rheum 32:665–670, 1989.

86. Describe the role of cytotoxic therapy in the treatment of lupus-associated nephritis.

Cytotoxic agents, such as cyclophosphamide and chlorambucil, are useful in the management of life-threatening rheumatic diseases. Because of their toxicity, they should be used only in situations in which careful clinical trials point to significant advantages. Clinical trials of cytotoxic agents have shown an advantage in patients with lupus nephritis. Patients with inflammatory renal lesions avoided or had a slower progression to end-stage renal disease and diminished mortality rates when the treatment regimen included cyclophosphamide.

87. What is the antiphospholipid antibody (APA) syndrome?

APA syndrome consists of one or more of the following: multiple miscarriages, arterial or venous thrombosis, and thrombocytopenia in association with a laboratory finding of antibodies directed against phospholipids. These antibodies can be specific (such as anticardiolipin antibodies), or they may be identified by their effect on the clotting cascade (lupus anticoagulant). Common laboratory tests indicating the presence of antibodies to various phospholipids include prolonged partial thromboplastin time, false-positive VDRL test for syphilis, or positive anticardiolipin antibodies. A less common example is the dilute Russell viper venom clotting time. APA syndrome may occur by itself (primary APA syndrome) or in association with an underlying connective tissue syndrome, primarily lupus (secondary APA syndrome).

88. How frequently do APAs occur in established SLE?

A biologic false-positive serologic test for syphilis occurs in 10% of patients with SLE. The lupus anticoagulant is reported in 6–10% and anticardiolipin antibodies in 15–40%.

89. Which rheumatic conditions are typically associated with Raynaud's phenomenon?

Raynaud's phenomenon is the eponym given to the color change (usually white, blue, then red) in the hands (or any distal part of the body) that is incited by intense emotion or exposure to cold. When one inquires about Raynaud's, it is sometimes difficult not to suggest a positive answer. Thus, one may ask, "While grocery shopping, do you notice any problems in the frozen food section?" or "If you look at your hands when you get cold, do they look any different to you?" Raynaud's phenomenon is part of the clinical presentation of many conditions, including the following:

- SLE
- APA syndrome
- CREST syndrome
- Drug-induced lupus
- Reflex sympathetic dystrophy
- Systemic sclerosis
- Idiopathic Raynaud's phenomenon
- Polymyositis
- Sjögren's syndrome
- Cold agglutinin disease
- Cryoglobulinemia (primary or associated with active hepatitis C)
- Systemic vasculopathies

90. What factors predict the development of systemic sclerosis in a patient presenting with Raynaud's phenomenon?

Patients presenting with Raynaud's phenomenon are at increased risk to develop a rheumatic disease. Positive serology, abnormal nail bed capillaries, or abnormal pulmonary function studies suggest an increased risk for development of disease.

91. List the noncutaneous features of scleroderma.

Arthritis, inflammatory muscle disease, GI dysmotility with resulting malabsorption, pulmonary interstitial pulmonary fibrosis with or without pulmonary hypertension, and scleroderma renal crisis.

92. Which autoantibodies are associated with polymyositis?

A positive ANA is not uncommon. Specifically, anti Jo-1 is found in patients with polymyositis, particularly those with concomitant pulmonary fibrosis. The antigen has been found to be histidyl-tRNA synthetase.

93. What further evaluation for an occult malignancy should be undertaken in an adult diagnosed with dermatomyositis?

The risk of malignancy is increased in patients with myositis. The data are strongest for patients with dermatomyositis, and the risk increases with age. Studies should include chest x-ray, mammography, stool guaiac, prostate-specific antigen, and full gynecologic examination. Depending on the results, follow-up evaluation may include endoscopy, colonoscopy, and biopsy.

94. What is Jaccoud's deformity?

Deformities of the hands secondary to chronic inflammation of the joint capsule, ligaments, and tendons. The changes may mimic those of RA (ulnar deviation of the fingers, MCP joint subluxation). Erosions are not present, although after several recurrences, notches may be seen in x-rays on the ulnar side of the metacarpal heads. Early in the course, patients can correct these changes voluntarily. Although originally described in rheumatic fever, this disorder has been extended to include the arthropathy in other conditions, most commonly SLE.

SPONDYLOARTHROPATHIES

95. What is a spondyloarthropathy? Which diseases are usually so classified?

Spondyloarthropathies are a group of diseases of uncertain etiology that have a predilection for inflammatory lesions of the spine and sacroiliac joints. In addition, they are characterized by the absence of RF or other autoantibodies. Other unifying features include peripheral oligoarthropathy, enthesopathy, extra-articular foci of inflammation, and an association with HLA-B27. Diseases classified as spondyloarthropathies include:

- Ankylosing spondylitis
- Reactive arthritis
- Arthropathy of psoriasis
- Arthropathy associated with inflammatory bowel disease

Arnett FC: Sero-negative spondyloarthropathies. Bull Rheum Dis 37(1):1–12, 1987.

96. Define enthesopathy.

The enthesis is the junction of ligament and bone. It is the site of inflammation in the spondyloarthropathies. In response to this inflammation, reactive new bone is formed. This process accounts for the formation of syndesmophytes in ankylosing spondylitis.

97. What mechanisms may explain the association of HLA-B27 with arthropathy?

The mechanism by which HLA-B27 predisposes to arthritis after urogenital or intestinal infection is unknown. Two hypotheses include:

1. B27 is involved directly in disease predisposition. It may act as a receptor for a microorganism, or it may be modified by an infecting microorganism to elicit an immune reaction against the new antigen. Alternatively, B27 may resemble the microbial epitopes; thus antibodies directed against the microorganism cross-react with host antigens (molecular mimicry).

2. Disease susceptibility may be conferred by a particular configuration of the T-cell receptor. Recent data using transgenic mice make a previous hypothesis—that a gene closely linked to HLA-B27 is the pathogenic culprit—very unlikely.

Careless DJ, Inman RD: Etiopathogenesis of reactive arthritis and ankylosing spondylitis. Curr Opin Rheum 7:290–298, 1995.

98. Describe the principal clinical features of ankylosing spondylitis.

Ankylosing spondylitis is one of the few inflammatory arthropathies that occurs more commonly in men than in women. The disease begins in late adolescence, usually with gradually worsening low back pain and stiffness. The pain typically improves with activity and worsens with rest, leading to the commonly experienced symptom of night-time awakening with pain and stiffness that require getting out of bed to stretch. Peripheral joints may be involved early in the course of the disease, mostly in the lower limbs. The disease is generally progressive, and extra-articular features may develop. The peripheral arthropathy occurs in both sexes, although sacroiliac and spinal involvement is more prominent in men.

Gran JT: An epidemiological survey of the signs and symptoms of ankylosing spondylitis. Clin Rheum Dis 4:161, 1985.

99. Name the extra-articular features of ankylosing spondylitis.

Anterior uveitis, aortitis, and pulmonary fibrosis.

100. What is the difference between a syndesmophyte and an osteophyte?

Syndesmophytes are thin, vertical outgrowths and represent calcifications of the annulus fibrosus. As syndesmophytes enlarge, ossification can involve adjacent anterior longitudinal and paravertebral connective tissue. Syndesmophytes predominate on the anterior and lateral aspects of the spine, particularly near the thoracolumbar junction, eventually bridging the disc space and connecting one vertebral body with its neighbor. **Osteophytes** are triangular and arise several millimeters from the discovertebral junction.

101. How is inflammation of the sacroiliac (SI) joint graded radiographically?

Grade I	Normal
Grade II	Sclerosis of bone adjacent to the SI joints
Grade III	Erosion at the SI joints
Grade IV	Bony fusion across the SI joints

Arnett FC: Seronegative spondyloarthropathies. Bull Rheum Dis 37:1–12, 1987.

102. Define reactive arthritis.

Reactive arthritis is an inflammatory arthropathy of at least 1 month's duration occurring after a bout of urethritis or dysentery. The mechanism for the development of the arthropathy is unclear.

103. Describe the mucocutaneous manifestations of reactive arthritis.

Skin and mucous membranes are commonly involved in reactive arthritis. Small painless areas of desquamation on the tongue may not even be noticed by the patient. Circinate balanitis, conversely, is rarely missed. It primarily affects the glans penis and can range from small erythematous macules to larger areas of dry, flaking skin. Keratoderma blennorrhagica is a thickening and keratinization of the skin that generally involves the feet, hands, and nails. The lesions resemble psoriasis both clinically and pathologically.

Fan PT, Yu TY: Reiter's syndrome. In Kelly WN, et al (eds): Textbook of Rheumatology, 4th ed. Philadelphia, W.B. Saunders, 1993, pp 961–973.

104. List the radiographic manifestations of reactive arthritis.

Periostitis at areas of tendinous insertions, frank articular erosions, and syndesmophyte formation.

105. List the five patterns of arthritis associated with psoriasis and their relative frequencies.

1. DIP joints of hands and/or feet	8%
2. Peripheral asymmetric oligoarthropathy	48%
3. Symmetric polyarthritis resembling RA	18%
4. Arthritis mutilans ("opera glass hands")	2%
5. Sacroiliitis with or without higher levels of spinal involvement	24%

Arnett FC. Sero-negative spondyloarthropathies. Bull Rheum Dis 37:1–12, 1987.

106. What percentage of people with psoriasis suffer from inflammatory arthritis?

From 6–20% of people with cutaneous psoriasis develop an inflammatory arthropathy. In 80% of cases, the arthritis develops after the skin disease is already present.

107. Discuss the two patterns of arthritis associated with inflammatory bowel disease.

Approxinmately 20% of patients with inflammatory bowel disease (IBD) have a **peripheral arthropathy,** which often is accompanied by fever, oral ulcers, and eye or skin lesions (erythema nodosum or pyoderma gangrenosum). The activity of this arthropathy usually parallels the gut disease, but occasionally the arthropathy precedes bowel symptoms. There is no increased frequency of HLA-B27 phenotype among patients with IBD and peripheral arthritis.

Sacroiliitis and spondylitis occur in approximately 10% of patients with IBD, and HLA-B27 is found more commonly in patients with this form of arthropathy. Spondylitis is independent of bowel disease activity; successful treatment of bowel disease does not influence its outcome.

Arnett FC: Seronegative spondyloarthropathies. Bull Rheum Dis 37:1–12, 1987.

108. What is pyoderma gangrenosum?

Pyoderma gangrenosum consists of skin lesions that begin as pustules or erythematous nodules and break down to form spreading ulcers with necrotic, undermined edges. It is associated with IBD but also occurs in chronic active hepatitis, seropositive RA (without evidence of vasculopathy), leukemia, and polycythemia vera. Differential diagnosis of the lesions includes necrotizing vasculitis, bacterial infection, and spider bites.

CRYSTAL ARTHROPATHY

109. What three principal crystals are associated with joint inflammation?

1. Urate (gout)   3. Hydroxyapatite
2. Calcium pyrophosphate (CPP; "pseudogout")

Dieppe P, Calvert P: Crystals and Joint Disease. London, Chapman and Hall, 1983.

110. What conditions have been associated with CPPD disease?

Hemochromatosis	Hypothyroidism	Neuropathic joint
Hyperparathyroidism	Hemosiderosis	Amyloidosis
Hypophosphatasia	Gout	Trauma, including surgery
Hypomagnesemia		

111. Why is the polarizing microscope important in the diagnosis of rheumatic diseases?

Use of a polarizing microscope allows the identification of specific etiologies in certain clinical syndromes. Its function is based on the relatively simple observation that crystals rotate light (i.e., they are birefringent). Polarized light passing through a crystal is no longer parallel to light not passing through the crystal. If a second polarizer is added so that its axis is rotated 90° (extinction) to the light as it emerges from the first polarizer but before it reaches the crystal, the only light reaching the observer's eye is the light that the crystal has rotated.

112. Where is chondrocalcinosis commonly demonstrated roentgenographically?

Chondrocalcinosis describes the radiographic appearance of CPP crystals in the joint cartilages. The prevalence in the general population (as assessed by multiple radiologic studies) is 10–15% in people aged 65–75 years but rises above 40% in people over 80 years old. They are generally punctate and linear densities in the articular cartilages: menisci of the knees, radiocarpal joints, annulus fibrosus of intervertebral discs, and symphysis pubis.

113. What is the most common pathogenic mechanism of hyperuricemia in gout?

Hyperuricemia can develop secondary to overproduction or underexcretion of urate. About 5–15% of patients with gout are urate overproducers. In the remaining patients, decreased renal clearance of urate accounts for hyperuricemia. Although nonrenal mechanisms for the removal of urate are known (e.g., GI tract), diminished clearance by these routes does not lead to hyperuricemia.

114. What are the four stages of gout?

Stage 1 consists of asymptomatic hyperuricemia. Serum urate levels are elevated without artic-ular disease or nephrolithiasis. Not all patients with asymptomatic hyperuricemia develop gout, but the higher the serum level, the greater the likelihood of developing articular disease. In most cases, 20–30 years of sustained hyperuricemia pass before an attack of nephrolithiasis or arthropathy.

Stage 2 is reached with the first attack of acute articular disease. It is exquisitely painful and usually occurs in a single joint. Fever, swelling, erythema, and skin sloughing may be associ-ated findings. Fifty percent of initial attacks occur as podagra, and 90% of patients with gout have podagra at some stage of disease without treatment.

Stage 3 is the period between attacks, described as intercritical gout. Most patients are completely asymptomatic. However, 62% of patients have a second attack of articular disease within 1 year of the first attack, 16% within 1–2 years, 11% within 2–5 years, 4% after 5–10 years, and 7% after > 10 years.

Stage 4, which is termed chronic tophaceous gout, occurs with the development of chronic arthritis and tissue deposition of urate. The principal determinant of the rate of urate deposition is the serum urate concentration.

Gutman AB: The past four decades of progress in the knowledge of gout with an assessment of present status. Arthritis Rheum 16:431, 1973.

115. Do women get gout?

Yes. Gout is recognized with increasing frequency in women. Some distinctions from gout in men have been observed. The onset is later in life, typically after menopause (not surprising given the hormonal influences on urate metabolism) in women not receiving supplemental estrogens. Diuretic therapy and renal insufficiency are also independent risk factors in women as compared with men. Alcohol is a significantly less common precipitating factor in women than in men.

OSTEOARTHRITIS

116. Is osteoarthritis (OA) a genetic disease?

The role of genetic factors in rheumatic disease is an area of vigorous research. OA clearly has a hereditary component. Perhaps the most recognized feature is the presence of Heberden's nodes in mothers and sisters. Recent studies have uncovered a mutation in a type II collagen gene (Arg519 to Cys) that predisposes to early OA.

Pun YL, et al: Clinical correlations of osteoarthritis associated with a single-base mutation (arginine 519 to cysteine) in type II procollagen gene: A newly defined pathogenesis. Arthritis Rheum 37:264–269, 1994.

117. Compare the biochemical changes of the aged joint with the osteoarthritic joint.

Although age is the single most significant epidemiologic factor associated with OA, there are biochemical differences between an old joint and an osteoarthritic joint. The major compo-nents of the joint are bone and cartilage. The major components of the cartilage include the chon-drocytes and matrix (which in turn is composed of collagen, water, and proteoglycans).

	AGING	OSTEOARTHRITIS
Bone	Osteoporosis	Thickened cortices, osteophytes, subchon-dral cysts, remodeling
Chondrocyte activity	Normal	Increased
Collagen	Increased cross-linking of fibrils	Irregular weave Smaller fibrils
Water	Slight decrease	Significant increase
Proteoglycan	Normal total content Decreased chondroitins Increased keratin Normal aggregation	Decreased total proteoglycan component Increased chondroitins Decreased keratin Decreased aggregation

From Brandt KD, Fife RS: Aging in relation to the pathogenesis of osteoarthritis. Clin Rheum Dis 12:117–130, 1986.

118. What is the prevalence of OA in the general population?

The prevalence of OA increases with age, but it also depends on which criteria are used to make the diagnosis. The prevalence of OA by autopsy in people over age 65 years is nearly 100%. Roentgenographic studies reveal a prevalence ranging from approximately 4% in patients aged 18–24 years to > 85% in people older than 75 years.

119. Describe the syndrome of spinal stenosis.

Progressive narrowing of the spinal canal leads to the syndrome of spinal stenosis, which results most commonly from OA of the lumbar or cervical spine. With cervical disease, patients typically present with pain and limitation of motion. Hyperreflexia is common. Other signs may include muscle weakness, spastic gait, and Babinski's sign. In the lumbar region, the clinical manifestations are mostly those of compression of the cauda equina (commonly claudication).

120. What is the difference between spondylolysis and spondylolisthesis?

Spondylolysis is an interruption of the pars interarticularis of the vertebra. **Spondylolisthesis** refers to displacement of one vertebra on another. The most common cause of spondylolisthesis is bilateral spondylolysis. Severe OA of the apophyseal joints can produce spondylolisthesis without spondylolysis.

121. What is the vacuum sign?

A radiographic sign of intervertebral osteochondrosis. Radiolucencies represent gas (nitrogen) that appears at the site of negative pressure produced by abnormal spaces or clefts. Clefts are produced by degeneration of intervertebral disc, especially the nucleus pulposus.

122. What is DISH?

Diffuse idiopathic skeletal hyperostosis (DISH) is a syndrome characterized by extensive ossification of tendinous and ligamentous attachments to bone. Involvement of the spine with flowing calcification over the anterior longitudinal ligament is among the most common findings. Extraspinal manifestations also are reported. Clinical symptoms are often mild and consist of morning stiffness and deep achiness of the affected portion. The following radiographic features help to distinguish DISH from ankylosing spondylitis, degenerative spine disease, and spondylosis deformans:

1. Flowing calcification along the anterolateral aspect of at least 4 contiguous vertebral bodies.

2. Relative preservation of intervertebral disc height in the involved vertebral segment and absence of extensive radiographic changes of "degenerative" disc disease (vacuum phenomena, vertebral body marginal sclerosis).

3. Absence of apophyseal joint ankylosis and sacroiliac joint erosion, sclerosis, and intraarticular osseous fusion.

123. List five classic radiographic findings of OA.

1. Subchondral cyst formation   4. Joint space narrowing
2. New bone formation (osteophytes)   5. Lack of osteoporosis
3. Sclerosis of bone

INFECTIOUS ARTHRITIS

124. Describe the mechanism for acute rheumatic fever.

Rheumatic fever occurs after group A streptococcal pharyngitis (which may be asymptomatic). Data indicate that the immune response initiated against the bacteria plays an important role. Antibodies cross-react with human antigens, leading to a persistent autoimmune reaction and tissue destruction (molecular mimicry). Development of immune complexes also has been documented.

125. What common viral illnesses are associated with arthropathy?

Common viruses associated with arthropathy include hepatitis B and C, parvovirus B19, rubella, and HIV. Chronic hepatitis B with persistent circulating B antigen has been associated with polyarteritis nodosa. Hepatitis C has a dramatically high rate of occurrence in patients with mixed cryoglobulinemia; this virus also has been documented in several cases of otherwise unexplained inflammatory polyarthropathy.

Active infection with parvovirus has been associated with a nondestructive RA-like picture, with RFs documented in the circulation. Of interest, the arthropathy clears with no chronic or destructive sequelae.

Some rare viral infections strongly associated with arthropathy include the group A arboviruses (Ross River virus, chikungunya, o'ynong-nyong, sindbis, Mayaro). Common viral infections that occasionally produce arthropathy include mumps, smallpox (vaccinia), Epstein-Barr virus, cytomegalovirus, and enteroviruses (ECHO and coxsackievirus). Rubella infection is associated with arthralgia and arthritis, especially in adult women. Joint symptoms usually begin within 1 week of the onset of the rash of German measles. In the past, arthritis and arthralgias often were seen after rubella vaccination, but they are less common since a less arthrogenic strain of virus is used for the vaccine.

Naides SJ: Viral arthritis including HIV. Curr Opin Rheumatol 7:337–342, 1995.

126. Which bacterial pathogens are most commonly responsible for septic arthritis?

Septic arthritis is usually classified as gonococcal or nongonococcal. Of the nongonococcal bacteria causing joint infections, staphylococci remain the most common. Species of streptococci are the next most common cause when grouped together. Finally, gram-negative bacilli may cause 20–30% of septic joints.

127. Describe the common clinical manifestations of gonococcal arthritis.

Gonococcal arthritis occurs in approximately 0.1–0.5% of patients with gonorrhea. Clinical manifestations may differ from those of other bacterial arthropathies. Even under optimal conditions, joint fluids are culture-positive in < 50% of cases. The arthropathy is commonly migratory and often accompanied by tenosynovitis. Skin lesions are often present, usually as a small macule or papule on a distal extremity.

128. Describe the classic skin manifestation of Lyme disease.

Erythema chronicum migrans (ECM) is an expanding erythematous ring (often asymptomatic) with central clearing beginning at the sight of the tick bite. The *Borrelia* organism can be cultured from the margin of the lesion. The rash occasionally is accompanied by flu-like symptoms (arthralgia, myalgia, and fever). In endemic regions ECM is the most common presenting feature of early Lyme disease. Recently, *Borrelia* spp. have been found in diffuse fasciitis. The disease caused by European ticks produces what is described as acrodermatitis chronica atrophicans.

Evans J: Lyme disease. Curr Opin Rheumatol 7:322–328, 1995.

129. What coinfections have been recently documented with Lyme disease?

Coinfections with *Babesia microti* and human granulocytic ehrlichiosis have been documented and probably occur because all three organisms use the *Ixodes* tick as a vector. *B. microti* may be fatal in splenectomized patients. Since leukopenia, thrombocytopenia, and high transaminases are not present in Lyme disease, coinfection should be considered when these features occur.

Nadelman RB, Horowitz HW, Hsieh T-C, et al. Simultaneous human ehrlichiosis and Lyme borreliosis. N Engl J Med 337:27–30, 1997.

130. Is the chronic arthritis of Lyme disease produced by active joint infection?

About 70% of untreated patients with Lyme disease in the U.S. develop arthritis. It may take the form of arthralgia, intermittent episodes of arthritis, or, in about 10% of patients, a chronic inflammatory synovitis. Treatment failure is associated with HLA-DR4. Some investigators hypothesize that an autoimmune response is produced; others have suggested persistent infection. Data, including those from PCR technology, suggest that acute arthritis is due to active infection, although viable organisms may not be necessary for the development of a chronic synovitis.

Evans J: Lyme disease. Curr Opin Rheumatol 7:322–328, 1995.

131. What is the common rheumatic problem associated with HIV infection?

Arthralgias are the most common rheumatic problem in patients infected with HIV and have been reported in 12–45% of cases. Painful articular syndrome usually occurs very late in the course of HIV infection. There is little outward sign of inflammation, and most diagnostic studies are negative. This syndrome is distinctly different from HIV-associated arthritis, a clearly inflammatory process that may affect up to 50% of HIV-infected patients. HIV-associated arthritis is usually asymmetric and may affect only a few joints, or it may be polyarticular. Patients are seronegative and lack HLA B27. Reactive arthritis remains a common rheumatic manifestation of HIV infection. Some patients have the complete triad (arthritis, urethritis, and conjunctivitis), but most have an incomplete form of disease. Extra-articular features such as nail pitting and onychodystrophy, aphthous ulcers, and skin changes are well described, as are systemic symptoms such as fatigue and malaise. Approximately 70% of such patients are HLA B27-positive. Psoriasis and psoriatic arthritis are also common in HIV infection. The rash and arthritis can predate the onset of disease or develop at any time during infection. The arthritis more commonly affects peripheral joints and often spares the SI joints and spine.

132. How does muscle involvement manifest in HIV infection?

Muscle involvement can take several recognized forms. Simple myalgias are rarely debilitating and most often transient. HIV infection has been associated with polymyositis and dermatomyositis. The clinical features and course of these illnesses do not differ significantly in non–HIV-infected patients. Muscular weakness associated with inanition secondary to medication (AZT) is well described. Nemaline rod myositis also has been described. Finally, myopathy associated with direct infection secondary to the severe immunosuppression has been recognized. The most common organisms include *Mycobacterium avium*, cryptococci, and microsporidia.

133. What is DILS?

Parotid gland enlargement caused by diffuse lymphocyte infiltration associated with symptoms of oral dryness mimics classic Sjögren's syndrome in HIV-infected patients and is commonly called diffuse infiltrative lymphocytosis syndrome (DILS). Differences from idiopathic Sjögren's disease include male predominance, absence of classic serologic markers, and its HLA association. DILS is associated with HLA-DR5 in African Americans and with HLA DR6 and HLA DR7 in Caucasians. Idiopathic Sjögren's disease is associated with HLA-B8, DR3, and DRw52. HLA-DR2 and DR4 are present in patients with Sjögren's secondary to SLE and RA, respectively.

134. Is the incidence of vasculitis syndromes increased in HIV-infected patients?

Yes. Examples include polyarteritis nodosa, Henoch-Schönlein purpura, and ANCA positive vasculidities.

135. How common is septic arthritis in HIV-infected patients?

The incidence of septic arthritis seems to be increased. Traditional organisms include *Staphylococcus aureus, Streptococcus pneumoniae*, and *Salmonella* spp.

136. What other rheumatic manifestations are associated with HIV infection?

Fibromyalgia, Raynaud's phenomenon, aseptic necrosis of bone, hypertrophic osteoarthropathy, and IgA nephropathy.

137. By what mechanisms does HIV infection cause rheumatic symptoms?

There are many possible mechanisms by which HIV infection can cause symptoms. Some data support the concept of direct HIV infection of joints and muscles. HIV has been found in synovial fluid aspirates, and HIV DNA has been found in the synovial tissue of infected patients with arthritis. A related retrovirus (simian immunodeficiency virus) induces polymyositis in about one-half of infected animals. Likewise, in patients with HIV-polymyositis, HIV-1 DNA and HIV-1 RNA are found in muscle tissue. Less directly, HIV infection may stimulate the production of proinflammatory cytokines that play a role in intensifying symptoms or increase tissue damage during opportunistic infections. Other immunologic factors may include, B- and T-cell hyperresponsiveness, increased serum immunoglobulins, circulating immune complexes, and the well described increase in the production of autoantibodies.

Espinoza LR, Cuellar ML: Retrovirus-associated rheumatic syndromes. In Koopman WJ (ed): Arthritis and Allied Conditions, 13th ed. Baltimore, Williams & Wilkins, 1997, pp 2361–2374.

MISCELLANEOUS RHEUMATIC CONDITIONS

138. What are the muscles of the rotator cuff? What syndromes are associated with their malfunction?

The muscles of the rotator cuff include supraspinatus, infraspinatus, teres minor, and sub-scapularis. Disease of the rotator cuff is a common cause of shoulder pain. Impingement syndrome occurs when the supraspinatus tendon is caught between the head of the humerus and the acromion, resulting in pain. The activity most likely to bring these structures into proximity (and thus cause pain) is overhead movement and internal rotation of the arm. Night pain is characteristic. If the tendon ruptures (rotator cuff tear), significant weakness may result. Impingement syndrome usually results from injury to the supraspinatus during repetitive elevation and forward motion of the arm. Rotator cuff tendinitis is often an acute problem and may be associated with calcification.

139. What are the most common causes of neuropathic joints in the upper extremity?

Without sensation and proprioception as regulators of joint function, gradual relaxation of supporting structure, abnormal mechanics, and ultimately joint destruction develop. Many diseases, including congenital pain insensitivity, amyloidosis, diabetes mellitus, alcoholism, and tabes dorsalis, can lead to neuroarthropathy. In the upper extremities, particularly the elbow, syringomyelia is a common cause of sensory abnormalities leading to arthropathy.

140. Describe the rheumatic manifestations of sarcoidosis.

Sarcoidosis is a systemic disease characterized by a noncaseating granulomatous reaction of unknown origin. Besides the lungs, involvement of the eyes, skin, and joints is not uncommon. Skin involvement, including erythema nodosum, occurs in approximately 30% of patients. Asymptomatic sarcoid granulomas have been found in muscle biopsy and may occur in bones, appearing radiographically as cysts. Osteolysis also has been described.

Articular symptoms are present in most patients with acute sarcoidosis (hilar adenopathy, fever, erythema nodosum), often affecting the ankles and knees. This articular syndrome is usually self-limited, lasting up to 4 weeks. When the disease is less acute in onset, articular involvement is less common. It can, however, be recurring and protracted, although joint destruction is infrequent. The articular involvement may predate pulmonary involvement or occur after 10 years of disease.

141. Which conditions are associated with Dupuytren's contracture?

Fibrosis and thickening of the palmar fascia can lead to the flexion contracture first described by Dupuytren. Associated diseases include diabetes mellitus, chronic liver disease, epilepsy, plantar fasciitis, carpal tunnel syndrome, RA, trauma to the hand, pulmonary tuberculosis, and alcoholism, to name a few.

142. Which conditions are associated with mononeuritis multiplex?

Mononeuritis multiplex is a peripheral neuropathy involving one or more nerves. It is sometimes difficult to distinguish from other mononeuropathies caused by local factors, such as trauma, compression (acoustic neuroma or peroneal palsy), and entrapment (carpal tunnel). Reported associations include diabetes mellitus, polyarteritis, SLE, RA, Lyme disease, Sjögren's syndrome, cryoglobulinemia, giant cell arteritis, scleroderma, leukemia, leprosy, AIDS, carcinoma, and lymphoma. One recent study found that even after extensive work-up, almost half of all nondiabetic patients with EMG evidence of mononeuritis multiplex had no established diagnosis.

> Hellmann CB, et al: Mononeuritis multiplex: The yield of evaluations for occult rheumatic disease. Medicine 67(3):145–153, 1988.

143. Describe the characteristic features of Wegener's granulomatosis (WG).

WG is one of the systemic necrotizing vasculopathies. The organs primarily affected are the respiratory tract (upper and/or lower) and kidneys. Respiratory tract involvement can manifest as recurrent sinusitis, otitis media, tracheobronchial inflammation and erosions, or pneumonitis with cavitation. With the inflammatory process unchecked, a saddle-nose deformity can occur. Additional symptoms, such as arthritis, neuropathies, and eye inflammation, may occur. Laboratory data are generally nonspecific, but recently an antibody to cytoplasmic components of the PMN leukocyte (c-ANCA) has been associated with active disease.

144. Compare polyarteritis nodosa (PAN), microscopic polyangiitis (MPA), WG, and Churg-Strauss syndrome (CSS).

	VESSELS AFFECTED	TARGET TISSUE	LABORATORY DATA
PAN	Predominantly medium-sized venules	Uniformly: peripheral nerve, sparing arterioles, capillaries, and GI tract. No glomerulonephritis or pulmonary involvement.	No ANCA; possible hepatitis B or C
MPA	Small to medium-sized vessels, including capillaries, venules, and arterioles	Uniformly: glomerulonephritis, skin. Commonly: pulmonary + alveolar hemorrhage. Less commonly: nerve, CNS, upper airway.	Usually p-ANCA (anti-MPO)
WG	Small to medium-sized vessels including capillaries, venules, and arterioles	Uniformly: glomerulonephritis, upper airway and pulmonary eye. Commonly: alveolar hemorrhage, peripheral nerve. Less commonly: skin, CNS.	Usually c-ANCA (anti-PR3)
CSS	Small to medium-sized vessels including capillaries, venules, and arterioles	Uniformly: pulmonary and peripheral nerve. Commonly: upper airway, skin, CNS, glomerulonephritis. Less commonly: alveolar hemorrhage.	Eosinophilia Usually p-ANCA (anti-MPO)

145. What are antineutrophil cytoplasmic antibodies (ANCAs)?

ANCAs are antibodies directed against enzymes found in azurophilic granules (proteinase-3 [PR-3] and myeloperoxidase). Immunofluorescence detects two principal staining patterns: a fine granular cytoplasmic staining (c-ANCA) and a perinuclear collection of antibody (p-ANCA). Despite the similar in vivo location of these enzymes, ethanol fixation produces an artifactual migration of the myeloperoxidase to a perinuclear location. There is no movement of the PR-3, which produces the cytoplasmic staining pattern. Although artifactual, the staining distinction is useful.

The p-ANCA is most associated with a microscopic polyarteritis or a pauci-immune crescentic glomerulonephritis. The PR-3 ANCA (usually staining as c-ANCA) is more sensitive and specific for WG. In fact, the antibody often allows earlier diagnosis and descriptions of what appear to be milder forms of the disease. There seems to be a correlation between disease activity and titers of c-ANCA in patients with WG.

Gross WL, Csernok E: Immunodiagnostic and pathologic aspects of antineutrophil cytoplasmic antibodies in vasculitis. Curr Opin Rheumatol 7:11–19, 1995.

146. Describe the characteristic features of CSS.

CSS, one of the systemic necrotizing vasculopathies, is associated with eosinophilia (circulating or tissue infiltration) and late-in-life onset of atopic disease (asthma or allergic rhinitis). CSS has been hypothesized to represent an overlap between the hypereosinophilic syndromes and vasculitides.

147. What is fibromyalgia (FM)?

FM is a chronic nondestructive illness characterized by fatigue, generalized pain, sleep disturbance (sometimes termed "nonrestorative" sleep), and tender points in a characteristic distribution (see figure below). FM replaced the term fibrositis because no inflammatory process has been objectively documented. Patients may have FM alone or concomitant diseases (e.g., RA, osteoarthritis, Lyme disease, and sleep apnea). The disease is often mimicked by hypothyroidism.

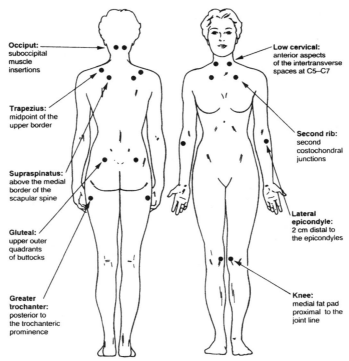

Location of tender points in fibromyalgia. (From Freundlich B, et al: The fibromyalgia syndrome. In Schumacher HR Jr, et al (eds): Primer on the Rheumatic Diseases, 10th ed. Atlanta, Arthritis Foundation, 1993, p 247, with permission.)

In addition to the generalized achiness, patients may have associated irritable bowel syndrome, tension headaches, irritable bladder, and even a chronic cough. Sleep is disturbed by alpha intrusion into delta sleep as documented by EEG. Eighteen reproducible tender points have been established, and diagnosis of FM requires the presence of at least 11.

Treatment is aimed at reconditioning muscles (slow but consistent physical training), restoration of more normal sleep patterns (tricyclic antidepressants in low doses are often helpful), and pain control (generally with nonnarcotic medications such as NSAIDs or acetaminophen and other techniques such as biofeedback).

Wolfe F, et al: The American College of Rheumatology 1990 criteria for the classification of fibromyalgia: Report of the multicenter criteria committee. Arthritis Rheum 33:160–172, 1990.

BIBLIOGRAPHY

1. Harris ED, Jr (ed): Rheumatoid Arthritis. Philadelphia, W.B. Saunders, 1997.
2. Kelly WN, et al (eds): Textbook of Rheumatology, 4th ed. Philadelphia, W.B. Saunders, 1993.
3. Koopman WJ (ed): Arthritis and Allied Conditions, 13th ed. Baltimore, Williams & Wilkins, 1997.
4. McCarty DJ, Koopman WJ (eds): Arthritis and Allied Conditions, 12th ed. Philadelphia, Lea & Febiger, 1993.
5. Resnick D, Niwayama G (eds): Diagnosis of Bone and Joint Disorders, 2nd ed. Philadelphia, W.B. Saunders, 1988.
6. Schumacher HR Jr, et al (eds): Primer on the Rheumatic Diseases, 10th ed. Atlanta, Arthritis Foundation, 1993.
7. Sheon RP, et al (eds): Soft Tissue Rheumatic Pain: Recognition, Management, Prevention, 2nd ed. Philadelphia, Lea & Febiger, 1987.
8. West SG (ed): Rheumatology Secrets. Philadelphia, Hanley & Belfus, 1997.
9. Wolfe F, Pincus T: Rheumatoid Arthritis: Pathogenesis, Assessment, Outcome, and Treatment. New York, Marcel Dekker, 1994.

12. ALLERGY AND IMMUNOLOGY

Roger D. Rossen, M.D.

> Some men also have strange antipathies in their natures against that sort
> of food which others love and live upon. I have read of one that could
> not endure to eat either bread or flesh; of another that fell in a swooning
> fit at the smell of a rose . . . . there are some who, if a cat accidentally
> come into the room, though they neither see it, nor are told it, will
> presently be in a sweat, and ready to die away.
>
> Increase Mather (1639–1723)
> *Remarkable Providence*

1. Name and explain the two major divisions of the immune system.

The **innate immune system** is phylogenetically the oldest and includes the phagocytic leukocytes, natural killer (NK) cells, complement proteins, and acute-phase reactants. All of these soluble
proteins and cells have in common genetically determined systems of pattern recognition; that is,
they bind to common motifs found on a wide variety of bacteria and viruses. The union of the mi-
crobe and an element of the innate immune system typically activates the innate immune system,
usually in a way that either kills the pathogen or nullifies its ability to injure the host. Innate immunity is the first line of defense against infection. Because elements of the innate immune system are
already present in the circulation, they can respond immediately to microbial invasion.

The **cognitive immune system** includes elements such as the B lymphocytes, which make antibodies, and T lymphocytes, which provide the effector elements of antigen-specific cell-mediated
immune responses. Elements of the cognitive immune system display a large repertoire of specific
antigen receptors. Because numerically there are very few cells at any one time that can recognize
newly introduced antigens, B cells and T cells must be appropriately stimulated and induced to
divide and produce multiple copies of themselves. The distinct advantage of the cognitive immune
system is its ability to select B cells and T cells that have high affinity receptors for new antigens and
to stimulate them to replicate and provide a specific, fine-tuned response to foreign invaders.

2. How do vaccines work?

The disadvantage of the cognitive immune response is that the required expansion process takes
time, in some cases more than 2 weeks. Many infectious agents can cause death or severe disability
in less time than it takes the cognitive immune system to mobilize a specific response. Vaccines have
been developed to fill this gap in the host defense system. They stimulate specific immune responses
in advance of an encounter with a pathogenic microorganism so that an appropriate immune recognition system is in place before the encounter takes place.

3. Explain immunologic memory.

Although the circulating antibodies and T cells produced during the initial response to a foreign substance may be lost with time, a second encounter with the same antigen typically induces a much more
vigorous response, which comes into play often within only a day or two after the second encounter. This
response is possible because of the immunologic memory of the cognitive immune system.

4. What are the major divisions of the cognitive immune system?

The two major limbs of the cognitive immune system are **humoral immunity** (HI), provided
by B lymphocytes, and cellular or **cell-mediated immunity** (CMI), provided by T lymphocytes.
Cells that produce antibodies are highly dependent on concurrent responses of T lymphocytes to the
same antigen and vice versa. Both are likewise dependent on cells of the innate immune response
system, most notably macrophages and dendritic cells, which take up antigens, process them, and

then present them to T cells and B cells in a way that stimulates them to divide, multiply, and differentiate in response to the signals provided by the antigen and the antigen-presenting dendritic cell or macrophage. Most antibodies are produced by terminally differentiated B lymphocytes called plasma cells. The complement system plays an important adjunctive or complementary role in humoral immunity. It binds to complexes created by the union of antibodies and antigens and generates substances that attract phagocytic leukocytes to the site of the antigen-antibody reaction and also simulates the phagocytes to ingest and metabolize the antigens that stimulated this reaction. CMI means essentially that the response is provided by specialized cells, not by soluble antibody proteins. Hence a key consideration is that these cells have to reach the site of the host response. The time it takes to mobilize these responses may be 24 hours or, more commonly, 36–48 hours. Thus, an alternative name for CMI is **delayed-type hypersensitivity**. The principal effector of CMI is the T cell, although macrophages and other cellular components also participate. CMI is critical for host defense against viral, fungal, and protozoan infections. It also helps to forestall development and expansion of clones of malignant cells, particularly in the lymphoreticular system, by recognizing and destroying cells that develop abnormal cell surface molecules.

5. What is the major histocompatibility complex (MHC)?

The MHC is a cluster of genes (located on chromosome 6 in humans) that play a critical role in directing the activities of T lymphocytes. For example, T cells of the CD8 subset bind only to antigenic peptides that are displayed within the antigen-presenting cleft of MHC class I molecules. Similarly, T cells that display CD4 molecules interact only with antigenic peptides that are bound within the cleft of MHC class II molecules. Humans have three major types of class I MHC molecules (HLA-A, HLA-B, HLA-C) and three major types of class II MHC molecules (HLA-DR, HLA-DQ, HLA-DP).

6. How do class I MHC molecules work?

MHC class I molecules are displayed on all somatic cells. They pick up the antigens that they display from within the cell's own endoplasmic reticulum; in effect, therefore, they display for the most part self molecules. If the metabolism of a host cell is taken over by a virus, viral proteins made within the cell's endoplasmic reticulum are also picked up by the developing MHC class I molecules. These novel, virus-encoded peptides are displayed on the cell surface in the antigen-presenting cleft of the somatic cell's own MHC class I molecules. As a result, virus-infected cells can be targeted for attack by CD8 T cells that can recognize the viral antigens in the context of self MHC class I molecules.

7. How do class II MHC molecules work?

Under resting conditions, class II MHC molecules are constitutively displayed only by professional antigen-presenting cells—that is, by monocyte/macrophages and dendritic cells. Newly synthesized class II MHC molecules reside within membrane-delimited vesicles inside the cytoplasm of quiescent antigen-presenting cells. Foreign materials taken up by these cells are enzymatically digested into small peptides that find their way into the vesicles that contain MHC II proteins. The peptides are captured within the antigen-presenting cleft of class II MHC molecules, which then migrate to the cell surface, where they stimulate exclusively CD4 T cells.

8. What mechanism ensures the specificity of the interactions of T cells with antigens?

To ensure the specificity of the interactions of T cells with antigens displayed by their respective MHC molecules, several additional molecules on the surfaces of CD4 and CD8 cells also must interact with homologous molecules on the antigen-presenting cells to induce T cells to multiply and differentiate. If these costimulatory molecules are not present, the T cell-MHC interaction may cause the T cell to undergo programmed cell death or apoptosis. Included within the stretch of chromosome 6 that contains the genes for MHC class I and class II molecules are genes for complement components C2, C4, and factor B and other molecules with immunoregulatory properties, including the genes for tumor necrosis factors alpha and beta (lymphotoxin). These additional genes on chromosome 6 are known in aggregate as class III MHC genes.

9. What are B lymphocytes (B cells)?

B cells are derived from hematopoietic stem cells and are the precursors of plasma cells, the antibody- or immunoglobulin-producing cells in the body. They differentiate from stem cells in the bone marrow, migrate through the blood, and eventually reside in the B-cell areas of the spleen, lymph nodes, and submucosal tissues of the respiratory tree and gut.

10. Describe the basic structure of an antibody.

An antibody or immunoglobulin (Ig) molecule is a protein produced by B cells that binds to antigens by means of a receptor structure created by the interaction of two long polypeptides, at their amino termini. The basic Ig structure (see figure) consists of two pairs of light and heavy polypeptide chains. The two heavy chains as well as the light chains and heavy chains are bound together by interchain disulfide bonds. The exception is IgA2, in which the light and heavy chains are not covalently linked to each other. There are two types of light chains, kappa (κ) and lambda (λ); all light chains of any individual Ig molecule are either κ or λ. The carboxy-termini of the light chain (C_L) and heavy chain (C_H) have relatively similar amino acid sequences within specific classes of Ig molecules that allow their classification as IgA, IgD, IgE, IgG, or IgM molecule. The C_H constant region contains three domains in IgG, IgD, and IgA and four domains in IgE and IgM. These constant regions are responsible for the functional aspects of the Ig molecules, including complement binding to the C_H2 region, half-life in the circulation, and ability to be transported across the placenta (IgG) or across mucous membranes (IgA). The amino-terminal half is the variable region. V_L and V_H have three regions in which the amino acid sequences are highly variable. Variation in sequence within these regions determines the ability of antibodies to bind to one but not to another antigen. In other words, the variable regions confer specificity. IgG, IgD, and IgE are monomeric in form. IgM is pentameric, and IgA is either monomeric or polymeric (some serum and all secretory forms of IgA are polymeric). The major characteristics and biologic functions of the five isotypes of Ig are shown in the table in question 7.

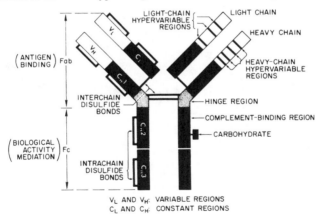

Structure of an Ig molecule. Schematic representation indicates the chain and domain structure of the Ig molecule and the existence of hypervariable regions within variable regions of both H and L chains. F*ab* and F*c* refer to fragments of the IgG molecule formed by papain cleavage. The former contains the the V_H and C_H1 H chain regions and an intact L chain; the latter consists of the C_H2 and C_H3 regions of two H chains, linked to one another by disulfide bonds. (From Wasserman RL, Capra JD: Immunoglobulins. In Horowitz MI, Pigman W (eds): The Glycoconjugates. New York, Academic Press, 1977, pp 323–348, with permission.)

11. What are the features of primary and secondary antibody responses?

A **primary** antibody response occurs after the first exposure to an antigen, whereas **secondary** antibody response occurs with the second and subsequent exposures. Major features of these two responses are illustrated on the following page.

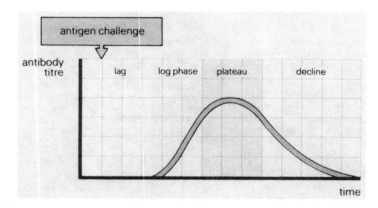

The four phases of a primary antibody response. After antigen challenge, the antibody response proceeds in four phases: (1) a lag phase when no antibody is detected; (2) a log phase in which the antibody titer rises logarithmically, (3) a plateau phase during which the antibody titer stabilizes, and (4) a decline phase during which the antibody is cleared or catabolized. (From Roitt IM, et al: Immunology. New York, Gower Medical, 1985, p 8.1, with permission.)

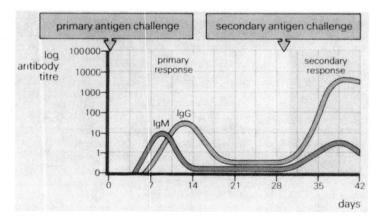

Primary and secondary antibody responses. In comparison with the antibody response to primary antivenin challenge, the antibody level after secondary antigenic challenge in a typical immune response (1) appears more quickly and persists for longer, (2) attains a high titer, and (3) consists predominantly of IgG. In the primary response the appearance of IgG is preceded by IgM. (From Roitt IM, et al: Immunology. New York, Gower Medical, 1985, p 8.1, with permission.)

12. Summarize the physical and biologic properties of the different classes of Ig.

Physical and Biologic Properties of Human Immunoglobulins*

PROPERTY	IGG	IGA	IGM	IGD	IGE
Molecular form	Monomer	Monomer, polymer	Pentamer	Monomer	Monomer
Subclass	IgG 1, 2, 3, 4	IgA 1,2	None	None	None
Molecular weight	150,000 for IgG 1, 2, 4 180,000 for IgG3	160,000 + polymers	950,000	175,000	190,000

Table continued on following page

Physical and Biologic Properties of Human Immunoglobulins *(Continued)*

PROPERTY	IGG	IGA	IGM	IGD	IGE
Serum level (mg/ml)	9, 3, 1, 0.5	2.1	1.5	4	0.03
Serum half-life (days)	23 for IgG 1,2,4 7 for IgG 3	6	5	3	3
Complement fixation	IgG 1, 2, 3+	–	+	–	–
Alternate pathway activation	IgG4	+	–	+	?
Placental transfer	+	–	–	–	–
Other properties	Secondary response	Mucous secretions	Primary response, rheumatoid factor	Class switching	Allergy

* The plus and minus signs indicate whether the molecules do or do not have the indicated property.
Modified from Paul WE: Fundamental Immunology, 2nd ed. New York, Raven Press, 1989, and Samter M, et al (eds): Immunological Diseases, 4th ed. Boston, Little, Brown, 1988, p 44, with permission.

13. Summarize the functions of the complement system.

The complement system functions as part of humoral immunity and also promotes inflammatory reactions. Specific functions of the complement system are summarized in the figure below.

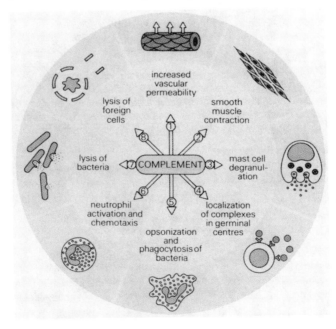

Summary of the actions of complement and its role in the acute inflammatory response. Note how the elements of the reaction are induced; increased vascular permeability (1) due to the action of C3a and C5a on smooth muscle (2) and mast cells (3) allows exudation of plasma protein. C3 facilitates both the localization of complexes in germinal centers (4) and the opsonization and phagocytosis of bacteria (5). Neutrophils, which are attracted to the area of inflammation by chemotaxis (6), phagocytose the opsonized microorganisms. The membrane attack complex, C5–9, is responsible for lysis of bacteria (7) and other cells recognized as foreign (8). (From Roitt IM, et al: Immunology. New York, Gower Medical, 1989, p 13.11, with permission.)

14. Compare the activation sequences of the classic and alternative complement pathways.

Initiation of classic complement pathway activation starts with binding of the C1 complex and proceeds through the activation cascade shown in the figure below. Activation of the alternative pathway is initiated by binding and activation of C3. Consequently, C5–9 are utilized, but C1, 2, and 4 are not involved.

An overview of the complement cascade showing the classic and alternative pathways. The central position of C3 in both pathways is indicated. (From Samter M (ed): Immunological Diseases, 4th ed. Boston, Little, Brown, 1998, p 205, with permission.)

15. What factors cause activation of the classic complement pathway?

The classic pathway is activated principally by antibody-antigen (immune) complexes. A single IgM or two IgG molecules (IgG doublet) of IgG subclasses 1, 2, and 3, but not 4, can bind C1, causing complement activation. Certain viruses, urate, DNA, and mitochondria that are released by damaged cells also activate the classical pathway.

16. What factors cause activation of the alternative complement pathway?

Substances that activate the alternative pathway are mainly components of bacterial or yeast cell walls. Aggregates of Ig and cells whose surfaces are poor in sialic acid residues also can activate the alternative pathway. Most bacteria, some parasites, and virtually all plant cells lack such residues. Healthy somatic cells express complement regulatory proteins such as decay-accelerating factor (DAF). As its name implies, DAF facilitates the breakdown of activated C3. This breakdown prevents the complement cascade from proceeding beyond C3 and thus protects the native somatic cells from injury by the products of the complement cascade.

17. In evaluating patients, does it help to measure serum complement levels?

Hospital clinical laboratories usually can measure serum levels of C3 and C4. When the differential diagnosis includes sepsis, active collagen vascular disease, or an allergic reaction, measurements of C3 and C4 are sometimes helpful. If the disease process is more than 24 hours old, the complement proteins are among the acute-phase reactants and biosynthesis is stimulated by an acute inflammation. Although complement may have been consumed in the first hours of the disease, new protein synthesis causes a prompt rebound in plasma levels to normal or even supernormal levels. Because these proteins are made in the liver, persistently low complement protein levels may be found only in patients with severe liver disease. Normal serum complement levels (C3 and C4) do not rule out either complement activation or complement-mediated tissue damage.

18. What patterns of serum C3 and C4 levels are seen with activation of the classic and alternative complement pathways? Name at least one disease associated with each pattern.

Serum Complement Levels in Disease

PATHWAY	C4	C3	DISEASE
Classic	↓	↓	Systemic lupus erythematosus, serum sickness
Classic (fluid phase)	↓	N	Hereditary angioedema
Alternative	N	↓	Endotoxemia (gram negative sepsis)
Alternative (fluid phase)	N	↓	Type II membranoproliferative glomerulonephritis (C3 nephritic factor)

↓ = decreased, N = normal.

19. What are the two major pathways of arachidonic acid metabolism? What effects do aspirin, nonsteroidal anti-inflammatory drugs (NSAIDs), eicosapentaenoic acid, and corticosteroids have on mediator production by these pathways?

Prostaglandin D_2 (PGD_2) and thromboxanes A_2 and B_2 are the major products of the cyclooxygenase (CO) pathway of metabolism. Leukotrienes (LTs), especially LTC4, LTD4, and LTE4, are major products of the lipoxygenase pathway. These eicosanoids exhibit an array of potent inflammatory and immunoregulatory properties. Aspirin and NSAIDs inhibit CO; that is, they inhibit PG and thromboxane but not LT production. Eicosapentaenoic acid (fish oil) inhibits both PG/thromboxane and LT formation by preferential fatty acid substitution for arachidonic acid in the cell membranes of eicosanoid-producing cells. Corticosteroids also inhibit both PG/thromboxane and LT generation by stimulating production of the intracellular protein, lipocortin, which inhibits the activity of phospholipase A.

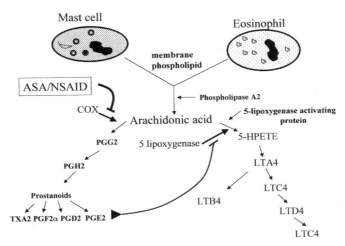

Effects of aspirin and NSAIDs on the two major pathways of arachidonic acid metabolism. (From Middleton E Jr, Reed CE, Ellis EF, et al (eds): Allergy: Principles and Practice, 5th ed, vol. II. St. Louis, Mosby, 1998, p 1229, with permission.)

20. What is aspirin hypersensitivity?

This condition is most dramatically evident in adults who have developed three manifestations of allergic disease (Samter's triad): (1) rhinitis, (2) nasal polyposis, and (3) asthma. The rhinitis and bronchospasm are greatly exacerbated by taking aspirin and other NSAIDS. Sometimes the bronchospasm is life-threatening. Among the explanations for aspirin hypersensitivity is the possibility that blockade of the CO pathway with NSAIDS increases delivery of substrate to the lipoxygenase pathway, but this theory is probably an oversimplification.

21. What are alpha, beta, and gamma interferons? How are they produced?

Interferons (IFNs) are divided into three classes: IFN-α, IFN-β, and IFN-γ. IFN-α and IFN-β were previously classified as type I and IFN-γ as type II. IFN-α has 20 or more subtypes, all of which have a high degree of homology. IFN-β has at least two subtypes. IFN-β_1 has about a 34% sequence homology with IFN-α, but the biologic effects of both are similar. IFN-β_2 has essentially no homology with IFN-α. IFN-γ is unrelated to the other IFNs in either structure or function. IFN-α is produced by leukocytes, fibroblasts (to a lesser degree), and other cells. IFN-β_1 is produced by fibroblasts, leukocytes (to a lesser degree), T cells, monocytes, and endothelial cells. IFN-γ is produced by activated T lymphocytes, NK cells, and lymphokine-activated killer (LAK) cells.

22. Summarize the function of alpha, beta, and gamma inteferons.

Both IFN-α and IFN-β_1 modulate antibody production, graft rejection, and delayed-type hypersensitivity (DTH) reactions. They can induce autoimmune and inflammatory reactions, and they have important antiviral, antibacterial, antifungal, and antitumor activities.

IFN-β_2 (interleukin [IL]-6) has important immunomodulatory activity and poor antiviral activity. It also has been called B-cell differentiation factor, because it stimulates mature B cells to differentiate into immunoglobulin-secreting plasma cells. It also plays a role in early hematopoiesis and may be an important autocrine growth factor for B-cell malignancies.

The biologic effects of IFN-γ include enhancing cytotoxic T cell and NK cell activity, induction of class II antigen expression on B cells and other antigen-presenting cells, and induction of IL-2 receptor expression on T cells. It downregulates collagen synthesis and inhibits IL-4–induced IgE synthesis.

23. What is the bursa of Fabricius? Which lymphoid organ is its equivalent in humans?

The bursa of Fabricius is the site of B-cell development in the chicken (*Gallus domesticus*). In humans, B-cell maturation occurs primarily in the bone marrow.

24. Outline B-cell ontogeny from stem cell to plasma cell.

Stem cell → pre-B cell → immature B cell → mature B cell → activated B cell → secretory B cell → plasma cell.

25. What is the role of surface Ig on B cells?

Before active secretion of Ig begins in B cells, the cell produces Ig with an added polypeptide tail at the carboxy terminus that anchors the Ig in the B-cell membrane. These cell surface Ig molecules provide antigen-binding sites. Binding of antigen to cell surface Ig molecules activates the B cells. If the B cell receives additional costimulatory signals via other cell surface molecules from T cells, the B cell differentiates into an antibody-producing cell. In the absence of costimulatory signals, it does not differentiate further or produce antibody.

26. What are the major subtypes of T cells? Describe the principal function of each.

T cells function both as effectors and regulators of the immune response. Like B cells, they are derived from the embryonic hematopoietic stem cells. They differ from B cells in that an important part of their early maturation occurs in the thymus; hence the name T cells. In the thymus cells that avidly recognize self-antigens are eliminated and die by apoptosis. The major types of T cells are:

1. CD4 T cells, which traditionally are considered to function primarily as helper/inducer T cells that provide (1) soluble and cognate signals to B cells to stimulate antibody production and

(2) cells that organize and promote cell-mediated delayed-type hypersensitivity responses. Recently it has been recognized that they also can act as killer cells or even as suppressor cells. They are stimulated to recognize and react against antigen presented by MHC class II molecules.

2. CD8 T cells, which classically are considered to kill virus-infected cells. They also may suppress cell-mediated immune responses. As noted with the CD4 T cell, many of these functional restrictions no longer apply because numerous exceptions have been noted. CD8 T cells recognize antigen only when presented by MHC class I molecules.

27. What is the CD nomenclature of phenotyping cells?

The CD (cluster designation) nomenclature is a system for identification of cell surface antigens that have been defined by monoclonal antibodies. Development of a monoclonal antibody to a cell surface protein is one important step in its characterization. These antibodies allow identification of target proteins on cell surfaces. They also help to purify the protein and illuminate their function. Thus far over 166 CD antigens have been recognized by international committees that assign these numbers. CD markers identify targets that can be used to remove whole classes of cells from the circulation by means of cytolytic monoclonal antibodies. For example, antibodies to CD3 and CD4 have been used to help control transplant rejection reactions by removing and inactivating the effector T cells. A few important CD markers are listed in the table below.

CD Markers, Isoforms, Sites of Expression, and Function

SURFACE MARKER	ISOFORMS	SITES OF EPRESSION	COMMENTS
CD2	50-kD protein	Thymocytes, T cells, NK cells (large granular lymphocytes)	Adhesion molecule that binds to LFA-3, a ligand on APC. Ligation with LFA-3 activates T cells.
CD3	γ: 25-kD glycoprotein δ: 20 kD glycoprotein ε: 20-kD protein	Thymocytes, T cells	Associated with T-cell antigen receptor (TCR). Required for cell surface expression of TCR
CD4	57-kD glycoprotein	Thymocytes, TH1 and TH2 T cells, monocytes, some macrophages	Coreceptor for MHC class II and for HIV-1 + HIV-2 and gp120.
CD8	α: 32-kd glycoprotein β: 32–34 kD	Thymocytes, CD8 T cells	Coreceptor for MHC class I; anti-CD8 blocks cytotoxic T-cell responses
CD16	50–80 kD	NK cells, granulocytes, macrophages	Low-affinity Fcγ receptor that plays a role in antibody-dependent cell-mediated cytotoxicity and activation of NK cells
CD19	95 kD	B cells	Coreceptor for B cells; involved in B cell activation.
CD28	44-kD homodimer	T cell subsets Activated B cells	Binding to CD80 (on B cells) or CD86 (on macrophages or dendritic cells) Sends costimulatory, differentiation-inducing signal.
CD45RO	180 kD glycoprotein	Memory T cells, B-cell subsets, monocytes	See CD45RA
CD45RA	205–220-kD glycoprotein	Naive T cells, B cells, monocytes	Role in signal transduction, tyrosine phosphatase

Table continued on following page

CD Markers, Isoforms, Sites of Expression, and Function (Continued)

SURFACE MARKER	ISOFORMS	SITES OF EPRESSION	COMMENTS
CD56	135–220-kD heterodimer	NK cells	Promotes adhesion of NK cells
CD80	60-kD protein	B cells subset	Ligand for CD28 on T cells, costimulator involved in antigen presenation
CD86	80-kD protein	Activated B cells Monocytes, dendritic cells	Costimulatory ligand for CD28 on T cells during antigen presentation.

From David J: Immunology. In Dale DC, Federman DD (eds): Scientific American Medicine. New York, Scientific American, 1996, p 6, and Janeway CA, Travers P, Walport M, Capra JD: (eds) Immunobiology, 4th ed. New York, Garland Publishing, 1999, with permission.

28. More than 38 cytokines have been identified. What are cytokines, where are they made, and what do they do?

A Few Cytokines and Their Biologic Activities*

CYTOKINES	CELL SOURCE			MAJOR ACTIVITIES
	T CELLS	MACROPHAGES	OTHER	
IL-1α and 1β		+	+	Fever; bone resorption; prostaglandin release; stimulate cytokine production by macrophages and T cells.
IL-2	+			Activates cytotoxic T cells and NK cells. Stimulates proliferation and differentiation of T cells, NK and lymphokine-activated killer (LAK) cells. Stimulates proliferation of B cells and antibody secretion.
IL-3	+		+	Supports proliferation and differentiation of stem cells, including pre-B cells. Activates mast cells.
IL-4	+		+	Activates resting B cells and induces IgG-to-IgE switch and Ig secretion by activated B cells. Stimulates proliferation of T cells and activates mast cells. Suppresses TNF-α, IL-1, IL-6 production in in monocytes.
IL-5	+		+	Induces IgA production and IgM secretion in activated B cells. Attracts and stimulates proliferation of eosinophils; stimulates differentiation of cytotoxic T cells.
IL-6	+	+	+	B-cell and T-cell growth and differentiation; causes fever and proliferation of megakaryocytes and myeloma cells. Mobilizes neutrophils during inflammation and synthesis of acute-phase reactants
IL-7			Thymic	Proliferation and differentiation of strand cells, pre-B and pre-T cells.
IL-8		+	+	Neutrophil chemotaxis.
IL-10	+	+	+	Suppresses macrophage functions

Table continued on following page

A Few Cytokines and Their Biologic Activities*

	CELL SOURCE			
CYTOKINES	T CELLS	MACROPHAGES	OTHER	MAJOR ACTIVITIES
IL-12		+	B cells	Proliferation of activated T cells and induction of T-cell differentiation to THI1-like cells.
TNF-α	+	+	+	Chemotactic for various leukocytes. Activates macrophages and endothelial cells. Induces or prevents apoptosis, depending on effects of other stimuli in microenvironment. Impairs cardiac muscle contractility. Causes fever, cachexia, and sometimes shock when released systemically.
TNF-β	+		+	Activates endothelial cells, principal cytotoxic molecule of killer T Cells.
IFN-γ	+		NK cells	Activates monocyte/macrophages, and induces expression of MHC and other molecules that promote antigen presentation.

IL = interleukin, TNF = tumor necrosis factor, IFN = interferon.
From Bennett JC: Approach to the patient with immune diseases. In Bennett JC, Plum F (eds): Cecil Textbook of Medicine, 20th ed. Philadelphia, W.B. Saunders, 1996, p 1395, and Janeway CA, Travers P, Walport M, Capra JD (eds): Immunobiology, 4th ed. New York, Garland Publishing, 1999, with permission.

29. What is anergy? What is its clinical significance?

Anergy is the lack of an immunologic reaction to common antigens under circumstances in which one would expect to see such a reaction. T-cell anergy, for example, is the lack of reaction to delayed-type hypersensitivity (DTH) recall antigens, as may be seen in patients with miliary tuberculosis, Hodgkin's disease, or HIV-infected people. B-cell anergy is failure to develop a specific antibody response in a person who has been immunized with antigens that routinely stimulate antibody responses in other members of the same species. Anergy may be temporary, as occurs during measles infection, or of indeterminate duration, as occurs in sarcoidosis, AIDS, and certain disseminated malignancies and overwhelming infectious diseases, including lepromatous leprosy. Anergic people have increased susceptibility to infections that require cell-mediated immune responses for adequate host defense.

30. How is anergy diagnosed?

To establish that a patient is T-cell anergic by DTH skin testing, it is customary to use 4 or 5 recall antigens to ensure a > 90% chance of using at least one antigen against which normal age-matched people would mount a delayed hypersensitivity response. Readily available antigens include trichophyton in a 1:30 dilution from Hollister Stier Labs; tetanus toxoid at 10 Lf/ml from Wyeth Labs; mumps antigen at 40 cfu/ml from Connaught Labs; candidal extract at 500 PNU/ml from Greer Labs, and purified protein derivative (PPD) at 50 TU/ml, also from Connaught Labs. To perform the test, 0.1 ml of each is injected intradermally at widely spaced sites, usually on the volar surface of the forearms. The mean diameter of induration is read at 48 hours. There is disagreement whether a 5- or 10-cm diameter represents a positive result. To assess nonspecific reactions, one can use 0.1 ml of saline as a negative control, but most forego this approach because there is nothing to observe at 48 hours unless the tester inadvertently triggers a capillary bleed at the site of the injection.

31. Explain the role of antigen-presenting cells (APCs) in the immune response.

APCs present antigens principally to T lymphocytes, as a result of which the T cells are activated and stimulated to perform one of their many functions. APCs present peptide fragments that are subunits of often much larger antigens either in the antigen-binding cleft of class I MHC molecules or in the antigen-binding cleft of class II MHC molecules. For example, viral antigens are presented by class I MHC molecules and are recognized by CD8 T cells. MHC class II molecules present extrinsic, environmental antigens to CD4 T lymphocytes. Antigen recognition requires costimulatory signals by other molecules physically associated with the T-cell antigen receptor. APCs may have constitutive antigen-presenting capability or acquire this capacity only after being stimulated to display MHC molecules on their surface, as occurs with fibroblasts (class I) , some types of macrophages (class II) and, rarely, somatic tissue cells. APCs include dendritic cells, Langerhans cells, B cells, macrophages, fixed tissue macrophages (e.g., Kupffer cells), microglial cells, and, less commonly, astrocytes, fibroblasts, and endothelial cells. Generally dendritic cells are the most effective APCs.

32. What is major basic protein (MBP)?

MBP is the principal bioactive protein in the cytoplasmic granules of eosinophils. It is the only protein localized to the crystalline core. It is also present in much smaller amounts in basophils.

33. Describe the biologic effects of MBP.

1. Highly toxic to many parasites (including *Schistosoma mansoni, Trichinella spiralis,* and *Trypanosoma cruzi*).
2. Toxic to a wide variety of mammalian cells (including human cells).
3. Stimulates histamine release from basophils and mast cells.
4. Neutralizes heparin.
5. Causes bronchospasm.

34. Describe the mechanism of immediate hypersensitivity reactions. Give clinical examples.

Type I (immediate hypersensitivity) reactions are classic allergic reactions initiated by the binding of an antigen to more than one IgE attached to Fc receptors on the surface of mast cells or basophils. This process results in cross-linkage of Fc receptors with high affinity for IgE, cell activation, noncytolytic degranulation, and release of potent mediators, including histamine, prostaglandins, and leukotrienes, from the granules. The reaction becomes clinically evident within seconds to minutes and is almost always apparent within 1 hour. Clinical examples include anaphylaxis, allergic rhinitis (hay fever), food allergy, extrinsic (allergic) asthma, immediate drug allergy (e.g., to penicillin), and acute urticaria (hives).

35. What are the four types of hypersensitivity reactions?

Coombs and Gell described four classic types of hypersensitivity reactions.

TYPE	ANTIGEN RECOGNIZED BY	SOLUBLE MEDIATOR	INFLAMMATORY RESPONSE	EXAMPLES
I. Reagenic, allergic	IgE	Basophil and mast cell products	Immediate flare and wheal, smooth muscle constriction	Atopy, anaphylaxis
II. Cytotoxic antibody	IgG or IgM	Complement	Lysis or phagocytosis of circulating antigens, acute inflammation in tissues	Autoimmune hemolytic anemia, thrombocytopenia associated with systemic lupus erythematosus (SLE)
III. Immune complex	IgG, IgM	Complement, leukotrienes, prostaglandins	Accumulation of polymorphonuclear leukocytes and macrophages	Rheumatoid arthritis, SLE
IV. Delayed hypersensitivity	T lymphocytes	Cytokines	Mononuclear cell infiltrate	Tuberculosis, sarcoidosis, polymyositis, granulomatosis, vasculitis

From Wyngaarden JB, Smith LH : Cecil Textbook of Medicine, 18th ed. Philadelphia, W.B. Saunders, 1988, p 1989, with permission.

36. Describe the mechanism of DTH reactions.

DTH (type IV) reactions are a reflection of cell-mediated immunity and are initiated by T cells. Unlike reaction types I–III, DTH can be transferred by T cells, but not by serum. When antigen-sensitized T cells are reexposed to the same antigen by APCs, they become activated. Activated T cells secrete IFN-γ, IL-2 and other cytokines, causing monocytes to accumulate at the site of the reaction and differentiate into macrophages. Over 90% of the T cells that accumulate at the site of a DTH reaction are not antigen-specific; they have been called to the site by the activity of the chemokines and cytokines produced by the infiltrating monocytes and few antigen-specific T cells that have localized in the vicinity of the APCs. Additional inflammatory mediators and cytokines are released that cause edema and sometimes necrosis of bystander cells. If the antigen persists or can be degraded only with difficulty (e.g., antigenic lipids of *M. tuberculosis*), lymphocyte and macrophage activation continues and may result in granuloma formation. DTH reactions differ in tempo, depending on the cells involved.

TYPE	INDUCING ANTIGEN	TIME TO PEAK	EXTERNAL SIGNS	HISTOLOGIC APPEARANCE
Tuberculin	Tuberculin	48 hr	Indurated, painful skin swelling	Intradermal lymphocyte and monocyte infiltration
Jones-Mote	Foreign proteins such as ovalbumin	24 hr	Slight skin thickening	Intradermal lymphocyte and basophil infiltration
Contact	Urushiol, the antigen of poison ivy	48 hr	Eczema	Same as tuberculin
Granulomatous	Talcum powder, silica, and other substances that stimulate phagocytosis but cannot be metabolized	4 wk	Skin induration	Epithelioid cell granuloma formation, giant cells, macrophages, fibrosis, necrosis

Modified from Klein J: Immunology. Oxford, Blackwell Scientific 1990, with permission.

37. Describe the mechanism of cytotoxic reactions, and give clinical examples.

Cytotoxic (type II) reactions occur when antibody binds to specific antigens on circulating cells or antigens fixed in tissues. Antibody binding activates complement. If the target site lacks decay-accelerating factor or other complement regulatory proteins, as is the case with red blood cells, the complement cascade can progress to completion, causing lysis of the target cell. Target cells that are coated with both antibody and bound complement fragments can be opsonized for phagocytosis by macrophages that reside within the reticuloendothelial system and by circulating phagocytes. Rarely, antigens localized in basement membranes can become a target of autoantibodies, as in Goodpasture's syndrome. In this case, the antigen is localized in the basement membranes of the renal glomeruli and lung. Deposition of antibody also binds and activates complement and induces leukocytes to localize at the sites of antigen-antibody and complement deposition, with the result that leukocyte proteases break down the basement membranes.

38. Describe the mechanism of immune complex reactions, and give clinical examples.

Immune complex-mediated reactions (type III) are caused by the formation of soluble or not-so-soluble antigen and antibody complexes in the circulation. They deposit preferentially in (1) fenestrated endothelia, as found in the choroid plexus and renal glomeruli, and (2) bifurcations of postcapillary venules, where eddy currents slow the flow of blood. Immune complexes usually activate complement in situ. As a result, neutrophils accumulate and cause tissue damage. Examples include the Arthus reaction (e.g., in hyperimmunized people who receive a tetanus toxoid booster) and generalized serum sickness (e.g., after injection of foreign protein into the circulation in people with preformed antibodies to that protein).

39. What is an Arthus reaction? When does it occur in a clinical setting?

Arthus reactions are caused by antigen-antibody complexes (immune complexes) and were first described by the French physiologist Nicolas-Maurice Arthus in 1903. The reaction is an acute inflammatory response at the site of deposition of antigen in tissue. The common site is skin near a site of subcutaneous injection of an antigen. Arthus reactions develop when there are high serum levels of complement-fixing antibodies. Immune complexes form in the blood vessel walls of the dermis and subcutaneous tissues, causing a localized vasculitis. Arthus reactions depend on both neutrophil and complement function. In humans, localized Arthus reactions have been reported at the sites of injection of second and subsequent tetanus and diphtheria immunizations and, rarely, at the site of injection of insulin in diabetics.

40. What is an allergen?

An allergen is a special type of antigen that commonly induces synthesis of IgE antibodies, which sensitize mast cells and basophils. Whether the host makes IgE depends on multiple factors, but most particularly on the type of cytokines that the T-helper cells make after injection of the antigen.

41. What are the major differences between mast cells and basophils?

PARAMETER	MAST CELLS	BASOPHILS
Life span	Weeks to years	Days
Origin	Probably bone marrow	Bone marrow
Location	Tissues, noncirculating	Normally circulating
Size	8–20 mm	5–7 mm
Nucleus	Round to oval, may be indented	Multilobulated
Cytoplasmic granules	Smaller, more numerous	Larger, fewer granules
High-affinity IgE receptor	Present	Present
Histamine release	Yes	Yes
Major arachidonic acid metabolites	PGD2; LTC4, -D4, -E4	LTC4
Staining characteristics		
Toluidine blue	Yes	Yes
Tryptase	Yes	No
Chloroacetate esterase	Yes	No

PG = prostaglandin, LT = leukotriene.

42. Are all mast cells alike?

No. Mast cell heterogeneity, which exists in both animals and humans, has been studied most extensively in mice, which appear to have two major populations: mucosal mast cells (MMCs) and connective tissue mast cells (CTMCs). MMCs are found principally at mucosal surfaces, whereas CTMCs are found within connective tissue, lining blood vessels, and at serosal surfaces. Humans also appear to have two major mast cell populations, which are identified by differences in neutral protease content of the cytoplasmic granules. Both populations contain tryptase, but only one contains both tryptase and chymase. The tryptase-only mast cells (MCTs) are located primarily at mucosal surfaces, whereas the tryptase and chymase-positive mast cells (MCTCs) are located primarily in connective tissue, around blood vessels, and at serosal surfaces. The factors responsible for human mast cell growth have not yet been clearly defined. Although human IL-3 appears to have some mast cell growth-promoting activity, its effects are less well defined. Of interest, MCTs, but not MCTCs, appear to be T-lymphocyte dependent, as suggested by a marked decrease in MCTs (but not MCTCs) in the tissues of patients with severe T-cell immunodeficiency disorders.

43. Which procedure is most useful in the diagnosis of systemic mastocytosis?

Bone marrow biopsy is the procedure of choice because of its high sensitivity and specificity. A positive skin biopsy does not indicate internal organ involvement. Plasma histamine levels may be normal or elevated, although very high levels are highly suggestive of systemic disease. Bone scan findings are nonspecific. Hepatomegaly and splenomegaly may or may not be seen and are not diagnostic. The bone marrow is characterized by prominent aggregates of mast cells in association with spicules, lymph tissue, or blood vessels. Eosinophils are often prominent, and variable degrees of fibrosis are present. If the diagnosis of systemic mastocytosis is suspected, the pathologist should be notified before the bone marrow biopsy is processed, because the standard bone marrow preparation involves decalcification, which results in poor staining of mast cell granules by metachromatic dyes such as toluidine blue. A Giemsa stain may be useful in identifying mast cells in such samples. Bone marrow aspiration without biopsy is insufficient to rule in or out systemic mastocytosis.

44. Which biologic functions are mediated via H_1, H_2, or a combination of H_1 and H_2 histamine receptors?

H_1 RECEPTORS	H_2 RECEPTORS	H_1 AND H_2 RECEPTORS
Smooth muscle contraction	Gastric acid secretion	Hypotension
↑ Vascular permeability	↑ Cyclic AMP	Tachycardia
Pruritus	Mucous secretion	Flushing
Stimulation of prostaglandin synthesis	Inhibits basophil but not mast cell histamine release	Headache
Tachycardia	Stimulates IL-5 production by TH2 cells.	
↑ Cyclic GMP production		

↑ = increased, ↓ = decreased, AMP = adenosine monophosphate, GMP = guanosine monophosphate.

45. What is the reticuloendothelial system (RES)? What are its principal functions?

The RES (mononuclear/phagocyte system) consists of a heterogeneous population of fixed-tissue phagocytic cells throughout the body. These cells remove particulate and soluble substances from the circulation and tissues, especially if the substances are coated with antibody and complement. Examples include immune complexes, bacteria, toxins, and exogenous antigens. These substances may be internalized by nonspecific endocytosis, nonimmune but receptor-mediated phagocytosis, or immunologic phagocytosis mediated by binding to Fc or complement receptors. Components of the RES include Kupffer cells of the liver, microglial cells of the brain, pulmonary alveolar macrophages, and macrophages in endothelial-lined channels in bone marrow, lymph nodes, lung, gut, and other tissues. Blockade of the RES is one postulated mechanism for prevention of platelet destruction by high-dose intravenous gammaglobulin (IVGG) in idiopathic thrombocytopenic purpura (ITP). The binding of IgG-sensitized platelets to the IgG-Fc receptors on RES cells, particularly in the liver and spleen, leads to phagocytosis and platelet destruction in ITP. This IgG-Fc receptor mechanism may be "blocked" or overwhelmed by the infusion of high-dose IVGG. IgG-Fc receptors are lost during phagocytosis and may take as long as several days to be reexpressed.

46. What maneuver elicits Darier's sign?

Darier's sign is the erythema and whealing that follows gentle stroking of the characteristic, reddish-brown skin lesions of urticaria pigmentosa. It is presumably caused by degranulation and mediator release from the large numbers of dermal mast cells.

47. What is cold agglutinin syndrome? How is it diagnosed?

Cold agglutinin syndrome is characterized by hemolytic anemia, usually secondary to IgM antibodies; low-affinity IgG antibodies also have been implicated. The IgM antibodies can cause red blood cell (RBC) lysis with decreasing temperature. IgG antibodies also can facilitate uptake of the antibody-coated RBC by phagocytes. Agglutination of normal RBCs at 20°C occurs with serum from virtually all patients with cold agglutinin syndrome. The direct Coombs' test is typically positive for complement and negative for immunoglobulin, reflecting the fact that the antibody involved has a high affinity for RBCs only in the cold. Warming the antibody causes it to dissociate. Hence, only RBCs in cold extremities (e.g., fingers, toes, tip of the nose) are likely to show a positive direct Coombs' test. Cold agglutinin syndrome is typically idiopathic, with the presentation of hemolytic anemia in the sixth or seventh decade of life. Despite the monoclonal nature of the antibody response, patients usually do not develop multiple myeloma or Waldenstrom's macroglobulinemia.

Cold agglutinin syndrome also may occur in association with lymphoproliferative disorders (e.g., non-Hodgkin's lymphoma), infections (mycoplasmal pneumonia, infectious mononucleosis), and, rarely, in connective tissue disorders (systemic lupus erythematosus [SLE]). The cold agglutinins in these disorders may be anti-I or directed at other RBC antigens. Determination of antibody specificity is not necessary for either diagnosis or as a prerequisite for blood transfusion.

48. List the general characteristics of antibody deficiency disorders.

Antibody deficiency disorders, whether acquired or congenital, have several general characteristics that are manifestations of the defect in antibody-mediated immune responses:

1. Recurrent infections with extracellular encapsulated pathogens.
2. Relatively few problems with fungal or viral (except enteroviral) infections.
3. Chronic sinusitis and pulmonary disease (some patients may develop bronchiectasis).
4. Growth retardation is not a striking feature.
5. Low antibody levels measured in serum and secretions but low antibody or Ig levels in body fluids are not sufficient evidence of an antibody deficiency syndrome.
6. Patients may or may not lack B lymphocytes. If B lymphocytes are present, they may lack surface immunoglobulins or complement receptors, indicating that they were arrested relatively early in ontogeny.
7. Absence of cortical follicles in lymph nodes and spleen are seen in X-linked agammaglobulinemia.
8. Scanty cervical lymph nodes and small or absent tonsils and adenoids are characteristic of X-linked agammaglobulinemia.
9. Replacement therapy with IV immunoglobulin G has greatly increased lifespan and reduced morbidity.

Wyngaarden JB, Smith LH: Cecil Textbook of Medicine, 18th ed. Philadelphia, W.B. Saunders, 1988, p 1943, with permission.

49. What is the most common immunoglobulin deficiency disorder?

Selective IgA deficiency has a frequency of approximately 1 in 500–700 persons. Many patients are asymptomatic, but some have recurrent infections, particularly of the respiratory tract. IgG_2 deficiency sometimes accompanies IgA deficiency, and such patients are particularly prone to infectious complications with encapsulated bacteria (e.g., *Streptococcus pneumoniae, Haemophilus influenzae*) because the principal IgG antibody response against bacterial polysaccharide is usually IgG_2. In selective IgA deficiency, the serum IgA level is < 5 mg/dl (0.05 mg/cc). IgA in secretions is almost always depressed. IgG and IgM levels are normal. A few patients have autoimmune disorders (including SLE and rheumatoid arthritis). Treatment is supportive. Even if patients have an increased incidence of infections, IVIG therapy should be undertaken with extreme caution because 50% of patients may have the ability to develop antibodies to the small quantities of IgA present in most IVIG preparations. Life-threatening anaphylaxis can occur with the second and subsequent infusion of IVIG. A similar risk is associated with blood transfusions. IgA-deficient patients can develop antibodies to plasma IgA that accompanies packed red blood cells. Subsequent transfusions, if needed, should be performed with well-washed RBCs to remove all traces of IgA.

50. What is common variable immunodeficiency disease (CVID)?

CVID is a heterogeneous group of disorders characterized by hypogammaglobulinemia (total IgG < 250 mg/dl and total immunoglobulin usually < 350 mg/dl), decreased ability to produce antibody after antigenic challenge, and recurrent infections. A significant fraction of patients whose serum IgG level is depressed but > 250 mg/dl may have a similar clinical presentation. The most common serum Ig pattern is panhypogammaglobulinemia with deficiency of IgG, IgM, and IgA.

CVID usually presents in late childhood or early adulthood but may present at any age. Recurrent infections of the upper and lower respiratory tract with encapsulated bacteria (e.g., *S. pneumoniae, H. influenzae*) are common, and bronchiectasis may develop. Patients also may have defective cell-mediated immunity and mycobacterial, fungal, and protozoal (e.g., *Giardia lamblia*) infections. Patients with CVID have an increased frequency of autoimmune disorders, including pernicious anemia, Coombs-positive hemolytic anemia, autoimmune thrombocytopenia, and thyroiditis. GI disorders are common, including diarrhea, malabsorption, and nodular lymphoid hyperplasia of the small intestine. Finally, there is an increased incidence of malignancy, particularly of the lymphoreticular system and GI tract.

51. Identify the principal immunologic defects in CVID.

The most commonly appreciated defect appears to be a defect in B-cell maturation. The B cells cannot terminally differentiate into antibody-producing plasma cells. Patients generally have normal numbers of circulating, surface Ig-positive B cells. Up to 20% of patients may have increased suppressor-cell activity, causing decreased antibody production. But a host of other immunologic defects is seen in some patients, including T-cell immunoregulatory defects. Depressed cell-mediated immunity, as demonstrated by cutaneous anergy, may be present in up to 30% of patients.

52. Is there a specific treatment for CVID?

The principal therapy for CVID is IVGG replacement and aggressive management of infections with appropriate antibiotics. IVGG is given every 3–4 weeks. The usual dose is 200 mg/kg, and the infusion is given slowly over several hours. Adverse reactions consisting of pruritus, headache, and nausea usually resolve with slowing or stopping of the infusion. IVGG often dramatically decreases the frequency and severity of infections and also may alleviate some of the symptoms, such as arthralgias, that may accompany CVID.

53. What are the clinical characteristics of disorders of cell-mediated immunity?

The manifestations of cellular immunodeficiency disorders, due to a partial or total defect in T-cell function, include:

1. Recurrent infections with low-grade or opportunistic infectious agents, such as fungi, viruses, or protozoa (e.g., *Pneumocystis carinii*).

2. T cell anergy (general lack of T cell-mediated immune responses).

3. Children have growth retardation, dramatically shortened life span, wasting, and diarrhea.

4. Graft-vs.-host disease (GVHD) may occur if patients are given fresh blood or unmatched allogeneic bone marrow.

5. Fatal infections after live virus vaccines and after vaccination with other attenuated microorganisms, including BCG.

6. High incidence of malignancy.

From Wyngaarden JB, Smith LH (eds): Cecil Textbook of Medicine, 18th ed. Philadelphia, W.B. Saunders, 1988, p 1945, with permission.

54. List the causes of secondary hypogammaglobulinemia.

CAUSE	MECHANISM
Drugs	
• Anticonvulsants (especially phenytoin)	Decreased B- and T-lymphocyte responses, often with hypogammaglobulinemia
• Cytotoxic agents	Decreased Ig production and T-cell activity
Multiple myeloma	Decreased Ig production
Chronic lymphocytic leukemia	Decreased Ig production and T-cell activity
Myotonic dystrophy	Selective hypercatabolism of IgG
Nephrotic syndrome	Ig loss in urine (particularly IgG)
Intestinal lymphangiectasia	Ig loss through GI tract, increased Ig catabolism
Radiation therapy	Decreased Ig production

55. How is the radioallergosorbent test (RAST) performed?

RAST is used for measurement of specific IgE antibody in serum. The test is only semi-quantitative. Purified allergen is coupled to a carrier (particles, paper discs, plastic wells) and incubated with the patient's serum. After washing, ^{125}I-labelled anti-IgE is added, and radioactivity present on the immunoabsorbent material (carrier) is measured. RAST is increasingly being converted to an an enzyme-linked immunsorbent assay (ELISA) that uses enzymatic color change rather than radioactivity. Recently Pharmacia produced quantitative antigen specific tests of IgE to selected allergens that may be more useful than the RAST in the diagnosis of allergic diseases.

56. How does RAST compare with skin testing in the diagnosis of allergy?

RAST is less sensitive, and its correlation with the clinical history of allergy to specific agents is less clear-cut than with skin testing. Furthermore, validity of RAST is highly dependent on proper controls and interpretation of the results by the reporting laboratory. However, RAST may be useful in patients in whom skin testing cannot be done, including patients with extensive skin diseases or dermatographism, urticaria pigmentosa, or cutaneous mastocytosis. It also may be useful in patients receiving H_1 antihistamines and patients in whom skin testing carries a high risk of severe anaphylaxis. By itself, no test of immediate hypersensitivity, whether skin testing or RAST, is diagnostic and cannot be taken as evidence of allergy to a specific agent unless the clinical history is supportive. In practice, although the specificity of the RAST and skin testing is low, sensitivity is relatively high. A negative RAST or, for that matter, negative intradermal testing is good evidence that the patient is *not* sensitive to a specific allergen.

57. Describe the basic technique for performance of ELISA.

To a great extent, ELISA has replaced the radioimmunoassay (RIA) in diagnostic testing. Compared with RIA, ELISA eliminates radioactive hazards and has a sensitivity that is comparable or better (sensitivity of 1 ng or less, depending on the test substance and various components used in the assay). ELISA is typically performed in plastic, flat-bottomed, 96-well, microtiter plates. The basic ELISA procedure used to test for antibody against specific antigen is outlined below. The concentration of the substance to be measured is determined by comparing the optical density of the test samples against negative controls and a standard curve.

ELISA Test Procedure

1. Coat wells with antigen (by incubating appropriate concentration of antigen in the wells), and then wash.	4. Add enzyme-linked antispecies immunoglobulin and incubate.
2. Add test sample and incubate.	5. Wash.
3. Wash.	6. Add developing substrate and measure optical density.

58. Which principal components of house dust have been implicated in allergic disease?

House dust, a frequent cause of allergic rhinitis and asthma, is a mixture of variable amounts of antigens from dust mites, cockroaches, cats, dogs, pollens, molds and other environmental substances. Dust mites and cockroach-related antigens are often the most important sources of offending allergens in the home and are particularly prevalent in clothing, carpets, and mattresses. Both species of dust mite (*Dermatophagoides pteronyssinus* and *D. farinae*) can be found in bedding, upholstered furniture, and carpets in offices and homes in the U.S.; the allergens are released into the excretions of the mites. Dust mites thrive optimally at 25°C and 80% relative humidity. Human epidermal scales are a major substrate for dust mite growth. Efforts to minimize exposure to dust and to decrease favorable environments for dust mite growth may be highly beneficial for allergic patients. Treatment with antiallergic medications and, when necessary, immunotherapy (allergy shots) is effective. In practice, symptoms of allergic rhinitis can be controlled in 90% of patients if the patients use prescribed medications regularly for prophylaxis as well as treatment and if proper attention is given to eliminating sources of dust mite and other allergens from the home.

59. What modes of therapy are available for allergic rhinitis?

1. Avoidance of the offending allergens
2. Medical therapy
   - H_1 antihistamines
   - Sympathomimetics (among the most effective is nasal inhalation of topical oxymetazo-line, but it must be used only intermittently)
   - Cromolyn sodium (in patients with ocular pruritus, cromolyn sodium eye drops are necessary to control the problem fully)
   - Corticosteroid nasal sprays must be used, often year round (systemic therapy is indicated only rarely for severe acute exacerbations and control of nasal polyps)
3. Allergen-specific immunotherapy

60. What immunologic changes occur in patients who undergo allergen-specific immunotherapy?

Allergen-specific immunotherapy involves the subcutaneous injection of extracts of the specific allergens responsible for the patient's symptoms. Immunologic changes reported in response to allergen-specific immunotherapy include:

1. Diminished seasonal increases of allergen-specific IgE
2. Increased allergen-specific IgG
3. Decreased basophil histamine release
4. Development of allergen-specific suppressor T cells

Despite these observations, the specific cause of the effectiveness of immunotherapy remains to be precisely determined.

61. Describe the mechanism of action of cromolyn sodium.

Cromolyn sodium is available for use via inhalational, intranasal, and topical ophthalmic routes. It inhibits the degranulation of mast cells, thereby preventing the release of the mediators of immediate hypersensitivity. The exact mechanism is unknown; inhibition of calcium influx is one of several proposed explanations. Cromolyn has no intrinsic antihistamine, bronchodilator, or anti-inflammatory activity. It is used as a prophylactic agent in patients with sufficiently frequent symptoms to justify continuous therapy, because it is most effective when administered before exposure to an allergen (i.e., before mast cell degranulation). Cromolyn inhibits both immediate hypersensitivity and late-phase reactions.

62. Describe the effects of 2 weeks of treatment with H_1 antihistamines, H_2 antihistamines, or corticosteroids on the results of allergy and DTH skin testing.

Allergy skin testing is used to evaluate patients for potential immediate hypersensitivity reactivity (type I reaction) to a specific allergen. Thus, if the mast cells have been sensitized with IgE antibody against the injected allergen, mast cell degranulation occurs, resulting in release of mediators such as histamine into the skin. The wheal and flare reaction of a positive skin test is due primarily to histamine stimulation of H_1 receptors. Thus, H_1 antihistamines markedly inhibit positive skin test reactivity and must be discontinued for a certain period (depending on the antihistamine) before skin testing. H_2 antihistamines typically do not have significant effects on skin test reactivity, but occasional effects have been observed. This emphasizes the importance of using a histamine standard as a positive control when allergy skin testing is performed. Corticosteroids do not affect mast cell degranulation, nor do they affect the biologic effects of histamine. Thus, corticosteroids do not alter allergy skin test results.

In contrast, **DTH skin testing** is a type IV reaction and is a sensitive measurement of T-cell function. Histamine does not play a significant role in DTH, and antihistamines (both H_1 and H_2) do not affect DTH skin testing. However, corticosteroids may substantially depress cell-mediated responses, including the mobilization of T cells to specific antigen depots. Thus, DTH reactions may be profoundly depressed by treatment with corticosteroids.

63. Which types of infections play a role in the exacerbation of asthma?

Strong evidence implicates upper respiratory infections (URI) caused by viruses and *Mycoplasma pneumoniae* as important exacerbating agents of asthma. The association is especially pronounced in children. Respiratory syncytial virus (RSV), parainfluenza, influenza A, rhinovirus, and adenovirus have been implicated. The severity of the exacerbation depends on multiple factors, including age, severity of the underlying asthma, concurrent medical problems, site and severity of the infection, and specific infectious agent. Bacterial infections of the respiratory tract, except as causative agents for chronic sinusitis, have not been commonly associated with exacerbations of asthma, but they may be a significant cause of exacerbation in patients with chronic obstructive pulmonary disease, in whom bronchospasm is triggered by allergenic stimuli. Empiric antibiotic therapy, while frequently used during exacerbations of asthma in children and adults, frequently does not result in remission of symptoms. More important in such cases is increased use of inhaled corticosteroids.

64. A 22-year-old patient complains of symptoms of asthma after playing basketball. What is the likely explanation?

The patient probably has exercise-induced asthma (EIA). Bronchoconstriction typically begins after cessation of exercise and usually peaks 3–12 minutes later. The severity varies, but the episode is almost always short-lived. The diagnosis of EIA is confirmed by a decrease in forced respiratory volume (FEV) after exercise or isocapnic hyperventilation, although the former is the preferred form of testing. The cause of EIA is believed to be water loss from the bronchial mucosa, resulting in hyperosmolarity in the bronchial tissue. This mechanism has been demonstrated by prevention of EIA during exercise with air that is fully saturated with water vapor at body temperature. Water content of the inspired air is probably the single most important factor affecting bronchospasm, but level of ventilation, temperature of inspired air, and interval since previous episode of EIA are also contributing factors. The last factor is important because a refractory period usually occurs for as long as 2 hours after the previous episode. During this period a second challenge will invoke less than half of the initial airway response. The severity of EIA cannot be predicted by baseline pulmonary function tests (PFTs).

65. What treatment is available for prevention of EIA?

Inhaled beta agonists are the most effective treatment, giving 90% or greater response rates. Approximately 60–70% of patients respond to inhaled cromolyn alone. Some patients require combination therapy, and ipratropium bromide (an anticholinergic agent) may offer additional relief. Patients should inhale medications from a hand-held nebulizer immediately before exercise. The protective effects of pharmacologic therapy may last for only 2 hours, even though in non–exercise-related bronchospasm benefits may continue for an additional 2–4 hours. Inhaled corticosteroids, taken over several weeks, may decrease both the severity of EIA and the doses of other medications required for control. Finally, nasal breathing may attenuate EIA, but it is not practical in strenuous exercise. Whenever possible, asthmatics should be encouraged to swim for exercise.

66. In patients who complain of nocturnal worsening of asthma, what potential factors should be considered?

Considerable attention has been directed at the role of circadian rhythms in nocturnal exacerbations of asthma (usually between 3 AM and 7 AM). Cortisol levels decrease, plasma histamine levels increase, and epinephrine levels decrease during the night. The decrease in plasma cortisol is not thought to be a major factor because administration of corticosteroids in the evening is ineffective in preventing nocturnal exacerbations. Plasma histamine levels do not correlate with changes in pulmonary function tests (PFTs). However, **epinephrine levels** do correlate, suggesting a possible important physiologic role.

Circadian changes in the airways themselves are also important. Both airway caliber and reactivity change at night, with an overall 5–10% decrease in flow rates in normal people, but up to a 50% decrease in asthmatics. Increased vagal tone, impaired mucociliary clearance, and airway cooling and drying also have been reported as contributing factors in nocturnal asthma.

Gastroesophageal reflux disease (GERD) also may exacerbate asthma at night by microaspiration or reflex bronchoconstriction caused by stimulation of nerve endings by acid in the lower esophagus. GERD may be exacerbated by theophylline, which decreases lower esophageal sphincter tone.

Potential **environmental and dietary agents** should be considered as exacerbating factors. For example, dust mites may cause immediate hypersensitivity reactions during the night. Allergen or irritant exposure several hours before going to sleep can also be important. The late-phase response that may occur after such exposure typically peaks 6–12 hours later and may cause severe, prolonged bronchospasm.

Nonasthmatic causes of wheezing, such as cardiac diseases, should be considered. Older patients who by other criteria are at risk for atherosclerotic cardiovascular disease should be systematically evaluated to be certain that the nocturnal asthma is not an early or subtle manifestation of paroxysmal nocturnal dyspnea.

Finally, what the patient perceives as nocturnal asthma in fact may be **sleep apnea**. Nocturnal asthma is not related to any particular stage of sleep. The patient's sleep partner should be interviewed to describe what type of sleep problems the patient is having. If indicated, a formal sleep study should be performed.

67. Describe the management of nocturnal asthma.

The patient's pharmacologic regimen should be carefully examined and compliance assured. Longer-acting, inhaled beta agonists are useful. Salmeterol, the long-acting form of albuterol, has a beneficial effect in some patients. Others appear to benefit from the use of leukotriene receptor antagonists. Theophylline absorption may be decreased at night, leading to lower serum levels. If necessary, the evening dose should be adjusted so that peak levels occur approximately 6 hours later. H_2 antihistamines and/or proton pump inhibitors may be helpful in patients with GERD. Possibly more important is a change in dietary habits to lengthen the interval between the last meal of the day and bedtime. High fat or protein content in food stimulates closure of the pylorus by a cholecystokinin-driven mechanism for as long as 4 hours in some people, resulting in prolonged retention of food in the stomach. Some patients with GERD are helped by raising the head of the bed on blocks by as much as 4–6 inches so that they may sleep with the head and thorax elevated.

Oral corticosteroids should not be given in the evening because the hypothalamic-pituitary-adrenal axis is more readily suppressed by exogenous corticosteroids. No evidence indicates that differences in time of administration either improve or reduce the benefits associated with their use.

Patients who have an allergic component to their asthma and who are on maximal pharmacologic therapy should be considered for immunotherapy.

68. Why is it critical that nocturnal asthma be treated aggressively?

The importance of the treatment of nocturnal asthma cannot be overemphasized, because most fatalities due to asthma occur during the early morning hours.

69. What are Charcot-Leyden crystals, Creola bodies, and Curschmann's spirals?

Charcot-Leyden crystals are composed of lysophospholipase. Their presence in tissue or secretions is considered a specific indicator of eosinophil activity. However, lysophospholipase is also found in basophils.

Creola bodies are clumps of epithelial cells and suggest a desquamating disease process.

Curschmann's spirals are plugs composed of mucus, proteinaceous material, and inflammatory cells in a swirling, spiraling pattern. They usually conform to the configuration of the involved airways.

These substances may be found alone or together as part of the clinical presentation of asthma. They are characteristically seen in patients who have died from status asthmaticus.

70. List the clinical manifestations of anaphylaxis.

General	Flushing, sense of foreboding
Skin	Urticaria/angioedema, flushing, pruritus
Eyes	Lacrimation, pruritus
Upper respiratory tract	Sneezing; nasal pruritus, discharge, and congestion; hoarseness, laryngeal edema, stridor
Lower respiratory tract	Bronchospasm, tachypnea, intercostal retractions, use of accessory muscles of respiration
Cardiovascular	Hypotension, tachycardia, arrhythmia
Gastrointestinal	Nausea, vomiting, abdominal pain, diarrhea
Neurologic	Headache, syncope, seizure

71. A 20-year-old patient presents with hypotension, wheezing, and urticaria 30 minutes after a bee sting. What is the appropriate treatment?
The presentation indicates systemic anaphylaxis, an immediate hypersensitivity reaction caused by mast cell/basophil release of multiple potent mediators, including histamine, prostaglandins, and leukotrienes, into tissues and the circulation. Prompt treatment is critical and should be directed toward maintaining cardiovascular and pulmonary function. Initial treatment should be administration of epinephrine either by subcutaneous or intramuscular routes (0.3–0.5 ml of a 1:1000 dilution). In the face of cardiovascular collapse, IV epinephrine may be indicated. Other immediate steps include applying a tourniquet proximal to the site of allergen inoculation (for example, a bee sting or allergen injection in the forearm). If the anaphylaxis is due to oral intake of an allergen (such as food ingestion), a nasogastric (NG) tube may be inserted and residual gastric contents removed to prevent further antigen absorption. The patient's legs should be elevated, oxygen and airway support provided as needed, and IV fluids (such as normal saline) given for blood pressure support. Parenteral H_1 and H_2 antihistamines also may be administered. Inhaled beta-1 agonists can be given prophylactically or if bronchospasm is present. Repeat doses of medication such as epinephrine should be given as needed, along with vasopressor agents when indicated. Although steroids do not alter the acute course of anaphylaxis, they may be given to attenuate a subsequent late-phase response. The aggressiveness of therapy depends on the severity of the anaphylaxis and response to treatment.

72. What are the major differences between Churg-Strauss syndrome (allergic angiitis and granulomatosis) and classic polyarteritis nodosa (PAN)?
Both diseases are systemic necrotizing vasculitides. Patients with characteristics of both Churg-Strauss and PAN are classified as having polyangiitis overlap syndrome. Patients who fail corticosteroid therapy or who have fulminant disease should receive cytotoxic drug therapy.

	CHURG-STRAUSS	POLYARTERITIS NODOSA
Pulmonary involvement	Yes	No
Histology	Necrotizing vasculitis with granulomas	Necrotizing vasculitis
Vessel involvement	Small-to-medium arteries	Medium muscular arteries; veins, venules with aneurysmal dilation
Asthma/atopic disease	Yes*	No
Eosinophilia (blood and/or tissue)	Yes	No
Association with serum hepatitis B surface antigen (HBsAg)	No	Yes

* Often present for years before onset of vasculitis.

73. What does palpable purpura indicate?
Cutaneous vasculitis.

74. What is the classic triad of Wegener's granulomatosis (WG)?

WG is a systemic necrotizing vasculopathy of unknown etiology. The classic triad includes (1) necrotizing granulomatous vasculitis of the upper respiratory tract and (2) lungs and (3) glomerulonephritis. Vasculitis of many other organs, including the skin, ears, eyes, joints, and central nervous system, also may be present. Vasculitis typically involves both small arteries and veins. The glomerulonephritis is usually focal or crescentic without vasculitis or granulomas. Since the original description by Wegener in Germany in 1939, many more limited forms of the disease have been recognized.

75. Describe the clinical presentation of WG.

The clinical presentation may include fever, chronic sinusitis, otitis media, cough, chest pain, hemoptysis, and arthralgias. Upper airway infections are common; *Staphylococcus aureus* is the most common pathogen. Such infections may mimic exacerbation or recurrence of disease after remission. With the inflammatory process unchecked, nasal septal perforation may occur, leading to a saddle-nose deformity.

76. What laboratory findings are associated with WG?

Laboratory data are generally nonspecific, although recently an antibody to cytoplasmic components of the polymorphonuclear leukocyte (antineutrophil cytoplasmic antibody [ANCA], also known as antibodies to proteinase 3) has been associated with active disease. The erythrocyte sedimentation rate (ESR) is markedly elevated (often > 100 mm/hr) and is a sensitive indicator of disease activity. Mild anemia, leukocytosis, and an increase in serum IgG and IgA levels are common. Chest x-ray patterns include multiple nodules (that frequently cavitate), infiltrates, and solitary nodules. The mean age of onset is 40 years with a male predominance.

77. How is WG treated?

Before the use of cytotoxic drugs, specifically cyclophosphamide, WG was an almost uniformly fatal disease, with a mean survival of 5 months. Corticosteroid therapy did not significantly alter the outcome. However, treatment with cyclophosphamide results in complete remission in over 90% of patients. Combination treatment with corticosteroids and cyclophosphamide should be given initially to gain benefits from the rapid anti-inflammatory effects of the steroid while the cytotoxic actions of the cyclophosphamide are taking effect. Prednisone may be started at 1 mg/kg/day, maintained for 1 month, tapered to alternate-day therapy, and then gradually discontinued, depending on the response. Cyclophosphamide should be started at 2 mg/kg orally and continued for at least 1 year. If, at the end of the year, clinical remission has been obtained, the cyclophosphamide may be tapered and discontinued. Hematologic parameters should be monitored closely for cyclophosphamide toxicity. The WBC count should be maintained above 3,000/mm^3, with a neutrophil count above 1,000/mm^3, to lessen the risk of infectious complications. Other cytotoxic drugs, such as azathioprine, are less effective than cyclophosphamide in the treatment of WG.

78. List the major differences between Wegener's granulomatosis and Goodpasture's syndrome.

	WEGENER'S	GOODPASTURE'S
Etiology	Unknown	Unknown, but hydrocarbon exposure increases risk
Patients	Male > female	Male >> female
	Fifth decade	Young adults
Histopathology	Necrotizing granulomatous vasculitis of upper/lower respiratory tract	Linear deposition of IgG along basement membrane of lung and kidney demonstrated by immunofluorescence, vasculitis absent

Table continued on following page

	WEGENER'S	GOODPASTURE'S
Target organs	Lung > kidney Also may affect CNS, eyes, ears, joints, skin, heart, others	Kidney > lung
Primary symptoms	Chronic sinusitis/rhinitis, fever, weight loss, cough, chest pain, hemoptysis may occur.	Hemoptysis, dyspnea, easy fatigability
Typical chest x-ray findings	Pulmonary nodule(s) with or without cavitation	Diffuse bilateral infiltrates
Diagnosis	Clinical picture with biopsy showing necrotizing vasculitis with granulomas of small arteries and veins	Demonstration of circulating or tissue-bound antibasement membrane antibodies, pulmonary hemorrhage, glomerulonephritis
Treatment	Cyclophosphamide, corticosteroids	Vigorous plasmapheresis, corticosteroids, cyclophosphamide

79. What clinical and laboratory findings are most important in determining the cause of angioedema?

In patients who present with recurrent angioedema, a careful history is of the utmost importance. For example, allergic angioedema may be suggested by a temporal relationship to exposure to specific allergens (such as food). Cold urticaria/angioedema is indicated by onset after exposure to cold temperatures. A number of findings may indicate hereditary angioedema (HAE), including a positive family history, low C4 during and between attacks, and low antigenic or functional activity of C1 esterase inhibitor. Most cases of angioedema are idiopathic, and an extensive evaluation fails to reveal a specific cause or associated underlying disease. The list of diseases associated with angioedema is exhaustive, but some of the most widely recognized are connective tissue diseases, malignancies, thyroid disease, and liver disease (such as hepatitis B). Not infrequently, angiotensin-converting enzyme inhibitors may increase the risk of angioedema. Consider an alternative drug to control hypertension.

80. What is the cause of angioedema in HAE?

HAE is caused by deficiency of C1 esterase inhibitor enzyme (C1INH). Eighty-five percent of patients have depressed serum levels of C1INH (by antigenic assay), whereas the remaining 15% have normal levels but enzymes lack functional activity. The clinical presentation and inheritance patterns are similar for both groups. Decreased C1INH leads to unchecked activation of the classical complement pathway and decreased inhibition of Hageman factor-dependent activation of the kinin and plasmin pathways. The result is increased generation of C2 kinin, bradykinin, and other molecules that can increase vascular permeability.

81. What are the most important clinical characteristics of HAE?

HAE is transmitted in an autosomal dominant pattern, although sporadic cases do occur. The age of onset is variable, and diagnosis can be hindered by a predilection for nonlaryngeal sites, such as the abdominal viscera. Inciting causes are not usually identified, although trauma, even if minor, can lead to attacks. Most patients have a high propensity for life-threatening laryngeal edema that is not characteristic of angioedema due to other causes. Urticaria, although commonly seen in association with other causes of angioedema, is not part of the HAE syndrome. Pain, not pruritus, is typical of HAE lesions. If pruritus is intense, the patient probably has urticarial angioedema. Patients typically have depressed serum C4 levels even when they are asymptomatic between attacks. Attenuated androgen (i.e., stanazolol) dramatically decreases the severity and frequency of attacks. Androgens should be tapered to the lowest dose that adequately controls disease activity to minimize potential adverse effects such as virilization and hepatic toxicity.

82. How do you begin the evaluation of a previously healthy 26-year-old patient who presents with an 8-week history of daily urticaria?

Urticaria persisting for longer than 6 weeks is deemed chronic. A careful history should be obtained to determine whether the urticaria is related to the ingestion of a specific food or liquid, environmental exposure, animal exposure, physical condition (e.g, heat, cold, water, sunlight, pressure, exercise), or stress. The history also should seek to rule out symptoms suggestive of an underlying systemic disease. A careful medication history should be obtained for both prescription and over-the-counter medications (particularly aspirin and aspirin-containing compounds). A thorough physical examination should be performed to identify potential underlying illnesses, such as thyroid disease, malignancy, infection, and rheumatic diseases.

83. What imaging studies may be appropriate?

A chest x-ray usually should be obtained, particularly if the patient has not had one within 6 months. CT scanning may help to detect malignancies that are more difficult to diagnose and treat, such as pancreatic cancer. If the patient has poor dental health or findings suggestive of a dental abscess, dental x-rays may reveal the source of an occult infection.

84. Which laboratory tests may be helpful?

Screening laboratory tests should include complete blood count with white blood cell count and differential, urinalysis, erythrocyte sedimentation rate, and liver function tests. In patients over the age of 40, a serum protein electrophoresis should be obtained to rule out paraproteinemia. Other tests that may be helpful in rare patients include cryoglobulins, screening for antinuclear antibodies, thyroid function studies, complement C3 and C4, and rheumatoid factor (RF). In patients who recently have traveled to third-world countries, stool for ova and parasites may be helpful; also to be considered is screening for hepatitis B and hepatitis C. In patients from South or Central America, American trypanosomiasis (Chagas' disease) should be considered. Whether these and other tests for the evaluation of systemic diseases are obtained depends on the degree of clinical suspicion based on the history, physical examination, and initial laboratory results. Tests for specific types of the physical urticarias can be performed as indicated. Some investigations attribute a significant fraction of chronic urticaria to the development of autoantibodies either to the mast cell receptor for IgE or to IgE itself.

85. What is the role of biopsy?

Typical urticarial lesions do not usually require biopsy. However, in particularly severe, persistent cases, especially when urticarial lesions are very painful (as opposed to pruritic) or very erythematous or persist longer than 24 hours, a skin biopsy may reveal urticarial vasculitis. Some of these cases are accompanied by hypocomplementemia and may require more aggressive medical therapy.

86. How should the patient be treated?

Despite extensive evaluation, more than 90% of the cases of chronic urticaria are ultimately classified as idiopathic. If an underlying treatable cause cannot be detected, it is appropriate to try empiric therapy with a combination of nonsedating H_1 and H_2 antagonists—for example, 60 mg fexofenadine and 150 mg ranitidine every 12 hours. In the great majority of patients, this treatment reduces the frequency and duration of urticarial episodes to a tolerable level. If combined H_1 and H_2 antagonist treatment is not sufficient, it may be necessary to add systemic corticosteroids at the lowest dose needed to control symptoms.

87. Discuss the usefulness of RFs in the diagnosis of rheumatoid arthritis (RA).

RFs are autoantibodies (most commonly IgM) that react with the Fc portion of IgG. The presence of RF is not diagnostic of RA and may not be detected in approximately 20% of patients with the disease. When present, RF may be detected in blood, synovial fluid, and pleural fluid. RF is also found in a long list of other illnesses, including other systemic inflammatory diseases, malignancies, infectious diseases (such as tuberculosis, viral infections, subacute bacterial endocarditis), and sarcoidosis. Furthermore, RF can be detected in a small percentage of normal people, particularly in the elderly population. Thus neither specificity nor sensitivity justifies the use of tests for RF as screening tools for collagen vascular disease. In patients with RA documented by clinical criteria, it may be useful to follow RF titers because high titers are found mainly in patients with more aggressive joint and extra-articular manifestations of disease.

88. What is the single best test for the diagnosis of Sjögren's syndrome?

Sjögren's disease is a chronic inflammatory disease of the exocrine glands characterized by keratoconjunctivitis sicca and xerostomia. The inflammatory infiltrate is composed primarily of lymphocytes and plasma cells. Primary Sjögren's disease is exocrine gland disease alone, whereas secondary Sjögren's disease occurs with another connective tissue disease, most commonly RA. Eye involvement may be confirmed by the Schirmer test, which measures tear production very simply. If the patient's tears wet only 10 mm of the filter paper in 5 minutes, the test is considered positive for poor tear production. Other ophthalmological tests include rose bengal staining of the conjunctivae and/or the finding of keratitis on slit lamp examination. Parotid salivary flow rates and salivary radionuclide scanning may be used to assess salivary gland function. Autoantibodies in sera may include Ro(SS-A), La(SS-B), RF, and Epstein-Barr–related nuclear antigen (RANA). All of these tests may be helpful in the evaluation of Sjögren's syndrome, but biopsy of the labial minor salivary glands is the most specific diagnostic procedure available.

89. What is the Prausnitz-Kustner (P-K) reaction?

The P-K reaction was used in the past to demonstrate the passive transfer of reaginic (IgE) antibodies in humans. Serum was removed from an allergic patient and injected into the skin of a person known not to be allergic to the specific allergen. Twenty-four hours later, the antigen (allergen) was injected intradermally into the sensitized skin and observed for a wheal-and-flare response. A positive response indicated passive transfer of IgE antibodies from the donor serum, which bound to the dermal mast cells in the recipient's skin, leading to an immediate hypersensitivity reaction. This procedure is no longer considered ethically justifiable because of the many infections that can be transferred with serum.

90. What do the direct and indirect Coombs tests measure? Explain the diagnostic usefulness of each.

Once the presence of hemolytic anemia has been confirmed, additional testing should be performed to determine whether an immune mechanism is causing the hemolysis. The **direct Coombs test** (direct antiglobulin test [DAT]) measures antibody or complement on the surface of RBCs. Titrations are performed to determine the degree of RBC sensitization. The test is performed by incubation of the patient's RBCs with anti-Ig or anti-C3 reagent. If surface-bound immunoglobulin or complement is present, agglutination occurs with the appropriate antisera.

The **indirect Coombs test** (indirect antiglobulin test [IAT]) measures the presence of antibody in the patient's serum. The serum is added to normal RBCs, and after incubation and washing, anti-Ig reagent is added. If the antibody from the patient's serum has bound to the RBCs, agglutination occurs.

91. When does a food allergy occur? What can mimic a food allergy?

True food allergy occurs when ingested food antigens bind to IgE on the surface of intestinal mast cells, causing an immediate hypersensitivity reaction. Basophils also may participate if food antigens appear in the circulation. The diagnosis is complicated by a bewildering array of other factors that may cause adverse reactions to food and that mimic allergic reactions. Examples include allergic as well as pharmacologic reactions to food additives, preservatives, dyes, and toxins. GI disorders such as eosinophilic gastroenteritis, malabsorption syndromes, enzyme deficiencies, gluten-sensitive enteropathy, gallbladder disease, peptic ulcer disease, and scrombroid poisoning are on the long list of important nonimmunologic causes of adverse food reactions. Finally, the psychological aspect of food intolerance may be important, particularly in patients who are convinced that allergy is the cause of their GI symptoms. Foods that commonly cause true allergies include peanuts, nuts, shellfish, eggs, milk proteins, and wheat. Cooking may destroy allergenic substances in some foods.

92. Describe the symptoms of food allergy.

Symptoms of food allergy may be localized to the GI tract, resulting in nausea, vomiting, diarrhea, bloating, and pain, or they may be systemic and include urticaria, angioedema, headache, wheezing, hypotension, and other symptoms of anaphylaxis.

93. How is a food allergy diagnosed?

A careful history and physical examination should be performed to rule out other potential causes of adverse reactions to food. In an allergic reaction, symptoms should occur after each ingestion of the specific food. This and the resolution of symptoms with elimination of the food from the diet support a diagnosis of food allergy. Onset of symptoms in most immediate hypersensitivity reactions occurs within 15–20 minutes, but it may be delayed for up to 2 hours. The longer time until onset of symptoms may be due to the need to transport the antigen into the GI tract or to other processes related to digestion and absorption. In practice, the patient's own experience is frequently the best guide. If the symptoms have been truly dramatic, the patient is likely to say, "Doctor I think I'm allergic to peanuts." If the history indicates an acute GI or systemic allergic response, further tests—for all practical purposes—are not necessary.

94. What tests may be used in doubtful cases?

The gold standard for diagnosing food allergens is a double-blind, placebo-controlled ingestion of the suspected food. To disguise its appearance, it is often desirable to put the food in gelatin capsules. Skin testing by means of a prick/puncture test with extracts of the suspected foods is also useful—mainly when the result is negative. Like skin testing for inhaled allergens, skin testing for food has a high sensitivity. If the result is negative it is unlikely that a particular food, at least in the form used for testing, is the offending agent. A positive skin test is not diagnostic of food allergy unless the history independently suggests that the particular food has caused allergic symptoms. Skin testing can be used to narrow the choices of foods to be used in a double-blinded, placebo-controlled trial of ingestion. The RAST and other more quantitative in vitro tests also may be used, but they should be reserved for patients in whom skin testing cannot be properly performed and interpreted and patients thought to be at particular risk of a severe anaphylactic reaction to skin testing.

Bock SA: Double-blind, placebo-controlled food challenge (DBPCFC) as an office procedure: A manual. J Allergy Clin Immunol 82:986, 1988.

95. Discuss the role of an open food challenge.

An open food challenge should be performed only in an appropriate medical setting, because life-threatening anaphylaxis may occur. In some patients, such as those with a low probability of a positive reaction, an open challenge may be useful. If the test is positive, a double-blinded, placebo-controlled challenge can be used to confirm the diagnosis.

96. Describe the treatment for food allergy.

The treatment for food allergy is avoidance. Treatment with antiallergic medications, such as antihistamines or oral cromolyn, cannot be expected to decrease the risk of life-threatening reactions. Anaphylaxis caused by food ingestion should be treated like any other anaphylactic reaction, except that nasogastric tube placement and lavage may be useful to remove residual food antigen. Immunotherapy has no place in the treatment of food allergy.

97. What is the difference between drug allergy, drug intolerance, and idiosyncratic drug reaction?

All three are types of adverse drug reactions. A true **drug allergy** is an immunologically mediated adverse reaction to a drug. It can occur with very small doses of the offending agent and accounts for only 54% of all adverse drug reactions. **Drug intolerance**, which also may occur with very small doses, results from an undesirable pharmacologic effect. An **idiosyncratic drug reaction** is based on an individual patient's biochemical alterations of drug metabolism. The listed drug is only one of many ingredients in a pill or capsule. Patients may develop allergic reactions to dyes, excipients, and other agents that stabilize the medication, slow its absorption, or make it resistant to stomach acids. The tip-off to this type of problem is the patient who confidently states that he or she is allergic to a long list of pharmacologically unrelated oral medications. Further investigation may reveal that they all use same colorant. One can test this hypothesis by giving the patient the intravenous form of the offending drug by mouth in a gelatin capsule.

98. What are the indications for skin testing for penicillin allergy?

Skin testing for penicillin allergy is indicated in patients with a possible or definite history of immediate hypersensitivity to penicillin in whom penicillin therapy is crucial because no effective alternative is available. Penicillin sensitization occurs by the haptenation mechanism and may involve a number of structural components (or "determinants") of the penicillin molecule. Penicilloyl is termed the major determinant, and other degradation products of penicillin G, including penicilloate, are termed the minor determinants. This "major" and "minor" nomenclature refers only to the abundance of the breakdown product and does not necessarily indicate relative clinical importance. However, reports suggest that the minor determinants may be responsible for most life-threatening anaphylactic reactions. The major determinant antigens can be purchased for immediate hypersensitivity skin testing as penicilloyl-polylysine. The minor determinants are not available except in a research setting. If the test with penicilloyl-polylysine is negative, the best strategy is to prepare dilutions of the particular formulation of penicillin that the patient requires and to proceed with serial dilutions for skin testing.

99. What is the "innocent bystander" mechanism of drug-induced hemolysis?

Some drugs (e.g., sulfonamides, phenothiazines, quinidine, quinine) can cause an immune hemolytic anemia even though they do not bind to RBCs. These drugs, bound to plasma proteins, stimulate the formation of complement-fixing antibodies that activate the classical complement pathway. The C3b generated by these reactions in the plasma binds covalently to nearby RBCs. Occasionally this process leads to full assembly of the terminal components of the complement cascade, causing intravascular hemolysis of "innocent bystanders."

100. Which class of medications should be used with particular caution in patients prone to develop anaphylaxis?

Beta blockers should be avoided whenever possible, because they may accentuate the severity of anaphylaxis, prolong its cardiovascular and pulmonary manifestations, and greatly decrease the effectiveness of epinephrine in reversing life-threatening manifestations.

101. What is C3 nephritic factor?

C3 nephritic factor (C3NF) is an IgG3 antibody that binds to the C3 converting enzyme (C3b,Bb), which is composed of activated C3 (C3b) bound to the activated alternative pathway protein, factor B (Bb). C3NF stabilizes C3b,Bb, preventing its inactivation. The result is accelerated breakdown of other available C3 molecules, which causes the serum levels of C3 to fall to very low levels. C3NF is found in partial lipodystrophy, some patients with systemic lupus erythematosus, and most patients with type II membranoproliferative glomerulonephritis. The pathologic significance of the antibody is unknown. The antibody level and degree of lowering of the serum C3 level do not correlate with the severity of tissue damage or disease activity.

102. Describe the mechanism of action of cyclosporine.

Cyclosporine inhibits calcineurin-dependent signal transduction. It binds to cytoplasmic immunophilins, and this interaction inhibits the phosphatase activity of calcineurin. The result is a reduction of IL-2 production and T-cell activation.

103. What are the principal side effects of cyclosporine?

Nephrotoxic (25–75% of patients)	Gingival hyperplasia
Hypertension	Central nervous system toxicity
Hirsutism	• Seizures (5% of patients)
Hepatotoxicity	• Tremor (> 50% of patients)

104. List the serum half-lives and relative potencies of commonly used glucocorticoids.

PREPARATION	POTENCY RELATIVE TO HYDROCORTISONE	RELATIVE SODIUM-RETAINING POTENCY	APPROXIMATELY EQUIVALENT DOSE OF ACTION (MG)	DURATION OF ACTION
Hydrocortisone	1	1	20	Short
Cortisone	0.8	0.8	25	Short
Prednisolone	4	0.8	5	Intermediate
Prednisone	4	0.8	5	Intermediate
6α-Methylprednisolone	5	0.5	4	Intermediate
Triamcinolone	5	0	4	Intermediate
Dexamethasone	25	0	0.75	Long
Betamethasone	25	0	0.75	Long

From Schleimer RP: Glucocorticosteroids. In Middleton E, et al (eds): Allergy: Principles and Practice, 3rd ed. St. Louis, Mosby, 1988, p 742, with permission.

105. Summarize the effects of corticosteroids on circulating leukocytes.

CELL TYPE	EFFECT ON NUMBERS	EFFECT ON FUNCTION	COMMENT
Neutrophil	Increase	Minimal effect on chemotaxis, phagocytosis, bactericidal activity; transendothelial migration in response to chemotactic stimuli is almost abolished	Decrease in numbers sequestered in marginating pools, increased production and release from bone marrow, increased half-life in circulation
Lymphocytes	Decrease	Decreased proliferative response, inhibition of mediator production and release, altered helper and suppressor function	Greater effect on T cells than on B cells. Priming for antibody formation to new antigens is unaffected.
Lymphocytes T cells	Decrease a. Helper/inducer (CD4): decrease b. Cytotoxic/suppressor (CD8): no change		
B cells	Minimal decrease or no change		
Monocytes	Decrease	Depressed chemotaxis, suppression of cytotoxic activity, decreased transendothelial migration	Possible sequestration
Eosinophils	Decrease	Inhibition of mediator production and release	Possible sequestration
Basophils	Decrease	Inhibition of degranulation	Possible sequestration
NK cells	No effect	No effect	
Null cells	No effect	Unknown	

106. What is Guillain-Barré syndrome (GBS)?

GBS is the acute form of the acquired demyelinating neuropathies. In patients who do not remit spontaneously within 4–6 weeks and develop chronic weakness, the disease is called

chronic inflammatory demyelinating polyradiculopathy (CIDP).The causes of these conditions remain obscure, but there is a growing consensus that they are immunologically mediated.

107. How are GBS and CDIP treated?

The principal therapy is supportive, particularly in regard to decreased respiratory function. Management involves a carefully orchestrated mix of anti-inflammatory and immunomodulatory therapy. Examples include azathioprine, cyclosporine, cyclophosphamide, plasmapheresis, and high-dose intravenous immunoglobulin. Dramatic but often unsustained remissions have been observed with these treatments, particularly if instituted within 7 days of onset of symptoms, when the disease process is still classified as acute GBS. Because plasmapheresis is an inefficient procedure for reducing circulating immunoglobulin levels, typically 6–10 or more procedures are performed at the rate of 2 or 3 per week. Each procedure consists of the exchange of total plasma volume (usually 2–3 liters in adults) with an albumin, saline, and electrolyte solution. The frequency of procedures varies with the patient's overall medical condition and availability of venous access. Plasmapheresis theoretically can be followed by intravenous infusions of immunoglobulin to prevent rebound synthesis of autoantibodies, but this approach adds significantly to the expense. At present it is not clear that the added cost would be worth it. A recent report suggests that IVIG treatment may be superior for the subset of patients who have IgG autoantibodies to GM1 gangliosides.

Kuwabara S, et. al: Intravenous immunoglobulin therapy for Guillain-Barre syndrome with IgG anti-GM1 antibody. Muscle Nerve 24:54–58, 2001.

108. What is Chinese restaurant syndrome?

A reaction to glutamate ingested as monosodium glutamate (MSG), a flavoring agent commonly used in Chinese cooking. It occurs within 15–30 minutes of ingestion and consists of a sensation of warmth and tightness on the face and anterior chest. It is occasionally confused with angina pectoris, but it is benign and requires no therapy except avoidance of foods cooked with MSG.

Kwok RHN: Chinese restaurant syndrome. N Engl J Med 278:1122, 1968.

109. What is the triad of Kartagener's syndrome?

Originally described by Kartagener in 1904, the syndrome consists of the triad of situs inversus, bronchiectasis, and chronic sinusitis. It is an autosomal recessive disorder resulting in a defect of the cilia, which lack dynein arms. Patients also suffer from chronic sinopulmonary infections, and sterility may occur in men (due to immotile spermatozoa).

Eliasson R. et al: The immotile cilia syndrome. N Engl J Med 297:1–6, 1977.

110. Chronic or recurrent meningococcemia or gonococcemia is commonly associated with which host immune defects?

Deficiencies of the late components of complement (C6, C7, and C8) are the predominant defects. Low C3, and absent C5 (properdin deficiency) also have been associated with such infections. In sexually active adults, acute monoarticular arthritis may be a consequence of bacteremia with *Neisseria gonorrhoeae*. Such patients must be worked up for complement deficiency after the septic joint is treated. The intense neutrophilic infiltrate triggered by these infections is considered an orthopedic emergency that requires immediate drainage of the pus and irrigation of the joint to reduce the residence time of the inflammatory leukocytes in the joint space and thus the damage to the articular cartilage caused by leukocyte proteases and reactive oxygen products.

Ross S, et al: Complement deficiency and infection: Epidemiology, pathogenesis and consequences of neisserial and other infections in an immune deficiency. Medicine 63:243–273, 1984.

111. Describe systemic reactions to the older radiocontrast media. What causes them?

Systemic reactions to the older hyperosmolar radiocontrast media occur in 1% of patients with a fatality rate of about 0.0009%. The reaction may begin just after the onset of the infusion or as late as 30 minutes after its completion. Cardiovascular collapse can result in death. The cause is unknown. It does not appear to be a true IgE-mediated immediate hypersensitivity reaction. It has been suggested that they are anaphylactoid reactions resulting from the ability of the dyes to initiate acute degranulation of mast cells and basophils. A method for detection of patients at risk is not available. Skin testing with IV contrast material or iodine is of no value.

112. A patient with a history of hypotension after an intravenous pyelogram (IVP) now requires a radiocontrast study. What procedure should be followed?

The considerable risk of a repeat reaction on reexposure can be minimized by use of the newer lower osmolar radiocontrast agents and by appropriate prophylaxis. Management includes careful evaluation and documentation of the essential nature of the procedure. Informed consent should be obtained from patient and family (especially with the small but definite risk of death). The presence of necessary personnel and supplies for emergency treatment, adequate patient hydration, and preprocedural prophylaxis are also necessary. The usual prophylactic regimen consists of steroids (usually methylprednisone, 32 mg orally, at 13, 7, and 1 hour before the procedure) and H_1 antihistamines (diphenhydramine, 50 mg parenterally or orally, 1 hour before radiocontrast media administration). When not contraindicated, ephedrine, 25 mg orally, may offer additional benefit. The usefulness of H_2 antihistamines and/or ephedrine is controversial.

Reactions after prophylactic therapy are usually mild. However, the procedure should be started at the scheduled time, or the efficacy of the prophylaxis may be decreased. It has been suggested that in patients with a history of radiocontrast media reactions, nonionic radiocontrast media do not seem to offer significant protective advantage over medical prophylaxis, but since the consequences of an adverse reaction are life threatening, it is wise to err on the side of caution and use prophylaxis as well as the newer low osmolar reagents.

Patterson R, et al: Drug allergy and protocols for the management of drug allergies. N Engl Reg Allergy Proc 7(4):325–342, 1989.

113. What clinical conditions are associated with deficiencies of the various components of the complement system?

DEFICIENT COMPONENT	NUMBER OF REPORTED CASES	ASSOCIATED DISEASES
C1	31	Autoimmune diseases, SLE-like syndromes
C4	20	Autoimmune diseases, SLE-like syndromes
C2	109	Autoimmune diseases, SLE-like syndromes
C3	20	Bacterial infections; mild glomerulonephritis
C5	28	Gram-negative coccal infections
C6	76	Gram-negative coccal infections
C7	67	Gram-negative coccal infections
C8	68	Gram-negative coccal infections
C9	18	Gram-negative coccal infections
Properdin	70	Gram-negative coccal infections
Factor I	17	Bacterial infections
Factor H	13	Bacterial infections
Factor D	3	Bacterial infections
C4-binding protein	3	—
C1 Inhibitor	100	Hereditary angioedema

SLE = systemic lupus erythematosus.
From David J: Immunology. In Dale DC, Federman DD (eds): Scientific American Medicine. New York, Scientific American, 1996, p 26, with permission.

114. What is the lupus band test?

It is a test that may be of value in questionable cases of systemic lupus erythematosus (SLE). It involves the demonstration of granular deposition of C3 and IgG along the dermal-epidermal junction in a biopsy of normal skin. The test is most likely to be positive in hypocomplementemic patients. However, the test rarely correlates with renal involvement.

115. What percentage of patients with SLE lack detectable antinuclear antibodies?

Five percent or less of patients with SLE have been reported to test negative for antinuclear antibodies (ANAs). Probably, however, they were tested with mouse kidney as the substrate, which does not readily detect antibodies against Ro/SSA, ssDNA, Jo, or centromere, which are found in some patients with SLE. Most patients with SLE (93–95%) show detectable ANA antibodies if the substrate contains either WIL-2 or HEP-2 cells. Antibodies specific for double-stranded DNA or anti-Sm antibodies are diagnostic for SLE. Other ANAs offer less assurance of a diagnosis.

116. What are the most common causes of drug-induced lupus?

Hydralazine and procainamide are the most common causes of drug-induced lupus. Up to 50–75% of patients receiving procainamide and a somewhat lower frequency of patients receiving hydralazine may develop a positive ANA test, although far fewer develop symptoms. Other drugs that cause a syndrome resembling SLE, albeit rarely, are isoniazid, chlorpromazine, methyl-dopa, quinidine, and interferon alpha. Slow acetylators of these drugs are particularly susceptible. Hydralazine-induced lupus is encountered most commonly when the total daily dose exceeds 400 mg; 10–20% of such patients develop a lupus-like syndrome. Other causes include D-penicillamine, and phenytoin. The ANA pattern in drug-induced lupus is usually homogeneous or speckled and is caused by antihistone antibodies. Antibodies to double-stranded DNA, as seen in SLE, are not found in drug-induced lupus.

117. Describe the clinical manifestations of drug-induced lupus. Which organs are characteristically spared compared with idiopathic SLE?

Drug-induced lupus manifests many of the same symptoms as idiopathic SLE, although they are generally milder. However, lupus nephritis and cerebritis rarely, if ever, complicate the syndrome. Drug-induced lupus is more frequent in women than men and in people with the HLA DR4 phenotype. Symptoms resolve shortly after discontinuation of the drug, although laboratory abnormalities may persist for months or years.

Clinical and Serologic Features of Drug-induced Lupus and Systemic Lupus Erythematosus

	DRUG-INDUCED LUPUS	IDIOPATHIC SLE		DRUG-INDUCED LUPUS	IDIOPATHIC SLE
Polyserositis	Yes	Yes	Nephritis	No	Yes
Arthritis	Yes	Yes	Cerebritis	No	Yes
Fever	Yes	Yes	Positive ANA	Yes	Yes
Rash	Yes	Yes	Positive anti-dsDNA	No	Yes
Photosensitivity	Yes	Yes	Reversible*	Yes	No
Hemolytic anemia	Yes	Yes			

• Within several months of drug discontinuation.
From Cush JJ, et al: Drug-induced lupus: Clinical spectrum and pathogenesis. Am J Med Sci 290:36, 1985, with permission.

118. Should patients with SLE receive live attenuated vaccines?

No. The major live attenuated vaccines currently available are rubella (measles), poliomyelitis, bacille Calmette-Guérin (BCG), mumps, and yellow fever. Vaccinia (small pox) is no longer given. People in whom live vaccination should be avoided include:

1. Patients with primary immunodeficiency disorders (especially those with defective CMI, such as severe combined immunodeficiency syndrome [SCID]).

2. Patients given immunosuppressive therapy (including corticosteroids, cytotoxic drugs, and radiation therapy).

3. Patients with malignancies that cause immunosuppression, including leukemia, lymphoma, and Hodgkin's disease.

4. Patients with systemic immunoregulatory, inflammatory, or infectious diseases associated with defective CMI (e.g., SLE, diabetes mellitus, sarcoidosis, HIV infection, atopic dermatitis).

5. Children less than 1 year of age.

6. Patients with severe malnutrition or burns.

7. Pregnant women (because of potential harm to the fetus). The exception is the yellow fever vaccine when the mother must travel to an endemic area. In this case, the risk of infection and detrimental effects without the vaccine are greater than the risk of immunization.

8. Household contacts of immunocompromised patients should not receive oral live polio vaccine, because the live attenuated strain may revert to the wild type in the GI tract and be spread by the fecal-oral route.

119. What is the Donath-Landsteiner antibody? In which disease is it found?

The Donath-Landsteiner antibody is an IgG cold-reacting antibody that binds to the p-antigen of the red blood cell. It was originally described in patients with syphilis who developed paroxysmal hemoglobinuria (Donath-Landsteiner hemolytic anemia) on exposure to cold temperatures. Now it is seen mainly in children after a virus infection. The clinical syndrome consists of paroxysmal chills, fever, headache, and diffuse pain in the abdomen, back, and legs, in addition to the hemoglobinuria.

120. Define erythema multiforme (EM).

EM is an immunologic reaction of the skin and mucous membranes to a variety of antigenic stimuli, but no such stimulus can be identified in up to 50% of cases. The lesions may be localized or widespread and consist of bullae, erythematous plaques, and epidermal cell necrosis. Usually they are distributed bilaterally and symmetrically on the extensor surfaces of the limbs, on the dorsal and volar aspects of the hands and feet, and on the trunk. The lesions, which resemble "targets" or "bull's eyes," are diagnostic. They appear as a central vesicle or dark purple papule, surrounded by a round, pale zone that is in turn surrounded by a round area of erythema.

121. What are the precipitating factors in EM?

1. Viral diseases: herpes simplex, hepatitis, influenza A, vaccinia, mumps
2. Fungal diseases: dermatophytoses, histoplasmosis, coccidioidomycosis
3. Bacterial diseases: hemolytic streptococcal infections, tuberculosis, leprosy, typhoid
4. Collagen vascular disease: RA, SLE, dermatomyositis, allergic vasculitis, PAN
5. Malignant tumors: carcinoma, lymphoma after radiation therapy
6. Hormonal changes: pregnancy, menstruation
7. Drugs: penicillins, sulfonamides, barbiturates, salicylates, halogens, phenolphthalein
8. Miscellaneous: rhus dermatitis, dental extractions, mycoplasma pneumonia infection

From Abel AE, Farber EM: Dermatology. In Dale DC, Federman DD (eds): Scientific American Medicine. New York, Scientific American Medicine, 1990, p 9, with permission.

122. What is Stevens-Johnson syndrome?

Stevens-Johnson syndrome is a severe form of EM associated with fulminant, disseminated, multisystem involvement. Patients appear toxic, with fever, chills, malaise, tachycardia, tachypnea, and prostration. Diffuse vesicular, bullous, and ulcerative lesions of the skin and mucous membranes develop and desquamate, leading to secondary infections, which in turn may lead to sepsis and even death. It is associated with all of the causes of EM.

123. Why is the Kviem test for sarcoidosis no longer performed?

The Kviem test was performed by intradermal injection of sarcoid spleen suspension into patients suspected of having sarcoidosis. The development of a skin reaction revealing non-caseating granulomas on biopsy was considered diagnostic of sarcoidosis. However, the test lacked specificity, and availability of the reagent was poor. Because of these problems and the risk of transmission of infectious diseases, the test is no longer performed.

124. Hepatitis B surface antigenemia is associated with which of the vasculitides?

Polyarteritis nodosa, which is seen in 40% of HBSAg-positive patients. The severity of the vasculitis does not correlate with the severity of the hepatitis.

125. What is the differential diagnosis of a positive blood test for RF?

Rheumatological diseases

Rheumatoid arthritis

Polyarticular juvenile rheumatoid arthritis

SLE

Mixed connective tissue disease

Behçet's syndrome

Sjögren's syndrome

Infectious diseases

Syphilis

Viral hepatitis

Parasitic infections

Granulomatous disease

Mononucleosis

Bacterial endocarditis

Pulmonary diseases

Bronchitis or asthma

Coal miner's disease

Asbestosis

Idiopathic pulmonary fibrosis

Sarcoidosis

Other diseases

Cirrhosis

Post myocardial infarction

Many neoplasms

Essential mixed cryoglobulinemia

Healthy elderly people

From Coffey R, et al: Immunologic tests of value in diagnosis. I: Acute phase reactants and autoantibodies. Postgrad Med 70:164,1981, with permission.

126. An 18-year-old man presents with abdominal pain, bloody diarrhea, peripheral neuropathy, and IgA deposition on biopsy of the GI tract. What is the most likely diagnosis?

The clinical presentation is characteristic of Henoch-Schonlein purpura (HSP), although the age of onset is younger. The disease is almost always limited to men. This type of hypersensitivity vasculitis principally involves the skin, joints, intestine, and kidney. The disease is usually self-limited, although in rare patients chronic renal failure may occur. A history of recent infection, usually of the upper respiratory tract, is often reported. Circulating IgA immune complexes are common. Serum IgA levels may be elevated, and IgA deposition can be demonstrated in the affected tissues.

127. Is skin testing useful for the diagnosis of histoplasmosis?

Skin testing is rarely useful in the diagnosis of histoplasmosis and should be limited principally to epidemiologic surveys. A positive skin test indicates prior exposure, not necessarily active infection. Furthermore, the histoplasmin reagent often causes a significant rise in antibody titers, thereby complicating interpretation of subsequent serologic studies. A negative skin test is highly suggestive of the absence of disease (even during dissemination stages), unless the patient is anergic.

128. How do anticentromere antibodies help differentiate between CREST syndrome and scleroderma (progressive systemic sclerosis)?

The anticentromere antibody is found by ANA testing in 60–80% of patients with CREST syndrome (**c**alcinosis, **R**aynaud's phenomenon, **e**sophageal involvement, **s**clerodactyly, and **t**elangiectasia) but is often undetectable in patients with diffuse scleroderma.

129. Which other laboratory and clinical findings distinguish CREST syndrome from diffuse scleroderma?

In CREST skin involvement is limited princially to the extremities, and internal organ involvement generally develops more slowly and is less severe than in diffuse scleroderma. Particularly noteworthy of the CREST syndrome (but rarely seen in diffuse scleroderma) is the development of pulmonary arterial hypertension in the absence of pulmonary fibrosis. This occurs in somewhat less than 10% of patients with limited systemic sclerosis or CREST. Intimal proliferation of the small and medium-sized pulmonary arteries is prominent. Pulmonary hypertension may be progressive and is almost uniformly fatal. Biliary cirrhosis also may occur in CREST syndrome but is uncommon in systemic sclerosis.

130. In a patient who complains of fatigue with hair-combing and stair-climbing, what are the most likely diagnoses?

Diseases characterized by proximal muscle weakness, such as myasthenia gravis, Eaton-Lambert (myasthenic) syndrome, polymyositis, dermatomyositis, and polymyalgia rheumatica.

131. Explain the importance of HLA and ABO typing in solid organ and bone marrow transplantation (BMT).

HLA compatibility of donor and recipient affects graft outcome in both solid organ transplantation (e.g., kidney, heart, lung, liver) and BMT. Matching for the HLA-D or MHC class II antigens is more important than matching for HLA-A or HLA-B (MHC type I antigens.) HLA compatibility is not a major factor in graft survival for first-time, nonvascularized corneal transplants. HLA incompatibility may lead to graft rejection and destruction in solid organ transplantation and to graft-vs.-host disease in BMT. In graft rejection, the graft is attacked by the recipient's immune system. In graft-vs.-host disease, the immunocompetent cells from the donor attack the recipient. ABO blood typing is critical in solid organ transplants, because ABO antigens are expressed on all tissue cells of the transplanted organ and because type O, type A or type B recipients almost always have preformed antibodies to these blood group antigens. Transplantation of a donor kidney from a type A donor into a type O recipient usually results in hyperacute rejection and immediate graft death.

132. What are the four types of graft rejection and their immunologic mechanisms?

TYPE	ONSET	MAJOR EFFECTOR MECHANISMS
Hyperacute	Minutes to hours	Humoral: preformed cytotoxic antibody against donor graft antigen(s) in recipient • ABO system • Anti-HLA class I
Accelerated	2–5 days	Cell-mediated: due to prior T-cell sensitization to donor antigen(s)
Acute	7–28 days	Principally cell-mediated immunity: allogeneic reactivity by recipient T cells against donor antigen(s) Humoral immunity to HLA antigens
Chronic	> 3 months	Principally cell-mediated immunity: allogeneic reactivity by recipient T cells against donor antigen(s) Humoral immunity to HLA antigens

133. What are the targets of the common autoantibodies that characterize specific autoimmune diseases?

DISEASE	TARGET OF ANTIBODY
Organ-specific diseases	
Myasthenia gravis	Acetylcholine receptors
Graves' disease	Thyroid-stimulating hormone receptor
Thyroiditis	Thyroid (often involves T cells as well)
Insulin-resistant diabetes with acanthosis nigricans	Insulin receptor
Insulin-resistant diabetes with ataxia telangiectasia	Insulin receptor
Allergic rhinitis, asthma, and autoimmune abnormalities	Beta$_2$-adrenergic receptors
Juvenile insulin-dependent diabetes	Pancreatic islet cells, insulin
Pernicious anemia	Gastric parietal cells, vitamin B12-binding site of intrinsic factor
Addison's disease	Adrenal cells
Idiopathic hypoparathyroidism	Parathyroid cells
Spontaneous infertility	Sperm
Premature ovarian failure	Interstitial cells, corpus luteum cells
Pemphigus	Intercellular substance of skin and mucosa
Bullous pemphigoid	Basement membrane zone of skin and mucosa

Table continued on following page

DISEASE	TARGET OF ANTIBODY
Organ-specific diseases (*cont.*)	
Primary biliary cirrhosis	Mitochondria
Autoimmune hemolytic anemia	Erythrocytes
Idiopathic thrombocytopenic purpura	Platelets
Idiopathic neutropenia	Neutrophils
Vitiligo	Melanocytes
Chronic active hepatitis	Nuclei of hepatocytes
Systemic (non–organ-specific) diseases	
Goodpasture's syndrome	Basement membranes of lung and kidney
Rheumatoid arthritis	IgG, Epstein-Barr virus-related antigens, types II and III collagen
Sjögren's syndrome	IgG, SS-A (Ro), SS-B (La)
Systemic lupus erythematosus	Nuclei, double-stranded DNA, single-stranded DNA, Sm, ribonucleoprotein, lymphocytes, erythrocytes, neurons, IgG, phospholipids such as cardiolipin, and other antigens
Scleroderma/CREST	Nuclei, Scl-70 (topoisomerase I), fibrillin SS-A (Ro), SS-B (La), centromere
Polymyositis	Nuclei, Jo-1, (histadyl-tRNA synthetase), PL-7 (threonyl-tRNA synthetase), PM-1, Mi-2
Rheumatic fever	Myocardium, heart valves, collagen of joints, renal glomerulus, caudate nucleus of brain

Adapted from David J: Immunology. In Dale DC, Federman DD (eds): Scientific American Medicine. New York, Scientific American, 1996, p 3, with permission.

134. What are the main immunologic defects associated with recurrent bacterial infections?

The principal defects are antibody deficiency, complement deficiency, and defective neutrophil function. Infections in patients with antibody deficiencies are most commonly due to encapsulated organisms (e.g., *Haemophilus influenzae, Streptococcus pneumoniae*).

135. How are patients screened for immunologic defects?

Screening for **antibody deficiency** begins with determination of serum immunoglobulin levels (IgG, IgM, and IgA) and IgG subclass levels if subclass deficiency is suspected. Further evaluation may include measuring serum isohemagglutinin titers (IgM antibodies) and serum IgG antibody levels against protein (tetanus toxoid) and carbohydrate antigens such as those found in the capsules of *S. pneumoniae* or *H. influenzae*. Ideally, antibody levels found in pre- and postimmunization sera are compared to measure accurately the antibody response to a specific antigen challenge. **Complement deficiency** can be evaluated by obtaining a CH50 (or CH100) assay and measuring levels of specific complement components as indicated. A nitroblue tetrazolium test can be performed to assess **neutrophil function** in patients with a clinical history suggestive of chronic granulomatous disease.

136. How do complement deficiences typically present?

Isolated C3 deficiency typically presents at a very early age, most often shortly after birth. Because C3 deficiency has such a profound negative effect on leukocyte phagocytic function, patients experience recurrent life-threatening pyogenic infections. Deficiencies of the terminal complement components, with the possible exception of C9, increase susceptibility to bacteremia with neisserial species, typically *N. gonorrhoeae*. Deficiency of properdin, an alternative complement pathway component, also may be accompanied by recurrent pyogenic and neisserial infections.

137. Discuss the epidemiology of defective neutrophil function. To which organisms are patients particularly susceptible?

Most defects of neutrophil function associated with recurrent infections occur in children. However, it is now recognized that some adults may have a variant of chronic granulomatous disease

(CGD) in which the defect in respiratory burst is qualitatively less than in typical CGD of childhood. Such patients are particularly susceptible to catalase-positive organisms. Bacterial infections are typically caused by *Staphyloccocus aureus, Escherichia coli,* and *Serratia marcescens,* whereas fungal infections are caused by *Candida albicans, Aspergillus,* and *Nocardia* species.

138. What causes rhinitis medicamentosa (RM)? How is it treated?

RM is caused by rebound vasodilation due to long-term use of topical vasoconstrictors, including over-the-counter medications such as oxymetazoline nasal spray (e.g., Afrin, 12-hr nasal spray) and illegal drugs such as cocaine. The nasal mucosa typically appears reddened, dry, and dull. Small areas may be covered with bloody crusts. Nasal septal perforations may be seen in some people who chronically inhale cocaine. Treatment consists of discontinuation of the offending drug. For severe cases it may be necessary to use a short course of oral corticosteroids. The risk of RM should not preclude the use of alpha-adrenergic topical vasoconstrictors, such as oxymetazoline, in treatment of allergic rhinitis. These agents help to open the nasal passages and increase nasal airflow temporarily to ensure that inhaled, topical corticosteroids are effectively delivered to the posterior nasopharynx. To be certain that there are no complications from the use of these potent vasoconstrictors, treatment must be interrupted by taking a drug holiday every 3 or 4 days.

139. List the major diseases associated with elevation of the total serum IgE level.

Atopic (allergic) diseases
  Allergic rhinitis
  Allergic asthma
  Allergic bronchopulmonary
    aspergillosis
Primary immunodeficiency disorders
  Hyper IgE syndrome
  Wiskott-Aldrich syndrome
  Nezelhof's syndrome (cellular
    immunodeficiency with Igs)
  Selective IgA deficiency (with
    concomitant atopic disease)
  Job's syndrome

Infections
  Parasitic infections
  Viral infections (infectious mononucleosis, others)
  Fungal infections (candidiasis, others)
Acute graft-vs.-host disease
Dermatologic disorders
  Atopic dermatitis
  Bullous pemphigoid
  Eczema and others
Malignancies
  Hodgkin's disease
  Bronchial carcinoma
  IgE myeloma

In many of these diseases, IgE levels may be normal, mildly elevated, or markedly elevated. The clinical usefulness of measurement of total serum IgE is usually limited to diagnosis and monitoring of exacerbations, remissions, and/or treatment of allergic bronchopulmonary aspergillosis, parasitic infections, and immunodeficiency disorders.

BIBLIOGRAPHY

1. Janeway CA, Travers P, Walport M, Capra JD: Immunobiology: The Immune System in Health and Disease, 4th ed. New York, Garland Publishing, 1999.
2. Klein J: Immunology. Oxford, Blackwell Scientific, 1990.
3. Middleton E, et al (eds): Allergy: Principles and Practice, 5th ed. St. Louis, Mosby, 1998.
4. Paul WE (ed): Fundamental Immunology, 4th ed. Philadelphia, Lippincott-Raven, 1999.
5. Roitt IM, et al: Immunology, 4th ed. St. Louis, Mosby, 1996.

WEBSITES

1. www.atallergy.com, a general site that is directed at physicians and informed lay people.
2. www.aaaai.org, the official web site of the American Academy of Allergy, Asthma and Immunology.
3. www.allergy.mcg.edu, the web site of the American College of Allergy, Asthma and Immunology as well as a much larger collections of web sites that deal with various aspects of Arthritis/Rheumatology.
4. www.docguide.com/news/content/nsf/PatientResAllCateg/Arthritis: One of the most comprehensive websites that deals largely with issues of concern to medical practitioners.

13. AIDS AND HIV INFECTION

Christopher J. Lahart, M.D.

*Dr. Rieux resolved to compile this chronical . . . to state quite simply
what we learn in a time of pestilence: that there are more things to
admire in men than to despise.*

Albert Camus
The Plague, Pt. V, translated by Stuart Gilbert

He is the best physician who is the best inspirer of hope.

Samuel Taylor Coleridge
Table Talk

1. Human immunodeficiency virus (HIV) is a retrovirus. What is a retrovirus?

A retrovirus, a member of the Retroviridae family, is an RNA virus that contains reverse transcriptase, an enzyme that is capable of transcribing DNA from the viral RNA. This process is the reverse of the normal DNA-to-RNA transcription; hence the name.

2. Do all patients who test positive for HIV have AIDS?

No. A positive test for HIV antibodies indicates infection with HIV, but HIV infection is a wide spectrum of illness, and the vast majority of patients are asymptomatic. AIDS, the final band in this spectrum of illness, is a syndrome of explicitly defined conditions that represent severe immunosuppression. A diagnosis of AIDS is made when a person with HIV infection develops a malignancy, opportunistic infection, other symptomatic illness, or a decreased CD4-lymphocyte count that meets the diagnostic criteria for AIDS. When a patient has tested positive for infection by HIV, a comprehensive history and physical examination are needed to identify symptoms and signs of immunosuppression and any comorbid conditions. A laboratory evaluation can help place the patient in a relative position on the spectrum.

Centers for Disease Control and Prevention: 1993 revised classification system for HIV infection and expanded case surveillance definition for AIDS among adolescents and adults. MMWR 41(RR-17):1–19, 1992.

NATURAL HISTORY AND TRANSMISSION

3. How long is a person with HIV infectious?

For life. There may be periods of increased infectiousness, such as during the initial infection with its high levels of viremia and at the later stages of disease. Some early evidence indicates decreased infectiousness during highly active antiretroviral therapy, but there is never a period of absolute noninfectiousness. This highlights the importance of changing high-risk behavior patterns. Such change must be consistent and permanent.

4. What is the risk of HIV transmission via needlestick?

The average risk of transmission in a large group of health-care workers suffering percutaneous exposure to HIV is approximately 0.3%. However, each exposure needs to be evaluated individually. There is tremendous variation in the degree of exposure, which affects the likelihood of infection.

Tokars JI, et al: Surveillance of HIV infection and zidovudine use among health-care workers after occupational exposure to HIV-infected blood. Ann Intern Med 118:913–919, 1993.

5. What variables increase the risk of occupational exposure?

Exposure to a large volume of infectious material (or material with a high viral load), a deep injury, visible blood on the device causing the injury, prolonged contact with the infectious material, and the body area exposed (portal of entry) are important factors. Mucosal splashes and exposure on intact skin are not routes of transmission (no transmission in > 12,500 exposures followed prospectively). Associated with increased risk are intramuscular injection, exposures via hollow needles (as opposed to suture needles and pins), and exposure to material from a viremic HIV-infected patient.

6. Does postexposure antiretroviral therapy prevent infection?

No controlled trial has been performed, and, most likely, none ever will be. However, a retrospective case-control study involving 31 exposed and infected health-care workers and 679 exposed, uninfected workers found that postexposure zidovudine reduced the risk of HIV infection by 79%. The study design is not the proper one for evaluating drug efficacy, but it does provide important information. Drug therapy must be part of a program that includes immediate availability of counseling as well as medication. Close follow-up should be provided and confidentiality guaranteed. Therapy recommendations include combination antiretroviral therapy based on the treatment status of the source patient. Consideration must be given to possible drug resistance.

Centers for Disease Control and Prevention: Case-control study of HIV seroconversion in health-care workers after percutaneous exposure to HIV-infected blood—France, United Kingdom, and United States, January 1988–August 1994. MMWR 44(50):929–933, 1995.

Centers for Disease Control and Prevention: Public Health Service guidelines for the management of health-care worker exposures to HIV and recommendations for postexposure prophylaxis. MMWR 47(RR-7):1–34, 1998.

7. Are heterosexuals at risk for HIV infection?

Most certainly. Although heterosexual contact does not appear to be as efficient a transmitter of infection as male homosexual contact, it clearly does transmit HIV. In many developing countries, the equal incidence of AIDS in males and females provides evidence for heterosexual transmission. As of December 31, 1999, in the U.S., 10.3% of 724,656 adult AIDS cases (74,476 cases)—4% of male cases (26,530 cases) and 40% of female cases (47,946 cases)—were attributed to heterosexual contact. If the temporal trends are examined, between 1981 and 1987, 2.5% of cases were attributed to heterosexual contact; between 1988 and 1992, 6.1%; and between 1992 and 1999, 12.1%. About 50% of the cases of heterosexually acquired AIDS result from sexual contact with an injecting drug user. In 1999, 23% of all AIDS cases were in females.

Centers for Disease Control and Prevention: HIV/AIDS Surveillance Report 11(No. 2):13-4, 1999.

8. How much time elapses between infection with HIV and the diagnosis of AIDS?

This period is not easily defined. Studies of large patient cohorts indicate that in the absence of treatment 50% of HIV-positive patients progress to AIDS in approximately 10 years. The rate of disease progression is not stable over this period, because few develop disease early after exposure and proportionally more develop AIDS with each passing year. It is not certain at this time that 100% of HIV-infected individuals will develop AIDS, even without specific antiretroviral therapy.

Litson AR, et al: The natural history of human immunodeficiency virus infection. J Infect Dis 158:1360–1367, 1988.

9. What is a CD4+-lymphocyte count? Why is it obtained?

A CD4+-lymphocyte count is a laboratory measurement of the number of CD4-positive (T4 or helper-inducer) lymphocytes present in peripheral blood. Since early in the HIV epidemic, it has been known that one of the most problematic effects of HIV infection is the depletion of CD4+-lymphocytes. By measuring these cells, a clinician can attempt to place a patient on the spectrum of HIV-related illness. The CD4+-lymphocyte count also is used to determine the timing of various interventions, such as antiretroviral therapy or prophylaxis against Pneumocystis carinii pneumonia (PCP). Thus, it is of prognostic and therapeutic value.

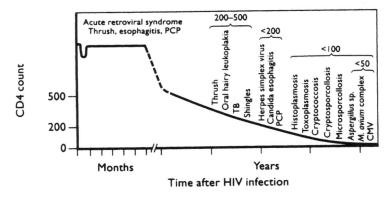

Onset of opportunistic infections with decreasing CD4+ count. (From Mildran D (ed): Atlas of Infectious Diseases: I. AIDS. Philadelphia, Current Medicine, 1995, p 15.2, with permission.)

10. What is a viral load?

Tests that measure HIV viral load by assaying for plasma HIV mRNA have recently been demonstrated to be the single best indicator of prognosis in HIV infection. The first such test was licensed in June 1996; thus, clinical experience is relatively short. The level of HIV mRNA reflects the level of HIV viral replication. It directly correlates with CD4+-lymphocyte level, rate of CD4 decline, development of disease, and death. HIV viral load levels also are used to assess the efficacy of therapy. CD4+-lymphocyte counts are still necessary to estimate immediate risk for the development of opportunistic infections.

Mellors JW, et al: Plasma viral load and CD4+ lymphocytes as prognostic markers of HIV-1 infection. Ann Intern Med 126:946–954, 1997.

11. What is the prognosis for patients infected with HIV-1?

In a review of 32 follow-up studies, Cooper and Jeffers reported the following:
• From the time of seroconversion, 10–20% of HIV-infected people progress to AIDS in 3–6 years.
• Once the patient has constitutional symptoms, herpes zoster, thrush, or a lowered CD4+-lymphocyte count, chances are > 40% of progressing to AIDS after 3 years of follow-up and > 50% after 5 years.
• These data are from untreated patients. Prognosis can be modified by antiretroviral therapy and general medical support.

Cooper GS, Jeffers DJ: The clinical prognosis of HIV-1 infection: A review of 32 follow-up studies. J Gen Intern Med 3:525–532, 1988.

12. How has HIV contributed to overall mortality in the U.S.?

In 1993, HIV infection became the leading cause of death among persons aged 25–44 years, accounting for 19% of all deaths in this age group. It became the most common cause of death for black men in 1991, for all men in 1992, and for white men in 1994. In 1994 it also became the third most common cause of death in women. Since 1995, however, there has been a dramatic decline in HIV-related mortality (over 60%) as a result of improvements in therapy and therapeutic monitoring. This decline has been seen across all age, gender, and ethnic groups, although its magnitude varies by group.

13. Is AIDS invariably fatal?

Certainly a large proportion of patients with AIDS die, but it is not yet clear whether all people infected will die from the disease. Of 733,374 patients with AIDS reported by the Centers for Disease Control and Prevention (CDC) through December 31, 1999, 59% have died.

Most experienced HIV clinicians now have some patients who have been in follow-up for over 10–15 years. Experience with the currently available therapeutics is 5 years old. It is premature to claim the end of HIV-related mortality based on these statistics.

Palella FJ, et al: Declining morbidity and mortality among patients with advanced human immunodeficiency virus infection. N Engl J Med 338:853–860, 1998.

DIAGNOSIS

14. Who should be tested for HIV?

- Gay or bisexual men
- Injecting drug users
- Prostitutes
- Patients in STD clinics
- Patients in tuberculosis (TB) clinics
- Persons who received blood products from 1978–1985
- Anyone having sex with a member of a high-risk group
- Anyone with a history of substance abuse, including alcohol

A clinician should recommend HIV testing for any patient with a high index of suspicion for infection. Several states now mandate that HIV testing be offered to pregnant women. In addition, the CDC recommends that hospitals with an HIV prevalence rate > 1% or an AIDS diagnosis rate of > 1/1000 discharges should offer HIV testing routinely to patients aged 15–54 years.

Centers for Disease Control and Prevention: Recommendations for HIV testing services for inpatients and outpatients in acute-care hospital settings. MMWR 42(RR-2):1, 1993.

McCarthy BD, et al: Who should be screened for HIV infection? A cost-effectiveness analysis. Arch Intern Med 153:1107–1116, 1993.

Freedberg KA, Samet JH: Think HIV: Why physicians should lower their threshold for HIV testing. Arch Intern Med 159:1994–1999, 1999.

15. Why are HIV ELISA tests confirmed by Western blot?

For various reasons, the enzyme-linked immunosorbent assay (ELISA) can yield a significant number of false-positive tests for the presence of anti-HIV antibodies. Most laboratories repeat a positive ELISA, but a repetitively positive result should be confirmed by Western blot to verify that the positive ELISA result is based on true HIV antibodies and not cross-reacting proteins. In populations with a low prevalence of HIV infection, as many as 29 of every 30 positive ELISAs are false-positives.

Meyer KB, Packer SG: Screening for HIV: Can we afford the false positive rate? N Engl J Med 317:238–241, 1987.

16. How should an "indeterminate" Western blot be followed up?

Assuming that the patient had an initial ELISA test repeatedly positive before the indeterminate Western blot, the Western blot should be repeated. If it is indeterminate again, both the ELISA and Western blot should be repeated in 3 months.

17. What are the diagnostic criteria for AIDS?

The diagnosis depends on the status of the patient's laboratory evidence for or against HIV infection:

1. For patients with laboratory evidence of HIV infection, a diagnosis of AIDS can be made if the patient has a presumptive or definitive diagnosis of one or more of a list of indicator diseases or a CD4+-lymphocyte count < 200/mm³.

2. For patients without laboratory evidence of HIV infection, a diagnosis can be made if there is no other cause for an underlying immunodeficiency state and the patient has a definitive diagnosis of one or more indicator diseases.

3. For a patient with laboratory evidence against HIV infection, a diagnosis can be made if the patient has had a definitive diagnosis of *P. carinii* pneumonia or has a definitive diagnosis of one or more indicator diseases with a CD4+-lymphocyte count < 400 cells/mm³.

Centers for Disease Control and Prevention: 1993 Revised classification system for HIV infection and expanded surveillance case definition for AIDS among adolescents and adults. MMWR 41(RR-17):1–19, 1992.

18. What are the AIDS indicator diseases?

Candidiasis of lungs, bronchi, trachea
Candidiasis, esophageal
Cervical cancer, invasive*
Coccidioidomycosis, disseminated or
  extrapulmonary
Cryptococcosis, extrapulmonary
Cryptosporidiosis, chronic intestinal
Cytomegalovirus (other than liver,
  spleen, nodes)
Cytomegalovirus retinitis
Herpes simplex, chronic ulcers or of
  bronchi, lungs, esophagus
Histoplasmosis, disseminated or
  extrapulmonary
HIV encephalopathy
HIV wasting syndrome
Isosporiasis, chronic intestinal
Kaposi's sarcoma
Lymphoid interstitial pneumonitis
Lymphoma, non-Hodgkin's
Lymphoma, primary CNS
Mycobacterium avium, disseminated
  or extrapulmonary
Mycobacterium kansasii, disseminated
  or extrapulmonary
Mycobacterium spp., disseminated or
  extrapulmonary
Mycobacterium tuberculosis, any site*
P. carinii pneumonia (PCP)
Pneumonia, recurrent bacterial*
Progressive multifocal leukoencephalopathy
Salmonella bacteremia, recurrent
Stronglyloidosis, non-GI
Toxoplasmosis of brain

* Newly added in the 1993 expansion of the AIDS surveillance case definition.

19. What classes of drugs are currently available to treat HIV infection?

GENERIC NAME	BRAND NAME	ALSO KNOWN AS	FDA APPROVAL DATE	FORM
Nucleoside analog reverse transcriptase inhibitors				
Zidovudine	Retrovir	ZDV, AZT	March 1987	
Didanosine	Videx	ddI	October 1991	
Zalcitabine	Hivid	ddC	June 1992	
Stavudine	Zerit	d4T	June 1994	
Lamivudine	Epivir	3TC	November 1995	
Abacavir	Ziagen	ABC, 1592	December 1998	
	Combivir	AZT/3TC		Fixed dose
	Trizivir	AZT/3TC/ABC		Fixed dose
Non-nucleoside reverse transcriptase inhibitors				
Nevirapine	Viramune	NVP	June 1996	
Delavirdine	Rescriptor	DLV	April 1997	
Efavirenz	Sustiva	EFV, DMP-266	September 1998	
Protease inhibitors				
Saquinavir	Invirase	SQV-HGC	October 1995	Hard-gel caps
Ritonavir	Norvir	RTV	March 1996	
Indinavir	Crixivan	IDV	March 1996	
Nelfinavir	Viracept	NFV	March 1997	
Saquinavir	Fortovase	SQV-SGC	November 1997	Soft-gel caps
Amprenavir	Agenerase	APV, 141W94	April 1999	
Lopinavir	Kaletra	ABT-378	October 2000	

20. How do the reverse transcriptase inhibitors (RTIs) work?

The RTIs act during the initial infection of a new host cell. They inhibit viral reverse transcriptase during the transcription of viral RNA to host complementary DNA. The RTIs are nucleoside analogs (NRTIs) or non-nucleoside analogs (NNRTIs). The analogs become phosphorylated to a triphosphate form and competitively interfere with native nucleosides during transcription, causing viral DNA chain termination. The non-nucleosides bind to reverse transcriptase, altering the active site and inactivating the enzyme.

21. How do the protease inhibitors work?

In host cells with established infection, after the synthesis of mRNA and then HIV polyproteins, HIV protease must cleave the polyproteins to result in the production of functional proteins. Protease inhibitors (PIs) act at this stage, preventing cleavage. Viral particles can still be formed and bud from the host cell, but they are nonfunctional and noninfective.

22. What are the dosing schedules and major side effects of the antiretrovirals?

DRUG	DOSING	TOXICITY	COMMENTS
Nucleoside analogs			
Zidovudine	300 mg bid	GI upset, headache, anemia, leukopenia	Marrow suppression more common in advanced disease
Didanosine	200 mg bid, avoiding food	Peripheral neuropathy, pancreatitis, diarrhea	Interaction of buffer with other drugs; early data on qd dosing
Zalcitabine	0.75 mg tid	Peripheral neuropathy, stomatitis	Most neurotoxic
Stavudine	40 mg bid	Peripheral neuropathy	
Lamivudine	150 mg bid	Minimal GI upset	May help maintain viral sensitivity to other nucleosides
Abacavir	300 mg bid	Hypersensitivity, GI upset	Never rechallenge after hypersensitivity
Non-nucleoside analogs			
Nevirapine	200 mg bid	Rash, hepatitis, Stevens-Johnson syndrome	200 mg qd × 14 days, then bid to decrease rash; class-wide resistance; inducer of cytochrome P-450
Delavirdine	400 mg tid	Rash, headache	Class-wide resistance; inhibitor of cytochrome P-450
Efavirenz	600 mg qhs	Dizziness, somnolence, confusion	Class-wide resistance; mixed effect on cytochrome P-450
Protease inhibitors			
Saquinavir	1200 mg tid (400 mg every 12 hr with ritonavir), with meal	GI upset, headache	
Ritonavir	600 mg every 12 hr (400 mg every 12 hr with saquinavir)	GI upset, emesis, paresthesias, hepatitis, elevated triglycerides	Strong cytochrome P-450 inhibitor, many drug interactions
Indinavir	800 mg every 8 hr on empty stomach or low-fat snack	GI upset, neprholithiasis, elevated bilirubin	Every 8 hr, not tid, dosing; hydration to prevent stones
Nelfinavir	1250 mg bid, with food	Diarrhea	Earlier dosing was 750 mg tid
Amprenavir	1200 mg bid	GI upset	
Lopinavir	400 mg bid		

bid = twice daily, tid = 3 times/day, qd = each day.

23. Does viral resistance to antiretrovirals develop?

Evidence indicates that HIV can develop decreased sensitivity to all of the available agents. In many cases, the virus develops outright resistance. Such changes in the viral sensitivities are associated with discrete and specific genetic mutations, which usually occur within 1–6 months of initiating therapy. Clinical correlation with these laboratory findings is, as yet, unknown.

Richman DD: Clinical significance of drug resistance in human immunodeficiency virus. Clin Infect Dis 21(suppl 2):S166–S169, 1995.

24. Can you test for the resistance that HIV develops to medication?

Yes. Both genotypic and phenotypic resistance tests are available, although not approved by the FDA. Such tests have demonstrated the transmission of resistant virus in people with acute HIV infection. In patients failing antiretroviral therapy, it may be possible to identify which drug in the multi-drug regimen is no longer effective because of HIV mutation, thereby preserving the concomitant drugs for future therapeutic use. Studies using resistance tests have demonstrated incremental improvements in HIV viral load levels, but no clinical outcomes have been demonstrated at this time.

25. How do you assess the efficacy of antiretroviral therapy?

Before starting or changing therapy, a baseline HIV viral load is obtained. Three to six weeks after the therapeutic change a repeat HIV viral load should be performed. The result should demonstrate a 1.0 or greater log (base 10) decrease in viral load. Therapy is then monitored in an ongoing fashion by reassessing HIV viral load every 2–3 months with the goal of attaining a level that is undetectable within 12 weeks. Prolonged follow-up in successfully treated patients can then be planned every 3–4 months.

26. When do you consider changing therapy?

Therapy can be changed at any time for toxicity or intolerance. In this setting only the offending drug need be discontinued and replaced. Therapy also should be changed for virologic failure. Failure can be defined as:

- < 1.0 log decrease in HIV viral load at 4 weeks, or
- Return of a detectable viral load after reaching an undetectable level, or
- Sustained 3-fold (0.5 log) increase in a detectable viral load or a decreasing CD4+ count despite apparent viral control.

27. How long does antiretroviral therapy work?

The durability of therapeutic efficacy is directly related to the nadir of the HIV viral load. With maintenance of viral suppression, some patients continue on therapy for over 5 years with no evidence of viral rebound.

28. When should antiretroviral therapy be started?

Since the first anti-HIV medication became available, this question has been debated. In patients with advanced disease (AIDS diagnosis or CD4+ count < 200/mm^3), antiretroviral therapy has been shown to prolong life. This result was found in the initial antiretroviral trial with zidovudine and also has been demonstrated with protease inhibitors. The study of patients in less advanced stages has been hampered by the limited efficacy of the RTIs when used alone. Clinically significant benefit in patients with CD4+ counts > 500/mm^3 has been difficult to demonstrate, but the newer prognostic information gained with viral load measurements and the promising strength of combination therapy have led authorities to recommend therapy in some of these patients.

Recommendations for When to Initiate Treatment

STATUS	RECOMMENDATION
Symptomatic HIV disease*	Therapy recommended for all patients
Asymptomatic, CD4+ cell count < 500 *or* viral load > 20,000	Therapy recommended†
Asymptomatic, CD4+ cell count > 500 *and* viral load < 20,000	Therapy may be deferred

* Includes symptoms such as recurrent mucosal candidiasis, oral hairy leukoplakia, and chronic and unexplained fever, night sweats, and weight loss.
† Some defer therapy in a subset of patients with stable CD4+ cell counts between 350 and 500.
From US Department of Health and Human Services, January 28, 2000.

29. How should medications be combined for antiretroviral therapy?

DHHS Recommendations for Initial Treatment of HIV Infection

Strongly recommended	One choice each from column A and column B	
	Column A	Column B
	Efavirenz	Stavudine+lamivudine
	Indinavir	Stavudine+didanosine
	Nelfinavir	Zidovudine+lamivudine
	Ritonavir+saquinavir	Zidovudine+didanosine
Alternative recommendations (less likely to provide sustained viral suppression or data inadequate)		
	Abacavir	Didanosine+lamivudine
	Amprenavir	Zidovudine+zalcitabine
	Delavirdine	
	Nelfinavir+saquinavir-SGC	
	Nevirapine	
	Ritonavir	
	Saquinavir-SGC	

Department of Health and Human Services (as of January 28, 2000).

30. Do patients taking antiretroviral therapy need PCP prophylaxis?

Maybe. In patients with advanced HIV infection on antiretroviral therapy but not on PCP prophylaxis, approximately one-half of the opportunistic infections are PCP. Therefore, it is recommended that patients also be given PCP prophylaxis once they meet the criteria (see question 53), regardless of other therapy that they may be taking. A patient's immune status may improve enough while on therapy to discontinue primary PCP prophylaxis in the future.

31. Can therapy prevent perinatal transmission of HIV infection?

Zidovudine therapy initiated between weeks 14 and 34 of gestation, continued intravenously during labor, and administered to the newborn for the first 6 weeks of life decreased the rate of transmission from 25.5% to 8.3%, a 67.5% reduction. Antiretroviral therapy for infected pregnant women is now recommended and has led to greater emphasis on prenatal HIV testing; some states mandate that the test be offered to all pregnant women. In general, therapy recommendations are the same as for nonpregnant patients, with the exception of the possible fetal toxicity of efavirenz.

Connor EM, et al: Reduction of maternal-infant transmission of human immunodeficiency virus type 1 with zidovudine treatment. N Engl J Med 331:1173–1180, 1994.

Centers for Disease Control and Prevention: Public Health Service Task Force recommendations for the use of antiretroviral drugs in pregnant women infected with HIV-1 for maternal health and for reducing perinatal HIV-1 transmission in the United States. MMWR 47:1–30, 1998.

CLINICAL MANIFESTATIONS

32. What are the symptoms of acute HIV infection?

SYMPTOM	FREQUENCY (%)
Fever	90+
Fatigue	80–90
Rash	50–80
Headache	40–75
Lymphadenopathy	40–70
Pharyngitis	40–70
Myalgia/arthralgia	40–70
Nausea, vomiting, diarrhea	30–50
Night sweats	30–50

33. What HIV-related manifestations are seen uniquely in women?

In addition to all the well-known manifestations of HIV infection seen in men, three conditions are specific to women: cervical neoplasia, pelvic inflammatory disease (PID), and vaginal candidiasis. The clinical course of all three is more aggressive because of HIV infection. Invasive cervical cancer was added to the list of AIDS-indicator diseases in the 1993 revision. Women with HIV infection need routine Pap smears at least every 6 months. Also common are menstrual irregularities with irregular periods, increased or decreased blood flow, increased premenstrual symptoms, and early menopausal symptoms.

Wofsy C: Care of women infected with the human immunodeficiency virus. J AIDS 9:361–70, 1995.

34. What is thrush?

Thrush is oropharyngeal pseudomembranous candidiasis, which often presages AIDS. It usually presents as white plaques (pseudomembranes), either scattered small plaques or large sheets, on any oral mucosal surface. Candidiasis also may present in an atrophic or erythematous appearance without plaques. Significant oral pain may be present along with altered taste. The diagnosis can be made clinically, with KOH smear or by culture. A clinician should not confuse thrush with oral hairy leukoplakia, a whitish corrugated growth along the margins of the tongue.

Thrush often indicates significant immune suppression, and if it is found during an initial exam, evaluation should begin for other HIV-related medical interventions, such as PCP prophylaxis.

35. How is thrush treated?

LIMITED INVOLVEMENT	EXTENSIVE INVOLVEMENT
Improved oral hygiene with peroxide rinses	Ketoconazole, 200 mg/day orally
Nystatin oral suspension	Fluconazole, 50–100 mg/day orally
Nystatin vaginal tablets, used oral	
Clotrimazole tablets	

36. What dermatologic conditions are common in HIV infection?

Besides Kaposi's sarcoma (KS), the multitude of skin findings may include seborrheic dermatitis, psoriasis, and ichthyosis. *Staphylococcus aureus* is the most common bacterial pathogen and typically manifests as folliculitis. Fungal infections such as candidiasis and tinea are common. Rarely, cryptococcosis and histoplasmosis are seen. Viral infections with herpes simplex type 2, varicella zoster, molluscum contagiosum, and condyloma acuminata are common. Rashes due to syphilis also must be considered in these high-risk patients.

Cockerell CJ: Human immunodeficiency virus infection and the skin: A crucial interface. Arch Intern Med 151:1295–1303, 1991.

37. What rheumatic conditions may occur in HIV-positive patients?

- Inflammatory myopathy
- Reiter's syndrome
- Psoriasis and psoriatic arthritis
- Sjögren's syndrome
- Vasculitis
- Oligoarticular arthritis
- Avascular necrosis

The arthritis does not seem to be responsive to NSAIDs. Also described are painful arthralgias of short duration that often require narcotics for relief. In addition to these clinical syndromes, lab evaluations often reveal low titers of rheumatoid factors, antinuclear antibodies, and anticardiolipin antibodies. Generalized hypergammaglobulinemia is also reported.

Calabrese LH: Rheumatologic aspects of acquired immunodeficiency syndrome. In Klippel JH, Dieppe PA, (eds): Rheumatology. 2nd ed. St. Louis, Mosby 6.7.1–6.7.12, 1998.

38. Do HIV-infected patients respond to the influenza vaccine?

Administration of the influenza vaccine has been recommended for all persons infected with HIV, although the antibody response to the vaccine is lower than in non–HIV-infected controls. A two-dose regimen is not superior in efficacy to the traditional single-dose regimen. CD4+ counts

< 100 are associated with poor antibody responses. Studies showing increased HIV viral load and decreased $CD4^+$ counts in study participants receiving influenza vaccine compared with placebo-injected controls have raised concerns, but no adverse clinical events have been demonstrated.

Tasker SA, et al: Effects of influenza vaccination in HIV-infected adults: A double-blind placebo-controlled trial. Vaccine 16:1039–1042, 1998.

39. Do HIV-infected patients respond to the pneumococcal polysaccharide vaccine?

The response is impaired compared with normal controls. HIV-infected patients mount an adequate antibody response to fewer of the serotypes contained in the 23-valent vaccine, and this response rate decreases with decreasing $CD4^+$ counts. As with influenza vaccination, there appears to be increased HIV viral activity after pneumococcal vaccination, but because morbidity due to pneumococcal disease is clearly and substantially increased in HIV-infected patients, the risk/benefit ratio supports vaccination.

Moore D, et al: Pneumococcal vaccination and HIV infection. Int J STD AIDS 9:1–7, 1999.

40. What is AIDS dementia complex?

Patients with AIDS may develop cognitive, behavioral, and motor dysfunction in the course of their illness. Although multiple opportunistic infections need to be ruled out (e.g., cryptococcosis, toxoplasmosis, tuberculosis), direct CNS infection by HIV seems to cause this complex of signs and symptoms. Early in its course, neuropsychologic testing may be needed to support a clinical suspicion of dementia, but the dementia can progress to a vegetative state. Patients may first complain of concentration difficulties, and family and friends may note personality changes. A thorough neurologic evaluation and investigation into other causes are needed. Zidovudine may be helpful in treating dementia, probably because of the high drug levels obtainable in cerebrospinal fluid.

McArthur JC, et al: Dementia in AIDS patients: Incidence and risk factors: Multicenter AIDS Cohort Study. Neurology 43:2245–2252, 1993.

41. Do neurologic conditions in AIDS appear only late in the course of the disease?

Not necessarily. Neurologic signs and symptoms may be the earliest manifestations of HIV infection in some patients. The most frequent cause of neurologic abnormality is subacute encephalitis, which may be a part of the initial HIV viral infection in many patients.

Simpson DM, Tagliati M: Neurologic manifestations of HIV infection. Ann Intern Med 121:769–785, 1994.

42. What is HIV wasting syndrome?

This AIDS-defining diagnosis includes profound weight loss of > 10% of body weight, with either chronic diarrhea or weakness and fever for > 30 days. These clinical events should be evaluated for other HIV-related illnesses; in the absence of other causes, a diagnosis of wasting can be made.

Grunfeld C, Feingold KR: Metabolic disturbances and wasting in the acquired immunodeficiency syndrome. N Engl J Med 327:329–337, 1992.

43. How often does HIV infection result in anemia or thrombocytopenia?

Patients with full-blown AIDS are frequently pancytopenic. Anemia occurs in up to 80%, neutropenia in 85%, and thrombocytopenia in 65% of cases. HIV-infected but asymptomatic patients are much less frequently cytopenic. Clinically significant thrombocytopenia indistinguishable from that seen in idiopathic thrombocytopenic purpura (ITP) may be a presentation of HIV infection. Typically, bone marrow is normal with adequate numbers of megakaryocytes. The disorder behaves much like classic ITP in that patients respond to steroids and splenectomy. It is appropriate to obtain an HIV blood test in most patients presenting with ITP.

Thrombocytopenic patients have improved on zidovudine therapy, although AZT may cause anemia. Of interest is the recent recognition of thrombotic thrombocytopenic purpura (TTP) in association with HIV infection.

Aboulafia DM, Mitsuyasu RT: Hematolic abnormalities in AIDS. Hematol Oncol Clin North Am 5:195–214, 1991.

44. What are the characteristic bone marrow aspirate and biopsy findings in AIDS?
- Decreased cellularity (rarely hypocellular), including dyserythropoiesis
- Increased lymphocytes and plasma cells
- Histiocytic hyperplasia with phagocytosis of red cells, platelets, and WBCs
- Granulomas, marrow fibrosis, serous fat atrophy
- Pure red cell aphasia with giant pronormoblasts (in parvovirus B19 infection)

In addition, patients receiving zidovudine often have ineffective hematopoiesis with megaloblastic maturation.

Namiki TS, et al: A comparison of bone marrow findings in patients with acquired immunodeficiency syndrome (AIDS) and AIDS-related conditions. Hematol Oncol 5:99, 1987.

45. What lymphomas are associated with AIDS? How often do they present with extralymphatic presentations?

AIDS is associated with high-grade B-cell lymphomas that arise most often in extralymphatic sites. The histologic types that are seen in 80–90% of patients include small noncleaved cell (resembling Burkitt's lymphoma) and immunoblastic lymphoma. Extranodal disease is the rule rather than the exception (68–98%). The most frequent extranodal sites are the bone marrow, liver, meninges, lung, soft tissue, primary CNS, rectum, and Waldeyer's tonsillar ring. In addition, B-type symptoms are extremely common in this patient group.

Primary CNS lymphomas occur most frequently in patients with a prior AIDS diagnosis and are associated with a median survival of < 3 months. Patients without prior histories of AIDS-related infections (such as PCP) and in good physical condition may respond to standard chemotherapy followed by institution of antiretroviral therapy. Patients who develop systemic lymphoma after other manifestations of AIDS typically do not fare well with chemotherapy. Supportive care only is a reasonable course.

Levine AM: Acquired immunodeficiency syndrome-related lymphoma. Blood 80:8–20, 1992.

46. Define lipodystrophy.

Lipodystrophy is a poor name for a poorly understood group of complications related to antiretroviral therapy. The complications include a body fat redistribution syndrome with intra-abdominal fat accumulation and wasting of subcutaneous tissue and fat on the extremities and face. Some patients develop a buffalo hump. Also seen are insulin resistance and dysglycemias with some overt cases of diabetes. Elevated levels of cholesterol and triglycerides are also seen, often necessitating lipid-lowering therapy. There are anecdotal reports of premature cardiovascular events associated with such changes. No clear underlying mechanism has been described, and no clear relationship with any particular medication or class of medications has been made, although some abnormalities, particularly lipid elevations, appear more common with protease inhibitor therapy.

Pneumocystis carinii INFECTION

47. What is PCP?

PCP stands for *Pneumocystis carinii* pneumonia. Before routine prophylactic treatments, PCP was the presenting diagnosis in 60% of patients with AIDS and eventually was seen in 80% of patients with AIDS at some time during their illness. With more active HIV testing and the initiation of effective primary PCP prophylaxis, the incidence of PCP should approach zero. Unfortunately, not enough patients receive early HIV testing, and a number progress asymptomatically to a point of immunosuppression at risk for PCP.

48. How does PCP present?

Cough, fever, and dyspnea on exertion are the most common presenting symptoms. The cough is usually nonproductive or productive of only scant, whitish sputum. Patients also may relate a sensation of chest tightness or an inability to take a full, deep inspiration. Other less common complaints include nonspecific weight loss, night sweats, and malaise. Findings on physical examination include fever, tachypnea, persistent cough, and dry rales. Rarely, a patient may endure symptoms at home long enough to present with cyanosis. Laboratory findings include hypoxemia with an elevated A–aO$_2$ gradient. Elevated serum lactate dehydrogenase levels are seen.

Moe AA, Hardy WD: Pneumocystis carinii infection in the HIV-seropositive patient. Infect Dis Clin North Am 8:331–364, 1994.

49. How is PCP diagnosed?

By pathologic demonstration of the organism in lung specimens. Several centers have reported success with examination of induced sputum, but most centers rely on bronchoscopy with bronchoalveolar lavage (BAL). Lavage alone has a sensitivity of > 95%; thus, transbronchial biopsy (TBB) is usually withheld except for cases not diagnosed by BAL. Open lung biopsy is rarely needed. An experienced HIV clinician may make an empiric diagnosis, but this approach should be reserved for patients known to be HIV-infected.

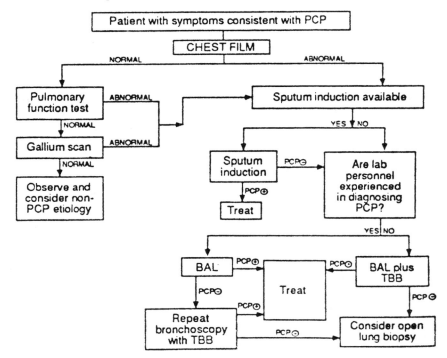

Diagnostic algorithm for PCP. (From Cohen PT, et al (eds): The AIDS Knowledge Base. Waltham, MA, Medical Publishing Group, 1990, with permission.)

50. What are the chest x-ray findings in PCP?

Typically seen is a diffuse, bilateral, interstitial infiltrate, often more pronounced in the hilar region (butterfly distribution). Areas of local consolidation are less common, as are cystic and cavitary changes. Normal chest x-rays are also seen, especially in patients presenting early in the illness. Pleural effusion is rare and, if present, should raise the suspicion of another diagnosis.

51. How is PCP treated?

Conventional treatment comes down to a choice among three agents: trimethoprim-sulfamethoxazole (TMP-SMX), pentamidine isethionate, or atovaquone. The first two agents seem to be equally effective in clinical use but differ in routes of administration. Both are available for IV use, but TMP-SMX also can be administered orally, enabling outpatient therapy. The usual daily dose is 20 mg/kg of TMP and 100 mg/kg of SMX in divided doses, 3–4 times/day for 21 days. A lower dose (15/75 mg/kg) may be equally effective with fewer side effects. Pentamidine usually is given at a dose of 4 mg/kg/day. The 3-mg/kg, once-daily dose may be effective in mild pneumonias.

Atovaquone is an alternative oral therapy for mild-to-moderate PCP (PO_2 > 60 mmHg, A–a O_2 gradient < 45 mm Hg) in patients who cannot tolerate TMP-SMX. In studies comparing it with TMP-SMX or pentamidine, atovaquone was less toxic and better tolerated. However, it is less effective than TMP-SMX, although equally as effective as pentamidine. The dosing regimen with the oral suspension is 750 mg twice daily, taken with a fatty meal, usually for 21 days. Because absorption depends on food intake, more acutely ill patients are not candidates.

Dohn MN, et al: Oral atovaquone compared with intravenous pentamidine for *Pneumocystis carinii* pneumonia in patients with AIDS. Ann Intern Med 121:174–180, 1994.

52. What are the expected side effects of treatment of moderate-to-severe PCP?

Drug-Associated Adverse Effects of TMP/SMX vs Pentamidine

	TMP-SMX (%)	PENTAMIDINE (%)
Fever (> 37° C)	78	82
Hypotension	0	27
Nausea, vomiting	25	24
Rash	44	15
Anemia	39	24
Leukopenia	72	47
Thrombocytopenia	3	18
Azotemia	14	64
Alanine aminotransferase	22	15
Alkaline aminotransferase	22	15
Alkaline phosphatase	11	18
Hypoglycemia	0	21
Hypocalcemia	0	3

TMP/SMX is very well tolerated in non-AIDS patients, but it produces side effects in 65–100% of patients with AIDS. Severe rash and neutropenia are often treatment-limiting but reversible with drug cessation. Progressive renal insufficiency and pancreatitis with dysglycemias are the most serious side effects of pentamidine infusion. Atovaquone is associated with treatment-limiting rash in only 4% of patients and no other adverse reaction in more than 1%.

Sattler FR, et al: TMP-SMX compared with pentamidine for treatment of PCP in AIDS: A prospective, noncrossover study. Ann Intern Med 109:280–287, 1988.

53. List the indications for PCP prophylaxis.

1. Prior episode of PCP (secondary prophylaxis)
2. CD4$^+$ count < 200/mm^3 (or CD4$^+$ < 14% of total lymphocytes)
3. Earlier initiation warranted for patients with:
   - Oral candidiasis
   - Unexplained fever
   - Rapid fall in CD4$^+$ count

54. What agents and regimens are recommended for PCP prophylaxis?
TMP-SMX
- TMP 160 mg/SMX 800 mg daily (one double-strength [DS] tablet)
- Side effects similar to but less common than with primary PCP treatment
- Decreasing dose by 50% (1 DS tablet 3 times/wk or single-strength daily) may limit side effects while preserving efficacy
- Also provides prophylaxis against CNS toxoplasmosis

Aerosolized pentamidine
- 300 mg once monthly via nebulizer
- Transient taste alterations and coughing or wheezing (can be minimized by pretreatment with inhaled bronchodilators)
- Evaluate patients for active TB before starting therapy

Dapsone (+ pyrimethamine)
- 50 mg twice daily or 100 mg/day
- Provides prophylaxis against toxoplasmosis with addition of pyrimethamine

Atovaquone
- 1500 mg/day
- Gastrointestinal discomfort is main adverse event
- Also covers toxoplasmosis

TMP-SMX appears virtually 100% effective in patients who can tolerate the side effects, whereas dapsone and pentamidine have a 5–10% failure rate per year. Failure means that PCP may be mild or atypical. In a practical, clinically pertinent study comparing the three agents, all had similar effectiveness when treatment-limiting toxicities were included.

Bozzette SA, et al: A randomized trial of three antipneumocystis agents in patients with advanced human immunodeficiency virus infection. N Engl J Med 332:693–699, 1995.

55. How does aerosolized pentamidine prophylaxis change the presentation of breakthrough PCP?

Because aerosolized pentamidine is not 100% effective, new episodes of PCP may occur during prophylaxis. These episodes may present with an atypical radiographic appearance, with more upper-lobe infiltrates rather than the traditional diffuse interstitial infiltrates. The yield of BAL for pathologic diagnosis also is decreased.

Jules-Elysee KM, et al: Aerosolized pentamidine: Effect on diagnosis and presentation of Pneumocystis carinii pneumonia. Ann Intern Med 112:750–757, 1990.

56. Should patients with PCP and respiratory failure be intubated?

Obviously the answer depends on the patient's previously expressed desires and the clinical setting of respiratory failure. One group of patients who may benefit from mechanical ventilation has been identified. They have a shorter duration of symptoms of PCP, a precipitous decline of respiratory status after bronchoscopy, and better arterial oxygenation on admission ($PO_2 > 60$ mmHg). Such patients may have a 1-year survival rate of up to 80%. To give critically ill patients proper advice about treatment options and outcomes, a practitioner must be aware of these data.

Franklin C, et al: Improving long-term prognosis for survivors of mechanical ventilation in patients with AIDS with PCP and acute respiratory failure. Arch Intern Med 155:91–95, 1995.

57. When should adjunctive steroids be used in therapy for PCP?

- Indicated in patients with $PaO_2 < 70$ mm Hg or $A–aO_2$ gradient > 35 mmHg on room air
- Corticosteroids are begun within 72 hr of initiating PCP treatment
- Improve clinical outcome and reduce mortality rate by 50%
- Avoid in presence of coincident pulmonary infection (TB, histoplasmosis) or process (KS)
- Recommended approach: oral prednisone given as follows:
    40 mg twice daily for 5 days, then
    40 mg once daily for 5 days, then
    20 mg once daily for 11 days (total duration 21 days)

Consensus statement on the use of corticosteroids as adjunctive therapy for pneumocystis pneumonia in the acquired immunodeficiency syndrome. N Engl J Med 323:1500–1504, 1990.

Bozzette SA, et al: A controlled trial of early adjunctive treatment with corticosteroids for Pneumocystis carinii pneumonia in the acquired immunodeficiency syndrome. N Engl J Med 323:1451–1456, 1990.

58. What is extrapulmonary pneumocystosis?

Pneumocystis infection can involve anatomic sites literally from head (otitis) to foot (vasculitis). The use of nonsystemic (i.e., inhaled) pentamidine therapy for PCP prophylaxis appears to be involved in such cases, although current clinical practice prefers systemic therapy with TMP-SMX or dapsone.

Telzalc EE, et al: Extrapulmonary *Pneumocystis carinii* infections. Rev Infect Dis 12:380–386, 1990.

59. Does the incidence of pneumothorax increase with pentamidine inhalation?

This question arose when patients enrolled in community trials of inhaled pentamidine had several episodes of pneumothorax. It appears that these episodes were related to recurrent episodes of PCP—not to the use of inhalation therapy.

CRYPTOCOCCAL INFECTION

60. How often does cryptococcus cause infection in AIDS?

Depending on which series is examined, cryptococcus may cause 5–10% of AIDS-defining opportunistic infections. Because patients also develop cryptococcal infections after a previous AIDS diagnosis, the overall estimate is 8–15%. Studies suggested a decreasing incidence of cryptococcosis, even before the era of more effective HIV therapy, possibly related to the more general use of fluconazole for either prophylaxis or treatment for other fungal diseases, such as oral and esophageal candidiasis.

61. How does cryptococcal infection present?

Meningitis is the most common presentation in AIDS. Extraneural disease is frequently seen with meningitis but is much less common in its absence. Meningismus is present in only 25–30% of patients with meningitis, but fever and headache are seen in 80–90%. Focal neurologic symptoms or signs are seen in a small minority of patients.

Features of Meningeal Cryptococcosis

Symptoms			
Fever	58 (65%)	Altered mentation	25 (28%)
Malaise	68 (76%)	Focal deficits	5 (6%)
Headaches	65 (73%)	Seizures	4 (4%)
Stiff neck	20 (22%)	Cough/dyspnea	28 (31%)
Nausea/vomiting	37 (42%)	Diarrhea	19 (21%)
Photophobia	16 (18%)		
Signs			
Fever	50 (56%)	Altered mentation	15 (17%)
Meningeal signs	24 (27%)	Focal deficits	13 (15%)

From Chuck SL, Sande MA: Infections with Cryptococcus neoformans in AIDS. N Engl J Med 321:795, 1989, with permission.

62. Which patients with cryptococcosis need a lumbar puncture (LP)?

All patients with a culture or a serum antigen titer positive for cryptococci require an LP, regardless of which site originally yielded the positive specimen. In any HIV-infected patient with an undiagnosed fever and/or headache in a medically urgent situation, an LP should be considered to assess the possibility of cryptococcal disease. If the situation is less urgent, a serum antigen titer can be obtained.

63. How often should an LP be done?

An LP is performed at the time of diagnosis of cryptococcal infection. If the LP is indicative of meningitis and the patient responds to therapy, a repeat LP should be performed by at least week 2 of therapy to help evaluate microbial response and to decide on the appropriateness of continued IV or oral therapy. Subsequent LPs should be done as clinically indicated until adequate microbial response is documented. If the clinical response is poor or if the initial opening pressure was elevated (> 25 cmH$_2$O), frequent LPs may be needed to relieve increased intracranial pressure and to guide therapy.

64. What cerebrospinal fluid (CSF) findings are seen in cryptococcal meningitis?

FINDING	NO. WITH FINDING/NO. TESTED	%
WBC < 20 cells/ml	96/128	75
Glucose > 40 mg/dl	87/127	68
Protein < 45 mg/dl	53/127	42
Positive India ink	92/125	74
Positive CSF antigen	116/126	92

From Chuck SL, Sande MA: Infections with Cryptococcus neoformans in the acquired immunodeficiency syndrome. N Engl J Med 321:794–799, 1989, with permission.

The CSF can appear remarkably normal. However, you should always perform an India ink test, which is usually positive and can yield an immediate diagnosis without waiting for other laboratory results.

65. What treatment is recommended for cryptococcosis in AIDS?
Trials comparing amphotericin B with fluconazole for treatment of cryptococcal meningitis have concluded that either therapy can be effective. There has been evidence of higher early mortality in patients assigned to fluconazole, and some studies may have used suboptimal doses of both amphotericin B and fluconazole. Because of concerns about early mortality, most clinicians now recommend an initial 2-week course of amphotericin B at 0.7 mg/kg/day, with or without flucytosine (100 mg/kg/day), followed by fluconazole at 400 mg/day.

Saag MS, et al: Comparison of amphotericin B with fluconazole in the treatment of acute AIDS-associated cryptococcal meningitis. N Engl J Med 326:83–89, 1992.

van der Horst C, et al: Randomized double-blind comparison of amphotericin B plus flucytosine to amphotericin B alone followed by a comparison of fluconazole to itraconazole in the treatment of acute cryptococcal meningitis in patients with AIDS [abstracts I216 and I217]. In Abstracts of the 35th Interscience Conference on Antimicrobial Agents and Chemotherapy, San Francisco, October 1995.

66. Is maintenance anticryptococcal therapy needed?
Cryptococcal infection in AIDS demonstrates a high relapse rate after primary therapy and a high mortality rate during relapse. The standard of care has been to give chronic maintenance or suppressive therapy. Intermittent infusions of amphotericin B and oral ketoconazole, itraconazole, or fluconazole have been used. Fluconazole (200–400 mg/day) is the agent of choice. All patients should be continued on maintenance therapy for life. There is no recommendation to discontinue because of immune reconstitution.

Powderly WG, et al: A controlled trial of fluconazole or amphotericin B to prevent relapse of cryptococcal meningitis in patients with the acquired immunodeficiency syndrome. N Engl J Med 326:793–798, 1992.

67. Are serum cryptococcal antigen levels good indicators of response to therapy?
No. Although the serum antigen test can be very helpful in the diagnosis of cryptococcal infection, it cannot be used to judge therapeutic response. In most cases of meningitis, the CSF antigen titer should be determined by repeat lumbar puncture. If after therapy the serum titer does revert to very low titer or negative, an increasing titer in the future should raise concern about a relapse.

68. How is a relapse of cryptococcal infection treated?
Depending on the patient's previous therapeutic course and compliance with maintenance therapy, relapse should be treated with a reinduction regimen of amphotericin B, followed by fluconazole. Development of resistance has not been demonstrated.

69. What are the poor prognostic indicators in AIDS-related cryptococcosis?

STUDY	NO. PATIENTS	POOR PROGNOSTIC INDICATORS	
Diamond (1974)	111	India ink-positive High opening pressure Low CFS glucose	CSF WBC < 20 Extra-CNS site of infection
Kovacs (1985)	27	No reliable factor identified	Pretreatment CSF antigen
Zugar (1986)	34	India ink-positive Post-treatment CNS antigen > 1:8	> 1:10,000
Chuck (1989)	89	Hyponatremia	Extra-CNS site of infection

In 1974, Diamond and Bennett described multiple prognostic factors in non-AIDS crypto-coccal meningitis. Several reports since have attempted to define similar factors in AIDS-related cryptococcosis but for the most part have been unsuccessful. Cryptococcal disease in patients with AIDS is a less predictable illness than in non-AIDS patients. Often an adequate response to anticryptococcal therapy is complicated by the development of new adverse clinical events related to the underlying HIV infection.

Diamond RD, Bennett JE: Prognostic factors in cryptococcal meningitis: A study of 111 cases. Ann Intern Med 80:176–181, 1974.

70. Is primary prophylaxis indicated against cryptococcosis?

Some clinicians have adopted primary prophylaxis because of the frequency of other fungal diseases (such as oral and esophageal candidiasis) as well as cryptococcosis. A study comparing fluconazole with clotrimazole troches found that fluconazole (200 mg/day) decreases the frequency of cryptococcosis and esophageal candidiasis, especially in persons at highest risk (i.e., $CD4^+$ count < 50/mm^3). However, no survival benefit was demonstrated, and it was estimated that > 11,000 doses of fluconazole were given to prevent 1 case of invasive fungal disease. Thus, fluconazole is not recommended at this time.

Havlir DV, et al: Prophylaxis with weekly versus daily fluconazole for fungal infections in patients with AIDS. Clin Infect Dis 27:1369–1375, 1998.

KAPOSI'S SARCOMA

71. What does Kaposi's sarcoma (KS) look like?

KS in HIV-infected patients is most often seen as cutaneous or oropharyngeal nodules ranging in size from 0.5–2.0 cm, although multiple nodules may coalesce. The nodules usually are raised and readily palpable, painless, and nonpruritic, with no evidence of inflammation or exudate. Rarely, lesions may become friable or verrucous (warty) and weep or bleed with trauma. Their color is usually blue or violet-to-purple; in darker-skinned patients, they often appear black. Nodules are often multiple when first diagnosed, reflecting the relatively aggressive nature of this malignancy in HIV infection. Any area of the body may be involved, although the palms of the hands are rarely affected despite the more common involvement of the soles of the feet.

72. Does a lesion suspicious for KS need to be biopsied?

In general, yes. If a patient with HIV infection has no previous diagnosis of KS or any opportunistic infection, suspicious lesions should be uniformly biopsied to establish a diagnosis. In a patient who has had previously diagnosed opportunistic infections and is under regular supervision and care, the need for confirming a clinical diagnosis by biopsy is less clear. However, there are other causes of pigmented cutaneous lesions in HIV infection. Patients with previously diagnosed KS do not need biopsy of new lesions unless they have been in remission after therapy.

73. Is KS sexually transmitted?

Investigators have demonstrated the presence of genetic material related to human herpesvirus 8 in KS tissue. This finding raises the possibility of the transmission of an infectious agent related to KS. No causative relationship has been established yet, but sexual transmission suggests clues as to why KS is more common in homosexual men than in other HIV risk groups.

Whitby D, et al: Detection of Kaposi's sarcoma associated herpesvirus in peripheral blood of HIV-infected individuals and progression to Kaposi's sarcoma. Lancet 346:799–802, 1995.

74. What treatment is recommended for KS?

There is no single therapeutic approach to KS in patients with AIDS. Often they have concurrent conditions that should receive priority because, with the exception of pulmonary KS, the disease is rarely threatening to the patient's immediate health. Although AIDS-associated KS is a more aggressive variant of KS, it is relatively benign compared with other AIDS-related processes. In addition, response rates of KS to systemic therapy have not been uniformly high, and myelosuppressive chemotherapy compromises other life-preserving antimicrobial or antiviral therapies. A general approach to AIDS-associated KS should start with an assessment of the possible course of disease and its effect on the patient's overall condition. The following table helps to distinguish between possible indolent disease from more aggressive KS.

Prognostic Variables in Kaposi's Sarcoma

PREDICTS INDOLENT COURSE	PREDICTS AGGRESSIVE COURSE
Few lesions (< 25)	Many lesions (> 25)
Low rate of growth	Rapid appearance of new lesions
No visceral KS identified	Intraoral or visceral lesions
No fevers, drenching night sweats, or weight loss	One or more constitutional symptoms
No prior opportunistic infection	One prior or concurrent opportunistic infection
Absolute $CD4^+$ count > $400/mm^3$	$CD4^+$ count < $200/mm^3$
Normal ESR	ESR > 40 mm/hr
HIV p24 antigen not detectable	HIV p24 detectable
Normal b2-microglobulin	b2-Microglobulin > 5
Normal blood counts	Leukopenia or anemia present

From Chaisson RE, Volberding PA: Clinical manifestations of HIV infection. In Mandell GL, et al (eds): Principles and Practice of Infectious Diseases, 4th ed. New York, Churchill Livingstone, 1995, p 1241.

75. What is the life expectancy for a patient with AIDS and KS?

There are no firm numbers with which to answer this question. Since survival statistics were first calculated for patients with AIDS, an AIDS-defining diagnosis of KS (as opposed to another malignancy or opportunistic infection) has carried the best prognosis because of the frequent appearance of KS at a less advanced point in the progressive immunosuppression. The exceptions are patients with pulmonary KS, which is a quickly progressive condition that often results in respiratory failure within 3–6 months.

76. Is KS always cutaneous?

Sites of Disease and Systemic Signs at Presentation in 49 Patients with Epidemic KS

Skin lesions		Lymph node involvement	
None	4 (8%)	None	19 (39%)
Generalized	13 (27%)	Generalized	30 (61%)
Locally aggressive	1 (2%)	Splenomegaly	5 (10%)
Visceral involvement		Systemic signs*	
Bone	1 (2%)	Fever and weight loss	9 (18%)
Hepatomegaly	5 (10%)	Fever only	4 (8%)
Lung	5 (10%)	Weight loss only	1 (2%)
GI tract	22 (45%)	Total with symptoms	14 (29%)

* Unexplained fever > 100°F (orally) and > 10% weight loss.
From DeVita VT, et al (eds): AIDS: Etiology, Diagnosis, Treatment and Prevention, 2nd ed. Philadelphia, J.B. Lippincott, 1988, p 252.

77. Does antiretroviral therapy treat KS?

In the more recent era of highly active antiretroviral therapy, regression of otherwise un-treated KS lesions has been widely described. It is now generally accepted practice, depending on the stage and severity of KS, to initiate effective antiretroviral therapy and observe the KS for any response. Suboptimal responses are then treated accordingly.

CYTOMEGALOVIRUS INFECTION

78. What is the cause of blindness experienced by some patients with AIDS?

Chorioretinitis caused by cytomegalovirus (CMV) is a vision-threatening infection formerly experienced by 5–10% of patients with AIDS during the course of their illness. It is an AIDS-defining diagnosis if it occurs as the initial opportunistic infection. Usually, however, this infec-tion appears later in the disease process, after a patient has already been diagnosed with AIDS. The incidence has declined dramatically during the era of more effective antiretroviral therapy.

Whitcup SM: Ocular manifestations of AIDS. JAMA 275:142–144, 1996.

79. How is CMV retinitis diagnosed?

Patients often present with nonspecific complaints of blurred vision, decreased visual acuity, or increasing "floaters," but occasionally CMV retinitis may present with a clear visual field cut. Ophthalmologic examination is essential and typically shows large white granular areas with he-morrhage. Diagnosis is based on this characteristic fundoscopic appearance because no tissue is obtained for pathologic examination. All patients with advanced HIV infection (CD4 counts < 100) should undergo routine retinal screening on a quarterly basis.

80. What drugs are available to treat CMV retinitis?

Ganciclovir, foscarnet, and cidofovir. The usual regimen consists of high-dose "induction" therapy for 2–3 weeks, followed by life-long suppressive therapy. Despite continued therapy, progression of retinitis is seen in most patients if no effective antiretroviral therapy is available.

Ganciclovir and foscarnet are both infused intravenously on a daily basis. A ganciclovir-im-pregnated bead can be implanted into the vitreous of the involved eye, allowing prolonged local therapy. Cidofovir is administered intravenously but is given only once weekly for the first 2 weeks, then every other week. Significant renal toxicity may limit its use. Despite this toxicity, its efficacy and infrequent dosing make it an attractive alternative.

SOCA Trial Group: Mortality in patients with the acquired immunodeficiency syndrome treated with either foscarnet or ganciclovir for cytomegalovirus retinitis. N Engl J Med 326:213–220, 1992.

SOCA Trial Group: Combination foscarnet and ganciclovir therapy vs monotherapy for the treatment of relapsed cytomegalovirus retinitis in patients with AIDS. Arch Ophthalmol 114:23–33, 1996.

81. What are the major toxicities of these medications?

The most common toxicity of **ganciclovir** is bone marrow suppression, usually seen as neu-tropenia and/or thrombocytopenia. Almost 40% of treated patients develop neutrophil counts < 1,000 cells/mm^3, and this side effect can become a dose-limiting toxicity. Also seen is CNS toxi-city manifested as confusion, headaches, or, rarely, seizures. Nausea, vomiting, and hepatitis also may be seen.

Foscarnet causes progressive renal dysfunction and potential renal failure. Over 25% of re-cipients have creatinine elevations > 2. Calcium, magnesium, phosphorus, and potassium bal-ances are upset and warrant close monitoring. Seizures can occur, and a fixed drug reaction with penile ulcerations has been described.

Cidofovir causes significant renal toxicity and must be administered in a controlled setting with probenecid and saline hydration.

82. Should all HIV-infected patients have eye exams?

Because CMV retinitis usually presents later in HIV infection, patients with less-advanced disease do not need an immediate referral to an ophthalmologist. However, a baseline exam should be performed, with subsequent exams as clinical symptoms and signs dictate. Patients with CD4+-lymphocyte counts chronically below 100/mm³ should be examined regardless of symptoms, with scheduled follow-up 2–3 times/year.

83. How else can CMV infection manifest in HIV infection besides chorioretinitis?

Interstitial pneumonia, colitis, esophagitis, adrenal insufficiency, and encephalitis.

84. Can anti-CMV and antiretroviral therapy be used in combination?

Most definitely. Because of overlapping toxicities, close observation must be maintained. Several studies have examined discontinuing CMV maintenance therapy in patients with retinitis whose CD4+ counts have increased to > 100–150 and whose HIV viral infection has been suppressed through effective antiretroviral therapy. Study participants have remained free of CMV relapse for up to 90 weeks. This approach should be considered only in close consultation with an experienced ophthalmologist.

HEPATITIS C AND AIDS

85. How do HIV and hepatitis C virus (HCV) interact?

HIV and HCV share mechanisms of transmission, particularly injecting drug use. It is estimated that 15–20% of HIV-infected patients are coinfected with HCV. Although HCV does not appear to alter the course of HIV infection, it appears to be facilitated, promoted, and exacerbated by HIV infection. In addition, several reports of increased hepatotoxicity of antiretroviral drugs in patients with HCV coinfection have been published, although this finding has not been uniformly seen. For the time being, coinfected patients should be monitored closely with more frequent transaminase assessments, especially after the initiation of a new medication regimen.

86. How is hepatitis C infection treated in HIV/HCV coinfection?

Few clinical studies have examined the response to HCV treatment in HIV infection. Some reports describe results similar to those in HIV-negative cohorts, whereas others describe a decreased response rate and increased intolerance. In select patients, combination therapy with ribavirin and interferon may be administered in consultation with an experienced HIV provider.

TUBERCULOSIS AND OTHER MYCOBACTERIOSES

87. Describe the relationship between AIDS and tuberculosis (TB).

Throughout most of the twentieth century, there was a steady, rapid decline in the morbidity and mortality attributed to TB. However, in the mid-1980s, this decline halted, and in 1986 the number of new TB cases increased for the first time since nationwide reporting was initiated in 1953. Several investigators cross-matched statewide public health registers for TB and AIDS cases and found a high number of patients on both lists. Multiple studies demonstrate the susceptibility of HIV patients to primary TB and the high rate of progression from latent to active TB in patients with preexisting latent TB and superimposed HIV immunosuppression. This finding is predictable from knowledge of the pathogenesis of each infection. Control of TB depends on cell-mediated immunity, precisely the most profound deficit in HIV infection. The incidence of TB in an HIV-infected population can be expected to mirror that population's previous exposure to *Mycobacterium tuberculosis*. Thus, immigrants, inner-city minorities, and IV drug users, with a high prevalence of both HIV infection and previous TB infection, develop a high number of active TB cases unless prophylaxis is used.

HIV is the strongest promoter of the development of active tuberculosis from latent infection. A person with latent TB is at a 5% lifetime risk of activation in the absence of HIV. With HIV infection, a person with latent TB is at a 5–9% risk per year of developing active disease.

Shafer RW, Edlin BR: Tuberculosis in patients infected with human immunodeficiency virus: Perspective on the past decade. Clin Infect Dis 22:683–704, 1996.

88. Does TB differ in presentation in HIV-infected patients?

TB in HIV-infected patients remains primarily a pulmonary disease, but the incidence of extrapulmonary disease is much higher in the HIV-infected population compared with the general population. Miliary and disseminated TB are seen more often, and "typical" apical or cavitary disease is less common. Although the symptoms of chronic productive cough and hemoptysis are less common, TB in HIV infection remains a progressive, febrile, wasting disease. The more "typical" TB cases appear in HIV-infected patients with a better preserved immune status, whereas the more "atypical" presentations are seen in patients further along in HIV-related illness. There appears to be a temporal clustering of TB cases around the time of an AIDS diagnosis.

Jones BE, et al: Relationship of the manifestations of tuberculosis to CD4 cell counts in patients with human immunodeficiency virus infection. Am Rev Respir Dis 148:1292–1297, 1993.

Long R, et al: The chest roentgenogram in pulmonary tuberculosis patients seropositive for human immunodeficiency virus type 1. Chest 99:123–127, 1991.

89. Is TB more contagious in patients with AIDS?

M. tuberculosis, a communicable pathogen in people with normal immunity, is the rare organism that may be transmitted from an HIV-infected person to a noninfected person. It may be that patients with AIDS are less contagious than non-AIDS patients, but the bottom line is that any patient capable of aerosolizing respiratory droplets containing *M. tuberculosis* is contagious. From the other perspective, patients with AIDS are much more susceptible to TB infection, and care should be taken to minimize new exposures.

90. Describe the treatment of TB in HIV infection.

Thus far, TB appears to be a curable infection in HIV-infected patients. The recommended treatment is currently the same for both HIV-infected and non-HIV-infected patients—isoniazid, 300 mg/day, plus rifampin, 600 mg/day, plus pyrazinamide, 20–30 mg/kg/day, for the first 2 months of therapy. Ethambutol, 25 mg/kg/day, is added initially to protect against the possibility of drug resistance. Directly observed therapy (DOT) is the standard of care. No further maintenance or suppressive therapy is advised.

Care must be taken, however, when TB and HIV are treated simultaneously. The metabolism of the drugs that have revolutionized HIV treatment (nonnucleosides and protease inhibitors) is affected by the cytochrome p450 system. Rifampin is one of the strongest known inducers of this system. Combining rifampin with these agents may result in subtherapeutic levels of the antiretrovirals and subsequent HIV treatment failure and drug-resistant HIV. Rifabutin may be substituted for rifampin, decreasing the induction of cytochrome p450. This combined therapy must be supervised by physicians experienced with both diseases.

Centers for Disease Control and Prevention: Prevention and treatment of tuberculosis among patients infected with human immunodeficiency virus: principles of therapy and revised recommendations. MMWR 47(RR-20), 1998.

91. Is purified protein derivative (PPD) testing of any use in HIV-infected patients?

The benefits derived from PPD skin testing depend on the prevalence of underlying TB infection in the screened population and the degree of immunosuppression already present. A PPD test currently is recommended in all patients shortly after the diagnosis of HIV infection. Patients with a reaction > 5 mm should receive isoniazid prophylaxis for 9 months, regardless of age at the time of diagnosis.

92. What about TB reporting and contact tracing?

TB remains a reportable disease in all states, and cases should be reported. This reporting is wholly independent from reporting of HIV infection or cases of AIDS. Because many localities have protocols to protect the confidentiality of HIV-infected patients, often the report of a TB case may not include HIV status. In areas where these protocols are not present, it is a good idea to add this information, which assists the local health department in prioritizing its cases.

93. Should patients with TB be screened for HIV infection?

Absolutely. Because a larger number of TB cases are now related to HIV infection and because early diagnosis of HIV infection has many benefits, all patients with TB should be asked to consent to HIV testing. In many large cities, the rates of HIV positivity are as high as 30–40%.

94. What other mycobacterial infections are seen in HIV-infected patients?

Very early in the HIV epidemic, a large number of patients had disseminated *M. avium* complex (MAC) infection. Autopsy series have demonstrated a prevalence of up to 50% at the time of death from AIDS, and clinical studies have shown an annual risk of approximately 20% in patients with AIDS. Multiple other mycobacteria have been found to cause infection in patients with AIDS, but the only one seen in significant numbers is *M. kansasii.*

Nightingale SD, et al: Incidence of *M. avium-intracellulare* complex bacteremia in human immunodeficiency virus-positive patients. J Infect Dis 165:1082–1085, 1992.

95. How does infection with MAC present?

MAC infection usually is associated with advanced HIV disease, and the patient often has multiple concurrent conditions. Thus, the individual contribution of MAC infection to the patient's overall condition can be difficult to ascertain. Usually seen are systemic symptoms such as fever, night sweats, weight loss, fatigue, and malaise. Laboratory exam may reveal increasing anemia or mild hepatitis. Chronic diarrhea with abdominal pain and/or malabsorption is also seen. The frequency of GI symptoms and pathologic changes suggest that the GI tract may be the portal of entry.

Diagnosis of MAC infection is made by culture of biopsy specimens or blood. The yield from blood cultures is excellent, and there is often only a short delay before results are available. Positive results can be reported in as few as 5–10 days. Specimens from biopsies quickly reveal acid-fast organisms on stains, thus facilitating the diagnosis.

96. Is there a standard therapy for MAC in patients with AIDS?

The development of the macrolides, clarithromycin and azithromycin, has opened a new door for treatment options in patients with MAC. For the first time, regimens containing these compounds have demonstrated high rates of blood culture sterilization and clinical improvement. The current recommendation is to include one of these agents in addition to at least one second drug—usually ethambutol.

Centers for Disease Control and Prevention: Recommendations on prophylaxis and therapy for disseminated *Mycobacterium avium* complex for adults and adolescents infected with human immunodeficiency virus. MMWR 42(RR-9):14–20, 1993.

97. Is there an effective prophylaxis against MAC?

Three drugs have been approved for prophylaxis against MAC: rifabutin, clarithromycin, and azithromycin. Rifabutin resulted in improved quality of life and decreased the rate of MAC from 18% to 9% in a group of patients with AIDS and a CD4[+] count < 200/mm^3. Clarithromycin decreased the rate of MAC from 12.6% to 4.5% in patients with AIDS and a CD4[+] count < 100/mm^3. This trial also demonstrated a survival benefit with clarithromycin prophylaxis.

Two concerns arise with prophylactic drugs. First, rifabutin may cause cross-resistance to rifampin in a patient with TB who is inadequately evaluated and then treated with this single drug inadvertently. Rifabutin also has significant pharmacologic interactions with antiretroviral drugs. Second, many MAC breakthroughs on clarithromycin prophylaxis have been shown to be clarithromycin-resistant, thus negating the efficacy of the most active drug used in treatment.

SYPHILIS AND AIDS

98. In which HIV-infected patients should a serologic test for syphilis (STS) be obtained?

Every HIV-infected patient needs an STS as well as a detailed history for all sexually transmitted diseases and past treatments. A growing body of literature suggests the possibility of an accelerated course and unusual progression of syphilis in patients also infected with HIV. With this finding in mind, along with the fact that the routes of transmission for HIV and syphilis are similar, all patients with a positive serology for one infection should be tested for the other.

Hook EW: Syphilis and HIV infection. J Infect Dis 160:530–534, 1989.

99. What if the STS is positive but the patient gives no history of syphilis?

Because of the concern about altered progression of syphilis in HIV infection, the discrimination between early syphilis, early latent syphilis, and late latent syphilis may be less important, because most practitioners aggressively treat early infection. A question does arise over the use of lumbar puncture (LP) to evaluate neurosyphilis. Currently LP is not recommended in early syphilis but is recommended in late latent syphilis (> 1-year duration). With no patient history to guide treatment decisions, it may be best to err on the side of caution and proceed with LP in HIV-infected patients, especially those with any neurologic signs or symptoms or a serum antibody titer > 1:32. An inquiry to the local public health office may provide additional history that the patient has not recalled.

Centers for Disease Control and Prevention: Recommendations for diagnosing and treating syphilis in HIV-infected patients. MMWR 37:600– 608, 1988.

100. Which HIV-infected patients with syphilis need a lumbar puncture (LP)?

Although a few authorities recommend an LP in all patients, most agree that patients with a clear episode of primary or secondary syphilis do not need an LP. Examination of the CSF should be done for all HIV-infected patients with syphilis of > 1 year's duration or any clinical signs or symptoms of CNS involvement. Patients with early syphilis whose serologic titers increase or fail to decrease appropriately (4-fold in 6 months) also should undergo an LP to evaluate CNS involvement before retreatment.

101. What is the treatment for neurosyphilis in HIV-infected patients?

It is the same whether or not the patient has HIV infection: aqueous crystalline penicillin G, 2.4 mU IV every 4 hours (12–24 mu/day) for 10–14 days. No non–penicillin-based therapy is considered wholly satisfactory. Patients with remote histories of unclear penicillin allergy may need skin testing.

102. If a chancre is present, is initial therapy changed?

The recommended regimen remains 1 dose of benzathine penicillin G, 2.4 mU IM, but many authorities treat primary syphilis more aggressively in patients coinfected with HIV and administer a total of 7.2 mU given as 2.4 mU weekly for 3 consecutive weeks.

Musher DM: How much penicillin cures early syphilis? Ann Intern Med 109:849–851, 1988.

103. How should patients with HIV infection and primary syphilis be followed up?

Patients should have repeat serologic testing at 1, 2, 3, 6, 9, and 12 months. If at any time there is a 4-fold increase in titer, an LP should be done. If by 3 months there has not been a 4-fold decrease in titer, the CSF should be examined.

104. Is HIV-related syphilis reportable to local health authorities?

Yes. The presence of concomitant HIV infection does not change the reporting requirement for syphilis.

105. Should all patients with syphilis be tested for HIV?

Absolutely. HIV infection may alter the course of syphilis or the response to treatment. Obviously, there are common risk factors for both infections. In addition, any condition that causes open sores in the genital area can facilitate the transmission of HIV.

TOXOPLASMOSIS

106. What are the most common causes of CNS mass lesions in AIDS?

Cerebral toxoplasmosis and primary CNS lymphoma. Other causes include progressive multifocal leukoencephalopathy (PML), cryptococcoma, tuberculoma, bacterial and fungal abscesses, and metastatic neoplastic disease. The increasing use of TMP-SMX as prophylaxis for PCP may coincidentially decrease the proportion of CNS mass lesions attributable to toxoplasmosis.

107. How is the differentiation between CNS toxoplasmosis and lymphoma made?

Most clinicians recommend empirical treatment for toxoplasmosis (pyrimethamine, 100-mg loading dose, then 25 mg/day, and sulfadiazine, 4–6 gm/day in divided doses). Response is judged clinically as well as on CT scanning. Response should be rapid (3–5 days). If it does not occur, an etiology other than toxoplasmosis is suggested.

108. What are the characteristic CT scan findings in CNS toxoplasmosis?

CT FINDING	TOXOPLASMOSIS	LYMPHOMA
Area involved	Deep gray matter and basal ganglia	White matter, periventricular areas
Mass effect	Yes	Yes
Enhancement	Ring-enhancement	Weakly, not ring-shaped
Number of lesions	Multiple	1–2

109. How long should patients with AIDS be treated for toxoplasmosis?

This AIDS-related infection appears to require life-long suppressive therapy. Chronic pyrimethamine and sulfadiazine therapy should be continued indefinitely. Clindamycin is used in sulfa-intolerant patients.

Porter SB, Sande MA: Toxoplasmosis of the central nervous system in the acquired immunodeficiency syndrome. N Engl J Med 327:1643–1648, 1992.

110. Should primary toxoplasmosis prophylaxis be given?

Yes. Patients positive for toxoplasma antibodies who also have a CD4+ count < 100 should receive primary prophylaxis. TMP, 160 mg, and SMX, 800 mg, is the preferred daily regimen, providing protection against both PCP and toxoplasmosis. If this regimen is not tolerated, dapsone-pyrimethamine or atovaquone can be given.

Podzamczer D, et al: Intermittent trimethoprim-sulfamethoxazole compared with dapsone-pyrimethamine for simultaneous primary prophylaxis of *Pneumocystis* pneumonia and toxoplasmosis in patients infected with HIV. Ann Intern Med 122:755–761, 1995.

BIBLIOGRAPHY

1. Centers for Disease Control: 1999 USPHS/IDSA guidelines for the prevention of opportunistic infections in persons infected with human immunodeficiency virus. MMWR 48(RR-10):1–66, 1999.
2. Holmes KK, et al: Sexually Transmitted Diseases, 2nd ed. New York, McGraw-Hill, 1990.
3. Mandell GL, Bennett JE, Dolin R: Principles and Practice of Infectious Diseases, 5th ed. New York, Churchill Livingstone, 2000.
4. Sande MA, Volberding PA: The Medical Management of AIDS, 6th ed. Philadelphia, W.B. Saunders, 1999.

Websites
1. www.HIVATIS.org: Web site with current and archived guidelines for HIV treatment and opportunistic infection treatment and prophylaxis.
2. www.medscape.com
3. http://hivinsite.ucsf.edu/

14. NEUROLOGY

Loren A. Rolak, M.D.

*This apoplexy, as I take it, is a kind of lethargy, an't please your lord-
ship; a kind of sleeping in the blood, a whoreson tingling. . . . It hath it
original from much grief, from study and perturbation of the brain. I
have read the cause of his effects in Galen. It is a kind of deafness.*
William Shakespeare (1564-1616)
Description of stroke, Henry IV, Part II

APPROACH TO THE PATIENT

1. What is the initial approach to evaluating patients complaining of neurologic symptoms?
The first step is to localize the lesion to a specific part of the nervous system. Only then
should an etiology be sought, since defining the anatomy usually implies certain causes. Because
each part of the brain, spinal cord, and peripheral nervous system has such specialized functions,
lesions in these areas produce specific clinical deficits. Therefore, symptoms can often be localized, sometimes to the millimeter, to discrete parts of the nervous system.

2. What are the most important regions for anatomic localization?
For clinical purposes, the most important neuroanatomy is limited to a few large regions.
The regions where lesions should be localized are (proceeding from distal to proximal):

1. Muscle
2. Neuromuscular junction
3. Peripheral nerve
4. Root
5. Spinal cord
6. Brainstem
7. Cerebellum
8. Subcortical brain
9. Cortical brain

3. How are symptoms localized to these neuroanatomic regions?
As in all aspects of medicine, the history guides the diagnosis. By asking the proper questions during the history, a clinician can accurately localize most neurologic lesions.
A useful system for diagnosis is to begin distally (with the muscle) and to ask the patient
questions about each part of the neurologic anatomy, working backward (proximally) from the
muscle, through the neuromuscular junction, peripheral nerve, root, spinal cord, cerebellum,
brainstem, subcortex, and ending with the cortex of the brain. By sequentially asking about each
of these areas, you can "examine" the patient thoroughly. Only after the lesion is localized by
means of history-taking should the physical examination begin. If localization of the lesion is
still unclear after a careful history, do not begin the physical examination—take a better history!

4. Which clinical features of muscle disease can be elicited by the history?
Muscle disease (myopathy) causes symmetric proximal weakness without sensory loss.
Therefore, questions should elicit these symptoms.
1. **Proximal leg weakness:** Can the patient arise from a chair, get out of a car, get off the
toilet, or go up stairs without using his hands?
2. **Proximal arm weakness:** Can the patient lift or carry objects, such as a briefcase, school
books, children, or grocery bags?
3. **Symmetric weakness:** Is the weakness relatively symmetric? Are both sides affected?
(Although most generalized processes are slightly asymmetric, weakness essentially confined to
one limb or one side of the body is unlikely to be a myopathy.)
4. **Sensory loss:** Is there numbness or other loss of normal sensation? (Pain and cramping
may occur with some myopathies, but actual sensory loss should not occur with disease that is
confined to the muscle.)

5. After a history of muscle disease is elicited, what findings can be expected on physical examination?

The examination should show proximal symmetric weakness without sensory loss. Tone is usually normal or mildly decreased, and reflexes are also normal or mildly decreased. There is seldom significant atrophy unless the process is advanced.

6. Which clinical features of neuromuscular junction disease can be elicited by history?

Neuromuscular junction diseases closely resemble myopathies, causing proximal symmetric weakness without sensory loss. However, the hallmark of disease of the neuromuscular junction is **fatigability**. The weakness worsens with use and recovers with rest. Since strength improves with rest, this fatigability does not usually present as a steady progressive decline throughout the day. Instead, it fluctuates as the muscle first fatigues, then recovers, then fatigues again, then recovers, etc. (Almost every medical symptom can be worse at the end of the day. Look for variability or fluctuation as the characteristic of neuromuscular junction fatigability.)

Another feature of neuromuscular junction diseases is that they are usually extremely **proximal**. They often involve muscles of the face resulting in drooping of the eyelids (ptosis), double vision, difficulty in chewing and swallowing, slurred speech, and facial weakness.

7. After a history of neuromuscular junction problems is elicited, what findings can be expected on physical examination?

Examination should show proximal symmetric weakness without sensory loss that results in fatigue. Repetitive testing weakens the muscles, which regain their strength with a minute or so of rest. Similarly, sustained muscular activity (such as upward gaze) leads to fatigability and progressive weakness (such as ptosis). Tone, reflexes, and muscle bulk are all normal.

8. Which clinical feature of peripheral neuropathies can be elicited by history?

Peripheral neuropathies cause distal, often asymmetric weakness with sensory changes. Atrophy and fasciculations may also appear. Questions should elicit these symptoms:

1. **Distal weakness in the legs:** Does the patient wear out the toes of his shoes or catch his toes and trip, as would be expected with a footdrop?

2. **Distal weakness in the hands:** Does the patient have trouble with his grip, or frequently drop things?

3. **Asymmetric weakness:** Is the process asymmetric? (Some neuropathies are distal, symmetric, stocking-and-glove neuropathies, but most are asymmetric, such as carpal tunnel syndrome or radial nerve palsy.)

4. **Denervation changes:** Has the patient noticed a shrinkage or wasting of the muscle (atrophy) or quivering, twitching muscles (fasciculations)?

5. **Sensory changes:** Is there numbness, tingling, or paresthesia?

9. After a history of peripheral neuropathy is elicited, what findings can be expected on physical examination?

Distal, often asymmetric weakness, with atrophy and fasciculations, and with sensory loss such as decreased pinprick, vibration, and occasionally position sense. Tone is normal or decreased, and reflexes are diminished. Sometimes, there are also trophic changes, such as loss of hair and nails and smooth, shiny skin.

10. Which clinical features of root diseases (radiculopathies) can be elicited by history?

The hallmark of root disease is pain. This pain is usually severe, described as sharp, hot, or electric, and commonly radiates down an arm or leg. In addition, radiculopathies usually have similar features to peripheral neuropathies: denervation (weakness, atrophy, fasciculations) with sensory loss. The weakness may be proximal (the most common radiculopathies in the arms involve C5/6 muscles, which are proximal) or distal (the most common radiculopathies in the legs involve L5/S1 muscles, which are distal). The history is therefore the same as for peripheral neuropathies, but with the added element of pain.

11. After a history of radiculopathy is elicited, what findings can be expected on physical examination?

The examination will show weakness in one myotomal group of muscles, such as C5/6 in the arm or L5/S1 in the leg, sometimes with atrophy and fasciculations. Tone is normal or decreased, and the reflex in those muscles is diminished or absent. There is sensory loss in a dermatomal distribution. Sometimes, maneuvers that stretch the root, such as straight leg raising, will elicit the pain.

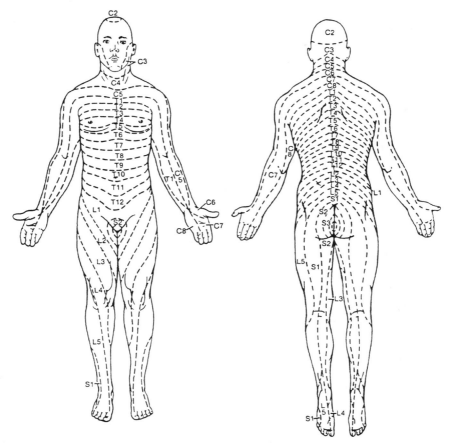

Map of the sensory dermatomes in the anterior and posterior aspects. (From Delong RN: The Neurologic Examination. Hagerstown, MD, Harper & Row, 1979, with permission.)

12. Spinal cord lesions cause a triad of symptoms. Name these.

1. **A sensory level.** This level, which may occur as a band of sensory change around the thorax or abdomen or as a sharp level below which sensation is lost, is the hallmark of spinal cord disease.
2. **Distal, usually symmetric weakness**
3. **Bowel and bladder changes** (sphincter dysfunction)

13. Which questions should be asked during the history to elicit the symptoms of spinal cord disease?

1. **Distal leg weakness:** Does the patient drag his toes or trip because of the leg weakness? Lesions in the pyramidal tract, also called the corticospinal tract or upper motor neuron, cause weakness that is usually greatest distally and thus can mimic a peripheral neuropathy.

2. **Spasticity:** Are the patient's legs stiff? Pyramidal tract weakness causes spasticity, and many patients report their legs are stiff and that their knees won't bend when they walk.

3. **Sensory level:** Patients sometimes describe this as feeling like a belt or band or "tight swimming trunks" around their waist or abdomen.

4. **Sphincter dysfunction:** Is there retention or incontinence of the bowel or bladder? The bladder is usually much more sensitive to spinal cord injury than the bowel.

14. After a history of spinal cord disease is elicited, what findings can be expected on physical examination?

Examination of a person with spinal cord disease shows distal weakness, usually worse in the legs than the arms, and usually worse in the extensors (dorsiflexors of the feet and extensors of the wrists and fingers) than in the flexors. Tone is increased, reflexes are brisk, and there are often extensor plantar reflexes (positive Babinski signs). Superficial reflexes, such as anal wink, sphincter tone, cremasteric reflex, and abdominal reflexes, are commonly lost. A sensory level can often be found, below which all sensory modalities are diminished.

15. Which clinical features of brainstem disease can be elicited by history?

Cranial nerve abnormalities are the hallmark of brainstem disease. The brainstem is essentially the spinal cord with cranial nerves embedded in it, so symptoms of brainstem disease generally consist of a combination of **long-tract findings** (such as weakness from the pyramidal tract, numbness from the spinothalamic tract, etc.) plus symptoms of cranial nerve impingement. Because the long tracts cross (decussate), the weakness and numbness are not in the distribution of a level, but rather in a hemiparesis or hemianesthesia. Because of the crossing of these long tracts, damage to one side of the brainstem, affecting the cranial nerves on that side, usually results in long tract symptoms that affect the opposite side of the body. These **crossed symptoms** are another hallmark of brainstem disease—e.g., weakness of one side of the face and the opposite side of the body.

16. What are the symptoms of cranial nerve lesions in the brainstem?

Cranial nerve (CN) lesions commonly cause the big "D's":

Diplopia—CN III, IV, VI
Decreased facial sensation—CN V
Decreased facial strength—CN VII
Dizziness—CN VIII
Deafness—CN VIII
Dysarthria and dysphagia—CN IX, X, XII

The history therefore should focus on eliciting these symptoms:

• Is there diplopia, facial weakness or numbness, dizziness, deafness, dysarthria, or dysphagia?
• Are there long-tract findings, such as hemiparesis or hemisensory loss?
• Are the findings crossed or bilateral?

17. After a history of brainstem disease is elicited, what findings can be expected on physical examination?

Examination shows a combination of cranial nerve and long-tract abnormalities.

Checking the **cranial nerves** may reveal ptosis, abnormalities of extraocular movements, diplopia, nystagmus, decreased corneal reflexes, facial weakness or numbness, decreased hearing, dysarthria, paralysis of the palate, decreased gag reflex, or tongue deviation.

Long-tract abnormalities may include hemiparesis, with a pyramidal pattern of distal weakness with increased reflexes, increased tone, and a positive Babinski sign. Hemisensory loss may include decreased sensation to one or more modalities.

18. Which clinical features of cerebellar disease can be elicited by history?

The cerebellum is responsible for smoothing out voluntary movements, and impairments produce abnormalities in the rate and rhythm of movements (clumsiness and lack of coordination). Questions should focus on incoordination in the legs and the arms:

1. **Legs:** Does the patient have a staggering, drunken walk? Most laymen use the term "drunken" walk to describe cerebellar disease. (Drinking alcohol does in fact impair the cerebellum, and the characteristic wide-based, ataxic, staggering gait of the intoxicated person is caused by cerebellar dysfunction.)

2. **Arms:** Does the patient have difficulty putting a key in a lock, lighting a cigarette, or performing other target-directed movements? The cerebellar tremor is worse with voluntary, intentional movements that require accurate placement. Fine, coordinated movements, such as extending a key and inserting it into the narrow slot of a lock, are perfect examples of difficult tasks for people with cerebellar lesions.

19. After a history of cerebellar disease is elicited, what findings can be expected on physical examination?

Patients with cerebellar disease usually have a staggering gait and difficulty with tandem walking. When they slide a heel down a shin, it wavers unsteadily. In the arms, there is a tremor and wavering when touching the examiner's finger, the patient's own nose, or other targets. Similarly, rapid alternating movements in the limbs are irregular in rate and rhythm.

20. How can the history and neurologic exam distinguish between subcortical and cortical brain disease?

Clinically, disease of the brain itself can affect either subcortical or cortical regions. The main features differentiating these are:

1. **Presence of specific cortical deficits:** Does the patient have aphasia (left hemisphere cortex) or visuospatial deficits (right hemisphere cortex)?

2. **Pattern of motor and sensory loss:** If the face and arm are involved, the lesion is cortical; if the face, arm, and leg are involved, it is subcortical.

3. **Type of sensory change:** Primary sensations, such as pain, temperature, touch, position, and vibration are registered in the thalamus (subcortex) and are not much affected by cortical lesions. Deficits seen with cortical damage are secondary sensory changes, such as astereognosis, agraphesthesia, and loss of two-point discrimination. (These are difficult to elicit by history.)

4. **Visual field deficits:** Because visual fibers run subcortically (in the optic tract, lateral geniculate, and optic radiations), cortical lesions do not cause field cuts. (Damage to the occipital cortex causes field cuts, but since there are no motor or sensory fibers there, it does not cause any other focal deficits.)

5. **Involuntary movements:** Most movement disorders are thought to arise from subcortical structures, such as the basal ganglia. A history of parkinsonism, chorea, dystonia, or hemiballismus thus suggests a subcortical lesion.

6. **Seizures:** Seizures arise from the paroxysmal discharge of neurons, almost exclusively in the cortex. Subcortical lesions seldom cause seizures.

21. How does the pattern of motor and sensory deficits differ between cortical and subcortical involvement?

Motor and sensory neurons corresponding to the various regions of the body are arranged across the cortex in a manner described as a **homunculus**. The parts of the body are draped upside-down over the surface of the outer cortex, with a large face and lips, small neck, a large hand and thumb, and a small trunk, such that a lesion localized to the cortex will result in a deficit in one or more of the anatomic regions. The leg, however, is not over the outside cortex but instead hangs down in the interhemispheric fissure, in the cortex deep between the two brain hemispheres. Most cortical processes, such as a stroke, affect the face and arm but cannot "get to" the leg fibers between the hemispheres, sparing involvement of the leg in these conditions.

Deeper in the brain, in subcortical regions, fibers from the face, arm, and leg lie close together in the pyramidal tract or spinothalamic tract. Even a small lesion in these tracts can affect the face, arm, and leg.

So, if the face and arm are involved, the lesion is cortical. If the face, arm, and leg are involved, it is subcortical.

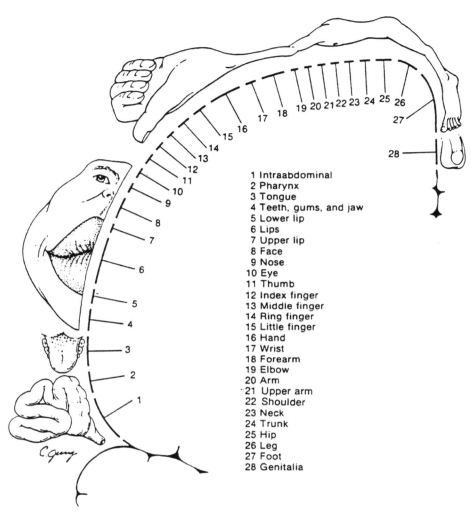

1 Intraabdominal
2 Pharynx
3 Tongue
4 Teeth, gums, and jaw
5 Lower lip
6 Lips
7 Upper lip
8 Face
9 Nose
10 Eye
11 Thumb
12 Index finger
13 Middle finger
14 Ring finger
15 Little finger
16 Hand
17 Wrist
18 Forearm
19 Elbow
20 Arm
21 Upper arm
22 Shoulder
23 Neck
24 Trunk
25 Hip
26 Leg
27 Foot
28 Genitalia

Homunculus showing sensory and motor representation over the cortex. (From Penfield W, Rasmussen T: The Cerebral Cortex. New York, Macmillan, 1950, with permission.)

MYOPATHIES

22. What are the most important myopathies?

- Muscular dystrophies: Duchenne's, myotonic, etc.
- Congenital myopathies: Kearns-Sayre, central-core, etc.
- Inflammatory myopathies: polymyositis, dermatomyositis, etc.
- Toxic myopathies: alcohol, zidovudine, clofibrate, steroids, etc.
- Endocrine myopathies: hypothyroidism, hypoadrenalism, etc.
- Infectious myopathies: trichinosis, AIDS, etc.

23. Which of the myopathies are most common on the medical ward?

Polymyositis is the most common. It is an inflammatory, probably autoimmune, disease of the muscles, characterized by the subacute onset of proximal weakness of the arms and legs, often with dysphagia. It may accompany connective tissue disease (such as systemic lupus erythematosus) or vasculitis but usually appears alone. It runs a variable course but can be severe or even fatal.

Dermatomyositis is a distinct clinical entity characterized by similar subacute proximal muscle weakness in association with a rash, often over the face and trunk. Like polymyositis, dermatomyositis may occur alone or in conjunction with other connective tissue diseases. There may also be an increased incidence of concomitant malignancies.

Treatment for polymyositis and dermatomyositis is the same and involves high-dose oral prednisone (at least 1 mg/kg body weight/day) as the mainstay of therapy. Azathioprine or methotrexate may be used in steroid-resistant cases or when complications develop from steroid use. IV immunoglobulin (IVIG), though expensive, may also be safe and effective, especially during acute exacerbations.

Piota PH, et al: Myositis: Immunologic contributions to understanding cause, pathogenesis and therapy. Ann Intern Med 122:715–724, 1995.

24. Which tests and procedures are used in the diagnostic evaluation of a patient with a myopathy?

The diagnostic evaluation of a myopathy generally entails a triad of tests:
1. Serum creatine kinase (CK)
2. Electromyography (EMG)
3. Muscle biopsy

Muscle destruction usually liberates **CK**, making elevation of this enzyme a good screening test for muscle disease. (The MM isoenzyme of CK is the most common.) An **EMG** is done by inserting a fine needle electrode into the muscle to record the electrical impulses related to contractions. Myopathies cause low-voltage, short-duration muscle contractions, and this test can thus confirm the presence of myopathy. Finally, a **muscle biopsy** is often needed to define the cause of a myopathy, since most myopathies are clinically similar. The tissue may show inflammation (polymyositis), mitochondrial abnormalities, or other specific diseases.

NEUROMUSCULAR JUNCTION

25. Name the most common neuromuscular junction disease seen on the medical ward.

Myasthenia gravis (MG). MG has a prevalence of 1 case/10,000 population and a bimodal age distribution, occurring in young women in their teens and 20s and old men aged 60 and above. It presents with proximal weakness, especially ptosis and diplopia, with fatigue on use and recovery with rest. Because MG can involve the respiratory muscles, pulmonary failure is the most feared complication.

26. How is MG treated?

MG is an autoimmune disease in which patients produce antibodies that destroy the acetylcholine receptors on muscle. Acetylcholine is the neurotransmitter that makes muscles contract. Treatment consists of acetylcholinesterase inhibitors, which block the enzymatic breakdown of acetylcholine, thus allowing for greater concentrations of acetylcholine at the receptor. **Pyridostigmine** (Mestinon) is the drug of choice, but immunosuppressive drugs, including prednisone, azathioprine, and cyclosporine, are often necessary to attack the underlying autoimmune process. Plasmapheresis and IVIG have also been shown to be helpful, usually to provide rapid (but transient) improvement during myasthenic crisis. Surgical thymectomy is probably beneficial, but its role in treating MG remains controversial.

Gronseth GS, Barohn RJ: Practice Parameter: Thymectomy for autoimmune myasthenia gravis. Neurology 55:7–15, 2000.

27. Are some drugs contraindicated for use in patients with neuromuscular junction diseases?
Some drugs can worsen these diseases, including
1. Aminoglycosides
2. Tetracycline antibiotics
3. Corticosteroids (acutely)
4. Thyroid hormone
5. Phenothiazines (i.e., chlorpromazine)
6. Quinidine
7. Lidocaine
8. Propranolol
9. Lithium
10. Dilantin

28. What is the second most common disease causing neuromuscular junction problems?
Lambert-Eaton myasthenic syndrome (LEMS). Like MG, LEMS is an autoimmune condition, although its target is the presynaptic voltage-gated calcium channel involved in acetylcholine release, not the receptor. It is commonly seen in association with occult carcinoma, especially small-cell carcinoma of the lung. LEMS clinically resembles MG because of fluctuating proximal weakness. It is generally treated by therapy for the underlying neoplasm, sometimes accompanied by plasmapheresis and other immune suppressors, especially in cases where no occult cancer can be found. Guanidine may provide symptomatic relief.
Sanders DB: LEMS: Pathogenesis and treatment. Semin Neurol 14(2):111–117, 1994.

29. How do we differentiate myasthenia gravis from Lambert-Eaton myasthenic syndrome?
1. Although MG and LEMS strongly resemble each other clinically, LEMS does not involve the extraocular muscles, so ptosis and diplopia, which are very common with MG, do not occur.
2. By EMG testing, repetitive stimulation of the nerve in MG shows a progressive decline in each muscle contraction, documenting the fatigability with repetitive stimulation. With LEMS, there is a paradoxical increase, rather than decrease, in successive muscle contractions when the nerve is repetitively stimulated. This is due to a progressive increase in the amount of acetylcholine released presynaptically by the stimulated nerve.
3. Blood tests are now available to detect antibodies against acetylcholine receptors (MG) or voltage gated calcium channels (LEMS).

30. What triad of tests is useful in the diagnostic evaluation of patients with neuromuscular junction problems?
1. Tensilon test
2. Serum antibody levels
3. Repetitive stimulation on EMG

31. Explain the Tensilon test.
The Tensilon test is performed by administering a small dose of intravenous **edrophonium** (Tensilon), which is a powerful but transient acetylcholinesterase inhibitor. This agent causes a reversal of weakness within 30 seconds to 2 minutes, which lasts approximately 10 minutes before returning to baseline. For example, ptosis of the eyes may transiently resolve after a Tensilon test.

PERIPHERAL NEUROPATHIES

32. Which peripheral neuropathies are seen most commonly on the medical ward?
Peripheral neuropathies are probably the most frequent neurologic problems seen on a medical ward, unlike myopathies and neuromuscular junction diseases, which are rare. The most common peripheral neuropathies can be remembered by the mnemonic DANG THE RAPIST:
D—Diabetes
A—Alcohol
N—Nutritional (vitamin deficiencies, etc.)
G—Guillain-Barré
T—Trauma (carpal tunnel, etc.)
H—Hereditary
E—Environmental (toxins, drugs)
R—Remote effects of cancer
A—Amyloid
P—Porphyria
I—Inflammation (collagen vascular disease, etc.)
S—Syphilis
T—Tumors

33. The evaluation of a patient with a peripheral neuropathy usually begins with which study?

An electromyogram and nerve conduction velocity (EMG/NCV) study. This test applies electrical current directly over the nerves and uses an electrode to record the speed with which the nerves conduct the current. It thus documents the extent and degree of slowing and impairment of nerve conduction. The EMG uses a needle electrode within the muscles to record muscle contractions and thus show denervation of the muscles.

Once a neuropathy has been confirmed, workup for the etiology focuses on the conditions listed in Question 32, requiring evaluation for diabetes, alcoholism, B_{12} deficiency, metabolic abnormalities such as thyroid disease or uremia, familial illnesses, toxic exposure, collagen vascular disease, etc. A spinal tap is often needed to detect inflammatory neuropathies. Only rarely is a nerve biopsy required. The neuropathy usually resolves with treatment of the underlying etiology.

Zochodne DW: Diabetic neuropathies. Curr Treat Options Neurol 2:23–29, 2000.

34. What is the most common entrapment neuropathy?

Carpal tunnel syndrome, caused by compression of the median nerve at the wrist. Most commonly the result of mechanical overuse, it usually presents with symptoms of pain and tingling in the hand (especially at night), weakness, and/or numbness. Pain in the hand at night is considered carpal tunnel syndrome until proven otherwise. There may be no objective neurologic findings in this condition. As with other peripheral neuropathies, EMG/NCV studies are helpful in making the diagnosis. Treatment is usually surgical, involving open or endoscopic release at the wrist, although conservative measures (such as wrist splinting) may be sufficient for mild cases.

Bracker MS, Ralph LP: The numb arm and hand. Am Fam Physician 31:103–116, 1995.

35. What is the Guillain-Barré syndrome (GBS)?

GBS is an acute inflammatory polyradiculopathy in which there is inflammation of the nerve roots and peripheral nerves. It is presumably autoimmune and often follows viral infections, surgery, pregnancies, and other immune-altering events. It runs a monophasic course, with weakness progressing for several days to weeks, reaching a plateau, and then recovering over a period of several weeks to months. The entire course may take up to 6 months.

Clinically, the diagnosis is confirmed by weakness, often but not always in an ascending pattern (from legs up the trunk to the arms and face). The weakness is hyporeflexive, but there is no significant sensory loss. *Rapidly progressive weakness with absent reflexes and no sensory change is almost always GBS.*

36. Treatment of Guillain-Barré syndrome is based on which of its abnormalities?

Although GBS is presumably autoimmune, no specific antigen or well-defined immune abnormality has been confirmed in this disease. Nevertheless, treatment is directed toward an immunologic cause, consisting of IVIG or plasmapheresis. If done early in the disease, these modalities do seem to shorten the overall course. Because autonomic dysfunction frequently complicates the syndrome and because respiration is often impaired by the weakness, patients usually require management in the intensive care unit. Management thus focuses on the day-to-day concerns of respirators, vital signs, nutrition, and other aspects of critical care.

Plasma Exchange/Sandoglobulin Guillain-Barré Syndrome Trial Group: Randomized Trial of Plasma Exchange, Intravenous Immunoglobulin, and Combined Treatments on Guillain-Barré Syndrome. Lancet 349:225–230, 1997.

RADICULOPATHIES

37. What is the most common cause of radiculopathies on the medical ward?

Mechanical compression, as from spondylosis or a herniated disc. The common manifestations are neck and low back pain radiating into a limb.

38. How should the patient with a radiculopathy be evaluated?

The diagnostic evaluation generally begins with an EMG/NCV to identify specifically which root is involved, and hence which muscles are denervated. The next step is often to image (MRI) the area where the root emerges from the spinal cord, since this is the most common site of disorders causing radiculopathies. If these studies are negative, showing no root compression, then nonmechanical causes such as tumor or infection should be considered.

39. Discuss the treatment for radiculopathies.

For most mechanical radiculopathies, the recommended treatment consists simply of analgesics, such as aspirin or other NSAIDs with avoidance of muscle relaxants and chronic opioid use. There are surprisingly few careful, controlled studies analyzing the value of bedrest, traction, spinal manipulation, or invasive procedures such as acupuncture or trigger point injection. At this time, these methods have no proven benefit in the treatment of radiculopathy.

Bigus S, et al: Acute Low Back Problems in Adults. [Clinical Practice Guideline 14.] Rockville, MD, Agency for Health Care Policy and Research, 1994. [AHCPR publ no. 95-0643.]

40. When is surgery appropriate for a radiculopathy?

One of the most controversial topics arises when radiculopathy due to spondylosis or a herniated nucleus pulposus (slipped disc) requires surgical treatment. Many experts believe that the presence of focal neurologic findings—findings such as weakness, atrophy, or fasciculations in the muscles affected, an absent reflex, or dermatome sensory loss—is a strong indication for surgery. Such hard findings are unlikely to improve spontaneously and may well progress unless pressure on the nerve is relieved.

Much more controversial is surgery for the relief of pain alone, without focal neurologic findings. Even in well-chosen patients with clear lesions and no overlying complications (such as litigation or secondary gain), surgery to alleviate pain is effective in only about half the cases. It is therefore often reserved for patients who have "failed medical management," which is a clinical decision and generally implies persistent, very severe pain after an adequate trial of analgesics.

41. What are the most common causes of back pain?

Only about 20% of back pain is caused by a slipped disc or root compression. There are many other causes, such as arthritis of the facet joints, but most back pain is felt to be musculoskeletal, from strain placed on the tendons, ligaments, and muscles of the back. Many experts feel that this pain is largely mechanical, secondary to the inherent instability of the lordotic spine required for the human upright posture and aggravated by the problems of obesity, lack of exercise, and other precipitating factors in the modern lifestyle. For most such pain, conservative therapy and patience are indicated.

Deyo RA, Rainville J, Kent DL: What can the history and physical tell us about low back pain? JAMA 268:760–765, 1992.

MYELOPATHIES

42. How does spinal cord compression present clinically? What are its most common causes?

Spinal cord compression causes the classic cord syndrome of a sensory level, bowel and bladder changes, and upper motor neuron weakness with spasticity, hyperreflexia, and a positive Babinski sign. Superficial reflexes, such as abdominal reflexes and the anal wink, may be diminished.

The most common cause of chronic spinal cord compression is cervical spondylosis. If there is no history of trauma, the acute syndrome is often due to compression by a neoplasm, usually metastatic. Such compression may develop almost instantaneously and may or may not cause back pain.

43. How is spinal cord compression best managed?

The first step is to localize the site of the lesion. Plain x-rays of the spine have a high yield for showing metastatic disease, as evidenced by lytic lesions and erosion of pedicles. Bone scans lack specificity and are generally of low yield. MRI has largely replaced myelography for the definitive documentation of compression.

Surgical intervention is indicated for compression due to cervical spondylosis or mechanical deformation, such as spondylolisthesis. For neoplastic compression, radiation therapy is increasingly favored over surgical decompression, since results are equally good in many studies. Otherwise surgery may be needed for diagnosis as well as treatment. In either case, high-dose IV steroids, such as 100 mg of dexamethasone daily, may provide additional relief.

Armstrong R: Myelopathies. In Rolak LA (ed): Neurology Secrets. Philadelphia, Hanley & Belfus, 1998, pp 103–111.

BRAINSTEM DISEASE

44. A patient presents with a primary complaint of dizziness. What characteristics of the dizziness should be ascertained during evaluation?

When evaluating a patient with dizziness, the first question should be whether this is true vestibular dizziness or "dizziness" because of near-syncope, ataxia, or another etiology. Patients with true vestibular dizziness complain of **vertigo**, which is a feeling of spinning.

The next step is to determine whether the vertigo is central (due to a brainstem lesion) or peripheral (due to an ear lesion). Although many accompanying signs and symptoms have been promulgated to differentiate central from peripheral vertigo, none has great sensitivity or specificity. The most useful way to diagnose vertigo is by the company it keeps: **brainstem vertigo** is almost always accompanied by other signs of brainstem dysfunction, such as double vision, weakness or numbness of the face, dysarthria, or dysphagia. **Peripheral vertigo** is usually accompanied by tinnitus or hearing loss, but no other neurologic abnormalities.

45. Name the common causes of peripheral vertigo and central vertigo.

Peripheral	**Central**
Menière's disease	Stroke
Vestibular neuronitis	Multiple sclerosis
Local trauma	Tumors
Drugs (antibiotics, diuretics)	
Acoustic neuroma	
Benign positional vertigo	

46. Which special procedures are helpful in the diagnostic evaluation of the dizzy patient?

The evaluation depends heavily on the history and physical examination. Audiograms are often useful to determine if there is any disease in the ear. Brainstem auditory evoked potentials can aid evaluation of both the peripheral eighth nerve in the ear and the CNS auditory pathways. Structural lesions, such as acoustic neuromas, are uncommon causes of dizziness, but when strongly suspected, they may be seen using MRI.

47. How is dizziness best treated?

Nonvertigo dizziness (including near-syncope, anxiety, and ataxia) should be treated by addressing the underlying cause. True vertigo can be treated symptomatically, almost regardless of the cause. **Scopolamine** has proved to be the best available treatment in comparative trials against other drugs and placebos. Sympathomimetics, such as ephedrine, also have proved to be helpful. Benzodiazepines and antihistamines are of some value, including meclizine (Antivert) and diazepam.

Ruckenstein MJ: A practical approach to dizziness. Postgrad Med 97:70–81, 1995.

CEREBELLAR DISEASE

48. What is the most common cause of cerebellar disease?

Alcoholism. Alcohol causes an anterior, midline (vermal) atrophy that leads to leg and truncal instability and thus to ataxic gait. Other metabolic causes of cerebellar disease include hypothyroidism and drugs such as 5-fluorouracil and phenytoin. Structural lesions, such as cerebellar infarcts, hemorrhages, and neoplasms (both primary and metastatic) are another cause.

49. What are the main clinical features of cerebellar diseases?

Cerebellar diseases comprise a disturbance of equilibrium, muscle tone, and execution of movement. The following findings can be present: hypotonia, ataxia, dysmetria, dysdiadochokinesia, nystagmus, rebound phenomenon, postural instability, scanning speech, and intention tremor. These findings vary in severity depending on whether the lesion is acute or chronic, bilateral or unilateral, hemispheric or midline. The common findings of cerebellar dysfunction can be remembered by the mnemonic **HANDS Tremor**:

H   Hypotonia (loss of muscle tone)
A   Asynergy (lack of coordination)
N   Nystagmus (ocular oscillation)
D   Dysarthria (speech abnormalities)
S   Station and gait (imbalance, gait ataxia)
Tremor = Tremor (coarse intention tremor)

50. Is there any treatment for cerebellar dysfunction?

Cerebellar tremor, dysmetria, and ataxia are among the most difficult symptoms to mask or treat effectively. Some studies have shown that high doses of isoniazid, 900–1200 mg/day, are superior to placebo for minimizing cerebellar dysfunction. However, the toxic effects on peripheral nerves, requiring pyridoxine supplementation, and on the liver, requiring constant blood monitoring, complicate use of this drug at these high doses. Other medications, such as propranolol, primidone, and trihexyphenidyl, have provided occasional success.

STROKE

51. What is a stroke?

A stroke is focal brain dysfunction due to ischemia. The ischemia may arise from atherosclerotic narrowing of a blood vessel, an embolus, hemorrhage, or other causes.

52. Name the four main kinds of stroke.

Types of Strokes

TYPE	% OF ALL STROKES	ONSET	PRECEDING TIAS (%)	ALTERED MENTAL STATUS (%)	MRI OR CT SCAN	OTHER FEATURES
Thrombotic	40	May be gradual	Up to 50	5	Ischemic infarction	Carotid bruit, stroke during sleep
Embolic	30	Sudden	10	1	Superficial (cortical) infarction	Underlying heart disease, peripheral emboli, or strokes in different vascular territories
Lacunar	20	May be gradual	30	0	Small, deep infarction	Pure motor or pure sensory stroke
Hemorrhagic	10	Sudden	5	25	Hyperdense mass	Nausea and vomiting, decreased mental status

53. What are the clinical features of a thrombotic stroke?

Thrombotic strokes are the most common type and account for approximately 40% of all strokes. They may have a gradual, stuttering, or stepwise onset rather than an abrupt deficit. The cause is generally atherosclerosis affecting large intracranial vessels. The large-vessel involvement explains why these strokes tend to cause considerable neurologic deficit. About one-third to one-half of thrombotic strokes are preceded by transient ischemic attacks (TIAs), which are focal but totally reversible deficits that last from a few minutes to 24 hours.

54. What are the major clinical features of an embolic stroke?

Embolic strokes generally arise from the heart with an underlying cardiac disease, such as atrial arrhythmias, valvular disease, or mural thrombus. They tend to be abrupt in onset, with more rapid resolution, and tend to cause smaller neurologic deficits than a thrombotic stroke. Because the embolus travels in the arterial stream until it reaches a blood vessel of sufficiently small caliber to occlude it, it often travels distally all the way to the cortex. Cortical deficits, such as aphasia, are thus characteristic of embolic strokes.

55. What are the mechanisms of a lacunar stroke?

Lacunar strokes are very small, discrete infarcts, < 1 cm^3 in size, occurring deep within the brain or brainstem (*lacune* means little lake or pond). These strokes are due to occlusion of tiny penetrating arterioles that supply the deep brain substance, usually in the region of the basal ganglia, thalamus, and internal capsule, as well as the brainstem. These small strokes may cause discrete clinical symptoms, such as a pure motor stroke (hemiparesis without sensory loss) or pure sensory stroke.

56. How do hemorrhagic strokes differ from the other three types?

An intracerebral hemorrhage is classified as a stroke because of its abrupt onset with focal neurologic deficits, but it is due to rupture of a blood vessel with subsequent bleeding and intracerebral mass, rather than to ischemia directly. Intracerebral bleeds have an abrupt onset and are usually accompanied by a significant headache and other signs of increased intracranial pressure, such as nausea, vomiting, and a diminished mental status. These are often devastating events with a poor prognosis. Bleeds tend to occur in the same deep locations as lacunas, i.e., the basal ganglia and brainstem.

57. What are the leading causes of death shortly after a stroke?

The three leading causes of death in the first 30 days after a stroke are not related primarily to the stroke itself or to neurologic deficits. They are:
1. Pneumonia
2. Pulmonary embolus
3. Ischemic heart disease

58. Discuss the medical management of the patient with acute stroke.

Medical management of the stroke patient should focus on the complications that develop after the stroke. Since the leading cause of death is **pneumonia**, care should be taken that the patient does not aspirate—keep the patient NPO until it is clear that swallowing is not impaired by neurologic damage. Fever should always be presumed to be pneumonia until proved otherwise. Measures to prevent **pulmonary embolus** should be instituted, including early mobilization. **Ischemic heart disease** commonly causes death, since atherosclerosis affecting the cerebral vasculature probably also involves the coronary arteries. Cardiac assessment should be individualized.

59. When should thrombolysis be used to treat acute ischemic strokes?

Recombined tissue plasminogen activator (TPA) is approved for the acute treatment of ischemic stroke, but only in certain settings. It must be given as soon as possible after the stroke and certainly within the first three hours. A CT scan of the head must not show any evidence of infarction (i.e., the tissue damage must not be severe) nor hemorrhage. The patient must have significant deficits (the drug would not be used if the patient would recover well without it), and there should be no other contraindications, such as active bleeding or severe hypertension. Few patients, in fact, meet all these requirements and are candidates for TPA.

60. How is thrombolytic therapy given?

Patients are treated with 0.9 mg/kg of TPA given over one hour after an initial 10% bolus. Studies suggest such patients show approximately 30% more recovery of function than untreated patients. The risk of intracranial hemorrhage is approximately 6%, however, and patients should be carefully monitored.

Chan BP, Albers GW: Acute ischemic stroke. Curr Treat Options Neurol 1:83–95, 1999.

61. When is anticoagulation indicated in cerebrovascular disease?

The role of anticoagulation in cerebrovascular disease is very controversial. The consensus among neurologists is that anticoagulation is mainly of benefit for embolic stroke from the heart. Following an initial brain embolus from a cardiac source, the risk of subsequent emboli is high, especially within the first few days and weeks, and evidence suggests that immediate anticoagulation dramatically reduces this risk. Although there is a chance that immediate anticoagulation will worsen a stroke by converting the ischemia into hemorrhage, data suggest that this worsening is minimal and more than outweighed by the benefits in preventing further emboli.

Brott T, Bogousslavsky J: Treatment of acute ischemic stroke. N Engl J Med 343:710–722, 2000.

62. Do antiplatelet agents have a role in the management of cerebrovascular diseases?

Aspirin, given at the time of a stroke, may have some protective effects. Antiplatelet agents, specifically aspirin, have been advocated for the secondary prevention of stroke. Patients with TIA or minor stroke are often treated with aspirin, usually one tablet (325 mg) per day, to prevent further episodes of cerebrovascular ischemia. There may be additional benefits to combining it with dipyridamole. Ticlopidine, like aspirin, acts as a platelet inhibitor and similarly decreases the risk of further cerebrovascular ischemia. Unlike aspirin, it does not affect the cyclo-oxygenase pathway and instead acts by interfering with platelet membrane interactions. Clopidogrel is another antiplatelet agent with similar properties. Their current role is primarily for the prevention of stroke in patients with cerebral ischemia for whom aspirin therapy has failed, has caused intolerable side effects, or is otherwise contraindicated.

63. What is the role of carotid endarterectomy in cerebrovascular disease?

For patients with symptomatic atherosclerotic stenosis of > 70% in the carotid artery, carotid endarterectomy is clearly beneficial, significantly decreasing the risk of ipsilateral stroke. In asymptomatic patients with atherosclerotic stenosis of the carotids, its role is less clear. Three large randomized trials done in the early 1990s detected no benefit of endarterectomy in these patients. However, the Asymptomatic Carotid Atherosclerosis Study (ACAS) demonstrated a reduction in cerebral infarction in asymptomatic patients with as little as 60% stenosis, provided perioperative morbidity was kept to a minimum. The benefits were sufficiently modest that not all experts were convinced of the utility of surgery, and considerable individual variation remains among physicians managing such patients. Clearly, any surgical intervention in the treatment of carotid artery stenosis must be used in addition to, not in lieu of, aggressive control of modifiable risk factors.

Executive Committee for ACAS Study: Endarterectomy for asymptomatic carotid artery stenosis. JAMA 273:1421–1428, 1995.

APHASIA

64. Define aphasia.

Aphasia is an acquired disturbance in language functions (i.e., the ability to manipulate sounds and symbols into concepts, words, and phrases). It must not be confused with dysarthria or slurred speech, which is strictly a problem with the motor control of talking. Aphasics not only have difficulty with talking but also with writing, reading, and all other forms of language production. The most common cause of aphasia in adults is cerebrovascular disease.

65. How do the fluent and nonfluent types of aphasias differ?

1. **Nonfluent aphasias** are generally produced by lesions in the cortex, in the anterior part of the dominant hemisphere around the sylvian fissure, and are often referred to by other expressions such as **Broca's**, motor, expressive, or anterior aphasia. Such patients have difficulty producing language and either cannot speak or do so only in monosyllables and short telegraphic phrases. Naming and repetition are also impaired, but comprehension is relatively preserved.

2. **Fluent aphasias** are due to lesions in the cortex in the posterior part of the dominant hemisphere, around the posterior temporal lobe. Such aphasias—also known as **Wernicke's**, sensory, receptive, or posterior aphasia—result in speech that is fluent and even loquacious, but senseless. These patients can talk but make no sense. They have many neologisms and paraphasic errors, inventing words and sounds as they go along and stringing words together in nongrammatical, meaningless fashions. Such patients usually have impaired naming, repetition, and severely impaired comprehension as well.

Comparison of the Main Types of Aphasia

TYPE	FLUENT	NAMES	REPEATS	COMPREHENDS
Broca's	No	No	No	Yes
Wernicke's	Yes	No	No	No

Damasio AR: Aphasia. N Engl J Med 326:531–539, 1992.

SEIZURES

66. What is an epileptic seizure?

An epileptic seizure is the abnormal discharge of a neuron or group of neurons that leads to excessive electrical activity in the brain, causing disruption of brain function sufficient to produce clinical symptoms such as staring spells or jerking of muscles.

67. What are the main kinds of epileptic seizures?

Generalized seizures
Generalized tonic–clonic (grand mal)
Generalized absence (petit mal)

Partial seizures
Partial simple (focal)
Partial complex (psychomotor)

68. Describe the clinical features of partial simple seizures.

Most partial simple seizures encountered in a medical setting consist of the focal jerking or twitching of an arm or leg on one side of the body. This is usually due to a structural lesion in the brain (such as a stroke, abscess, or tumor) that leads to local irritation and an epileptic discharge. If this discharge spreads, the focal seizure also spreads, sometimes involving the other side of the brain and causing twitching or jerking of both arms and legs (generalized tonic–clonic or grand mal seizure). Occasionally, metabolic lesions, especially hyperglycemia and hyperosmolar states, can cause focal lesions and focal partial seizures.

69. What are the clinical features of partial complex seizures?

Partial complex seizures may be preceded by an aura of abnormal smells or tastes, visual sensations, or mental phenomena, such as *deja-vu*. The seizure itself may consist of an episode of staring, lip smacking, and automatic, semipurposeful movements, such as picking at clothes. Often there is no jerking of muscles, no loss of tone, and no falling down. Patients, however, are in a state of significantly altered mental status and often completely unresponsive. After a minute or two the seizure passes, leaving a postictal state of confusion and lethargy.

70. Which group is most likely to develop generalized absence seizures?

Generalized absence seizures, sometimes referred to as petit mal, are seen almost exclusively in children. These seizures usually do not have a significant aura or postictal state but may consist of just a few seconds of staring and altered mental status. This may be so brief as to escape detection by untrained observers. At other times, children are thought to be daydreaming rather than experiencing a seizure.

71. How do generalized tonic–clonic seizures present?

Generalized tonic–clonic seizures, the so-called grand mal seizures, consist of the sudden onset, often without any preceding aura, of jerking tonic and clonic activity of both arms and both legs, with a generalized increase in muscle tone and loss of consciousness. There may be tongue biting or incontinence. Seizures usually last a minute or two and then resolve, often with a period of postictal lethargy and confusion.

72. How do the identifiable causes of seizures vary by age?

Common Causes of Seizures by Age

NEONATE TO 3 YRS	3–20 YRS	20–60 YRS	> 60 YRS
Prenatal injury	Genetic predisposition	Brain tumors	Vascular disease
Perinatal injury	Infections	Trauma	Brain tumors, esp. metastatic tumors
Metabolic defects	Trauma	Vascular disease	
Congenital malformations	Congenital malformations	Infections	Trauma
CNS infections	Metabolic defects		Systemic metabolic derangements
Postnatal trauma			Infections

73. What are the most common causes of seizures seen in the emergency department or on the medical ward?

Anticonvulsant withdrawal. Most patients seen here are known epileptics who have been taking medicine and, for one reason or another, are noncompliant with their drugs. Alcohol withdrawal, drug overdose, and metabolic derangements such as hyponatremia are other common causes. Structural brain disease, including stroke and meningitis, is a less common cause of seizures.

74. How do alcohol withdrawal seizures present?

These seizures generally occur 12–48 hours after cessation or abrupt reduction in the intake of alcohol. These seizures are always generalized tonic–clonic seizures, without locality. They are often single, isolated seizures, but sometimes patients may have two or more over a span of < 6 hours. Status epilepticus is rare after alcohol withdrawal but does occasionally occur. Alcohol withdrawal seizures seldom persist and are self-limited.

75. What are the most important principles of seizure management?

Most seizures can be controlled completely, or nearly so, by following a few basic principles:

1. Pick the most appropriate anticonvulsant for the type of seizure the patient is experiencing.

2. Steadily increase the dose of that drug, guided by serum anticonvulsant levels, until seizures are controlled. If drug toxicity develops before the seizures stop, then the drug is not the appropriate one; try a different one. Obviously, increase the new anticonvulsant to therapeutic levels before tapering off the old drug.

3. Monotherapy is preferable. Good therapeutic levels of one drug are preferable to subtherapeutic levels of multiple drugs.

76. Which drugs are the most useful anticonvulsants for the different types of seizures?

	PHENY-TOIN	CARBA-MAZEPINE	PHENOBAR-BITAL	ETHO-SUXIMIDE	VAL-PROATE	GABA-PENTIN	LAMO-TRIGINE
Partial simple	+	+	+		+	+	
Partial complex	+	+	+			+	+
Generalized absence			+	+			
Generalized tonic–clonic	+	+	+		+		

Adapted from Brodie MJ, French JA: Management of epilepsy in adolescents and adults. Lancet 356: 323–329, 2000.

77. How is status epilepticus treated?
1. Rapid history and physical examination, including airway, breathing, circulation.
2. Start IV and draw blood for complete blood count (CBC), electrolytes, anticonvulsant levels. Administer thiamine and glucose.
3. Infuse phenytoin by slow IV push at 50 mg/min to a dose of ~20 mg/kg (1500 mg). To break a continuous seizure, give diazepam up to 20 mg or lorazepam up to 8 mg.
4. Infuse IV phenobarbital, 100 mg/min up to 600 mg.
5. Institute general anesthesia.

Experts disagree about when to intubate the patient. Some do it in step 2, others wait until step 4. You should always be prepared to immediately intubate any patient in status epilepticus.

Treiman DM: Convulsive status epilepticus. Curr Treat Options Neurol 1:359–369, 1999.

MOVEMENT DISORDERS

78. List the four cardinal features of Parkinson's disease.
1. Tremor
2. Rigidity
3. Bradykinesia
4. Postural instability

Parkinson's disease is a gradual, progressive, degenerative disease of the basal ganglia (extrapyramidal) motor system. It is a very common condition, probably affecting 1% of people over age 60. The **tremor** is usually a to-and-fro, pronation-supination, resting tremor that diminishes with voluntary movement. It is coarse and slow and most prominent in the hands and head. Patients have **rigidity**, with a diffuse increase in muscular tone and sometimes a "cog-wheeling" property to their joints when passively moved. **Bradykinesia** refers to slowness of movement. The patients also have a paucity or lack of movement and tend to show minimal axial expression—they often sit quite immobile, almost like statues.

79. What is the differential diagnosis of Parkinson's disease?
A few conditions can cause parkinsonism, a symptom complex that mimics idiopathic Parkinson's disease. The most common causes are the neuroleptic drugs, including phenothiazines (such as chlorpromazine, thioridazine, etc.) and butyrophenones (such as haloperidol). Similar symptoms also can be mimicked by multiple strokes, hydrocephalus, and degenerative conditions such as Alzheimer's disease.

80. How is Parkinson's disease treated?
The best treatment is a combination of L-dopa plus carbidopa (Sinemet). The main cause for the symptoms of Parkinson's disease is a deficiency of dopamine within the pathway running from the substantia nigra to the basal ganglia. Since dopamine cannot be given directly (because it does not cross the blood-brain barrier), it is given as L-dopa. To prevent L-dopa from being decarboxylated and metabolized before it reaches the brain, carbidopa is given in combination.

Other dopamine agonists are sometimes used to supplement Sinemet. The main one is bromocriptine. Anticholinergic agents, which suppress the overactive cholinergic system and bring it into balance with the diminished dopamine system, can alleviate symptoms. A CT scan of the head must not show any evidence of infarction (i.e., the tissue damage must not be severe) nor hemorrhage. The patient must have significant deficits (the drug should not be used if the patient would recover well without it), and there should be no other contraindications, such as active bleeding or severe hypertension. Few patients, in fact, meet all these requirements and are candidates for TPA.

81. What are the other important types of tremors?

Parkinson's disease is a common form of **resting tremor** and can often be recognized by the accompanying rigidity and bradykinesia. Other important types of tremors include:

1. **Essential tremor.** This rapid, fine tremor involving the head and arms especially is present at rest but becomes more noticeable with sustained postures or intentional movement. A family history, with an autosomal dominant inheritance, is seen in about half the cases. Treatment may include a β-blocker (propranolol, 80 mg/day) or primidone (starting at 50 mg/day).

2. **Cerebellar tremor.** Damage to the cerebellum disturbs motor control by causing a tremor. This is absent at rest and only appears with intentional or voluntary movements. It is a slow, coarse, dyssynergic tremor. Other evidence of cerebellar dysfunction may be present. Pharmacologic treatment is generally unsatisfactory.

Lambert D, Waters CH: Essential tremor. Curr Treat Options Neurol 1:6–13, 1999.

82. What are dystonias?

Dystonias, as the name suggests, are disorders of muscle tone that result in involuntary, sustained muscle contractions. These can lead to abnormal posturing or unique repetitive movements. Examples include spasmodic torticollis, blepharospasm, and oromandibular dystonia.

83. How is botulinum toxin used in the treatment of dystonias?

Botulinum toxin type A (Botox), one of the most potent toxins found in the environment, has become the treatment of choice for focal dystonias such as blepharospasm and torticollis. Carefully localized intramuscular injections act to block the release of acetylcholine at the presynaptic membrane of the neuromuscular junction, thereby decreasing excessive muscle activity.

Treatment has been quite successful, with improvement noted in 70–90% of patients. The effects can last up to 4 months. Botulinum toxin has proven to be quite safe if administered properly, with temporary localized weakness as the only major side effect.

Hughes AJ: Botulinum toxin in clinical practice. Drugs 48:888–893, 1994.

HEADACHE

84. What are the key principles in evaluating headache?

1. The brain is anesthetic. This means that most causes of head pain do not arise from the brain itself but rather from surrounding structures, such as blood vessels, periosteum, etc. Since most headaches are not caused by brain disease, most are benign.

2. The more severe the headache, the more benign the disease. The exception to this is intracranial hemorrhage, but, in general, most severe headaches are due to self-limited causes.

3. Eye problems and sinus disease seldom cause headaches. Patients tend to blame their headaches on eye strain or sinusitis, but, in fact, these are rare etiologies.

85. What are the common types of headache?

1. Common migraine (without aura)
2. Classic migraine (with aura)
3. Tension headaches

Other less common or rare types of headaches include cluster headaches and headaches from brain tumor, meningeal irritation, and temporal arteritis.

86. Which serious diseases capable of causing permanent neurologic dysfunction can present as headaches?

Most processes causing headache are benign, but some are serious, as follows:

Serious Diseases that May Present as a Headache

1. Primary brain tumor	7. Meningitis
2. Metastatic brain tumor	8. Temporal arteritis
3. Abscess	9. Hypertension
4. Subdural hematoma	10. Hydrocephalus
5. Intracerebral hemorrhage	11. Glaucoma
6. Subarachnoid hemorrhage	

87. How can you tell if your headache is due to a brain tumor?

Brain tumors generally cause a mild-to-moderate headache, seldom severe, that is rather nonspecific in its symptoms. It is dull, chronic, and throughout the whole head. Often, it is not localized to the region of the tumor. The headache is usually worse with maneuvers that cause the tumor to shift around, such as changes in position (e.g., getting out of bed, bending over). Valsalva maneuvers, which increase intracranial pressure, also worsen the headache. Most brain tumors produce abnormal findings on physical examination, such as altered mental status, papilledema, or focal weakness or numbness. A headache with a normal neurologic examination is unlikely to be a brain tumor.

88. What clinical features are seen with increased intracranial pressure (ICP)?

Because the brain is completely surrounded by the hard bony skull, any increase in ICP can impair brain function. The most sensitive indicator of increased ICP is an altered mental status, and it is usually the first symptom to change as the pressure rises. With increased pressure, the brain can herniate downward through the foramen magnum, compressing and destroying the brainstem. Herniation can be recognized by the development of brainstem signs as the top of the brainstem (midbrain) becomes impaired. In addition to altered mental status, these signs include dilatation of one or both pupils ("blown pupil"), hyperventilation, and focal neurologic signs such as hemiparesis. Herniation can progress to coma and death.

89. How can intracranial pressure be lowered?

Lowering ICP requires reduction of the intracranial contents to make room for the mass lesion and increased pressure. The intracranial contents consist essentially of the brain, cerebrospinal fluid (CSF) filling the ventricles, and blood within the blood vessels.

1. **Lowering blood pressure** lowers the ICP and can be accomplished with a diuretic such as furosemide. Osmotic diuresis is particularly effective, and therefore mannitol is the mainstay of therapy. It is given IV in a dose of 100 mg, followed, if necessary, by 50 mg boluses every 2 hours.

2. **Incubation and hyperventilation** cause vasospasm that reduces the blood volume intracranially. This temporarily lowers ICP, but because of compensatory reequilibration, it provides only a few hours of relief.

3. **Steroids** can reduce swelling secondary to vasogenic edema, such as occurs with neoplasms, but they are not useful for edema that is cytotoxic, such as develops after a stroke or intracerebral hemorrhage. They may take hours or days to work and have little value acutely.

4. **Shunting** can be used in emergency situations to remove CSF and so lower ICP.

90. How do subarachnoid and intracerebral hemorrhage differ in clinical presentation?

Intracranial hemorrhage causes the abrupt onset of an extremely severe headache. Patients report that it is "the worst headache in my life." The bleeding may result from the rupture of a vessel outside the brain (subarachnoid hemorrhage) or inside the brain (intracerebral hematoma).

Subarachnoid hemorrhage is usually due to the rupture of a small intracranial aneurysm, called a berry aneurysm, often located on the anterior communicating artery, middle cerebral artery, or their branches. Approximately half of these patients die at the time of the bleed. The remainder usually present to an emergency department with an altered mental status but may not have significant focal neurologic findings.

Intracerebral hemorrhage also causes collapse, coma, and death in a high percentage of patients, but since it occurs within the parenchyma of the brain, there are almost always focal neurologic findings, such as hemiparesis. Most patients also have altered mental status. It is strongly associated with hypertension.

91. What are the clinical features of headache due to meningitis?

The headache of meningitis, as in other severe illnesses, is often mild-to-moderate rather than extremely intense. It is a diffuse pain throughout the head, sometimes accompanied by photophobia, and shows signs of irritation of the brain and meninges, such as a stiff neck.

Meningitis is unlikely to be overlooked in the differential diagnosis of headache because of the accompanying signs of fever, elevated white blood cell (WBC) count, and other evidence of infection. It usually presents as an infectious, toxic process rather than as a headache.

92. What is temporal arteritis?

Temporal arteritis is the confusing term used to describe a **giant cell arteritis** which may present as a headache. It is confusing because the process is not confined to the temporal arteries, but rather is a systemic illness with generalized symptoms such as fevers, myalgias, arthralgias (polymyalgia rheumatica), anemia, and elevated liver function tests. The headache is a mild-to-moderate diffuse pain, not necessarily confined to the temples or frontal region of the head. The disease should be suspected in elderly people, over age 55, who develop new headaches. The erthrocye sedimentation rate (ESR) is usually very elevated, >100 mm/min, and is a good screening test. The confirmatory test is a temporal artery biopsy showing granulomatous arteritis.

93. How do you treat temporal arteritis?

High-dose steroids for a period of 1–2 years are often required, sometimes in doses of 60 mg/day of prednisone equivalent or more. This is effective in controlling most symptoms of temporal arteritis, including the most tragic symptom, which is blindness from vasculitic involvement of the ophthalmic blood supply. Approximately 15% of these patients, if left untreated, develop significant visual loss.

MIGRAINE AND TENSION HEADACHE

94. At what age do migraine headaches have their onset?

Migraines typically begin in the teenage years, sometimes even in childhood, and diminish in both frequency and intensity of attacks in later adulthood. About half of all patients with migraine have a family history of the problem.

95. How frequently do migraine headaches occur?

Migraine headaches are paroxysmal, intermittent headaches occurring on an average of once a month and lasting from 4–12 hours or more. The frequency is highly variable, with some patients reporting multiple attacks per month and others only a few in their lifetime.

96. What are the common symptoms of migraines?

1. About one-third of patients have hemicranial pain, but in two-thirds of patients the headache is diffuse over the entire head.

2. Some patients have a preceding aura for 20–40 minutes before the headache. This often consists of visual changes, such as flashing lights.

3. Gastrointestinal disturbances are very common, including nausea, vomiting, and anorexia. If you can eat during your headache, it is probably not migraine!

4. Photophobia and phonophobia
5. Mood changes
6. Visual or sensory loss

97. What triggers migraine headaches?

Some patients notice factors associated with the onset of their headaches. Hormonal triggers are common, and many women have headaches at the time of menstruation or ovulation. Alcohol, emotional stress, and some foods such as chocolate can also trigger headaches.

Some Precipitating Factors in Migraine Headaches

1. Head trauma	5. Diet: Chocolate, alcohol, MSG
2. Psychological stress	6. Hormonal changes
3. Sleep	7. Physical exertion
4. Changes in weather (barometric pressure)	

98. Is the cause of migraine headaches known?

Not entirely. Probably low serotonin levels in the brain trigger certain brainstem neurons to fire, which alters cerebral function and blood flow. The nausea, neurologic deficits, and head pain result from low brain serotonin levels, aggravated by concomitant vascular changes.

99. What is the best treatment for a migraine headache?

For symptomatic relief from mild-to-moderate migraines, simple analgesics or NSAIDs such as aspirin or naproxen may be sufficient. For more severe attacks, triptans are the drugs of choice. Sumatriptan, a 5-hydroxytryptamine receptor agonist, was the first triptan to be used and is a more effective antimigraine agent. Patients should be warned of the flushing, sweating, and chest tightness that can occur as a side effect. The oral preparation, in doses of 50 mg, provides good relief, but it is also available as a nasal spray and an injection. Other similar drugs are naratriptan, rizatriptan, and zolmatriptan.

100. Which agents are useful as prophylactic therapies?

For patients having very frequent headaches (2–3/month or more) or for the occasional patient whose headache is complicated by persistent neurologic deficits, prophylactic treatment may be indicated. A variety of drugs from different classes are helpful:

1. **Amitriptyline**, a tricyclic compound. Doses of 100 mg/day or more may be necessary. Most other tricyclics are not effective.

2. **Propranolol**, a β-adrenergic blocking agent. Again, doses of 100 mg/day or more may be needed. Most other β-adrenergic blockers are not effective.

3. **Calcium channel blockers**. Both nifedipine and verapamil are useful.

Ferrari MD: Migraine. Lancet 351:1051–1093, 1998.

101. What are the clinical features of tension headaches?

Tension headaches are diffuse headaches, often described as a band around the head, usually bifrontal but sometimes occipital. Patients with chronic, persistent, tension headaches report that the pain is very severe (though it seldom seems so to the physician). Unlike migraine, these headaches are usually not paroxysmal but are constant and chronic. Like migraine, they are more common in women and generally begin early in life. About half of the patients have a family history. Usually, there are no associated neurologic symptoms (such as visual changes) or nausea and vomiting. Tension and migraine headaches commonly coexist in the same patient.

102. What causes tension headaches?

The cause is not known. There is no convincing evidence that they are due to psychological factors or emotional stress, nor are there good data showing they are related to muscle contraction.

103. How should tension headaches be treated?

Amitriptyline, up to 75–150 mg/day, works independently of its antidepressant effects. NSAIDs are useful for common headaches but are seldom successful in chronic persistent tension headache. Muscle relaxants also are not effective (not surprising, since muscle contraction is not the cause of the headache).

DEMENTIA

104. What is dementia?

Dementia is a progressive decline in cognitive and intellectual functions in the presence of a clear sensorium. Dementia implies that the person has lost intellectual function from a baseline state—i.e., he or she was not born mentally retarded (this is an acquired process) and is not delirious, lethargic, or otherwise suffering from an impaired level of consciousness.

105. What causes dementia?

Etiologies of Dementia

Senile dementia of Alzheimer's type	50–60%
Multi-infarct dementia (MID)	10–20%
Combination Alzheimer's and MID	10–20%
Other disorders	5–10%
Reversible or partially reversible	20–30%

Other causes of dementia include neurosyphilis, hypothyroidism, HIV infection, neoplasm, subdural hematoma, and head trauma. The old belief that generalized atherosclerosis and global reduction in blood flow can cause dementia has proven correct in only rare cases. Cerebrovascular disease essentially does not cause dementia except by actual destruction (infarction) of brain tissue, as in MID.

Small GW, Rabins PV, Bary PP, et al: Diagnoses and treatment of Alzheimer's disease and related disorders. JAMA 278:1363–1371, 1997.

106. What is the diagnostic approach to the patient with dementia?

Most dementias, such as Alzheimer's disease, have no effective treatment, so the evaluation of any patient presenting with dementia generally focuses on finding the treatable causes, even though these are uncommon.

Reversible Causes of Dementia

D—Drugs
E—Emotional disorders (pseudodementia or depression)
M—Metabolic and endocrine disorders (hepatic encephalopathy, hypothyroidism, chronic renal failure)
E—Eye and ear dysfunction
N—Nutritional deficiencies, normal pressure hydrocephalus (NPH)
T—Tumor, trauma (including chronic subdural hematoma)
I—Infections (neurosyphilis, chronic meningitis)
A—Alcohol, arteriosclerotic complications

Screening for Reversible Dementias, in Addition to History and Physical Examination

Thyroid function tests	Vitamin B_{12} level
Serum chemistries (including CA^{21})	Head CT or MRI
Examination of CSF for possible NPH	Syphilis serology
or if RPR positive or if cranial nerve abnor-	CBC
malities are present (consistent with meningitis)	Serum folate level

A workup includes CT scan or MRI to image the brain, an electroencephalogram (EEG) to show metabolic encephalopathies (diffuse slowing) or some specific dementias (e.g., periodic sharp waves seen in Creutzfeldt-Jakob disease), and sometimes lumbar puncture to rule out neurosyphilis, cryptococcal meningitis, or other chronic infections. Blood studies detect most other causes of dementia, such as hypothyroidism, B_{12} deficiency, and vasculitis.

Morris JC: Differential diagnosis of Alzheimer's Disease. Clin Geriatr Med 10(2):257–276, 1994.

107. What is Alzheimer's disease?

Alzheimer's disease is a degenerative dementing process of unknown etiology. Most elderly patients who were once termed "senile" probably had Alzheimer's disease, which is now felt to be a specific, distinct disease entity rather than the mere loss of intellectual function with normal aging.

Pathologically, Alzheimer's disease is characterized by degenerative changes in the brain, especially senile plaques, neurofibrillary tangles, and granulovacuolar degeneration. These degenerative changes are seen in great concentration in the hippocampus.

108. How is Alzheimer's disease diagnosed?

There is no biological marker or specific test for Alzheimer's disease, so the clinical diagnosis is largely one of exclusion. The criteria for the diagnosis of Alzheimer's disease, short of a brain biopsy, are summarized below:

Clinical Diagnosis of Alzheimer's Disease

1. Proof of dementia by neuropsychologic testing
2. Deficits in 2 or more areas of cognition (i.e., not just memory loss)
3. Progressive worsening
4. No disturbance of consciousness
5. Onset between ages 40–90 (usually after age 65)
6. Absence of other causes of dementia

109. Is there any treatment for Alzheimer's disease?

Tacrine, a cholinesterase inhibitor, was the first drug accepted for use in the treatment of Alzheimer's disease. While it does not seem to alter the course of the underlying disease, tacrine was shown to slow the rate of cognitive decline when compared with placebo in multiple clinical trials. Tacrine therapy carries with it a risk of hepatotoxicity, with significant (albeit temporary) elevations of serum enzymes in half of patients receiving the drug. Other cholinesterase inhibitors have largely replaced tacrine, including **donepezil** and **rivastigmine**, but still without clear effect on the underlying disease.

American Psychiatric Association: Practice guidelines for the treatment of patients with Alzheimers disease and other dementias of late life. Am J Psychiatry 154:1–39, 1997.

MULTIPLE SCLEROSIS

110. What is multiple sclerosis (MS)?

MS is the most common disabling neurologic disease of young people under age 40, affecting approximately 250,000 Americans. It is probably an autoimmune disease, characterized by relapsing and remitting episodes of inflammation in the brain and spinal cord. This inflammation destroys the myelin, which is the insulating sheath around nerve cells, and hence destroys the ability of the nerves to conduct electrical impulses (action potentials).

111. What are the clinical symptoms of MS?

Clinically, MS may affect almost any part of the brain or spinal cord. Generally, symptoms come on fairly abruptly, over a period of hours to days, persist for several weeks, and then resolve over a period of several more weeks, often returning completely to normal. On average, patients have one attack per year, although about 20% of patients have a chronic progressive course with steady worsening deficit, without abrupt attacks.

The highly variable presentation of MS reflects the fact that it may involve the optic nerves, spinal cord, pyramidal tracts, spinothalamic tracts, brainstem, or cerebellum. Common symptoms include:

Most Common Symptoms of Multiple Sclerosis

Focal weakness	45%	Cerebellar ataxia	30%
Optic neuritis	40%	Diplopia and nystagmus	25%
Focal numbness	35%	Bowel and bladder changes	20%

112. How is the diagnosis of MS made?

Schumacher Criteria for Definite Multiple Sclerosis

1. Two separate CNS lesions	4. Objective deficits on examination
2. Two separate attacks of symptoms	5. Age 10–50 years (usually 20–40)
3. Symptoms must be consistent with a white matter (myelin) lesion	6. No other disease to explain symptoms

The diagnosis of MS is often difficult given the great variability in signs and symptoms. Generally, young people who have had two separate lesions in the CNS at two separate times have a strong likelihood of having MS.

113. Does laboratory testing or imaging have any role in diagnosing MS?

Although the Schumacher criteria are quite accurate, it is not possible to use them to diagnose MS when the first symptom appears. A definitive diagnosis requires two separate symptoms. For this reason, patients suspected of having MS often undergo further testing to provide some laboratory confirmation of the diagnosis.
- MRI of the head is very sensitive for showing the white matter lesions of MS, but not very specific.
- Spinal fluid usually shows immunologic abnormalities, specifically the presence of multiple polyclonal concentrations of IgG.
- Evoked potentials is a technique in which visual, auditory, or electrical stimulation is flashed to the brain, whose reactions are recorded using electrodes, similar to an EEG. A delay in the impulses evoked by the stimuli often indicates an underlying lesion in patients with MS.

114. How are the symptoms of MS best managed?

Because the cause of MS is not known, there is no cure. Steroids often help alleviate attacks by reducing inflammation. However, they do not appear to alter the natural history of the disease.

Symptomatic management consists of medications to improve spasticity, management of the neurogenic bladder, and braces or other aids to ambulation.

115. Can any treatments alter the natural course of MS?

While a cure for MS remains elusive, some therapies may actually alter the natural course of MS. Beta Interferon-1a (Avonex), Beta Interferon-1b (Betaseron), and glatiramer acetate (Copaxone) all decrease the number of yearly relapses in patients with MS, as demonstrated in large clinical trials. The drugs seem equally effective, cutting attacks by approximately one-third. Major side effects of β-interferon include flulike symptoms and leukopenia. Copaxone has relatively few side effects, mild injection site inflammation being the only one of note.

Despite their apparent benefit in decreasing relapses of MS, none of the drugs has shown much benefit in patients with chronic progressive MS, nor is it clear how well they prevent ultimate disability.

Johnson KP, et al: Copolymer-1 reduces relapse rate and improves disability in relapsing-remitting MS. Neurology 95:1268–1275, 1995.

The IFNB MS Study Group: IFNB-1b in the treatment of MS. Neurology 95:1277–1285, 1995.

116. How long do patients survive after the onset of MS?

Most patients live 40 years or longer. MS may be disabling but is seldom fatal.

COMA

117. What are the most common causes of coma?

1. Drugs (including alcohol, illicit drugs, accidental or intentional overdose, etc.)
2. Hypoxia
3. Hypoglycemia
4. Other metabolic derangements (sepsis, uremia, hepatic failure, etc.)
5. Structural brain disease (stroke, intracranial hemorrhage, etc.)

Most etiologies of coma are medical problems, not primary neurologic diseases.

118. What is the approach to the patient in coma?

1. ABCs—protect the airway, breathing, and circulation.
2. Draw blood to check for metabolic derangements, infection, and drugs.
3. Infuse glucose, thiamine, and naloxone.
4. History and physical exam for clues to the cause of coma. Focus on pupils and extraocular movements for evidence of brainstem dysfunction.
5. Definitive diagnosis (and therapy) may require CT scanning, lumbar puncture, EEG, and other studies depending on the situation.

119. What is the prognosis of coma?

Almost 70% of patients admitted to a hospital in a coma die. Brainstem abnormalities—absent extraocular movements, gag reflex, or spontaneous respirations, or unreactive pupils—carry an especially grim prognosis.

Hamel MB, et al: Identification of comatose patients at high risk for death or severe disability. JAMA 273:1842–1848, 1995.

OTHER MEDICAL CONDITIONS

120. How does alcohol affect the nervous system?

Alcohol can affect virtually any part of the nervous system:

- Alcoholic myopathy—occurs in heavy drinkers in a fashion analogous to alcoholic cardiomyopathy.
- Acute rhabdomyolysis—rare, associated with heavy alcohol consumption.
- Peripheral neuropathy—usually a distal, symmetric, stocking-and-glove sensory and motor polyneuropathy.
- Nerve compression—increased susceptibility in alcoholics (e.g., "Saturday night" palsy).
- Fulminant necrotic myelopathy—rare, associated with heavy alcoholic intake.
- Wernicke's encephalopathy—due to thiamine deficiency secondary to alcoholism.
- Cerebellar ataxia—alcohol leads to degeneration of the anterior (dermis) region of the cerebellum, causing a very ataxic gait.
- Alcoholic dementia—amnesia (Korsakoff's syndrome) and generalized dementia.

Diamond I, Messing RO: Neurologic effects of alcoholism. West J Med 161:279–287, 1994.

121. What triad of findings is seen in Wernicke's encephalopathy?

Alcohol can affect the brainstem in the classic Wernicke's encephalopathy, which causes a triad of:

1. Nystagmus with extraocular abnormalities
2. Cerebellar ataxia
3. Confusion

Wernicke's is really due to a thiamine deficiency rather than to alcohol ingestion itself. The brainstem signs reverse readily with parenteral thiamine infusion, but the confusion resolves more slowly.

122. Does HIV affect the nervous system?

HIV can cause widespread damage in the nervous system, probably entering through macrophages that cross the blood–brain barrier. Approximately 10% of all AIDS patients present initially with neurologic symptoms, and up to 50% develop neurologic complications at some point during their illness.

- Inflammatory myopathy—similar to polymyositis, with symptoms of slowly progressive proximal weakness. Zidovudine may also cause a similar reversible myopathy.
- Peripheral neuropathy—distal symmetric (glove-and-stocking) pattern, with distal burning and other dysesthesias, seen in approximately 30% of patients.
- Acute inflammatory demyelinating polyneuropathy—like Guillain-Barré syndrome but with CSF pleocytosis.
- AIDS myelopathy—vacuolar degeneration resembling B_{12} deficiency, a chronic progressive spinal cord syndrome.
- HIV encephalopathy—progressive dementia manifested by apathy, personality change, and/or loss of higher cognitive functions.
- Aseptic meningitis—due to HIV itself.

Klepser ME, Klepser TB: Drug treatment of HIV-related opportunistic infections. Drugs 53:40–73, 1997.

123. What two conditions should be suspected when a CT scan reveals CNS mass lesions in a patient with AIDS?

Cerebral toxoplasmosis and primary CNS lymphoma.

124. What are the effects of diabetes mellitus (DM) on the peripheral nervous system?

The primary effect of DM on the nervous system is on the peripheral nerves. The most frequent problem is a distal, symmetric, stocking-and-glove sensory and motor **polyneuropathy**. This usually begins in the feet, generally with numbness, and then ascends to the hands. Often, there are burning, painful paresthesias. In severe cases, proprioceptive loss may be sufficiently significant to cause Charcot joints. A motor neuropathy frequently accompanies the sensory changes.

Mononeuropathy can occur because the small vessel disease that accompanies DM frequently leads to infarction of nerves by occlusion of the vasa nervorum. Femoral neuropathies and cranial nerve palsies are particularly common. Another type of neuropathy is thoracoabdominal neuropathy, in which a thoracic root is damaged, again possibly by infarction, leading to severe chest or abdominal pain that is often mistaken for a visceral crisis.

Finally, the autonomic peripheral nervous system may be affected, leading to impotence, bowel and bladder dysfunction, gastroparesis, orthostatic hypotension, or arrhythmias.

125. In what ways does diabetes affect the CNS?

Involvement of the CNS by diabetes is more indirect than its effects on the peripheral nerves. Because diabetes is a risk factor for atherosclerosis, there is an increased incidence of stroke. **Hypoglycemia** from overmedication can lead to focal neurologic findings, such as hemiparesis or aphasia, or, if severe, altered mental status including coma. **Hyperglycemia**, from diabetic ketoacidosis or from nonketotic hyperosmolar states, also causes altered mental status, sometimes accompanied by seizures.

126. How does renal failure affect the nervous system?

1. Uremia is one of the most common metabolic abnormalities affecting the nervous system, especially the peripheral nerves, where there is a stocking-and-glove distal, symmetric, **sensorimotor neuropathy.**

2. Patients with renal failure are prone to **metabolic encephalopathies** causing confusion, lethargy, and even coma. This may be aggravated by fluid and electrolyte shifts during dialysis.

3. Because of the anticoagulation necessary for dialysis, there is an increased incidence of **intracerebral hemorrhage**, such as subdural hematomas.

4. A special type of mental status change is the syndrome of **dialysis encephalopathy**, which is a progressive deterioration in mental status, with hyperreflexia and dysarthria, usually accompanied by myoclonus and seizures. This syndrome is often irreversible and progressive until death.

127. How does metastatic cancer present in the nervous system?

Cancer affects the nervous system primarily by direct invasion. Metastases to the brain occur in 10–30% of patients with primary neoplasms, most commonly in lung and colon cancer in males and breast cancer in females. Metastatic cancer usually presents as a focal neurologic deficit, such as hemiparesis, but may also cause seizures. As the tumor enlarges, it produces increased ICP, leading to headache, altered mental status, and ultimately herniation and death.

Cancer may metastasize or spread locally to the spinal cord, leading to acute spinal cord compression. Usually, this is accompanied by back pain from vertebral body destruction. The onset of symptoms may be sudden with paraparesis, sensory level disturbances, and bowel and bladder disturbances.

128. What other effects of cancer may be seen?

Carcinomatous meningitis is most common in lymphomas and leukemias, but can be seen with solid tumors as well. Usually this presents as altered mental status, sometimes with fever, and sometimes with focal neurologic deficits as the cancer invades cranial nerves and roots as they emerge from the CNS.

Involvement of the peripheral nervous system by direct extension is sometimes seen, such as when a Pancoast tumor invades the brachial plexus. Peripheral neuropathies are uncommon.

Paraneoplastic syndromes, or remote effects of cancer, are quite rare. They may include myopathy (polymyositis), neuromuscular junction deficit (Lambert-Eaton myasthenic syndrome), and a peripheral neuropathy, predominantly sensory.

There is also a condition of diffuse cerebellar ataxia, likely caused by circulating immunologic proteins or antibodies that cross-react with neurologic tissues.

BIBLIOGRAPHY

1. Aminoff M: Neurology and General Medicine, 2nd ed. New York, Churchill-Livingstone, 1995.
2. Asbury AK, Thomas PK: Peripheral Nerve Disorders, 2nd ed. New York, Butterworth-Heinemann, 1995.
3. Bradley WG, Daroff RB, Fenichel GM, Marsden CD: Neurology in Clinical Practice, 3rd ed. Boston, Butterworth-Heinemann, 2000.
4. Caplan LR: Stroke: A Clinical Approach. New York, Butterworth-Heinemann, 1995.
5. Feldmann E: Current Diagnosis in Neurology. St. Louis, Mosby, 1994.
6. Johnson RT, Griffin JW: Current Therapy in Neurologic Disease, 5th ed. St. Louis, Mosby, 1997.
7. Rolak LA: Neurology Secret, 3rd ed.. Philadelphia, Hanley & Belfus, 2001.
8. Victor M, Ropper AH: Principles of Neurology, 7th ed. New York, McGraw-Hill, 2001.
9. Wyllie E: The Treatment of Epilepsy: Principles and Practice, 2nd edition, Philadelphia, Lea & Febiger, 1999.

Useful websites
www.neuroguide.com
www.aan.com (American Academy of Neurology)
www.medmatrix.org
www.internets.com/mednets/sneurolo.htm
www.medwebplus.com/subject/Neurology.html

15. MEDICAL CONSULTATION

Jane M. Geraci, M.D., M.P.H.

Physicians who meet in consultation must never quarrel or jeer at one another.

Hippocrates
Precepts VIII

Whenever he [Thomas Jefferson] saw three physicians together, he looked up to discover whether there was not a turkey buzzard in the neighborhood.

Quoted by Dr. Everett, private secretary to James Monroe

The delivery of medical care is to do as much nothing as possible.

Shem S.
13th Law of The House of God, Putnam, 1978, p 420, with permission

1. What are the ten commandments of effective medical consultation?

1. Determine the question.
2. Establish the urgency of the consultation.
3. Personally assess the patient (do not rely on others' assessments of the chest pain history, for example).
4. Be as brief as appropriate (this is why you determine the question).
5. Be specific in your recommendations.
6. Provide contingency plans.
7. Honor thy turf.
8. Teach with tact.
9. Talk is cheap—and effective.
10. Follow-up is essential.

Goldman L, Rudd P: Ten commandments for effective consultations. Arch Intern Med 143:1753–1755, 1983, with permission.

2. List eight strategies that improve the referring physician's compliance with recommendations of a medical consultant.

1. Perform the consult within 24 hours of the request.
2. Frequent, regular follow-up, with notes in the chart.
3. Verbal contact and a positive, professional interaction with the referring physician/service.
4. Limit recommendations to no more than five.
5. Recommendations are related to the reason for the consultation.
6. Phrase recommendations as definitive statements.
7. Assert the importance of the recommendation.
8. Give precise information about how to order the recommended diagnostic test or dose and how to administer any recommended treatment.

Adapted from Gross RJ, Caputo GM: General Medical Consultation Service: The Role of the Internist. In Gross RJ, Caputo GM (eds): Kammerer and Gross' Medical Consultation, 3rd ed. Baltimore, Williams & Wilkins, 1998, p 7, with permission.

PREOPERATIVE RISK ASSESSMENT

3. What are the essential "dos" and "don'ts" of preoperative risk assessment?

1. *Do* interview and examine the patient with respect to major organ-system disease, and describe the extent, severity, and stability of each disease in your assessment.

465

2. *Don't* tell the anesthesiologist which type of anesthesia and anesthetic agent to use; this determination is the anesthesiologist's job. The anesthesiologist relies on you for adequate characterization of the patient's burden of medical disease.

3. *Do* explain to the patient your estimate of his or her risk of complications of anesthesia and surgery, and document the explanation in your consultation note.

4. *Don't* "clear" the patient for surgery—such a step implies complete freedom from risk of adverse events, and we can never guarantee that a patient will not suffer an adverse outcome.

5. *Do* specify how the patient's current medications should be handled in the perioperative period (see also questions 54–61).

6. *Don't* directly try to change a patient's mind about proceeding with surgery—you are interfering in a patient-doctor relationship! Encourage patients to ask the surgeon questions about the proposed procedure. If you have serious concerns about surgery for a particular patient, call the referring surgeon and speak with him or her in a confidential manner and setting.

7. *Do* make recommendations for venous thromboembolism prophylaxis in patients who may benefit (see also question 46).

4. Describe general anesthesia (GA), regional anesthesia (RA), and monitored anesthesia care (MAC).

GA provides a loss of sensation with the loss of consciousness. Patients under GA may receive inhaled agents, inhaled plus intravenous drugs, or intravenous drugs alone. Ventilation may be managed through a mask, with or without an oropharyngeal or laryngopharyngeal airway, or through an endotracheal tube.

RA uses local anesthesia to produce loss of sensation to part of the body. Examples include epidural, spinal, axillary, and other regional blocks. Patients receiving RA also may receive some sedation. A patient undergoing RA may need to receive GA if the block is not adequate.

MAC involves an anesthesiologist's management of the patient during a procedure and may include provision of IV sedation, antiemetics or narcotics, and other pharmacologic treatments. MAC sometimes resembles GA in the amount of sedation produced in the patient.

5. Induction, maintenance, and reversal are the three phases of general anesthesia. Define induction, and list some of the potential problems.

Induction of anesthesia consists of administering medication to the conscious, perceiving patient to produce a state of unconsciousness and lack of perception. Although inhalational agents can be used to induce anesthesia, in current practice induction usually is accomplished by the intravenous (IV) route. Although it is advisable to intubate some patients before induction, endotracheal intubation usually is carried out immediately after induction. Potential problems include retching, vomiting, aspiration, cough, laryngospasm, hypotension, and cardiac dysrhythmias.

6. Which anesthetic technique is safer for patients—spinal/epidural or general?

This is a trick question. The few available well-designed studies that have compared RA with GA found no difference in cardiac outcomes. GA with inhalational agents directly suppresses myocardial contractility and reduces functional residual capacity in the lungs, with increased mismatch of ventilation and perfusion. Hence, inhalational GA may not be optimal for patients with severe cardiac or pulmonary insufficiency. Although spinal and epidural blocks do not have these effects, patients receiving RA can develop hypotension and bradycardia. In addition, the patient's airway is not as easily protected with RA. The higher the level of the spinal/epidural block, the more prominent the hypotension. Spinal and epidural blocks can be administered somewhat more quickly than GA.

7. What hemodynamic changes occur with spinal anesthesia?

Spinal anesthesia (the injection of local anesthetic into the subarachnoid space) blocks transmission of impulses from the sympathetic nervous system as well as impulses mediating motor and sensory functions. The sympathetic nervous system controls the caliber of the blood vessels.

At basal levels of sympathetic tone, the vessels are maintained at about half their maximal diameter. Sympathetic stimulation causes vasoconstriction, whereas sympathetic enervation, as in spinal anesthesia, causes vasodilatation. Vasodilatation causes a drop in systemic vascular resistance and consequent pooling of blood in the lower extremities. Arterial blood pressure usually decreases with administration of spinal anesthesia, and the drop is more severe in patients who are volume-depleted before the anesthetic is given. Patients with hypertension (controlled or not) also tend to have exaggerated hypotensive responses to spinal anesthesia.

8. What are the major, intermediate, and minor clinical predictors of perioperative adverse cardiovascular events after noncardiac surgery?

Major Predictors	Intermediate Predictors	Minor Predictors
Unstable coronary syndromes	Mild angina pectoris	Advanced age
Decompensated congestive heart failure	Prior myocardial infarction	Abnormal electrocardiogram
	Compensated/prior congestive heart failure	Rhythm other than sinus
Serious arrhythmias		Low exercise tolerance
Severe valvular disease	Diabetes mellitus	History of stroke
Acute myocardial infarction		Uncontrolled hypertension

Eagle KA et al: ACC/AHA guidelines for perioperative cardiovascular evaluation for noncardiac surgery. Circulation 93:1280–1317, 1996, with permission.

9. List the surgical procedures considered to place the patient at low, intermediate, and high risk of cardiac complications.

Low risk (< 1%)	Intermediate risk (< 5%)
Endoscopic procedures	Carotid endarterectomy
Superficial procedures	Head and neck surgery
Cataract surgery	Intraperitoneal and intrathoracic surgery
Breast surgery	Orthopedic surgery
	Prostate surgery

High risk (> 5%)

Emergent, major surgery, especially in elderly patients
Major vascular surgery, including aortic surgery
Peripheral vascular surgery
Prolonged surgery, with expected large fluid shifts and/or blood loss

Eagle KA, et al: ACC/AHA guidelines for perioperative cardiovascular evaluation for noncardiac surgery. Circulation 93:1280–1317, 1996, with permission.

10. Discuss the relationship of patient functional status to postoperative complications.

Poor functional status increases a patient's risk of both cardiac and noncardiac complications of surgery. Assessment of functional status is an essential part of the American College of Cardiology/American Heart Association (ACC/AHA) perioperative assessment guide. Cardiologists express functional status in terms of metabolic equivalent (MET) levels. One MET is equal to the oxygen consumption (3.5 ml/kg/min) of a 70-kg, 40-year-old man in a resting state. With this benchmark, functional capacity is excellent in patients who can perform at a level of > 7 METs; moderate at 4–7 METs; and poor if patients cannot meet a 4-MET demand during most daily activities. The 4-MET cut point is used in the ACC/AHA guideline. Patients who can do the following on a regular basis will pass this test:

- Brisk walks of at least several blocks
- Climb at least one flight of stairs
- Heavy housework such as scrubbing tiles and floors and moving furniture
- Golfing (without a cart), participation in team sports such as doubles tennis or pitching in baseball
- More strenuous activities (which approach 10 METs or more in energy consumption) include swimming, singles tennis, basketball, and skiing.

Eagle KA, et al: ACC/AHA guidelines for perioperative cardiovascular evaluation for noncardiac surgery. Circulation. 93:1280–1317, 1996, with permission.

11. Summarize the ACC/AHA approach to perioperative risk assessment.

Patients with *major clinical predictors* of cardiac risk (see question 8) should be evaluated and stabilized before elective surgery.

Patients with *intermediate clinical predictors* of cardiac risk who have poor functional status (< 4 METs) or moderate or excellent (> 4 METs) functional status but who are undergoing high surgical risk procedures (see question 9) should undergo noninvasive cardiac testing to refine risk assessment. Patients with intermediate clinical predictors who are undergoing low surgical risk procedures and patients with moderate to excellent functional status who are undergoing procedures of no more than intermediate risk may go to the operating room without further cardiac evaluation.

Patients with *minor or no clinical predictors* should undergo noninvasive testing only if they have both poor functional status (< 4 METs) and are scheduled to undergo a high surgical risk procedure. All other patients with minor or no clinical predictors may go directly to the operating room.

Eagle KA, et al: ACC/AHA guidelines for perioperative cardiovascular evaluation for noncardiac surgery. Circulation 93:1280–1317, 1996, with permission.

12. What two scoring systems are used by the American College of Physicians (ACP) to assess perioperative cardiac risk in patients undergoing noncardiac surgery?

The ACP Guidelines for Assessing and Managing the Perioperative Risk from Coronary Artery Disease Associated with Major Noncardiac Surgery are depicted in the figure on the facing page. The ACP algorithm first stratifies patients by a point system originally developed by Goldman and colleagues in the 1970s and modified and validated by Detsky and colleagues in the 1980s. In patients considered at high risk (10–15%) for cardiac complications according to this scoring system, the specific nature of the risk should be characterized as largely due to ischemic heart disease, other major cardiac disease, or nonmodifiable factors such as age. The decision to proceed with elective noncardiac surgery can then be reconsidered in light of these high-risk factors.

Because the low-risk stratum of the Modified Cardiac Risk Index does not adequately identify patients who are truly at low risk for perioperative cardiac complications, the ACP recommends a second risk assessment with the "Low-Risk Variables" of either Eagle or Vanzetto:

Eagle	**Vanzetto**
Age > 70 yrs	Age > 70 yrs
History of angina	History of angina
Diabetes mellitus	Diabetes mellitus
Q waves on electrocardiogram	Q waves on electrocardiogram
History of ventricular ectopy	History of myocardial infarction
	ST-segment ischemic abnormalities during resting electrocardiography
	Hypertension with severe left ventricular hypertrophy
	History of congestive heart failure

The presence of none or one of these risk factors identifies patients who are at low risk (< 3%) of perioperative cardiac complications and can proceed to surgery. The presence of two or more of these risk factors identifies patients at intermediate risk (3–15%) for perioperative cardiac complications. Patients in this group who are being considered for vascular surgery should undergo a noninvasive test for ischemic heart disease, such as dipyridamole thallium imaging or dobutamine stress echocardiography. Patients considered for vascular surgery in whom noninvasive testing shows evidence of reversible perfusion defects are at increased risk for perioperative cardiac events and should be managed as other high-risk patients. Patients considered for vascular surgery who show no reversible perfusion defects are at low risk for cardiac complications and may proceed to surgery.

13. What is the major difference between the ACC/AHA and the ACP guidelines?

The chief difference between the two guidelines is that the ACC/AHA recommends more frequent use of noninvasive tests for patients considering elective noncardiac surgery. The ACP recommends against noninvasive testing for ischemic heart disease in intermediate-risk patients undergoing noncardiac, nonvascular surgery, based on the results of studies indicating that positive results of noninvasive tests do not reliably identify patients who will have perioperative cardiac

Modified Cardiac Risk Index*

VARIABLE	POINTS
Coronary artery disease	
MI < 6 mo earlier	10
MI > 6 mo earlier	5
CCS angina class[†]	
Class III	10
Class IV	20
Alveolar pulmonary edema	
Within 1 wk	10
Ever	5
Suspected critical aortic stenosis	20
Arrhythmias	
Rhythm other than sinus or sinus plus atrial premature beats on EKG	5
> 5 premature ventricular contractions on EKG	5
Poor general medical status, defined as any of the following: PO_2 < 60 mmHg, PCO_2 > 50 mmHg, K^+ < 3 mmol/L, BUN > 50 mmol/L, creatinine > 250 μmol/L, bedridden	5
Age > 70 yr	5
Emergency surgery	10

* Class I = 0–15 points, class II = 20–30 points, class III = > 30 points.

† Canadian Cardiovascular Society classification of angina: 0 = asymptomatic, I = angina with strenuous exercise, II = angina with moderate exercise, III = angina with walking 1–2 level blocks or climbing 1 flight of stairs or less at normal pace, IV = inability to perform any physical activity without development of angina.

Adult facing surgery

Very young, very minor surgery, no systemic disease? → **Proceed directly to surgery**

strong evidence → **Collect variables from Modified Cardiac Risk Index**

Is the noncardiac surgery an emergency?

Class II (20–30 points) or Class III (> 30 points)?

Class I (0–15 points)?

strong evidence → **Collect low-risk variables**

0 or 1 factor? → **Low risk (< 3%)**

2 or more factors? → **Intermediate risk (3%–15%)**

High risk (> 15%) → **Determine nature of risk as per Figure B**

Undergoing nonvascular surgery? — *weak evidence* → **No further testing**

Undergoing vascular surgery? — *strong evidence* → **Perform DTI or DSE**

Negative Low risk / Positive High risk

Proceed directly to surgery

Author's addendum: For all patients, determine eligibility for beta-blocker use‡

† See question 12
‡ See question 53

A

ACP algorithm for assessment of perioperative cardiac risk. DTI = dipyridamole thallium imaging. DSE = dobutamine stress echocardiography. (From American College of Physicians: Guidelines for assessing and managing the perioperative risk from coronary artery disease associated with major noncardiac surgery. Ann Intern Med. 127:309–312; 1997, with permission.)

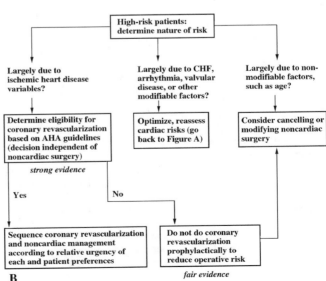

High-risk patients: determine nature of risk

Largely due to ischemic heart disease variables? → **Determine eligibility for coronary revascularization based on AHA guidelines (decision independent of noncardiac surgery)** *strong evidence*

Largely due to CHF, arrhythmia, valvular disease, or other modifiable factors? → **Optimize, reassess cardiac risks (go back to Figure A)**

Largely due to nonmodifiable factors, such as age? → **Consider cancelling or modifying noncardiac surgery**

Yes → **Sequence coronary revascularization and noncardiac management according to relative urgency of each and patient preferences**

No → **Do not do coronary revascularization prophylactically to reduce operative risk** *fair evidence*

B

complications. In contrast, the ACC/AHA recommends noninvasive testing for the following groups of elective surgery patients:

- Patients with intermediate clinical predictors who also have poor functional capacity (< 4 METs), regardless of the risk of the planned surgical procedure
- Patients with moderate-to-excellent functional capacity (> 4 METs) being considered for high-risk surgical procedures.
- Patients with minor or no clinical predictors of perioperative cardiac complications who have poor functional capacity and are to undergo a high surgical risk procedure.

American College of Physicians: Guidelines for assessing and managing the perioperative risk from coronary artery disease associated with major noncardiac surgery. Ann Intern Med 127:309–312; 1997.

14. What is the prevalence of underlying coronary artery disease (CAD) among patients with peripheral vascular disease?

Patients with peripheral vascular disease are highly likely to have CAD. Among 1000 consecutive patients with vascular disease but no clinical evidence of CAD who underwent coronary angiography, 37% had at least one coronary artery stenosis > 70%. This can be considered the minimal pretest probability of CAD in a population of patients under consideration for peripheral vascular surgery. However, many patients with vascular disease may have some clinical evidence of CAD, and in such patients the prevalence is far higher. Thus, for the patient population as a group the incidence is approximately 60%.

Gersh JB, et al: Evaluation and management of patients with both peripheral vascular and coronary artery disease. J Am Coll Cardiol 18:203–214, 1991.

Hertzer NR, et al: Coronary artery disease in peripheral vascular patients: A classification of 1000 coronary angiograms and results of surgical management. Ann Surg 199:223–233, 1984.

15. What is the leading cause of death after carotid endarterectomy?

Myocardial infarction (MI).

16. Discuss the major complications of the cross-clamping procedure and related maneuvers in repair of an abdominal aortic aneurysm.

Ischemia can result in the territories that are served by the clamped arteries. For obvious reasons, this problem is a major concern when the aorta is clamped. Decreased blood flow during the cross-clamping can result in a number of complications caused by ischemia, including acute renal failure, bowel infarction, and spinal cord damage that may result in paraplegia.

A rare complication is embolization of cholesterol and atheromatous fragments from the diseased aorta into the peripheral circulation. Although embolization can result from any angiographic procedure in which an atheromatous blood vessel is cannulated, a study obtained through a femoral artery seems to pose the highest risk. A shower of cholesterol emboli causes ischemic damage to the skin, extremities, and visceral organs (e.g., intestines and kidneys). Small emboli to the kidneys can cause progressive renal failure; large emboli can obstruct the main renal arteries and cause fulminant acute renal failure. Clues to the diagnosis of cholesterol emboli syndrome include a predisposing procedure in a patient with extensive vascular disease; the presence of leukocytosis and especially eosinophilia in the peripheral blood film; and cholesterol crystals in tissue specimens and retinal arteries.

17. Why do general anesthesia and surgery carry a higher risk for perioperative cardiac complications in patients with asymptomatic but significant aortic stenosis (AS)?

AS presents a fixed obstruction to the outflow of blood from the left ventricle (LV). In other words, the stenotic orifice limits maximal cardiac output (CO). In early AS, CO is maintained and the pressure gradient across the stenotic valve during systole increases with increased flow (i.e., increased CO). As the valve orifice decreases in diameter, the LV hypertrophies in response to the chronic pressure overload. As outflow obstruction worsens, CO cannot increase appropriately with exercise, although it is normal at rest.

In normal people, when tissue demands for oxygen go up (as with exercise), CO is increased by three mechanisms: (1) arterial dilatation with a drop in LV afterload; (2) enhanced myocardial contractility; and (3) a drop in venous capacitance with increased return to the heart and thus increased preload. In patients with moderately severe AS, arterial dilatation has little effect on improving CO, because the stenotic valve remains the major obstruction to outflow. Because such patients do not have an appropriate response to peripheral dilatation, they are prone to hypotension with exercise or other situations in which peripheral dilatation is induced (e.g., anesthesia). Furthermore, because of LV hypertrophy such patients have stiff ventricles so that, for any given intracavitary volume, the pressure is higher than normal. When cardiac return is increased in an effort to augment CO, there is the potential for rapid rises in filling pressures with resultant pulmonary edema.

At the time of surgery, patients with AS are at risk for hypotension, pulmonary edema, and MI. Ischemia can develop in patients with AS for several reasons. First, atherosclerotic coronary disease frequently coexists with AS. In addition, the pathophysiologic features of AS also affect myocardial oxygen balance unfavorably. Myocardial hypertrophy is associated with an increase in myocardial oxygen demand, and decreases in aortic pressure, especially during diastole, lead to decreases in myocardial oxygen delivery.

18. What are the risk factors for perioperative MI with noncardiac surgery?

In theory, anything that increases myocardial oxygen demand or decreases oxygen supply to the myocardium so that irreversible cell injury occurs is a risk factor for perioperative MI. In practice, however, because of the remarkable range of the autoregulation of perfusion across the coronary bed in people with normal coronary arteries and myocardium, the most important risk factor is heart disease (e.g., stenotic coronary arteries, hypertrophied muscle, dilated chambers). These conditions make the heart less able to compensate for the perturbations of myocardial oxygen demand and supply that may occur with anesthesia and surgery. In other words, they abbreviate cardiac reserve.

The occurrence of sustained hypotension intraoperatively seems to be the most important extraneous risk factor. Sustained intraoperative hypertension does not seem to be as important.

Ashton CM: Perioperative myocardial infarction with noncardiac surgery. Am J Med Sci 308:41–48, 1994.

19. How do you make the diagnosis of MI in postoperative patients?

As in other settings, the diagnosis rests on the triad of typical symptoms, typical pattern of change in cardiac enzymes, and EKG changes. However, the postoperative patient presents some diagnostic challenges. Up to one-half may not have the chest pain typical of MI. Instead, they present with unexplained hypotension, dysrhythmias, pulmonary congestion, mental status changes, and restlessness. Although the symptoms are atypical for MI, the truly asymptomatic perioperative MI is an uncommon event.

Secondly, of the so-called cardiac enzymes, only the MB fraction of creatine kinase (CK) is not elevated by the muscle trauma associated with anesthesia and surgery. Thus, although the total CK may be "falsely" elevated in postoperative patients, CK-MB retains its excellent sensitivity and specificity for acute MI. Because EKG changes are common in the postoperative setting, the EKG by itself is of little utility in diagnosing infarction. Up to 20% of postoperative patients have new EKG abnormalities, usually minor changes such as T-wave inversion or flattening. In any setting, Q waves pathognomonic for infarction develop in only 60% of patients with documented MIs.

20. Summarize the principles of evaluation and management of patients with congestive heart failure (CHF) who must undergo noncardiac surgery.

Whether CHF results from systolic impairment or diastolic dysfunction, determining the state of compensation is the most important component of the preoperative evaluation—even more important than the ejection fraction. The ejection fraction tells nothing about the state of compensation, and no consistent relationship has been found between ejection fraction and exercise tolerance as determined on a treadmill. Dyspnea on exertion is the earliest and most reliable symptom of CHF. Recent declines in exercise tolerance, increasing fatigue, orthopnea, and paroxysmal nocturnal dyspnea are the symptoms of decompensation. The signs of decompensation are weight increase, jugular venous distention, S3 gallop, hepatomegaly, and edema. It is important to have the patient as well compensated as possible before surgery. CHF seems to be an independent risk factor for perioperative cardiac complications. Monitoring right atrial or pulmonary wedge pressure intraoperatively and, even more importantly, postoperatively can help in the management of intravascular volume.

21. What is the significance of postoperative atrial fibrillation? How is it treated?

Atrial fibrillation is common after intrathoracic or cardiac procedures, which may directly irritate the atria and precipitate fibrillation. Patients with chronic pulmonary or cardiac disease also may develop atrial fibrillation becaue of the combination of the disease and the high catecholamine state that exists after surgery. The evaluation and management of patients with postoperative atrial fibrillation are similar to those for nonsurgical patients. One difference is that, wherever possible, beta blockers or calcium channel blockers are preferred over digoxin for ventricular rate control. These drugs counter the excessive postoperative catecholamines and have anti-ischemic effects, which also may be beneficial. Atrial fibrillation often resolves relatively quickly, but if it persists, the patient should be anticoagulated, if possible, to prevent development of atrial thrombus and embolic stroke. Eventually the patient should undergo elective cardioversion.

Bach DS: Management of specific medical conditions in the perioperative period. Prog Cardiovasc Dis 40:469–476, 1998.

22. What are the clinically significant pulmonary complications of surgery?

Any pulmonary abnormality that affects the clinical course of the surgical patient is considered clinically significant. Examples include:
- Atelectasis
- Infection, including bronchitis and pneumonia
- Prolonged mechanical ventilation and respiratory failure
- Exacerbation of chronic obstructive pulmonary disease
- Bronchospasm

23. What are the risk factors for postoperative pulmonary complications?

Definite risk factors	Probable risk factors
• Upper abdominal or thoracic surgery	• General anesthesia (vs. spinal or epidural anesthesia)
• Surgery lasting more than 3 hours	• Obesity
• Poor general health status, as defined by high ASA class	**Possible risk factors**
• Chronic obstructive pulmonary disease	• Current upper respiratory tract infection
• Smoking history within the past 8 weeks	• FEV_1 < 70% predicted
• $PaCO_2$ > 45 mmHg	• Abnormal chest radiograph

Smetana GW: Evaluation of preoperative pulmonary risk. In UpToDate, vol. 8 no. 3, 2000, with permission.

24. Which surgical patients should undergo preoperative spirometry? Arterial blood gas (ABG) analysis?

The only group for whom preoperative pulmonary function tests (PFTs) are mandatory is the group under consideration for lung resection. For all other types of surgery, there is no absolute minimal lung function, as assessed by PFTs, for avoidance of postoperative pulmonary complications. In other words, even patients with severe chronic obstructive pulmonary disease can be managed perioperatively with a satisfactory outcome. Of course, patients with unexplained pulmonary symptoms may benefit from preoperative PFTs.

Patients with a $PaCO_2$ > 45 mmHg are at increased risk for postoperative complications. Such patients usually have underlying severe chronic obstructive pulmonary disease. The ACP recommends preoperative ABG testing for patients undergoing coronary bypass surgery or upper abdominal surgery with a history of smoking or dyspnea and for patients undergoing lung resection.

25. Which strategies help to reduce the risk of postoperative pulmonary complications in patients with chronic pulmonary disease?

Preoperative strategies
- Smoking cessation 8 or more weeks before surgery
- Inhaled beta agonists for patients who wheeze or are dyspneic

- Preoperative systemic corticosteroids for patients who are not optimized to baseline at the time of surgery
- Antibiotics for definite pulmonary infection
- Teaching lung expansion maneuvers to patients before the surgery

Introperative strategies
- Limit the surgical procedure and anesthesia to less than 3–4 hours in duration
- Surgery other than upper abdominal or thoracic, when possible
- Regional anesthesia for very high-risk patients

Postoperative strategies
- Lung expansion maneuvers (deep breathing or incentive spirometry) in high risk patients
    Smetana GW: Evaluation of preoperative pulmonary risk. In UpToDate, vol. 8 no. 3, 2000 with permission.

26. For how long must a surgical patient completely abstain from cigarette smoking to gain the benefit of a decreased risk of postoperative pulmonary complications?

Several studies have demonstrated that patients must stop smoking cigarettes completely at least 8 weeks before surgery to decrease the risk of postoperative pulmonary complications.

27. Describe the principles of management for asthmatic patients who must undergo non-pulmonary surgery.

The two major principles of managing asthmatic patients are control of bronchospasm and control of secretions. Tracheal intubation can exacerbate bronchospasm and also is associated with increased sputum production. This problem is minimized by ensuring that bronchospasm is under optimal control before the patient goes to the operating room. Inhaled bronchodilators should be administered on a regular schedule, and if the patient is receiving theophylline, the serum level should be kept in the therapeutic range. Secretions can be managed by a pulmonary toilet program perioperatively. Such a program includes incentive spirometry in addition to inhaled bronchodilators. Steroid-dependent asthmatics, in whom adrenal function is often suppressed, should receive IV corticosteroids in the perioperative period to cover the stress of anesthesia and surgery.

28. Are patients with obstructive sleep apnea (OSA) at increased risk for postoperative complications?

Virtually no data are available to answer this question. When patients undergo surgery, such as uvulopalatopharyngoplasty, to correct OSA, the most common complications are airway-related, but the complication rate is still low. There are no data about outcomes of other noncardiac surgical procedures in patients with OSA. In evaluating a patient with known OSA who is treated with continuous positive airway pressure (CPAP), the consulting physician should determine whether the patient is compliant. Noncompliance with CPAP is quite common. The physician should assess the patient for signs and symptoms of right heart failure. Room-air arterial blood gas and electrolyte analyses reveal CO_2 retention consistent with inadequately treated OSA.

The patient with OSA who is most likely to have a postoperative complication is the patient whose syndrome is not yet diagnosed. As is always the case with potentially life-threatening medical disease, this problem should be addressed before the patient goes to the operating room whenever possible.

    Gupta RM, Gay PC: Perioperative cardiopulmonary evaluation and management: Are we ignoring obstructive sleep apnea syndrome? Chest 116:1843, 1999.

29. What is the fat embolism syndrome (FES)? Which patients are most likely to develop it?

FES is most often seen 24–72 hours after major orthopedic trauma and manifests classically as hypoxemia, altered mental status, and a petechial rash. In its severest form, patients may develop respiratory failure requiring mechanical ventilation and seizures or focal neurologic deficits. The petechial rash is highly useful for diagnosis, when present. It occurs on the head, neck, anterior thorax, subconjunctiva, or axillae and is not associated with thrombocytopenia. The rash is attributed to obstruction of dermal capillaries by fat globules, with resultant extravasation of red blood cells.

FES is most commonly associated with long-bone or pelvic fractures but has been reported in other patient populations, including those with soft tissue injuries, burns, liposuction, and bone marrow harvesting and transplant. Medical conditions that rarely may be associated with FES include pancreatitis, diabetes mellitus, osteomyelitis, bone tumor lysis, steroid therapy, sickle cell hemoglobinopathies, alcoholic liver disease, lipid infusion therapy, and cyclosporine solvent.

30. How is FES diagnosed, treated, and prevented?

FES must be diagnosed based on clinical findings, because no tests are highly specific or sensitive. For example, chest radiographs are frequently normal, and fat globules can be found in the sputum or serum of many fracture patients who have no clinical signs and symptoms of FES. Bronchoscopy with bronchoalveolar lavage is currently under investigation to detect fat droplets in alveolar macrophages. Treatment of clinically evident FES is supportive. Prevention of FES may be achieved with the following:

- Early immobilization of fractures
- Operative vs. nonoperative management
- Consideration of steroid prophylaxis for patients at highest risk (long-bone or pelvic fractures): methylprednisolone, 1.5 mg/kg IV every 8 hours for 2 days.

Surgeons are also exploring modifications of operative techniques for fracture repair, such as use of cementless fixation of hip prostheses.

31. What is the "lesion" in postoperative adult respiratory distress syndrome (ARDS)?

ARDS is a type of pulmonary edema. Pulmonary edema is of two types: cardiogenic, in which alteration of Starling forces is responsible for increases in water content of the interstitium and alveoli, and noncardiogenic, in which Starling forces are not deranged, but interstitial and alveolar water accumulates because of inflammatory injury to alveoli. Thus, the "lesion" in ARDS is alveolar damage, caused by proinflammatory cytokines, such as tumor necrosis factor, and activated neutrophils. Both alveolar and capillary epithelia are damaged, with resultant flooding of alveolar spaces with fluid. (Starling forces include the hydrostatic pressure inside the capillary, hydrostatic forces in the interstitium, oncotic pressure inside the capillary, and oncotic pressure in the interstitium.)

It is impossible to distinguish noncardiogenic pulmonary edema (ARDS) from cardiogenic pulmonary edema on the basis of clinical presentation and radiographic findings. The two conditions can be differentiated by measurement of the pulmonary capillary wedge pressure (PCWP), which reflects LV filling pressures and is normally 6–12 mmHg. PCWP is elevated in cardiogenic pulmonary edema, reflecting the elevated LV filling pressures. It is normal in ARDS, because LV filling pressures are normal since the defect is at the alveolocapillary membrane.

32. How can the risk of general medical complications be assessed in patients with chronic liver disease?

Patients with chronic liver disease are at increased risk for medical complications of surgery and anesthesia. The medical consultant should identify the nature of the liver disease (acute or chronic hepatitis and whether cirrhosis is present) and describe its severity. Most studies examining surgical outcomes have evaluated patients with cirrhosis. The Child-Pugh classification of cirrhotic severity has been shown to predict morbidity and mortality:

RISK FACTOR	POINTS ASSIGNED		
	1	2	3
Ascites	Absent	Slight	Moderate
Bilirubin (mg/dl)	≤ 2	2–3	> 3
Albumin (gm/dl)	> 3.5	2.8–3.5	< 2.8
Prothrombin time			
Seconds over control	1–3	4–6	≥ 6
International normalized ratio	< 1.7	1.8–2.3	> 2.3
Encephalopathy	None	Grade 1–2	Grade 3–4

Score interpretations:	5–6 points = grade A (well-compensated disease)
	7–9 points = grade B (significant functional compromise)
	10–15 points = grade C (decompensated disease)
Predicted mortality rate:	Grade A $\cong$ 10%
	Grade B $\cong$ 30%
	Grade C $\cong$ 80%

Thus, patients with grade B or grade C cirrhosis are at increased risk for morbidity and mortality after surgery. In the absence of definite cirrhosis, patients with chronic hepatitis have a surgical risk that is proportional to the severity of the disease, as manifested by the derangements in the Child-Pugh classification system. Finally, patients with acute alcoholic or viral hepatitis, fulminant hepatic failure, or severe and uncorrectable hypoprothrombinemia are not candidates for elective surgery.

Friedman LS: Assessing surgical risk in patients with liver disease-II. In UpToDate, vol. 8 no. 3, 2000, with permission.

33. What measures should be undertaken to prepare patients with chronic liver disease for surgery?

- Treatment of hypoprothrombinemia with vitamin K or fresh frozen plasma to achieve a prothrombin time within 3 seconds of normal
- Platelet transfusion to maintain a count of at least 100,000/ml
- Cessation of all alcohol intake (For patients with alcoholic hepatitis, this may improve liver function indices; some experts recommend serum gamma glutamyl transferase [GGT] as a useful marker of hepatic inflammation due to alcohol. GGT levels should return to normal 3–5 weeks after cessation of alcohol intake.)
- Treatment and control of ascites with diuretics to reduce the risk of wound dehiscence in the abdomen
- Correction of electrolyte abnormalities, such as hypokalemia
- Consideration of perioperative nutritional support for malnourished patients who must undergo major surgery (i.e., hepatic resection/transplant)

34. What tests should be performed before cataract surgery?

Schein and colleagues randomized over 18,000 patients at nine medical centers to undergo or not to undergo a standard set of preoperative tests (EKG, serum electrolytes, renal function, complete blood count) in addition to the history and physical examination. They found no difference in complication rates between the two groups overall, nor did specific subgroups based on characteristics such as age or medical history benefit from preoperative tests. Based on these results, it appears reasonable to forego routine blood work and EKG for patients whose history and physical examinations reveal no need for such evaluation.

Schein OD, Katz J, Bass EB et al: The value of routine preoperative medical testing before cataract surgery. N Engl J Med 342:168–175, 2000.

35. How can asymptomatic patients at risk for perioperative bleeding due to hereditary hemorrhagic or coagulation disorders be identified?

Patient history is the most useful screening tool for disorders that may cause perioperative hemorrhage, such as von Willebrand's disease or hemophilia. All patients should be questioned about excessive bleeding after prior surgeries, procedures, or childbirth; history of transfusions; and medication use that may be associated with acquired coagulation defects.

36. How should you determine the cause of new-onset renal insufficiency in postoperative patients?

In postoperative patients, as in other populations, it is useful to classify new-onset renal insufficiency as prerenal, renal, or postrenal. **Prerenal azotemia** results from decreased renal perfusion. Its causes include intravascular volume depletion due to hemorrhage, GI losses (as with nasogastric suction or ileostomy), or third-spacing of fluids (as with peritonitis); decreased cardiac function due to pump failure, valvular abnormalities, dysrhythmias, or pericardial tamponade; excessive peripheral vasodilatation as seen in sepsis or with afterload-reducing agents; and obstruction of blood flow through renal arteries or veins. To evaluate prerenal causes, a careful history and physical examination should be performed, with special reference to the cardiovascular system. The blood urea nitrogen (BUN):creatinine ratio approaches 20:1 (normal = 10:1). Urinary sodium measures also are extremely helpful. Because the kidney has only one stereotypical response to what it perceives as a threat to intravascular volume (i.e., conservation of sodium and hence water), the urinary sodium level is very low (≤ 10 mEq/L).

Obstruction to urine flow causes **postrenal azotemia**. In the work-up of postoperative renal insufficiency, obstruction at or below the bladder neck should be ruled out by the insertion of a catheter. For obstruction above the bladder to cause renal failure, it must be bilateral. Inadvertent ligation of the ureters during abdominopelvic surgery occasionally occurs. The presence of hydronephrosis/hydroureter can be ascertained by renal ultrasonography.

Causes of postoperative **renal azotemia** include ischemia, as may occur with abdominal aortic aneurysm surgeries, and exposure to nephrotoxins, such as contrast agents and aminoglycosides. The diagnosis is suggested by a BUN:creatinine ratio $\geq 20:1$ and a urine sodium ≤ 10 mEq/L. The urine sodium is elevated because the injured parenchyma is unable to conserve sodium.

37. What is the incidence of perioperative acute renal failure? What patient- and surgery-specific characteristics are associated with its occurrence?

Perioperative acute renal failure occurs in 1.2% of all surgical patients. Elderly patients and patients with jaundice, chronic renal failure, congestive heart failure, or diabetes are at increased risk. Cardiac and aortic surgical procedures are associated with higher rates of perioperative renal failure. The mechanism of the renal failure is most commonly ischemic injury to the kidney, which can be caused by intraoperative hypotension and cardiopulmonary bypass and aortic cross-clamping procedures related to cardiac and aortic surgeries. Another important cause of acute renal failure in patients undergoing aortic surgery is renal artery cholesterol embolism after clamping and unclamping of the atherosclerotic aorta during repair of aortic aneurysm. In the most severe cases, patients develop sudden, complete anuria during the release of the cross-clamp, as a manifestation of bilateral renal artery embolism. A careful skin and ophthalmologic exam may reveal cholesterol emboli, which provide essential evidence for the diagnosis.

Kellerman PS: Perioperative care of the renal patient. Arch Intern Med 154:1674–1688, 1994.

38. Are dialysis patients who undergo surgery at increased risk for adverse outcomes?

Yes. Dialysis patients appear to have an increased likelihood of postoperative complications compared with surgical patients with normal renal function and to require longer hospital stays, pressor support, and intensive care. Causes of postoperative complications in dialysis patients include:
• High incidence of underlying coronary artery disease and myocardial dysfunction
• Lack of physiologic maintenance of volume and electrolyte status, leading to perioperative volume overload or sodium or potassium disturbances
• Underlying bleeding diathesis, leading to perioperative hemorrhage
• Poor blood pressure control
• Retarded excretion/metabolism of some anesthetics and analgesics

Kellerman PS: Perioperative care of the renal patient. Arch Intern Med 154:1674–1688, 1994.
Soundararajan R, Golper TA: Medical management of the dialysis patient undergoing surgery. In UpToDate, vol. 8 no. 3, 2000, with permission.

39. When should dialysis be performed in relation to elective surgery?

Most nephrologists recommend that patients with end-stage renal disease (ESRD) should undergo dialysis immediately before surgery to optimize volume status and electrolyte levels.

40. Many patients with ESRD have a bleeding tendency. Should bleeding time be assessed before surgery?

No. Experts do not recommend using the bleeding time to screen patients because (1) a normal bleeding time does not predict the safety of surgery, and (2) a prolonged bleeding time does not predict hemorrhage. This finding may be due in part to the effect of technical factors in test performance. However, nephrologists do recommend assessment of the bleeding time before renal biopsy. Platelet dysfunction in uremia is probably multifactorial; causative factors include uremic toxins (hence performance of dialysis immediately before surgery is advisable), anemia, excessive parathyroid hormone, and aspirin use. Some patients with chronic renal disease are hypercoagulable; therefore, one should not assume that all dialysis patients are safe from acute venous thromboembolism.

41. How does perioperative bleeding due to uremia typically present? How is it treated?

Uremic bleeding usually develops as hemorrhage in the skin or oozing at sites of trauma or surgery. Therefore, bleeding from an organ should be evaluated with the appropriate diagnostic tests to identify a cause, such as peptic ulcer disease. Treatment options for uremic bleeding include:

- Transfusion to increase the hematocrit to 25–30%
- Desmopressin (DDAVP) at a dose of 0.30 µg/kg either intravenously (IV) or intranasally (onset of action = 1 hour, duration = 4–24 hours)
- Cryoprecipitate, 10 units IV every 12–24 hours (duration of effect = 8–24 hours)
- Conjugated estrogens, 0.6 mg/kg/day IV for 5 days; Premarin, 2.5–5.0 mg/day orally, or 50–100-µg transdermal estradiol twice weekly (onset at 1 day after initiation, peak effect 5–7 days later, duration of effect up to 1 week or more after cessation of therapy)
- Dialysis

Rose BD: Platelet dysfunction in uremia. In UpToDate, vol. 8 no. 3, 2000.

Soundararajan R, Golper TA: Medical management of the dialysis patient undergoing surgery. In UpToDate, vol. 8 no. 3, 2000, with permission.

42. What is the correct diagnostic approach to patients with postoperative hyponatremia (serum sodium of 127 mEq/L)?

The plasma concentration of sodium, the primary determinant of serum osmolality, is maintained within a narrow normal range by means of a balance of water intake, regulated by the thirst mechanism, and water excretion by the kidney. The normal kidney can excrete up to 10 L/day of water. Consequently, hyponatremia is rarely caused by excessive water intake. The most common cause of hyponatremia is a defect in renal excretion of water. The following is a time-honored approach to the hyponatremic patient. The first step is to assess the patient's volume status by performing a physical examination. Three possibilities exist, each with its own differential diagnosis:

1. The **volume-depleted patient** is salt- and water-depleted, with the salt deficit exceeding the water deficit. The deficits result from either renal losses (e.g., diuretic excess) or extrarenal losses (e.g., GI losses).

2. The **edematous patient** has an excess of total body water and salt, with the water excess greater than the salt excess. The excesses result from the kidney's retention of salt and water in conditions, such as cardiac failure and cirrhosis, in which it perceives a decrease in the "effective arterial blood volume." Salt and water excesses also are seen in nephrosis and advanced renal failure, although the inciting causes are different.

3. The **hyponatremic patient** who appears to be euvolemic is usually modestly volume-expanded and has an excess of total body water, although this excess is not detectable on examination. The most likely explanation for "euvolemic" hyponatremia is prolonged release of antidiuretic hormone (ADH) in the face of persistent water intake. Postoperative pain is one stimulus for ADH release.

Measurement of urinary sodium concentration is a useful adjunct in distinguishing among the diagnostic possibilities in the three categories. Hyponatremia is quite common in postoperative patients. Usually it results from a combination of hypotonic fluid administration and release of ADH. Hyperglycemia can cause a "factitious" hyponatremia (called factitious because plasma osmolality is normal or high, although sodium is low). This is an important consideration in postoperative diabetics with hyponatremia.

Berl T, Schrier RW: Disorders of water metabolism. In Schrier RW (ed): Renal and Electrolyte Disorders, 5th ed. Philadelphhia, Lippincott-Raven, 1997, pp 32–72.

43. What is the TURP syndrome?

Altered mental status due to postoperative hyponatremia in a patient who has undergone transurethral resection of the prostate (TURP). During the TURP procedure the operative field is continuously irrigated, and hypotonic fluid may be absorbed into the bloodstream, causing hyponatremia. Most patients are asymptomatic, but some develop delirium progressing to hypertension, seizures, intravascular hemolysis, and fatal cardiac rhythm abnormalities. TURP syndrome may be prevented or detected early through the use of regional anesthesia, which allows communication with the patient to detect signs of change in mental status.

44. What are the symptoms and signs of postoperative adrenal insufficiency?

Adrenal insufficiency in the perioperative period is rare. Although it is an eminently treatable condition, clinicians often omit it from the differential diagnosis of intra- or postoperative deterioration. Surgery is a physiologically stressful situation that may unmask chronic adrenal insufficiency. The first sign may be persistent intraoperative hypotension. Postoperatively, the patient may be febrile (to 103°F) with nausea, vomiting, and severe abdominal pain—findings that often are misdiagnosed as an intra-abdominal catastrophe. Hypotension and shock can develop. Whenever the diagnosis is entertained, a serum cortisol level should be drawn, and corticosteroids should be administered without waiting for the result.

The patient with chronic adrenal insufficiency is at risk for an adrenal crisis precipitated by surgery. The symptoms and signs of chronic adrenal insufficiency are asthenia, fatigue, muscle weakness, postural hypotension, nausea, vomiting, anorexia, weight loss, abdominal pain, hyperkalemia, hyponatremia, anemia, and eosinophilia. Hyperpigmentation may or may not be present. Although very helpful if elicited as part of the preoperative evaluation, these findings in postoperative patients are difficult to interpret because they can be attributed to iatrogenic causes, such as anesthesia, surgery, and fluid and electrolyte administration.

45. What is the incidence of postoperative delirium? What risk factors may lead to its occurrence?

In a prospective cohort study, Marcantonio and colleagues identified postoperative delirium in 9% of patients undergoing general, orthopedic, or gynecologic surgery at a single institution. Multivariate analysis revealed the following independent predictors of delirium:

- Age > 70 years
- Alcohol abuse
- Poor cognitive status, as measured by the Telephone Interview for Cognitive Status (a score of 30 correlates with a score of 24 on the Mini-Mental Status Exam).
- Poor physical functional status, as measured by a class IV assessment according to the Specific Activity Scale (patients are unable to walk 4 km/hr for one block, make their bed, or dress themselves without stopping to rest)
- Preoperative electrolyte abnormalities: serum sodium < 130 or > 150 mmol/L, serum K < 3.0 or > 6.0 mmol/L, or serum glucose < 60 or > 300 mg/dL.
- Aortic aneurysm surgery
- Noncardiac thoracic surgery

These factors can be used to score the patient's risk. Each item above is scored with 1 point with the exception of aortic aneurysm surgery, which is scored with 2 points. In the validation study set, no patients with scores of 0 developed delirium, whereas 11% of patients with scores of 1 or 2 and 50% of patients with scores > 3 developed postoperative delirium.

Marcantonio ER, et al: A clinical prediction rule for delirium after elective noncardiac surgery. JAMA 271:134–139, 1994.

46. How can the risk of perioperative venous thromboembolism (VTE) be assessed?

There are numerous risk factors for VTE. They may occur in combination in a single patient, in which case their effect is cumulative. The risk assessment for each surgical patient must be comprehensive, taking into account past medical history, current illness, and planned surgical procedure. The VTE risk factors can be grouped as follows to facilitate the choice of prophylactic treatment:

Negligible risk	Increased risk	Moderate-to-high risk
Age under 40 years	Age over 40 years	Knee or hip replacement
No chronic medical illnesses	General (nonorthopedic) surgery	Hip fracture
	Acute MI admission	Pelvic/lower extremity trauma
	Congestive heart failure	Spinal cord injury
	Acute cerebrovascular accident with lower extremity paralysis	
	Pneumonia admission	
	Pregnancy	
	Malignancy	
	Use of oral contraceptives	
	Prior VTE	
	Obesity	

In general, patients with negligible risk who are not undergoing a moderate-to-high risk (right column) surgical procedure do not need VTE prophylaxis. Patients at highest risk for VTE are those who are undergoing major orthopedic procedures or have suffered pelvic or lower extremity trauma. Such patients warrant aggressive VTE prophylaxis with low-molecular-weight heparin or warfarin compounds, as do patients with multiple risk factors listed in the middle column. Patients who combine high-risk surgery with several or more other risk factors should be considered for combined-modality prophylaxis (i.e., intermittent pneumatic compression plus low-molecular-weight heparin).

47. List the nine treatment modalities that have been evaluated as prophylaxis against venous thromboembolism.

1. Aspirin
2. Elastic stockings (use with or without IPC in lower-risk general surgical and medical patients)
3. Intermittent pneumatic compression devices (IPC), which provide rhythmic compression to the lower extremity (use in neurosurgery, moderate-risk general surgery, and total knee replacement)
4. Low-dose, unfractionated heparin (5000 U 2–3 times/day subcutaneously)
5. Low-molecular-weight (LMW) heparin (enoxaparin, 30 mg twice daily or 40 mg/day subcutaneously)
6. Adjusted-dose unfractionated heparin
7. Dextran (rarely used)
8. Warfarin ("mini-dose"= target INR 1.5; adjusted dose = target INR 2.0–3.0)
9. Vena cava filter (may prevent pulmonary embolism only in the short term; use only if anticoagulant-based prophylaxis is not feasible)

48. What is the optimal duration of VTE prophylaxis in patients undergoing total hip or knee replacement? For patients who have had repair of a hip fracture?

This is an area of ongoing inquiry. Such patients continue to be at risk for postoperative VTE after discharge from the hospital. In 2001, the Sixth American College of Chest Physicians Consensus Conference recommended that patients who have had total knee or hip replacement should receive 7–10 days of postoperative warfarin or LMW heparin but noted that optimal prophylaxis may actually be longer in duration. Newly published data suggest a benefit to extending prophylaxis with LMW heparin in hip replacement patients to 35 days postoperatively. Warfarin is stopped with discharge. Unfortunately, no such data exist for patients who have undergone surgery for hip fracture. The best course is to treat such patients with VTE prophylaxis until they are fully ambulatory.

Greets WH, et al: Prevention of venous thromboembolism. Chest 119:132S–175S, 2001.

Hull RD, et al: Low-molecular-weight heparin prophylaxis using dalteparin extended out-of-hospital vs in-hospital warfarin/out-of-hospital placebo in hip arthroplasty patients. Arch Intern Med 160:2208–2215, 2000.

49. Two days after repair of a hip fracture, an elderly patient develops sudden dyspnea and tachypnea. He has been receiving LMW heparin for VTE prophylaxis. What diagnosis must be ruled out first?

Despite VTE prophylaxis, there is a good possibility that the patient has sustained a pulmonary embolism. In randomized, controlled trials of interventions to prevent VTE in patients with hip fracture, the groups that received prophylaxis (low-dose or LMW heparin or low-intensity warfarin) had a DVT prevalence of 24–27% by venogram (compared with 48% for the control/placebo groups). Thus, some patients who have received prophylaxis develop VTE, and the medical consultant and orthopedist must maintain a high index of suspicion.

Greets WH, et al: Prevention of venous thromboembolism. Chest 119:132S–175S, 2001.

50. What is malignant hyperthermia?

Malignant hyperthermia is a rare genetic disorder that develops in response to treatment with certain anesthetic agents, most commonly succinylcholine and halothane. The onset is within a few hours of anesthetic administration. Clinical findings include muscle rigidity, sinus tachycardia, cyanosis, and mottling of the skin, closely followed by marked hyperthermia with temperatures possibly as high as 45°C. Hypotension, arrhythmias, rhabdomyolysis, electrolyte disorders, and disseminated intravascular coagulation may ensue rapidly. The full syndrome can develop without hyperthermia, although this occurrence is rare.

51. How is malignant hyperthermia treated?

Dantrolene is the treatment of choice and should be administered as quickly as possible to ensure survival. Dantrolene is a nonspecific skeletal muscle relaxant that acts by blocking release of calcium from the sarcoplasmic reticulum. It should be given as a 2-mg/kg IV bolus and then repeated every 5 minutes until the symptoms resolve to a maximal dose of 10 mg/kg. This protocol may be repeated every 10–15 hours. Once the patient has responded, oral therapy may be initiated at 4–8 mg/kg/day in 4 divided doses for 3 days.

MANAGEMENT OF CHRONIC MEDICAL AND OTHER DISEASES IN THE PERIOPERATIVE PERIOD

52. What are the important issues in the perioperative care of patients with a permanent cardiac pacemaker?

Two issues must be addressed: the cardiac status of the patient, including assessment of adequacy of pacemaker function, and safety in the operating room. In general, the adequately functioning pacemaker (1) senses the patient's own intracardiac signals and (2) delivers an electric stimulus to depolarize the myocardium at a time when it is excitable and at an appropriate rate. Pacemaker function should be assessed during the month before elective surgery at the usual source of pacemaker care.

In the operating room, electromagnetic interference (usually from electrocautery) may cause failure of the demand pacemaker. This problem can be solved by converting the pacemaker from a demand mode to a fixed-rate mode by placing a high-powered magnet over the generator. The possibility of electromagnetic interference can be minimized by placing the ground plate as far from the generator as possible and by using electrocautery in short bursts. In patients with a temporary pacemaker, the pacemaker leads provide a direct pathway by which extraneous external electrical impulses can go directly to the heart. The contact points between the leads and the generator should be covered with a surgical glove, and gloves should be worn when the unit is handled.

53. Which patients undergoing noncardiac surgery are candidates for perioperative beta blockade to prevent adverse postoperative cardiac outcomes?

Two studies have demonstrated that perioperative beta blockade reduces adverse cardiac outcomes, including cardiac death, in high-risk patients undergoing noncardiac surgery. Thus, indications for such treatment include the following:

- Established coronary artery disease
- Peripheral vascular disease
- Presence of multiple cardiac disease risk factors: tobacco use, hypertension, diabetes mellitus, hyperlipidemia, age > 65 years

Mangano DT, Layug EL, Wallace A, et al: Effect of atenolol on mortality and cardiovascular morbidity after noncardiac surgery. N Engl J Med 335:1713–1720, 1996.

Poldermans D, Boersma E, Bax JJ, et al: The effect of bisoprolol on perioperative mortality and myocardial infarction in high-risk patients undergoing vascular surgery. N Engl J Med 341:1789–1794, 1999.

54. In which patients on chronic or life-long warfarin therapy may warfarin be withheld before surgery without use of preoperative intravenous heparin?

There is an emerging consensus that ambulatory patients taking warfarin for prevention of stroke due to chronic atrial fibrillation may stop the drug 4–5 days before surgery (to achieve an international normalized ratio [INR] ≤ 1.5). This practice has been inspired in large part by an analysis published by Kearon and Hirsh, who noted that most patients have partial protection against thromboembolism for several more days after the cessation of warfarin because of the slow decline in the anticoagulation effect. The argument against preoperative heparin also includes the fact that patients receiving heparin have a risk of hemorrhage that more than offsets the decrement in thromboembolism risk.

Warfarin also may be withheld without preoperative heparin treatment in patients who suffered an acute arterial or venous thromboembolic event longer than 1 month before. For patients with more recent thromboembolic events, Kearon and Hirsh recommend avoiding elective surgery if possible; if avoidance is not possible, patients should receive intravenous heparin and/or a vena caval filter.

Kearon and Hirsh also suggest that patients with mechanical heart valves do not warrant either preoperative or postoperative intravenous heparin while off warfarin for surgery. However, the physicians providing longitudinal or primary care for such patients often are averse to leaving them "unprotected" against thromboembolic events. In patients with mechanical valves and patients on lifelong warfarin therapy with multiple prior arterial or venous thromboembolic events, the author defers the decision about perioperative heparin to the patients and their primary care physicians.

Kearon C, et al: Management of anticoagulation before and after elective surgery. N Engl J Med 336:1506–1511, 1997.

55. Which patients who have stopped warfarin before surgery should have postoperative intravenous heparin while awaiting therapeutic oral anticoagulation?

The risk of thromboembolism in the postoperative period is the sum of the patient's baseline risk plus risks associated with the surgery. Kearon and Hirsh recommend that patients within 3 months of an acute venous or 1 month of an acute arterial thromboembolic event receive postoperative heparin to prevent another such event while they are awaiting full oral anticoagulation. The risk of venous or arterial thromboembolism in untreated patients outweighs the risk of bleeding associated with postoperative intravenous heparin. Other patients should receive the appropriate therapy to prevent postoperative venous thromboembolism while resuming warfarin.

Kearon C, et al: Management of anticoagulation before and after elective surgery. N Engl J Med 336:1506–1511, 1997.

56. What are the adverse consequences of hyperglycemia (serum glucose > 300 mg/dl) in postoperative diabetics?

Despite the difficulty of proving the assertion, most physicians believe that wound healing is impaired in patients with poorly controlled diabetes. A second adverse effect may be a predisposition to infection. Although the clinical ramifications are not yet known, several defects in host defense mechanisms have been shown in poorly controlled diabetes, including impaired leukocyte chemotaxis, decreased intracellular bactericidal activity, and impaired cell-mediated immune response.

A third, often forgotten, adverse effect is the osmotic diuresis that hyperglycemia induces. In the renal tubule, the maximum tubular transport capacity (T_m) for glucose is about 375 mg/min. Once the filtered load of glucose exceeds the T_m, no more glucose can be reabsorbed, and glucose appears in the urine. The osmotic presence of glucose in the renal tubular fluid retards water and salt reabsorption. In postoperative patients (as in other settings), this process may lead to volume depletion and prerenal azotemia.

57. How should the blood sugar of type I diabetics be managed in the perioperative period?

Type I diabetics, who account for 10% of all diabetics, have an absolute deficiency of insulin and therefore require regular administration for survival. The physiologic stress induced by induction of anesthesia and surgery leads to increased blood glucose concentrations. Surgery induces release of catecholamines, adrenocorticotropic hormone, glucagon, and growth hormone, all of which cause gluconeogenesis. Without insulin to counteract this process, diabetic ketoacidosis may result.

One approach is to give the patient one-half to two-thirds of the usual morning dose of intermediate-acting (NPH) insulin, monitor blood sugars throughout the early postoperative period, administer sliding-scale regular insulin as needed, and then resume the patient's usual regimen when he or she is able to eat. Alternatively, a patient may be treated with a continuous insulin infusion with concomitant intravenous dextrose.

58. How should the treatment regimens of type II diabetics be managed perioperatively?

Type II diabetics who are treated with insulin may be managed as described above, particularly if time in the operating room is expected to be long. For surgical procedures of minor or intermediate complexity, and especially for day surgery, patients may withhold the morning dose of insulin, have periodic checks of blood glucose during recovery, and resume their usual regimen the same evening when they are able to eat.

Type II diabetics are currently treated with a variety of oral medications that remedy one or more of the specific defects associated with type II diabetes: target-tissue resistance to insulin, low insulin secretion by islet cells, and increased hepatic gluconeogenesis. These agents should be withheld before surgery. The manufacturer of metformin recommends that it be held 48 hours before a contrast-dye procedure is performed because of concerns that lactic acidosis may occur in a patient who develops acute renal failure. The longer-acting, older sulfonylureas (chlorpropamide and tolbutamide) should be discontinued at least 3 days before surgery because of their long half-lives. The second-generation sulfonylureas may be stopped on the day of surgery. Patients with chronic liver or renal disease should stop sulfonylureas at an earlier point because of their prolonged activity in such disease states. All diabetics should have preoperative and postoperative glucose checks, and hyperglycemia can be treated with sliding-scale insulin. Oral antidiabetic drugs can be resumed with resumption of oral intake.

Newer Antidiabetic Agents

DRUG	COMMERCIAL NAME	MECHANISM/ SITE OF ACTION	WHEN TO DISCONTINUE PREOPERATIVELY
Acarbose	Precose	Limits intestinal absorption of glucose	With last meal
Glimepiride	Amaryl	Increases β-cell sensitivity to insulin	24–36 hr
Glipizide GITS	Glucotrol XL	Increases β-cell sensitivity to insulin	72 hr
Metformin	Glucophage	Increases insulin action	24–36 hr; stop earlier for contrast dye procedures
Repaglinide	Prandin	Insulin secretagogue	With last meal
Rosiglitazone	Avandia	Increases peripheral glucose uptake	48 hours

59. What are the two reasons for strict continuation of medications for comorbid diseases during the perioperative period?

1. Uninterrupted administration of medications minimizes the chance that patients will develop an acute exacerbation of the chronic disease in the perioperative period. Patients with serious chronic disease should receive medications on the day of surgery and throughout the perioperative period. Such conditions include but are not limited to coronary artery disease, congestive heart failure, hypertension, seizure disorders (particularly if the seizure is generalized tonic-clonic), Parkinson's disease, and chronic obstructive pulmonary disease.

2. Continued administration of medications avoids the development of a withdrawal syndrome with abrupt cessation.

MEDICATION	WITHDRAWAL SYNDROME
Alpha blockers (clonidine)	Rebound hypertension
Benzodiazepines	Rebound anxiety and insomnia
Beta blockers	Rebound hypertension
Short-acting SSRI antidepressants (sertraline, venlaxafine)	Headache, nausea, dizziness

SSRI = selective serotonin reuptake inhibitor.

60. When should antiplatelet agents be discontinued before surgery?

AGENT	EFFECT ON PLATELETS	WHEN TO DISCONTINUE PREOPERATIVELY
Aspirin	Irreversible defect	7 days
Cilostazol	Reversible inhibition of platelet aggregation	3 days
Clopidogrel	Irreversible defect	7 days
NSAIDs	Reversible defect	4–5 half-lives before surgery
Ticlopidine	Irreversible defect	7 days

61. How should patients on chronic corticosteroid therapy be managed in the perioperative period?

Although it is possible to assess the reserve of the hypothalamic-pituitary-adrenal (HPA) axis in response to stress, this assessment is rarely done in clinical practice. Instead, it is assumed that most patients on chronic corticosteroid therapy are at risk for developing secondary adrenal insufficiency due to the stress of surgery and therefore should receive stress doses of steroids. Included are patients taking daily prednisone for more than 3 weeks and patients with Cushing's syndrome. In patients taking < 10 mg each morning, the HPA axis is unlikely to be suppressed, but many experts nevertheless recommend that they receive stress doses of steroids for surgery. A suggested steroid regimen for illness or surgery is summarized below:

- For moderate illness: hydrocortisone, 50 mg twice daily orally or intravenously; taper rapidly to maintenance dose.
- For severe illness: hydrocortisone, 100 mg IV every 8 hours; decrease dose by half each day, keeping in mind the course of the illness.
- For minor procedures under local anesthesia and most radiologic studies: no corticosteroid supplementation is needed.
- For moderately stressful procedures (e.g., barium enema, endoscopy, arteriography): single 100 mg dose of hydrocortisone IV just before the procedure.
- For major surgery: hydrocortisone, 100 mg IV just before induction of anesthesia and every 8 hours for the first 24 hours; then taper rapidly by decreasing the dose by half each day to maintenance level.

Note: if IV access cannot be obtained, hydrocortisone can be administered rectally.

Orth DN, Kovacs WJ: Pharmacologic use of glucocorticoids, and Orth DN: Treatment of adrenal insufficiency. In UpToDate, vol. 8, no. 3, 2000, with permission.

CARE OF THE PSYCHIATRIC PATIENT

62. Define somatization disorder.

According to the DSM-IV-TR, it is a psychiatric condition characterized by multiple, recurrent physical complaints for which no organic basis can be found. The disorder begins before age 30 and is more common in females. Common physical complaints include vomiting, pain in the extremities, shortness of breath, amnesia, pain in the sexual organs or rectum, and dysmenorrhea. The patient makes frequent visits to physicians because of the physical symptoms, often seeing several physicians concomitantly. Patients undergo extensive, repetitive diagnostic work-ups, take many prescription drugs, and often undergo surgical procedures. None of these interventions reveals an organic basis for the symptoms. There is no known effective therapy for somatization disorder.

63. How should the internist approach the patient with somatization disorder?

Because the cycle in somatization disorder (or any somatoform disorder) often is physical complaint → unrevealing work-up → empiric therapy → unsatisfying outcome → return to doctor, the danger of iatrogenic disease is quite real. The physician who can establish a long-lasting relationship with the patient is occasionally able to break the cycle. To be successful, the physician must have confidence in his or her history-taking and physical examination ability and must be able to exercise diagnostic and therapeutic restraint. Even more important is that the patient trusts the physician— often patients develop substantial mistrust of health care providers after repeated encounters are fruitless and they are labelled "crocks." A dedicated primary care physician may be able to identify underlying emotional or mental health issues (i.e., sexual abuse) that may be amenable to psychiatric consultation and treatment. Care of the somatizing patient is extremely difficult in public hospital or clinic settings, because a new physician may see the patient at each visit.

64. What is a personality disorder?

A personality disorder is an enduring pattern of maladaptive behavior that interferes with a person's ability to achieve success and satisfaction in interpersonal and work relationships. At present the DSM-IV-TR divides 10 personality disorders into three groups:

Cluster A: "odd or eccentric" (paranoid, shizoid, schizotypal)
Cluster B: "dramatic" (histrionic, narcissistic, borderline, antisocial)
Cluster C: "anxious" (avoidant, dependent, obsessive-compulsive)

This classification is likely to change; many experts believe that the definitions are not as clinically useful as they should be for a variety of reasons. Nevertheless, patients with personality disorders meeting DSM-IV-TR criteria more frequently sustain injuries, attempt suicide, abuse substances, and have poorer outcomes for depression treatment than the general population.

American Psychiatric Association: Diagnostic and Statistical Manual of Mental Disorders, 4th ed., Primary Care Version (DSM-IV-PC). American Psychiatric Association, Washington, DC, 1995, with permission.

65. When should a clinician suspect that a patient has a personality disorder?

Such patients often pose severe challenges to a physician's professionalism and empathy. They often do not see a connection between their behavior and its outcomes, and pointing out such relationships can lead to considerable anger. It may be impossible to establish a mutually satisfying patient-physician relationship; the patient alternates between glowing approval and open distrust of the physician. A physician's own discomfort within a particular patient-physician relation may signal the presence of a personality disorder. Patients with severe behavioral difficulties should be referred to mental health professionals for treatment. In addition, patients presenting with depression or anxiety disorders who also have symptoms suggestive of a coexistent personality disorder should be referred to mental health professionals, because the personality disorder frequently complicates the treatment of the mood disorder.

66. What is a panic attack?

A panic attack is a sudden feeling of extreme fear or terror. The DSM-IV-TR criteria stipulate that the panic attack and the associated physical symptoms start abruptly and reach a peak within

10 minutes. Furthermore, sufferers should manifest at least four of the following symptoms:
- Cardiopulmonary: chest pain/discomfort, shortness of breath, palpitations
- Neurological: trembling/shaking; paresthesias; dizziness; lightheadedness
- Autonomic: sweating, chills, hot flashes
- Gastrointestinal: nausea, abdominal pain, feeling of choking
- Psychiatric: feelings of unreality or of being detached from oneself, fear of losing control, fear of dying

Panic disorder is diagnosed when a person has recurrent panic attacks and, after at least one of the attacks, one month or more of worry about the attack or a change in behavior related to the attack (e.g., avoidance of the place of occurrence).

American Psychiatric Association: Diagnostic and Statistical Manual of Mental Disorders, 4th ed., Primary Care Version (DSM-IV-PC). American Psychiatric Association, Washington, DC, 1995, with permission.

67. List the differential diagnoses for panic attack.

Alcohol withdrawal	Electrolyte abnormalities
Amphetamine abuse	Hyperparathyroidism
Asthma	Hyperthyroidism
Caffeinism	Hypoglycemia
Cardiac dysrhythmias	Hypothyroidism
Cardiomyopathies	Marijuana-induced palpitations
Cocaine abuse	Menopausal symptoms
Complex partial seizures	Mitral valve prolapse
Coronary artery disease	Pheochromocytoma
Cushing's syndrome	Pulmonary embolism
Drug withdrawal	Vertigo

Katon W: DHHS Pub. No (ADM) 89-1629, U.S. Government Printing Office, Washington, DC, 1989.

68. How do you differentiate between delirium and dementia?

Both are associated with impairment of the three main aspects of cognition: thinking, perception, and memory. In dementia, however, the cognitive impairment develops insidiously and is enduring, whereas in delirium the impairment has an abrupt onset and is short-lived. Moreover, delirious patients are frequently not completely alert, whereas patients with dementia maintain alertness until the disease is quite advanced.

CHARACTERISTIC	DELIRIUM	DEMENTIA
Onset	Sudden	Insidious
Course over 24 hours	Fluctuating, worse at night	Stable
Consciousness	Reduced	Clear
Attention	Disordered	Normal except in severe cases
Cognition	Disordered	Disordered
Hallucinations	Visual or auditory	Often absent
Delusions	Poorly systematized	Often absent
Orientation	Usually impaired	Often impaired
Psychomotor activity	Variable	Often normal
Speech	Often incoherent	Difficulty in word-finding, perseveration
Involuntary movements	Asterixis/coarse tremor	Often absent
Physical illness or drug toxicity	One or both present	Often absent

Adapted from Lipowski ZJ: Delirium in the elderly patient. N Engl J Med 320:578–582, 1989.

69. What is "steroid psychosis"?

Corticosteroid use is frequently associated with changes in mood (euphoria, dysphoria, or emotional lability), sleep pattern (insomnia, weird dreams, nightmares), and appetite (usually increased). Corticosteroids also can have important effects on behavior and thought processes, inducing frank psychosis in persons without a prior history of psychiatric disturbance or decompensation in known psychotics.

70. How should diagnosis and treatment of hypertension be handled in patients with a major psychiatric disorder?

In patients with major depression, schizophrenia, or bipolar disorder, elevated blood pressure should be evaluated in the same way as for patients without these disorders. According to the Joint National Commission for Hypertension Detection and Treatment, hypertension should be diagnosed after the mean of multiple readings on three separate occasions demonstrates a systolic pressure > 140 mmHg and/or a diastolic pressure > 90 mmHg. Patients in whom the diagnosis is made should be educated about the beneficial effects of exercise, reduction of dietary salt intake, and limited use of alcohol. If these measures do not reduce blood pressure, pharmacologic therapy should be recommended.

Diuretics must be used with caution in patients treated with lithium because they may cause volume depletion, lithium toxicity, coma, and even death. Beta blockers and central alpha agonists may not be advisable for patients with depression, and reserpine is contraindicated in depressed patients. With these provisos, reasonable medications for treatment include:

• Thiazide diuretics (for patients not on lithium therapy)
• Beta blockers
• Long-acting calcium channel blockers (e.g., verapamil, felodipine)
• Angiotensin-converting enzyme (ACE) inhibitors (monitor serum creatinine in patients taking lithium)

Beta blockers and central alpha agonists are best avoided if compliance is a problem, because sudden cessation of these medications is associated with rebound hypertension.

National Institutes of Health: The Sixth Report of the Joint National Committee on Prevention, Detection, Evaluation, and Treatment of High Blood Pressure. Washington, DC, NIH Publication No. 98-4080, 1997.

71. What renal lesions may be caused by chronic lithium treatment?

Up to 20% patients on chronic lithium therapy develop resistance to antidiuretic hormone (ADH), resulting in polyuria and polydipsia. Lithium accumulates in the collecting tubule cells and interferes with the ability of ADH to increase water permeability. Nocturia not accompanied by fluid ingestion before sleep suggests a urinary concentrating defect. However, polyuria in a patient on lithium therapy cannot be automatically ascribed to the lithium. Psychiatric patients also may have primary polydipsia or central diabetes insipidus. Other renal complications of chronic lithium treatment are type I (distal) renal tubular acidosis and nephrotic syndrome due to minimal change disease or glomerulosclerosis.

72. What conditions and drugs can cause lithium retention and hence toxicity?

1. Any condition that causes or predisposes a patient to volume depletion or renal ischemia can cause decreased lithium excretion and hence toxicity: gastrointestinal losses, congestive heart failure, and cirrhosis.

2. Certain types of drugs, if not monitored carefully, can disturb lithium excretion: diuretics, NSAIDs, and ACE inhibitors.

73. What are the symptoms of lithium toxicity? How is severity of toxicity graded?

Symptoms include coarse tremors, muscle weakness, ataxia, delirium, nausea, vomiting, diarrhea, leukocytosis, sinus bradycardia, hypotension, seizures, and, in the most severe cases, coma. Severity of toxicity is graded as follows:

Mild: lithium level of 1.5–2.5 mEq/L
Moderate: lithium level of 2.5–3.5 mEq/L
Severe: lithium level > 3.5 mEq/L

74. How is lithium toxicity treated?

- Volume repletion if the patient is hypovolemic
- Oral charcoal in cases of acute overdose (to adsorb other ingested drugs)
- Hemodialysis (treatment of choice in severe cases)

Hemodilaysis should be initiated if the serum lithium level is > 4 mEq/L, regardless of symptoms. With lower lithium levels, hemodialysis should be initiated if patients have severe symptoms or concomitant conditions (i.e., congestive heart failure, cirrhosis) that limit urinary excretion. Effective dialysis is likely to require several sessions or a long session of 8–12 hours, because the movement of lithium from within to outside cells is slow. In addition, there may be a rebound in the serum lithium level after cessation of a short hemodialysis session.

75. Define serotonin syndrome. What are the symptoms?

Serotonin syndrome can result when a patient takes two or more serotonergic agents with different mechanisms of action, either concurrently or in close succession. Symptoms include altered mental status, altered muscle tone (hyperreflexia, myoclonus, tremor, ataxia), autonomic instability with wide fluctuations in vital signs, hyperthermia, and diarrhea.

76. Which drugs may cause serotonin syndrome?

Any two agents from the list below may cause the syndrome. Of note, because some agents have very long half-lives, great caution must be used in starting a second agent in patients who have just stopped another serotonergic agent.

Serotonin precursor: tryptophan.

Serotonin release at the synapse: some amphetamines, selective serotonin-reuptake inhibitors (SSRIs: citalopram, fluoxetine, paroxetine, sertraline) and other newer antidepressants (e.g., venlaxafine), tricyclic antidepressants, trazodone, dextromethorphan, meperidine, tramadol.

Decreased serotonin metabolism: monoamine oxidase (MAO) inhibitors; St. John's wort (has MAO inhibitor activity in vitro).

Other serotonergic activity: buspirone, lithium, sumatriptan, dihydroergotamine.

To date, most reported cases appear to have resulted from the combination of SSRIs and MAO inhibitors. If a patient is to begin therapy with an MAO inhibitor after treatment with an SSRI, at least 2 weeks should be allowed for wash-out of the SSRIs. The exception is fluoxetine, which may require up to 5 weeks. Treatment of serotonin syndrome chiefly involves withdrawal of the inciting drug(s); there are some reports of rapid resolution of symptoms with cyproheptadine.

77. Define neuroleptic malignant syndrome (NMS). How is it treated?

NMS is a clinical state of high fever, muscle rigidity, altered mental status and dysautonomias that is thought to arise from depletion of dopamine in the central nervous system. The chief causative agents are the major tranquilizers (e.g., haloperidol), which are antidopaminergic in nature. Some patients develop the syndrome suddenly, after years of treatment with major tranquilizers; it also has been reported after sudden cessation of treatment with dopaminergic agents. Although NMS seems to resemble the serotonin syndrome in some of its features, experts currently believe that they are two distinct entities. Treatment of NMS consists of cooling, bromocriptine for mild or dantrolene for severe cases, and, most importantly, withdrawal of the offending agent.

78. Describe the medical complications of anorexia nervosa.

Anorexia nervosa is a psychiatric disorder that predominantly affects young women. Because of disordered body image. patients labor to stay extremely thin by eating little; purging with induced vomiting, laxatives or enemas; and sometimes exercising excessively. In addition to abnormal body image, the DSM-IV-TR requires the following three findings for a diagnosis of anorexia nervosa: (1) refusal to maintain a body weight within 15% of the ideal for age and sex, (2) amenorrhea, and (3) fear of weight gain.

Anorectic patients develop numerous laboratory abnormalities and medical complications. Low electrolyte levels may lead to sinus bradycardia or arrhythmias. Amenorrhea is common and may persist after the weight gain that is a sign of successful treatment. Relative hypothyroidism may occur, with low serum T3 but normal serum T4 levels. Dry skin and hair and cold intolerance may be seen. The left ventricle may become thin, and anorectic patients may develop congestive heart failure with aggressive refeeding. Thus increased oral intake must be monitored carefully. Anorectics are prone to the development of osteoporosis because of estrogen deficiency and poor intake of calcium and vitamin D.

BIBLIOGRAPHY

1. Carey CF, Lee HH, Woeltje KF (eds): The Washington Manual of Medical Therapeutics, 29th ed. Philadelphia, Lippincott Williams & Wilkins, 1998.
2. Desai SP, Isa-Pratt S (eds): Clinician's Guide to Laboratory Medicine: A Practical Approach. Cleveland, OH, Lexi-Comp, 2000.

16. AMBULATORY CARE

Mary P. Harward, M.D.

Here, at whatever hour you come, you will find light and help and human kindness.
Albert Schweitzer (1875–1965)

The sooner patients can be removed from the depressing influence of general hospital life the more rapid their convalescence.
Charles H. Mayo (1865–1939)
Lancet, 1916

Education is a lifelong process, in which the student can make only a beginning during his college course.
Sir William Osler (1849–1919)

1. What are the most common reasons that patients are seen in ambulatory care clinics?

Reasons named by patients	Reasons named by physicians
General medical examination	Essential hypertension
Hypertension	Diabetes mellitus
Progress visit, no other symptoms	Chronic ischemic heart disease
Chest pain and related symptoms	Acute upper respiratory infection
Cough	General medical examination
Blood pressure test	Osteoarthritis and allied diseases
Diabetes mellitus	General symptoms
Symptoms referable to throat	Chronic airway obstruction
Abdominal pain, cramps, spasms	Asthma
Headache, pain in head	Bronchitis
Upper respiratory infection (head cold, coryza)	Neurotic disorders
	Angina pectoris
Back symptoms	Chronic sinusitis
Vertigo, dizziness	Acute pharyngitis
Shortness of breath	Cardiac dysrhythmia
Tiredness, exhaustion	Miscellaneous (diagnosis missing or illegible)
Leg symptoms	Other disorders of soft tissue
Shoulder symptoms	Other respiratory symptoms
Neck symptoms	Congestive heart failure
Ischemic heart disease	Peripheral enthesopathies

National Ambulatory Medical Care Survey.

Barker LR: Curriculum for ambulatory care training in medical residency: Rationale, attitudes and generic proficiencies. J Gen Intern Med 5(Suppl 1):S3–S14, 1990.

2. Describe the initial evaluation of a 45-year-old black man whose blood pressure, measured on several occasions, has ranged between 140/95 and 155/105 mmHg.

The initial evaluation of a recently identified and confirmed hypertensive patient must uncover treatable causes of secondary hypertension. Recent medication use, including recreational drugs, appetite suppressants, cold remedies containing sympathomimetics, thyroid supplements, nonsteroidal anti-inflammatory agents (NSAIDs), oral contraceptives, and estrogens, should be reviewed. Extensive evaluations are not useful, however, if the treatment will not change. Baseline evaluation of any systemic effects of hypertension and end-organ damage also is useful in evaluating future therapies.

The history and physical evaluation, when thoroughly done, and limited diagnostic tests suggest the presence of most secondary causes, assess organ function, identify other risk factors for heart disease, and establish baseline for monitoring of future effects of hypertension or medication side effects. In general, causes of secondary hypertension are more likely in patients whose hypertension begins during adolescence or after age 50 or who have hypertension resistant to therapy.

Diagnostic Evaluation of the Newly Diagnosed Hypertensive Patient to Identify Secondary Causes and End-organ Effect and to Establish Baseline

DIAGNOSTIC TEST	SECONDARY CAUSE OR END-ORGAN EFFECT	RESULTS OR FINDINGS
Urinalysis	Renal parenchymal disease	Proteinuria
Blood urea nitrogen, creatinine	Renal parenchymal disease	Azotemia, renal insufficiency, renal failure
Fasting glucose	Diabetes mellitus	Hyperglycemia
Calcium	Hyperparathyroidism	Hypercalcemia
Potassium	Hyperaldosteronism	Hypokalemia
Uric acid	Not applicable	Hyperuricemia
Total cholesterol and high-density lipoprotein	Additional risk factor for heart disease	Hypercholesterolemia
Thyroid-stimulating hormone	Thyrotoxicosis	Hyperthyroidism
Complete blood count	Increased cardiac output	Anemia
Electrocardiogram	Presence of left ventricular hypertrophy	

3. What findings on history and physical examination suggest secondary hypertension?

FINDING	IMPLICATION
Positive CAGE questionnaire*	Alcoholism
History of drug use	Stimulant use
Medication history	Use of oral contraceptives (OCP), cyclosporine, antidepressants, decongestants, appetite suppressants, nonsteroidal anti-inflammatory agents, monoamine oxidase inhibitors
Obesity, facial hair, striae	Cushing's syndrome
Anxiety, tremor, tachycardia	Pheochromocytoma, hyperthyroidism
Goiter, exophthalmos	Hyperthyroidism
Diaphoresis	Pheochromocytoma
Pallor	Anemia
Diastolic murmur	Aortic insufficiency
History of amenorrhea	Pregnancy
Muscle cramps, weakness	Hyperaldosteronism
Hypersomnolence, snoring, obesity	Sleep apnea
Diminished femoral pulses, heart murmur, bruit best heard over back	Aortic coarctation
Periumbilical bruit	Renovascular disease
Fatigue, confusion, constipation	Hyperparathyroidism

*For CAGE, see question 88.

4. Can licorice ingestion cause elevated blood pressure (BP)?

Yes. Excessive ingestion of confectioner's black licorice (but not red licorice) can elevate BP > 10 mm Hg. Black licorice contains glycyrrhizic acid. Glycyrrhizic acid is also found in chewing tobacco.

5. How often should you screen for hypertension in normotensive adults?

In normotensive adults (diastolic BP < 85 mmHg and systolic BP < 140 mm Hg), BP should be measured at least every 2 years. Adults with diastolic BPs between 85–89 mm Hg should be screened annually.

6. List nonpharmacologic treatments for hypertension.
- Weight loss
- Smoking cessation
- No-added salt diet
- Regular exercise
- Decreased alcohol intake
- Biofeedback/relaxation techniques
- Stress reduction
- Low-saturated-fat diet rich in fruits and vegetables

7. What level of systolic hypertension should be treated?

Patients, particularly the elderly, with systolic BP > 140 mmHg have an increased risk of stroke and cardiovascular disease.

8. What level of elevated cholesterol should be treated?

INDICATION FOR THERAPY	NO. OF RISK FACTORS*	CHOLESTEROL LEVEL	GOAL OF THERAPY
Any CAD, carotid disease, or PVD	NA	LDL > 100 mg/dl	LDL < 100 mg/dl
No CAD, carotid disease, or PVD	2 or more	LDL > 160 mg/dl	LDL < 130 mg/dl
No CAD, carotid disease, or PVD	1	LDL > 190 mg/dl	LDL < 160 mg/dl

CAD = coronary artery disease, PVD = peripheral vascular disease, NA = not applicable.
* Male > 44 years old; female > 55 years old and not receiving estrogen replacement therapy; family history of CAD, including father or first-degree relative with sudden death from CAD before 55 years or mother or first-degree female relative with sudden death from CAD before 65 years; cigarette use; hypertension (including BP controlled by therapy); diabetes mellitus; high-density lipoprotein < 35 mg/dl.
From Grundy SM: Second Report of the Expert Panel on Detection, Evaluation, and Treatment of High Blood Cholesterol in Adults. (Advisory Treatment Panel II). Circulation 89:1309, 1994.

9. Is a fasting sample required for lipid measurement?

Cholesterol and high-density lipoprotein (HDL) cholesterol can be measured in the non-fasting state. Low-density lipoprotein (LDL) cholesterol is calculated from the triglyceride, HDL, and total cholesterol levels. Because triglycerides rise quickly after eating, a fasting sample is required for triglyceride measurement in order to calculate the LDL. Cholesterol measurement may vary by as much as 14% between laboratories and can vary as much as 10% within the same patient. Cholesterol levels are affected by acute-phase reactants, which are elevated in infection, acute myocardial infarction (MI), and surgery. The effect after MI may persist for up to 2 months.

10. Describe the physical findings of an innocent murmur and the murmur of mitral valve prolapse (MVP).

FINDING	INNOCENT MURMUR	MITRAL VALVE PROLAPSE
Location	Base	Apex (left lateral decubitus position)
Intensity	< 3/6	≥ 3/6
Timing	Early systole	Mid-to-late systole
Response to maneuvers	Decreases with standing and Valsalva	Begins earlier in systole with standing and Valsalva; may increase with handgrip or Valsalva
Associated signs	Normal S2	Midsystolic click

11. What prophylactic antibiotics are recommended in patients with MVP scheduled for an elective dental procedure? For patients with a prosthetic aortic valve?

Antibiotic prophylaxis against endocarditis is recommended for patients with congenital heart disease (except uncomplicated secundum atrial septal defect), rheumatic or acquired valvular disease, hypertrophic cardiomyopathy, MVP with mitral insufficiency, prosthetic heart valves, or a history of previous endocarditis when they undergo procedures that are likely to lead to bacteremia with pathogenic organisms. *Streptococcus viridans* is the most common cause of endocarditis after dental or upper respiratory procedures; enterococci are the most common cause of endocarditis after gastrointestinal (GI) or genitourinary (GU) procedures.

Prophylactic Antibiotics for Adults Undergoing Invasive Procedures

PROCEDURE	ORAL REGIMEN	PARENTERAL REGIMEN
Upper respiratory or dental procedures	Amoxicillin, 2 gm PO 1 hr before procedure	Ampicillin, 2 gm IV or IM within 30 min of procedure
If allergic to penicillin	Clindamycin, 600 mg PO, *or* cephalexin* or cefadroxil,* 2 gm, *or* azithromycin or clarithromycin, 500 mg 1 hr before procedure.	Clindamycin, 600 mg IV, or cefazolin.* 1 gm IV or IM within 30 min before procedure
GU/GI procedures		
Moderate-risk patients	Amoxicillin, 2 gm PO 1 hr before procedure	Ampicillin, 2 gm IV within 30 min of procedure
If allergic to penicillin		Vancomycin, 1 gm IV over 1–2 hr, completed within 30 min of procedure
High-risk patients		Ampicillin, 2 gm IM or IV, plus gentamicin, 1.5 mg/kg, within 30 min of procedure; ampicillin, 1 gm IM or IV, or amoxicillin, 1 gm PO, 6 hr later
If allergic to penicillin		Vancomycin, 1 gm IV over 1–2 hr, plus gentamicin, 1.5 mg/kg IV or IM, within 30 min of procedure

PO = orally, IV = intravenously, IM = intramuscularly.
* Do not use cephalosporins if the patient has history of reaction to penicillin, including urticaria, angioedema, or anaphylaxis.
From American Heart Association: Prevention of bacterial endocarditis: Recommendations by the American Heart Association. Circulation 96:358–366, 1997.

12. What types of dental procedures require preventive treatment for bacterial endocarditis in at-risk patients?

Extractions, periodontal procedures, dental implant placement, replacement of avulsed teeth, root canals, sublingual placement of antibiotic fibers or strips, initial placement of orthodontic bands (but not brackets), intraalimentary local anesthetic injections, and prophylactic teeth cleaning when bleeding is likely.

13. How do you evaluate an asymptomatic patient with new-onset atrial fibrillation (AF)?

The evaluation should look specifically for the causes of AF and evidence of cardiac dysfunction. Because patients with AF are at risk of embolization and may need systemic anticoagulation, risk factors for excessive bleeding due to anticoagulation should be sought, including excessive alcohol use, history of previous central nervous system bleeding, active bleeding, recent neurosurgery, severe hypertension, history of frequent falls likely to lead to head trauma, tendency to bleed, pregnancy, or high-risk occupations in which trauma may occur. Patients with diabetes mellitus and hypertension also have an increased risk of systemic embolization.

Evaluation for the Causes of Atrial Fibrillation

CAUSE	HISTORY	PHYSICAL EXAM	LABORATORY TESTS
Alcohol use	Daily use, binging	Jaundice, spider angiomata, palmar erythema, hepatomegaly	Liver function tests
Medications	Digoxin	—	Digoxin level, EKG
Drug use	Stimulant use	—	Toxin screen
Congestive heart failure	Dyspnea on exertion, paroxysmal nocturnal dyspnea, peripheral edema, nocturia	Jugular venous distention, rales, edema, S3	Chest x-ray
Pulmonary embolism	Chest pain, dyspnea, calf pain, predisposing factors (recent surgery, immobilization)	Calf swelling, pleural rub	ABG, chest x-ray; consider V/Q, venous duplex exam
MI	Chest pain	S4	EKG, cardiac enzymes
Cerebrovascular accident	Paresis, paralysis, aphasia, visual loss, numbness	Muscle weakness, sensory loss, dysarthria, reflex changes	Head CT scan or MRI
Mitral valve disease	Rheumatic fever or valvular disease	Heart murmur	Echocardiogram
Organic heart disease	Hypertension or heart disease	S3, S4, elevated BP	Chest x-ray, EKG, echocardiogram
Hyperthyroidism	Weight loss, depression	Goiter	Thyroid function tests
WPW syndrome	Palpitations	—	EKG
Tachy- or brady-cardia (sick sinus syndrome	Syncope	—	Holter or event monitor

EKG = electrocardiogram, ABG = arterial blood gas analysis, V/Q = ventilation/perfusion scan, MI = myocardial infarction, WPW = Wolff-Parkinson-White.

14. How is anticoagulant therapy with warfarin monitored in patients with AF?

The prothrombin time (PT) and international normalized ratio (INR) are checked regularly with medication adjustment to maintain an INR of 2 .0–3.0. In general, the anticoagulant weekly dosage should not be adjusted by more than 10% unless the INR is markedly elevated or decreased.

15. What are the LEOPARD and LAMB syndromes?

These acronyms refer to constellations of findings, but both are characterized as hyperpigmentation disorders because of the presence of lentigines.

L = Lentigines (hundreds covering the body, developing in childhood)
E = EKG abnormalities, primarily conduction disorders
O = Ocular hypertelorism
P = Pulmonary and subaortic valvular stenosis
A = Abnormal genitalia
R = Retardation of growth
D = Deafness

L = Lentigines
A = Atrial myxomas
M = Mucocutaneous myxomas
B = Blue nevi

16. Describe the therapeutic plan for an adolescent with a moderate case of acne vulgaris.

1. Avoid oily cosmetics and frequently rubbing the face.
2. Use mild cleansing soap.

3. For obstructive acne (whiteheads and blackheads), use topical 0.025% or 0.05% retinoic acid cream or gel at bedtime. Use sunscreen.

4. For inflammatory acne (erythematous papules and pustules), use topical 2.5% benzoyl peroxide gel once or twice daily, topical antibiotic (erythromycin or clindamycin), or both. Combination products with benzoyl peroxide and antibiotic are available.

5. Use oral tetracycline or derivative (doxycycline or minocycline) or erythromycin. After inflammation improves, the antibiotic dose can be decreased slowly. Chronic antibiotic use may cause vaginitis in women.

6. Refer to a dermatologist if intralesional steroids or 13-cis-retinoic acid is needed.

7. Avoid oral contraceptive pills (OCPs) containing norgestrel or norethindrone.

8. Consider use of an OCP containing norgestimate (Ortho Tri-Cyclen) in women requiring OCP because it has been shown to decrease acne, as have OCPs containing levonorgestrel or norethindrone acetate.

17. What is hidradenitis suppurativa? Erythrasma?

Hidradenitis suppurativa is an infection of the apocrine sweat glands that leads to chronic inflammation and scarring. It occurs in the axilla, groin, and buttocks and under women's breasts. Antibiotic therapy (erythromycin or dicloxacillin) can be useful, but sometimes surgical excision is required. Erythrasma is a skin infection caused by *Corynebacterium minutissimum;* it occurs mostly in intertriginous areas such as toes, groin, and axillae. It is treated with topical benzoyl peroxide or topical or systemic erythromycin.

18. Describe the typical locations and appearance of psoriasis.

Psoriasis typically occurs on the extensor surfaces (elbows and knees), waistline, umbilicus, external genitalia, and gluteal fold. The typical lesions are elevated, reddish-brown plaques and papules with silvery scales. Bleeding points occur where the scale is removed (Auspitz's sign). In addition, the nails may be pitted. Some patients have arthritic involvement of the distal interphalangeal (DIP) joints.

19. List the major causes of alopecia.

Androgenetic alopecia
Alopecia areata (associated with pernicious anemia, autoimmune disorders, and vitiligo)
Medications (anticoagulants, beta blockers, HMG CoA reductase inhibitors ["statins"])
Infections (secondary syphilis, tinea capitis)
Trichotillomania (nervous hair pulling)
Discoid lupus erythematosus
Telogen effluvium (associated with significant traumatic event)
Iron deficiency anemia
Hypo- or hyperthyroidism
Chemical hair products
Mechanical traction (due to hair style)

20. Describe the characteristic appearance of tinea versicolor (pityriasis versicolor). How is it treated?

Tinea versicolor, caused by infection with the fungus *Malassezia furfur*, has various colors (red, pink, brown) and is usually macular with slight scaling. The involved areas of skin do not tan well, and the infection becomes particularly obvious in the summer, when the involved areas are hypopigmented. The lesions fluoresce orange and gold under Wood's light.

Tinea versicolor should be treated with 2.5% selenium sulfide suspension or pyrithione zinc shampoo, applied with a rough washcloth to the entire body and left in place for 10 minutes before rinsing. Recurrences are common. Topical antifungal agents (clotrimazole, miconazole) can be used for small areas. Systemic antifungal agents (ketoconazole) can be used in severe cases or immunocompromised patients.

21. Describe the routine follow-up for a patient with diabetes mellitus.

Diabetics should be seen at least semiannually if glycemic control is stable. If their regimen requires a change, more frequent visits are needed. Individualized goals for glycemic control should be established with the patient. At the visit, obtain historical information about the frequency, cause, and severity of hypoglycemic or hyperglycemic episodes; home glucose monitoring records; current medications; other illnesses; lifestyle changes; life stressors; and difficulty with compliance with treatment recommendations. Weight and blood pressure, optic fundi, and any symptom-directed organ system should be examined thoroughly. A foot examination is especially important and should include inspection for trauma, callouses, and nail and skin conditions; palpation of pedal pulses; and sensory exam. Annual dilated ophthalmologic exams are necessary. Patients should receive counseling about depression, smoking cessation, nutrition, physical activity, foot care, medication management during illness, and management of hypo/hyperglycemia, when indicated.

Regular lab tests include glycohemoglobin (Hgb A1C) at least quarterly or as often as needed to establish control. Fasting glucose may provide additional information. Lipid profiles (including fasting total cholesterol, triglycerides, and HDL) should be tested at least annually. Additional monitoring may be needed if therapeutic changes are made. An annual urinalysis is recommended, as is testing for microalbuminuria if urine protein testing is negative. Diabetics require pneumococcal vaccine (every 5 years), influenza vaccine (annually), and tetanus/diphtheria toxoid (every 10 years).

22. Name the two most frequent causes of mild, asymptomatic hypercalcemia in ambulatory patients.

Thiazide drugs and hyperparathyroidism.

23. What are the major adverse consequences of obesity?

Obese patients are more likely to have hypertension and coronary artery disease than patients who are not overweight. Obese patients also have increased mortality from all causes, including cancer. They may have impaired glucose tolerance or overt diabetes mellitus. Obesity can complicate chronic obstructive pulmonary disease, sleep apnea, and osteoarthritis. Obese patients have difficulty following a regular exercise program. They may have a depressed mood and poor self-esteem.

24. What should be included in a treatment regimen for patients with chronic, idiopathic constipation?

1. Regular bowel habits with attempted bowel movements at the same time each day (15–20 minutes after breakfast when the gastrocolic reflex is the strongest).
2. High-fiber diet (approximately 15 gm/day) , including beans (navy, lima, kidney), baked potato with skin, broccoli, peas, corn, apple with peel, oranges, peaches, raspberries, wheat bread, and bran cereals.
3. Adequate fluid intake (at least eight 8-oz glasses of water each day).
4. Bulk laxative (psyllium, polycarbophil, or methylcellulose).
5. Nonabsorbable saccharide laxative (sorbitol or lactulose), if needed.
6. Daily exercise.
7. Evaluation of medications to avoid constipating agents when possible.
8. Use of commode instead of bedpan in patients confined to bed during acute illness.

25. What are the causes of chronic constipation?

Medications: calcium channel blockers, antihistamines, opiates, iron, tricyclic antidepressants, anticholinergics, aluminum and calcium antacids, laxatives (if abused), sucralfate, disopyramide.

Endocrine/metabolic disorders: hypothyroidism, diabetes mellitus, hyperparathyroidism, hypokalemia, pregnancy, hypercalcemia.

Mechanical obstruction: tumors, strictures, adhesions.

Neurogenic disorders: spinal cord disease, multiple sclerosis, scleroderma.

Rectal disease: hemorrhoids, anal fissure.

Psychological disorders: major depression, personality disorder, anxiety, phobias, situational stress.

GI disease: irritable bowel syndrome, diverticular disease, colon carcinoma.
Physical inactivity: obesity, excessive television watching or computer use.
Diet: inadequate dietary fiber intake.

26. Describe the office evaluation of a patient with acute diarrhea for less than 24 hours.

Most causes of acute diarrhea are infectious, resulting from viruses, bacteria, and parasites; many are self-limited. The history and physical exam help to guide further evaluation. In the history, inquire about recent travel; antibiotic use; food and beverage ingestion (particularly raw meats and poultry, seafood, unpasteurized milk and juices, rice, bean sprouts, herbal teas, caffeinated beverages, alcohol, and custards); exposure to animals or people with similar symptoms; frequency, volume, and appearance of stool; associated symptoms (including fever, abdominal pain, tenesmus, skin rash, and blood, mucus, or pus in the stool); history of lactose intolerance; and current medications. During the physical exam, check the temperature, abdomen, and rectum (including a test for fecal occult blood). The examination should include a check for the presence of orthostatic changes in the BP and pulse and skin rash.

Patients with few associated symptoms need no further evaluation unless the diarrhea does not resolve within 1 week. In patients with severe systemic symptoms or bloody diarrhea, a search for and treatment of specific pathogens is needed and is best accomplished by flexible sigmoidoscopy. In addition to direct visualization of the mucosa, samples can be obtained for fecal leukocytes and cultures. If flexible sigmoidoscopy cannot be performed, stool samples may be collected by the patient for leukocytes, Gram stain, bacterial cultures, and *Clostridium difficile* toxin.

27. Describe the office evaluation of a patient with diarrhea persisting for 2–3 weeks.

Fecal blood and leukocytes should be rechecked and cultures repeated, with a specific request for ova and parasite examination and *C. difficile* toxin. *C. difficile* infection is associated with recent antibiotic use, especially clindamycin, but also can be found in outbreak situations, such as nursing homes. Sometimes, as many as three specimens are needed for identification of the pathogen and detection of *C. difficile* toxin. The diagnostic yield can be increased if the examination is done on a fresh stool specimen.

Complete blood count, serum electrolytes, calcium, glucose, liver function tests, and amylase may indicate a systemic illness. Sigmoidoscopy is indicated. In certain patients with evidence of malabsorption such as weight loss, a Sudan stain for fat, followed by quantitative 72-hour fecal fat collection, is useful. If no cause is determined, additional evaluations guided by a gastroenterologist are needed.

28. Describe the symptoms of irritable bowel syndrome (IBS). How is it treated?

Because it is the most common GI disease seen in clinical practice, most physicians are all too familiar with IBS. However, its management can be frustrating. Patients with IBS often complain of diarrhea alternating with constipation for months to years. The stools may contain excessive mucus but no blood. Frequently audible bowel sounds, left lower quadrant or generalized abdominal pain, and urgency to defecate accompany the diarrhea or constipation. Patients may even describe left arm or shoulder pain with the splenic-flexure syndrome. Associated symptoms include anxiety, depression, and signs of vasomotor instability (e.g., palpitations, hyperventilation, sweating, headaches).

The treatment of IBS includes acknowledgment of the symptoms, identification of and counseling for any underlying psychiatric stress or illness, education about the benign nature of the disorder, and therapy for chronic constipation or diarrhea (increased dietary fiber). Increased physical activity is also beneficial. Short-term limited use of anticholinergic medications is useful in a few patients but should not be the sole therapy. New medications available for IBS include alosetron, a serotonin antagonist, which is indicated for women with predominant symptoms of diarrhea. However, alosetron has been associated with colitis and severe constipation.

29. How do you manage an anal fissure?

Patients with an anal fissure usually complain of severe pain with defecation, sometimes associated with bleeding. Most fissures are located in the midline and are visible. Conservative management with warm sitz baths, stool softeners, and bulk laxatives improves ease of defecation. Systemic analgesics may be needed. Drugs that cause constipation should be avoided. If this therapy fails, the patient should be referred for consideration of surgical repair.

30. Define proctalgia fugax.

A fleeting, deep pain in the rectum, probably caused by muscle spasm that may be associated with chronic rectal trauma due to poor posture. Digital rectal examination shows muscle tenderness.

31. Which tests are most useful in determining whether acute hepatitis is viral in etiology?

If one suspects viral hepatitis based on history, physical exam, and elevated liver transaminases, a test for hepatitis B surface antigen (HBsAg) should be ordered first. If it is negative, a test for IgM hepatitis B core antibody-IgM (IGM anti-HBc) will pick up additional cases of acute hepatitis B that are antigen-negative. Hepatitis A can be detected through hepatitis A antibody-IgM (IgM anti-HAV). Antibody to hepatitis C virus (HCV) can be detected through commercially available enzyme-linked immunosorbent assays (ELISA) or polymerase chain reaction (PCR) methods (anti-HCV).

Block ER, Bordley DR, Tape TG, Panzer RJ: Diagnostic Strategies for Common Medical Problems, 2nd ed. Philadelphia, American College of Physicians, 1999.

32. How do you diagnose cervicitis due to chlamydial infection?

Chlamydiosis is diagnosed by a variety of immunologic techniques that use direct immunofluorescence techniques, ELISA, or PCR. Chlamydial cervicitis is suspected in a sexually active woman when a mucopurulent discharge with cervical erythema, ulceration, and friability (easy bleeding) are seen during speculum examination of the vagina. Chlamydial infections also may be asymptomatic. Screening is effective in high-risk populations, including women who attend sexually transmitted disease (STD) or family planning clinics; are less than 25 years old and sexually active; or have a history of previous STDs, multiple sexual partners, or a new sexual partner.

33. How should you evaluate a 20-year-old, sexually active woman who complains of acute dysuria?

The multiple causes of dysuria include urethritis, cystitis, vaginitis, and cervicitis. A history of sexual activity (particularly with a new partner) may point to vaginitis or cervicitis. The history should focus on the presence of hematuria, vaginal discharge, flank pain, fever, and chills. The physical exam should include temperature, pulse, BP (with orthostatic changes, if symptoms are severe), and bimanual pelvic examination. Any vaginal discharge should be examined microscopically. Appropriate testing for *Neisseria gonorrhoeae* and *Chlamydia* spp. should be done if a mucopurulent cervicitis is present. Mucopurulent cervicitis is diagnosed by the presence of a yellowish discharge (mucopus) on a clean, cotton swab inserted into the cervix. If the history and physical exam suggest acute uncomplicated cystitis, the patient may be empirically treated with a fluoroquinolone without urine testing. If she remains symptomatic after 3–7 days of treatment, urinalysis and urine culture should be done.

34. List the common causes of abnormal vaginal bleeding in premenopausal women.

Dysfunctional uterine bleeding: idiopathic, Stein-Leventhal syndrome.

Pregnancy: threatened or complete abortion, ectopic pregnancy.

Medical conditions: thrombocytopenia, qualitative platelet disorder, hypothyroidism, bleeding diathesis, excessive androgens, hypercortisolism, polycystic ovary syndrome.

Medications: anticoagulants, oral contraceptives.

Anatomic causes: perineal (bladder pathology, hemorrhoids), vulvar (infection, laceration, tumor, atrophic vaginitis), vaginal (infection, laceration, tumor, foreign body), cervical (infection, erosion, polyp, carcinoma), uterine (infection, polyp, leiomyomata, carcinoma, intrauterine device), ovarian (infection).

Normal variant: ovulation.

35. How do you manage a woman with postmenopausal vaginal bleeding?

The woman should be referred to a gynecologist for consideration of a dilatation and curettage (D&C) of the uterus to detect endometrial carcinoma.

36. Describe the characteristic vaginal discharges caused by *Candida albicans*, *N. gonorrhoeae*, *Gardnerella vaginalis*, overgrowth of lactobacilli (cytolytic vaginosis), and *Trichomonas vaginalis*.

ORGANISM	DISCHARGE CHARACTERISTICS
C. albicans	Thick, white, curdlike, adherent to vaginal wall with erythema or perineal satellite lesions
N. gonorrhoeae	Mucopurulent with cervicitis
G. vaginalis	Foul-smelling ("fishy" odor with KOH), thin, scanty, nonpruritic, adherent to vaginal wall
Lactobacilli	White, frothy with pH > 3.5 and < 4.5
T. vaginalis	Copious, yellow-green, frothy

37. What are clue cells?

Clue cells are seen in the discharge of vaginal infections caused by *G. vaginalis*. Microscopically, they appear on a wet mount of vaginal secretions as epithelial cells covered with coccobacilli or curved rods.

38. What are the absolute contraindications to the use of oral contraceptives?

Pregnancy, lactation
Estrogen-dependent neoplasms
  (breast or endometrium)
Thromboembolic disease
Undiagnosed genital bleeding
History of subacute bacterial endocarditis
Atrial fibrillation
Diabetes mellitus with nephropathy,
  retinopathy, neuropathy or vascular
  disease
Smoking > 20 cigarettes/day

Severely impaired liver function
Prolonged immobility
Migraine headaches with focal symptoms
Cardiovascular disease with pulmonary
  hypertension
Active thrombophlebitis
Cerebrovascular accident
Viral hepatitis, severe cirrhosis, hepatic
  adenomas
Severe hypertension

Hatcher RA, Trussell, J, Stewart F, et al: Contraceptive Technology. New York, Aradent Media, 1998.

39. How would you evaluate a new breast nodule discovered during routine physical examination of a woman?

The characteristics of the nodule (size, firmness, mobility) are not predictive of the likelihood of malignancy. Nipple discharge and axillary adenopathy should be evaluated. If multiple, cystic nodules are present and the woman is premenopausal, she should be followed through several menses for any changes in the nodules. Any dominant, solitary nodule requires referral for biopsy. A mammogram may be useful for localization of the nodule, but a normal mammogram should not preclude the need for biopsy of a solitary nodule. Needle aspiration biopsy may be appropriate for cystic nodules.

40. What treatments are available for premenstrual syndrome (PMS)?

Many agents have been used in the management of PMS, including antidepressants, bromocriptine, danazol, evening primrose oil, spironolactone, progesterone, and prostaglandin synthetase inhibitors. The selective serotonin reuptake inhibitors (SSRIs) and alprazolam have been shown to be effective. The SSRIs may be used intermittently during the luteal phase of the cycle. Vitamin B6 may be useful.

41. What pharmacologic therapies are available for osteoporosis?

Adequate calcium intake (1500 mg/day for postmenopausal women not taking estrogen and 1200 mg/day for those receiving estrogen) and adequate vitamin D (400 IU/day) are necessary treatment for osteoporosis, either through the diet or as nutritional supplements. Many calcium preparations are combined with vitamin D. Now that many foods (e.g., juices, breads, cereals) are fortified with calcium, women may ingest excessive calcium if too many supplements are taken. In addition, estrogen, bisphosphonates (etidronate, pamidronate, alendronate, risedronate), salmon calcitonin (available as nasal spray), and slow-release sodium fluoride can be useful in combination with calcium.

42. What are the clinical symptoms of influenza?

Influenza typically presents with the sudden onset of high fever, malaise, myalgia, coryza, headache, and sore throat. GI symptoms (nausea, vomiting, diarrhea) also may be present. With complications, symptoms of pneumonia, encephalitis, hepatitis, pancreatitis, or myositis may develop. Persistent cough, easy fatigability, and asthenia can persist after the initial symptoms have abated.

43. How do you differentiate influenza from other acute respiratory illnesses?

It is difficult to distinguish influenza on clinical grounds alone, but combining clinical evidence with epidemiologic surveys of influenza activity in the community can confirm a likely diagnosis of influenza. Although a patient presenting with characteristic symptoms during an outbreak of influenza in the winter months most probably has the disease, laboratory diagnosis is the only way to be certain and can be made during acute illness from sputum samples, throat swab, or nasopharyngeal washes. Rapid diagnostic tests for ambulatory care use are available. With the availability of medications to treat influenza, a high level of suspicion based on clinical symptoms during a documented outbreak of influenza A or B in the community may be sufficient to initiate treatment. Treatment must be started within 30–48 hours of symptoms.

Streptococcal pharyngitis, infectious mononucleosis (IM), and early bacterial pneumonia can resemble influenza. Unlike influenza, bacterial pneumonia is generally not self-limited. Streptococcal pharyngitis can be identified through commercially available rapid antigen detection kits or throat culture. IM is characterized by marked cervical adenopathy, particularly the posterior cervical and posterior auricular nodes. The heterophil antibody test (Monospot) may confirm IM, but a negative result does not rule out the disease.

44. Who should receive the influenza vaccine?

The inactivated, trivalent influenza vaccine is recommended annually for the following groups:

1. People at increased risk for the complications of influenza (including death, influenza pneumonia, and secondary bacterial pneumonia):
   - Adults and children with chronic pulmonary or cardiovascular illnesses (including asthma)
   - Residents of nursing homes or other chronic care facilities with any chronic medical condition
   - Adults 50 years of age and older
   - Adults or children with chronic medical conditions requiring regular medical follow-up or hospitalization during the preceding year (e.g., diabetes mellitus, renal dysfunction, hemoglobinopathies, HIV infection, immunosuppression)
   - Children and teenagers (aged 6 months to 18 years) who are receiving long-term aspirin therapy and are therefore at increased risk for developing Reye's syndrome after an influenza infection
   - Women who will be in the second or third trimester of pregnancy during the influenza season
2. People capable of transmitting influenza to high-risk persons:
   - Physicians, nurses, students, and other personnel in both inpatient and outpatient settings who have extensive contact with high-risk patients in all age groups

- Providers of home care to high-risk patients
- Household members (including children) of high-risk persons

3. Other groups:
   - Anyone, especially people providing essential services, who wishes to reduce his or her chance of acquiring influenza infection
   - All HIV-infected persons
   - People embarking on foreign travel during the influenza season at their destination

Update: Influenza activity—United States and worldwide, 1999–2000 season, and composition of the 2000–01 influenza vaccine. MMWR 49(17):375–381, 2000.

45. What treatments are available for influenza?

Zanamivir (Relenza) and oseltamivir phosphate (Tamiflu) are neuraminidase inhibitors, available to treat influenza A and B. If started within 30 hours of the first symptoms, both drugs can reduce the duration of symptoms. Zanamivir is given through an inhalational device and may precipitate bronchospasm; therefore, it probably should not be used in patients with asthma or chronic obstructive pulmonary disease. Oseltamivir is taken as a pill. Amantadine and ramantidine can be used to treat influenza A only, but resistance has developed to amantadine and both drugs can cause significant central nervous system side effects. The mainstay of treatment of influenza is prevention through vaccination.

Two neuraminidase inhibitors for treatment of influenza. Med Lett 41:91, 1999.

46. When are combined tetanus/diphtheria toxoid (Td) and tetanus immune globulin (TIG) indicated in wound management?

If a patient does not have a definite history of at least three previous doses of Td, TIG should be given if the wound is contaminated with dirt, feces, or saliva or results from puncture or sharp object penetration, frostbite, or burn.

47. What organisms commonly cause nongonoccal urethritis (NGU) in men?

Chlamydia trachomatis, Mycoplasma genitalium, T. vaginalis, and *Ureaplasma urealyticum.* Reiter's syndrome (urethritis, conjunctivitis, iritis, fever, polyarthritis, balinitis, and ulcerations) can present with a urethral discharge suggestive of NGU. Chlamydial infection is the most common cause.

48. What organisms commonly cause epididymitis?

C. trachomatis, N. gonorrohoeae, and *U. urealyticum* are the most common causes in men younger than 35 years. Older men are more likely to have epididymitis as a complication of prostatitis and gram-negative rod infection. Rarely, testicular carcinoma or mumps can cause epididymitis, as can fungal and tubercular infections. Appropriate antimicrobial therapy is guided by cultures.

49. How do you differentiate acute epididymitis from testicular torsion?

	EPIDIDYMITIS	TORSION
Age	Older	Prepubertal
Pyuria	+	–
Bacteriuria	+	–
Urethritis symptoms	+	–
Physical exam	Palpable epididymis	Firm, tender mass

50. What are the causes of community-acquired pneumonia (CAP)?

The most common cause remains *Streptococcus pneumoniae.* Other causes include *Staphylococcus aureus,* group A streptococci, *Haemophilus influenzae, Legionella pneumophila, Klebsiella pneumoniae, Moraxella catarrhalis,* and *Bordetella pertussis.* Other nonbacterial causes include *Mycoplasma pneumoniae,* viruses (influenza A and B, adenovirus, respiratory syncytial, cytomegalovirus and parainfluenza), *Chlamydia psittaci* (psittacosis), *Chlamydia pneumoniae* (TWAR strain), *Coxiella burnetti* (Q fever), fungi (histoplasmosis, coccidioidomy-cosis), and *Pneumocystis carinii*.

51. What are the prodromal symptoms of herpes zoster (shingles)?

Before the vesicles appear, infected patients experience headache and malaise. Pain and paresthesia may be felt in the involved dermatomes. If the involved dermatome is on the anterior chest wall, the pain may be confused with anginal or MI pain.

52. How can the history and physical exam predict whether acute pharyngitis in adults is due to streptococcal infection?

The presence of fever, pharyngeal and/or tonsillar exudates, and cervical lymphadenopathy suggests an approximately 40% probability of streptococcal pharyngitis. The diagnosis can be confirmed by rapid streptococcal test or culture.

Komaroff AL: Sore throat and acute infectious mononucleosis in adult patients. In Black ER, Bordley DR, Tape TG, Panzer RJ (eds): Diagnostic Strategies for Common Medical Problems, Philadelphia, American College of Physicians, 1999.

53. Which adults should receive measles vaccine?

Adults (over age 18) born after 1956 should receive at least one dose of live measles vaccine if adequate documentation of live virus vaccination or physician-diagnosed measles is unavailable and there is no serologic proof of immunity. Adults born after 1956 should receive a second dose of vaccine if they work in health care fields where exposure to measles is likely, travel to an endemic area, or are entering a secondary educational institution. College entry and beginning of employment in a medically related field are important times to ensure completion of both vaccine doses. Measles vaccine is preferably given in the combined form of measles-mumps-rubella (MMR) and is administered subcutaneously. Adults born before 1957 are generally considered to have immunity.

54. Who should receive meningococcal vaccine?

Students entering college and educational institutions should consider meningococcal vaccine.

Meningococcal disease and college students. Recommendations of the Advisory Committee on Immunization Practices (ACIP). MMWR 49(RR-7):11–29, 2000.

55. Who should receive hepatitis A vaccine?

People who frequently travel to Mexico, the Caribbean, Asia (excluding Japan), eastern Europe, South America, and Africa should consider hepatitis A vaccine. It also should be considered in patients with chronic liver disease (e.g., cirrhosis, hepatitis B, hepatitis C). People under 40 may benefit from hepatitis A vaccine in areas of the U.S. with high prevalence (e.g., California).

Prevention of hepatitis A through active or passive immunization: Recommendations of the Advisory Committee on Immunization Practices (ACIP). MMWR 48(RR12):1–37, 1999.

56. What form of polio vaccine should be given to adults?

Adults should receive an injection of inactivated polio vaccine. Polio is endemic in all countries other than the Americas, Australia, New Zealand, Japan, and most European countries. Travelers to endemic countries should consider polio vaccine.

57. Which immunizations should a person with a splenectomy receive?

Pneumococcal (every 5 years), meningococcal, and *H. influenzae* vaccines.

58. What are the common causes of meralgia paresthetica?

Meralgia paresthetica is caused by localized entrapment of the lateral femoral cutaneous nerve that produces pain over the anterolateral thigh. It may occur with diabetes mellitus and pregnancy (during the final weeks of gestation) or during sudden weight loss or gain. Tight girdles, gun belts, and other accessories have been implicated.

59. Describe the typical symptoms of migraine, tension, and cluster headaches.

SYMPTOM	CLUSTER	MIGRAINE	TENSION
Location	Unilateral	Hemicranial	Entire head or bitemporal
Quality of pain	Burning	Throbbing	Pressure-like ache, tightness
Duration	1–2 hr	2–6 hr	Days
Frequency	Flurry of frequent attacks for several weeks	Episodic	Daily
Associated symptoms	Ipsilateral sweating, flushing, lacrimation, and rhinorrhea	Prodrome (scotoma, paresthesia, confusion or behavioral changes)	Neck and shoulder ache

60. What are the symptoms of a transient ischemic attack (TIA) in the anterior (carotid) distribution? Posterior (vertebrobasilar) distribution?

ANTERIOR	POSTERIOR
Transient paresis of face and/or arm	Transient global amnesia
Paresthesia	Ataxia
Aphasia	Dysarthria
Amaurosis fugax (sudden loss of vision in eye)	Weakness, dizziness
Homonymous hemianopia	Hearing loss

61. List the triad of symptoms associated with Ménière's syndrome.

Paroxysmal vertigo, hearing loss, and tinnitus, possibly accompanied by nausea and vomiting.

62. What are the leading causes of acute impairment or loss of the sense of smell?

Head trauma, especially in children and active young adults, and viral infections, especially in older adults.

63. What are the characteristics of bacterial conjunctivitis? Viral conjunctivitis? Allergic conjunctivitis?

CHARACTERISTIC	BACTERIAL	VIRAL	ALLERGIC
Foreign body sensation	–	+/–	–
Itching	+/–	+/–	++
Tearing	+	++	+
Discharge	Mucopurulent	Mucoid	–
Preauricular adenopathy	–	+	–

Adapted from Goroll AH, Mulley HG: Primary Care Medicine: Office Evaluation and Management of the Adult Patient, 4th ed. Philadelphia, Lippincott Williams & Wilkins, 2000, p 1079, with permission.

64. What is a wrist ganglion? How is it treated?

The ganglion is the most common tumor of the hand and wrist and occurs more frequently in women. The most common site is the dorsum of the wrist between the extensor tendons of the thumb and index finger. Most ganglia do not require treatment, but aspiration and/or corticosteroid injection may be useful. If the ganglion recurs after treatment, surgical excision may be necessary.

65. How do you treat a coccygeal fracture?

A coccygeal fracture is treated conservatively with analgesia and seating cushions. Inflatable "donut" cushions should not be used because they can lead to areas of increased pressure and subsequent ulceration. The fracture most often results from a direct blow, usually a fall onto the buttocks.

66. What is Phalen's maneuver? Tinel's sign?

In carpal tunnel syndrome, forced flexion or hyperextension of the wrist (Phalen's maneuver) reproduces the symptoms of pain and paresthesia as well as numbness in the palm and first three or four fingers. In Tinel's sign the symptoms are reproduced when the median nerve is tapped lightly over the wrist.

67. What should be included in the exam of a patient complaining of a "sprained ankle?"

The history should include the details of the injury, particularly whether the ankle was inverted or a tearing sensation was felt. The initial exam should check for tenderness along the anterior talofibular ligament (located slightly anterior to the lateral malleolus), fibulocalcaneal ligament (immediately below the lateral malleolus), and posterior talofibular ligament (posterior to the lateral malleolus). The latter two structures usually are tender only in more severe strains. The degree of swelling should be noted. If ecchymosis is present, the patient has at least a second-degree injury.

Ankle stability is tested by the anterior drawer sign. With the patient relaxed, the lower leg is firmly grabbed anteriorly with one hand. The heel and calcaneus are grasped with the other hand, and the foot is pulled forward. The ankle should be held in 20° flexion. The examiner notes how far the ankle can be moved in comparison with the uninvolved ankle. Foot strength, sensation, and blood flow are noted. An x-ray is needed in almost all strains to check for a fracture.

68. What is a second-degree ankle sprain? How is it treated?

In a second-degree ankle sprain, a portion of a ligament is torn without complete disruption. The exam reveals ecchymosis and slight asymmetry between the involved and uninvolved ankle on the anterior drawer sign. Second-degree sprains are treated with elevation, bulky dressing or elastic bandage, and ice packs for 20 minutes every 3–4 hours for 2–3 days. The patient should avoid weight-bearing and use crutches. He or she can begin plantar- and dorsiflexion exercises after 48 hours. Weight-bearing is allowed after 5–10 days if pain and swelling are decreased.

69. Where are the locations of muscle weakness, sensory loss, and reflex absence associated with an L4 root compression?

ROOT	DISC	MUSCULAR	SENSORY	REFLEX
L4	L3–4	Leg extensors (quadriceps)	Anterolateral thigh, medial lower leg	Patellar
L5	L4–5	Large toe dorsiflexion (extensor hallucis longus), heel walking (tibialis anterior)	Dorsum of foot	None
S1	L5–S1	Toe walking (gastrocnemius)	Lateral foot and fifth toe	Ankle

70. Which toe fractures should be referred to an orthopedist?

Fractures of the proximal phalanx of the first toe. A fracture that involves the distal phalanx and extends into the interphalangeal joint also should be referred.

71. Describe the physical exam findings in a patient with rotator cuff tendinitis.

With rotator cuff tendinitis, there is subacromial tenderness and pain on passive elevation (usually to a certain point). Specific findings include:

- Positive impingement signs
- Rotator cuff and biceps weakness
- Positive supraspinatus test
- Pain with abduction from 70° to 120° (painful arc)
- Possible atrophy of shoulder muscles (compare with opposite side)
- Possible tenderness over corocoacromial ligament

Julian MJ, Mathews M: Shoulder injuries. In Mellion MG: The Team Physician's Handbook. Philadelphia, Hanley & Belfus, 1990, p 326.

72. How do you manage a patient with lumbosacral strain?

Patients with acute back strain should remain at strict bedrest on a firm mattress or hard floor for at least 2 days. If needed, a bed board may be inserted between the mattress and box spring. Controlled physical activity after 2 days of rest promotes recovery, and prolonged bedrest is discouraged. Ice or dry or moist heat (depending on patient preference) for 20 minutes 3–4 times/day may be beneficial. NSAIDs are most useful for pain control. If significant muscle spasm is found on physical exam, muscle relaxants such as cyclobenzaprine are useful.

73. What is Reiter's syndrome?

Reiter's syndrome is common in young, white men and produces arthritis of the lower extremities (knees, ankles, small joints of the feet). Accompanying symptoms include urethritis (dysuria with mucopurulent penile discharge) and mild conjunctivitis. There may also be plantar fasciitis (heel pain), diffuse swelling of the toes (sausage digits), shallow painless oral ulcers or penile lesions, and onychodystrophy (crumbling of the nails). The characteristic skin rash is called keratoderma blennorrhagica and appears as discrete papules. The illness may develop after an acute, diarrheal illness.

74. What conditions may present as chronic fatigue?

Psychologic disorders: depression, anxiety, somatization disorders.

Endocrine-metabolic disorders: hypothyroidism, diabetes mellitus, apathetic hyperthyroidism of the elderly, pituitary insufficiency, hyperparathyroidism or hypercalcemia of any origin, Addison's disease, chronic renal failure, hepatocellular failure.

Drugs: hypnotics, antihypertensives, antidepressants, tranquilizers, drug abuse and withdrawal.

Infections: endocarditis, tuberculosis, infectious mononucleosis, hepatitis, parasitic disease, chronic Epstein-Barr virus infection, cytomegalovirus, HIV infection.

Neoplasm: occult malignancy.

Hematologic disorders: severe anemia.

Cardiopulmonary disorders: chronic congestive heart failure, chronic obstructive pulmonary disease.

Connective tissue disorders: rheumatoid arthritis, chronic fatigue syndrome, fibromyalgia.

Sleep disturbances: sleep apnea, esophageal reflux, allergic rhinitis.

Adapted from Goroll AH, Mulley HG: Primary Care Medicine: Office Evaluation and Management of the Adult Patient, 4th ed. Philadelphia, J.B. Lippincott, 2000, p. 43, with permission.

75. To which clinical syndrome does "hay fever" refer?

Seasonal allergic rhinitis, which incidentally is not caused specifically by hay or associated with fever. This perennial rhinitis has symptoms of sneezing, nasal passage obstruction, rhinorrhea, itching, and lacrimation. It is caused by entrapment of airborne pollens in the nasal folds, with digestion of the outer coat by mucosal enzymes and release of protein allergen. There is usually a family history of similar allergic conditions. Vasomotor rhinitis is a kindred symptom complex without a known allergic basis.

76. What is Tietze's syndrome?

Mild inflammation of the costochondral junction that produces localized warmth, swelling, erythema, and pain. The symptoms are reproduced by palpation of the involved area.

77. What are the diagnostic criteria for major depression?

At least five of the following symptoms must have been present nearly every day for 2 weeks:
1. Depressed mood most of the day
2. Markedly diminished interest or pleasure in nearly all activities
3. Weight loss or gain (> 5% of body weight in 1 month) or decrease or increase in appetite
4. Insomnia or hypersomnia
5. Psychomotor agitation or retardation

6. Fatigue or loss of energy
7. Feelings of worthlessness or inappropriate guilt
8. Decreased ability to think or concentrate
9. Recurrent thoughts of death, suicidal ideation, or suicide attempt
American Psychiatric Association: Diagnostic and Statistical Manual of Mental Disorders, 4th ed. Washington, DC, APA, 1994, p 237.

78. Which medical illnesses can cause depression?

Endocrine disorders: hyperthyroidism, hypothyroidism, Cushing's syndrome, Addison's disease, hypercalcemia, hyperparathyroidism.

Rheumatic disorders: rheumatoid arthritis, systemic lupus erythematosus, fibromyalgia.

Neurologic disorders: temporal lobe epilepsy, chronic hematoma, cerebrovascular accident, multiple sclerosis, frontal lobe tumor, Alzheimer's dementia.

Infections: hepatitis, infectious mononucleosis, Lyme disease, HIV infection, tuberculosis, syphilis.

Nutritional deficiency: vitamin B12.

Toxic syndromes: alcoholism, drug withdrawal.

Neoplasm: pancreatic carcinoma, occult malignancy.

Unknown etiology: chronic fatigue syndrome.

79. Which antidepressants are sedating?

DRUG	SEDATION	DRUG	SEDATION
Amitriptyline	Marked	Nefazodone	Mild
Desipramine	Mild	Bupropion	None
Doxepin	Marked	Fluoxetine	None
Imipramine	Moderate	Paroxetine	Mild/moderate
Nortriptyline	Mild	Sertraline	None
Trazodone	Marked	Venlafaxine	Mild
Citalopram	Mild		

From Depression Guideline Panel: Depression in Primary Care. Vol. 2: Treatment of Major Depression, Clinical Practice Guideline, Number 5. Rockville, MD, Agency for Health Care Policy and Research, 1993 [AHCPR publ no. 93–0551.]

80. Which antidepressant causes priapism?

Trazodone (Desyrel).

81. Which antidepressants cause sexual dysfunction? How can this side effect be managed?

Selective serotonin reuptake inhibitors (SSRIs) and some tricyclic antidepressants may cause sexual dysfunction independently of the decreased libido associated with depression. Men may experience delayed ejaculation and women, anorgasmia or delayed orgasm. Withholding the medication a day or two before anticipated sexual activity may help patients taking SSRIs other than fluoxetine. Changing to an antidepressant in a different class may be needed.

82. What is agoraphobia? How is it treated?

Agoraphobia is the fear of being in public places. The patient with agoraphobia may live a reclusive life. It usually appears in women in their late teens or early 20s and may be associated with panic attacks. During panic attacks, the patient has at least four of the following symptoms, in addition to apprehension or fear: dyspnea, palpitations, chest discomfort, choking sensation, dizziness, feelings of unreality, paresthesia, hot and cold flashes, sweating, faintness, trembling, or fear of dying or going crazy. Severe agoraphobia is best treated in consultation with a therapist skilled in behavioral therapies such as desensitization. If the patient has panic attacks without the avoidant behavior (panic disorder), an SSRI antidepressant (sertraline, paroxetine, or fluoxetine), alprazolam, or imipramine may be useful.

American Psychiatric Association: Diagnostic and Statistical Manual, 4th ed. Washington, DC, APA, 1994.

83. Define hyperkinetic heart syndrome.

A syndrome found in asymptomatic young males who present with increased cardiac output of no discernible cause. They usually seek medical attention because of palpitations, tachycardia, and atypical chest pain. The diagnosis is uncertain and has been variously listed as neurasthenia, anxiety neurosis, DaCosta syndrome, effort syndrome, and soldier's heart.

84. List the common causes of impotence.

Hormonal disorders (testosterone deficiency, hypothyroidism, hyperprolactinemia)
Depression
Medications (spironolactone, clonidine, methyl-dopathiazide diuretics, antidepressants, cimetidine, ketoconazole)
Peripheral vascular disease
Peyronie's disease
Diabetes
Prostate surgery
Drugs (alcohol, heroin, cocaine)

85. What are some of the early signs and symptoms of anorexia nervosa?

Anorexia nervosa should be suspected in a female adolescent with amenorrhea, weight loss, and distorted body image (feeling "fat" in the face of emaciation). It also may occur in women in their 30s.

86. List the risk factors for suicide.

1. Male sex
2. Single or widowed marital status
3. Unemployment
4. Social isolation
5. Urban residence
6. Recent loss of health or surgery
7. History of impulsive behavior or suicide attempts
8. Chronic pain syndrome, major depression, psychosis, alcoholism, substance abuse, organic brain syndrome, or chronic illness
9. Family history of suicide

87. What is an anniversary reaction?

A bereaved patient frequently experiences a depressed mood or somatic symptoms on the anniversary of the death of a close friend or relative. An anniversary reaction may occur after any significant loss, such as job loss, amputation of a limb, or divorce.

88. How do you make the diagnosis of alcoholism?

Alcoholism is persistent, heavy drinking that interferes with the person's health, interpersonal relationships, position in society, or means of livelihood. The consequences of drinking define alcoholism. Internists and family physicians often miss or choose to ignore the diagnosis. Unfortunately, this avoidance behavior interferes with the physician's ability to get at the real cause of common complaints, such as insomnia, nonspecific GI symptoms, and depression. It also makes the doctor an unwitting accomplice in the patient's destructive behavior. A rapid, simple, and reliable screening test for alcoholism is the **CAGE** test. A positive answer to at least two of the questions warrants an in-depth review of drinking habits.

C = Have you ever felt the need to **c**ut down on drinking?
A = Have you ever felt **a**nnoyed by criticism of your drinking?
G = Have you ever felt **g**uilty about your drinking?
E = Have you ever taken a morning **e**ye-opener?

Johnson B, Clark W: Alcoholism: A challenging physician-patient encounter. J Gen Intern Med 4:445–452, 1989.

89. How is the nicotine patch used in smoking cessation? What other medications are available?

The nicotine patch should be used by patients who have already stopped smoking to maintain smoking cessation. The nicotine patch should not be used by patients who continue to smoke. Typically, an initial dose of 14–21 mg/day of nicotine is used, depending on previous cigarette use. After 4–6 weeks of initial therapy, the dose is decreased and eventually discontinued. Nicotine substitution therapy is usually ineffective unless combined with behavioral therapy. Bupropion (Zyban) may be used in addition to nicotine patch or gum to assist patients in smoking cessation.

90. List the differential diagnoses of chronic cough.

Environmental irritants: cigarette smoking, pollutants, dusts, lack of humidity.

Lower respiratory tract problems: lung cancer, asthma, chronic obstructive pulmonary disease, interstitial lung disease, congestive heart failure, pneumonitis, bronchiectasis.

Upper respiratory tract problems: chronic rhinitis, chronic sinusitis, disease of the external auditory canal, pharyngitis, allergic rhinitis.

Extrinsic compression: adenopathy, malignancy, aortic lesions, aneurysm.

GI problems: reflux esophagitis.

Psychogenic factors

Medications: angiotensin-converting enzyme (ACE) inhibitors.

Adapted from: Goroll AH, et al: Primary Care Medicine: Office Evaluation and Management of the Adult Patient, 4th ed. Philadelphia, J.B. Lippincott, 2000, p 273, with permission.

91. What are the health consequences of smoking?

Smoking is associated with increased morbidity and mortality from chronic obstructive pulmonary disease, malignancy (including lung cancer), and cardiovascular disease. Smokers also have an increased incidence of recurrent respiratory infections, peptic ulcer disease, cerebrovascular disease, sudden death, death from abdominal aortic aneurysm, and graft occlusion after lower extremity vascular reconstruction. The overall morbidity and mortality rates among smokers after any type of surgery are also increased.

92. What is the characteristic history of most patients with occupationally related asthma?

The history reveals a cyclical pattern of:
1. Wellness on arrival at work
2. Symptoms that appear toward the end of the shift period
3. Symptoms that increase in severity for a period after departing from the worksite
4. Symptoms that gradually regress over time away from the worksite
5. Holidays and weekends that are free from asthma

93. Describe the findings of acute arterial occlusion.

With acute peripheral arterial occlusion, the patient complains of the sudden onset of severe pain. Some patients may have a more insidious onset over several hours. They also may complain of numbness, paresthesia, and muscle weakness or paralysis. On exam, the involved limb is pale and cold with no pulses distal to the occlusion.

94. How does arterial insufficiency typically present?

Patients are frequently elderly and have a history of smoking. Typical symptoms include pain or muscle tightness in the calf, predictably reproduced after a certain amount of exercise. The pain or tightness is relieved by rest. Other symptoms include numbness and paresthesia. With progressive disease, the patient may develop ulcerations of the feet and pain at rest. Patients also describe pain that awakens them from sleep and is relieved by dangling the feet over the bed.

95. What should be included in a foot care plan for patients with arterial insufficiency?

1. Inspect both feet daily, particularly the soles, for trauma.
2. Wash daily with lukewarm water (test water temperature with the hand or elbow before immersing the feet).

3. Avoid prolonged soaking.
4. Use a moisturizing cream daily.
5. Use an antifungal powder as needed.
6. Place lamb's wool between the toes at areas of pressure.
7. Cut toenails straight across, preferably with podiatric supervision.
8. Wear properly fitting shoes at all times.
9. Treat corns and calluses with physician supervision.
10. Avoid trauma.

96. When would you refer a patient with claudication for surgery?

Patients with rest pain, nonhealing distal ulcers, or early gangrene should be referred for surgical evaluation. Patients with disabling symptoms that interfere with their lifestyle should be referred. Counsel all patients with claudication to stop smoking.

97. What are the physical findings of deep venous thrombosis (DVT)? How sensitive are these findings?

One may find unilateral swelling, warmth, pitting edema, or engorged superficial veins in the involved extremity. The patient may complain of aching pain. The occurrence of DVT, particularly in the postoperative period, may be asymptomatic. The physical findings may be present in as few as 50% of cases. Although frequently cited as a sign of DVT, Homan's sign (calf pain with forced dorsiflexion) is not useful. There may be a palpable cord. Because the physical findings are not that useful in predicting the presence or absence of DVT, venous duplex scanning should be performed immediately whenever DVT is suspected. Delay in diagnosis and treatment of DVT may lead to death from pulmonary emboli. Pulmonary emboli are more likely to result from proximal rather than distal DVT.

98. When can low-molecular-weight heparin (LMWH) be used to treat DVT?

Reliable patients with localized DVT may be treated as outpatients with self or supervised injection of LMWH and warfarin. The LMWH should be continued for 4–7 days until the warfarin has achieved an appropriate INR of 2–3. Patients with pulmonary emboli, documented hypercoagulable state, or extensive DVT may benefit from hospitalization and intravenous heparin.

99. What are the characteristics of an ulcer due to venous stasis disease? How is it treated?

A venous stasis ulcer is usually pigmented with hemosiderin and is located on the medial leg. It should be treated with debridement, either surgical or enzymatic. A moist wound environment and compression should be provided with multilayer wraps of dressings and overlying compression wrap.

100. What are the causes of a nonhealing ulcer? How are they diagnosed?

CAUSE	DIAGNOSIS
Arterial insufficiency	Complete arterial exam, including segmental arterial BP measurements including toe pressures; continuous-wave Doppler waveform analysis and duplex scanning; arteriography
Venous valvular insufficiency, deep and/or superficial	Venous reflux exam with duplex scanning
Malignancy	Skin biopsy
Diabetes	Fasting blood sugar, fructosamine, glycosylated hemoglobin
Collagen vascular disease	Antinuclear antibody, erythrocyte sedimentation rate, rheumatoid factor, skin biopsy
Medications	History of corticosteroid use
Pressure or recurrent trauma	History of decreased mobility, improperly fitting shoes
Infection	Wound culture, including fungal cultures

101. What is an advanced directive?

An advanced directive is a person's written or oral statement indicating his or her preferences for end-of-life therapies. A living will is an example of an advanced directive. Living wills typically state that a person does not want life-sustaining treatments such as artificial ventilation or resuscitation started or continued if he or she has a terminal illness without effective treatments. A durable power of attorney for health care (DPAHC) designates the medical decision-maker for a person who is unable to make his or her own decision because of incapacity or severe medical illness.

BIBLIOGRAPHY

1. ACP Task Force on Adult Immunization: Guide for Adult Immunization, 3rd ed. Philadelphia, American College of Physicians, 1994.
2. Barker LR, Burton JR, Zieve PD: Principles of Ambulatory Medicine, 4th ed. Baltimore, Williams & Wilkins, 1995.
3. Dale DC, Federman DD: Scientific American Medicine. New York, Scientific American, 1994.
4. Goroll AH, Mulley AC (eds): Primary Care Medicine: Office Evaluation and Management of the Adult Patient, 4th ed. Philadelphia, J.B. Lippincott, 2000.
5. Mladenovic J: Primary Care Secrets. Philadelphia, Hanley & Belfus, 1995.

Websites

www.cdc.gov: up-to-date information on immunizations, travel, infectious diseases, and health and safety issues from the Centers for Disease Control and Prevention.

www.acponline.org: website for the American College of Physicians-American Society of Internal Medicine.

www.nof.org: information about osteoporosis.

17. GERIATRIC CARE

Sarah E. Selleck, M.D.

But when old age has silver'd o'er thy head,
When memory fails, and all thy vigour's fled,
Then may'st thou seek the stillness of retreat,
Then hear aloof the human tempest beat,
Then will I greet thee to my woodland cave,
Allay the pangs of age, and smooth thy grave.
James Grainger (1723–1767)
Solitude

GENERAL TOPICS

1. Why is geriatrics an increasingly important area of research and clinical practice?

Although some clinicians may choose practices that inherently limit their contact with older adults, it is a rare case in which a clinician is able to entirely avoid elderly patients, younger patients with aging parents, or younger patients whose lives are touched by issues of aging family members. The American population in 2030 is expected to increase by 32% from the population in 1995, and the elderly are expected to more than double to 69 million by 2030. Despite public and personal efforts to remain healthy as we age, this trend unavoidably will be associated with increasing numbers of elderly people deserving specialized medical care for disability and chronic disease.

2. What are some principles that might assure the delivery of quality medical care for this aging population?

William Reichel and Joseph J. Gallow list the following eleven principles as essential to the delivery of good care:

1. The role of the physician as the integrator of the biopsychosocial-spiritual model
2. Continuity of care
3. Bolstering the family and home
4. Good communication skills
5. Building a sound doctor-patient relationship
6. The need for thorough evaluation and assessment
7. Prevention and health maintenance
8. Intelligent treatment with attention to ethical decision making
9. Interdisciplinary collaboration
10. Respect for the usefulness and value of the aged individual
11. Compassionate care

A twelfth principle might include honest communication about dying and attention to palliative and end-of-life care.

3. What is a Comprehensive Geriatric Assessment (CGA)? When should it be employed?

A CGA involves a medical, psychosocial, and functional evaluation of an older adult, often performed by an interdisciplinary team possibly consisting of (but by no means limited to) physicians, nurses, social workers, pharmacists, and therapists. A CGA is most effective in terms of scarce resources of time and money when it is used for targeted patients for whom screening raises concerns of frailty, memory loss, depression, falls, anorexia or weight loss, or a functional decline.

4. What are some of the "tools" commonly employed in a CGA in addition to thorough history taking and a physical exam?

Although every assessment is tailored to a patient's specific needs, most CGAs include at least some of the following screening tests: (1) the Mini Mental State Exam (MMSE), (2) the Geriatric Depression Scale (GDS), (3) Activities of Daily Living (ADL), (4) Instrumental Activities of Daily Living (IADL), and (5) an assessment of stability and mobility such as the Tinnetti or "Get up and Go." Each tool generally takes less than five minutes to perform and score. Scores may be used to identify a disorder, to gauge the progression of a dementia or resolution of a delirium, or to assess the utility of an intervention (such as therapy for a gait disorder or medication for depression). All of these tests are used as screening tools only and are neither 100% sensitive nor specific. The results should be used in conjunction with more advanced evaluation when warranted.

5. Discuss the three major theories of aging.

1. **Cellular theory:** Proposes that genetic instability (such as accumulated errors in DNA replication) and progressive cellular damage (from both internal and environmental factors such as oxidative stress) cause the aging process.

2. **Autoimmune theory:** Proposes that aging is the result of progressive "self-destruction" through autoimmune mechanisms. This process may be mediated by genetic, environmental, endocrine, or other factors.

3. **Neuroendocrine theory:** Proposes that changes in the neural and endocrine systems cause aging. These changes may lead to the development of diseases that limit lifespan (cancers, atherosclerotic cardiovascular diseases, etc.).

6. Name three genetic diseases characterized by accelerated aging.

1. **Hutchison Gilford syndrome** (childhood progeria) is an autosomal recessive condition characterized by accelerated physical appearance of aging and cardiac disease that generally results in death by age 30.

2. **Werners syndrome** (adult progeria) is autosomal recessive and caused by a gene on chromosome 8 which codes for a helicase involved in DNA unwinding. Affected individuals suffer skin and hair changes typical of aging, cardiac disease, diabetes, osteoporosis, and an increased risk of sarcomas. They generally die by age 50.

3. **Down's syndrome** (trisomy 21) may result from the B amyloid gene and results in accelerated aging and early onset of dementia with a decreased life expectancy.

7. Name some general and organ-specific changes in human morphology and function associated with aging.

Organ-specific Changes Associated with Aging

SYSTEM	MORPHOLOGY	FUNCTION
Skin	↑ wrinkling Atrophy of sweat glands	—
Cardiovascular	Elongation and tortuosity of arteries ↓ maximum cardiac output ↑ intimal thickening of arteries ↑ fibrosis of the media of arteries ↓ rate of cardiac hypertrophy Sclerosis of heart valves	↓ maximum cardiac output ↓ heart rate response to stress ↓ compliance of peripheral blood vessels
Kidney	↑ number of abnormal glomeruli	↓ creatinine clearance ↓ renal blood flow ↓ maximum urine osmolarity

(Table continued on next page.)

Organ-specific Changes Associated with Aging (cont.)

SYSTEM	MORPHOLOGY	FUNCTION
Lung	↓ elasticity ↓ cilia activity	↓ vital capacity ↓ maximal O_2 uptake ↓ cough reflex
GI tract	↓ hydrochloric acid ↓ saliva flow ↓ number of taste buds	—
Bones	Osteoarthritis Loss of bone substance	—
Eyes	Arcus senilis ↓ pupil size Growth of lens	↓ accommodation Hyperopia ↓ visual acuity ↓ color perception ↓ depth perception
Hearing	Degenerative changes of the ossicles ↑ obstruction of eustachian tube Atrophy of external auditory meatus Atrophy of cochlear hair cells Loss of auditory neurons	↓ high-frequency perception ↓ pitch discrimination
Immune	—	↓ T-cell function
Nervous	↓ brain weight ↓ cortical cell count	↑ motor response time Slower psychomotor performance ↓ complex learning ↓ hours of sleep ↓ hours of REM sleep
Endocrine	↓ free testosterone ↑ insulin ↑ norepinephrine ↑ parathyroid hormone (PTH) ↑ vasopressin	—

From Kane RL, et al: Essentials of Clinical Geriatrics, 2nd ed. New York, McGraw-Hill, 1989, p 7, with permission.

8. What percentage of persons over age 65 are fully independent in activities of daily living (ADLs)?

The ADLs consist of bathing, toileting, dressing, walking, and eating. Despite the prevalent image of dependent, frail old people, 90% of people over age 65 do not require any assistance in performing their ADLs.

9. What changes are seen on a glucose tolerance test in older patients? Why?

Fasting glucose changes very little with increasing age, perhaps 1 mg/dl for each decade over age 30. The impairment in glucose tolerance is much larger. At 1 and 2 hours after the challenge meal (usually 100 gm of glucose), the plasma glucose increases 5–6 mg/dl for each decade above 30. The same impairment is seen with a standard meal. If the normal 30-year-old has a 2-hour postprandial glucose of 140 mg/dl, then the normal 70-year-old might reach 160 or more (diabetic by some criteria). Insulin release is delayed, and its maximum serum concentration is higher in the elderly. Insulin resistance at the tissue level is thought to be a predominant mechanism in the impaired glucose tolerance of the elderly, and this may be explained by increased fat mass in the older person.

Cefalu WT, et al: Contribution of visceral fat mass to the insulin resistance of aging. Metab Clin Exp 44:954–959, 1995.

10. What is known about sexuality as people age?

The frequency of sexual intercourse decreases for most men and women as they age but not to zero! For many, interest in the expression of intimacy remains high. The need for this expression should be considered when assessing the quality of life among community dwelling and institutionalized elders. Physiologically, all four main phases of the sexual response—arousal, plateau, orgasm, and resolution change with aging in both men and women. These changes often combine with physical conditions (such as cardiac disease or arthritis) and with medications affecting libido and sexual enjoyment. Clinicians must be comfortable taking a sexual history and asking about symptoms such as dyspareunia, depression secondary to the loss of a partner (be it because of death or illness), and homosexuality. Even the possibility of hypersexuality is not uncommon in dementia.

11. Why are older people more prone to accidental hypothermia and hyperthermia?

More than half of patients hospitalized with accidental hypothermia are over age 65. This is due in part to the impairment in temperature regulation seen in normal elderly people. The "thermostat" within the hypothalamus is less responsive to changes in both skin temperature and core temperature and therefore signals shivering to begin at a lower temperature. Shivering in the elderly does generate normal amounts of heat, but the loss of subcutaneous tissue with aging produces a loss of insulation, leading to more rapid loss or gain of heat. Additionally, the basal metabolic rate of the older person is lower than in the young, so there is less heat to conserve in the first place. Finally, the older person has a reduced drive to micro-acclimatize (put on warm clothing) when the surroundings are cold. All of these small changes (especially in the presence of impaired cognition or sedative medications) add up to a large risk of accidental hypothermia.

Hyperthermia may result from the increased threshold to produce sweat combined with a lower maximum sweating rate due to either a decrease in the number of glands and/or a decrease in the maximum production of sweat by both eccrine and apocrine sweat glands.

12. Why are old people more likely to become dehydrated?

Water and salt homeostasis are well maintained in the healthy elderly in the absence of stress. With stress, however, this may not be the case. The elderly have a decreased thirst drive, and it takes a larger change in plasma osmolarity to stimulate water intake. Even then, the amount of water ingested is less than that in the young and is often less than necessary. The amount of sweat produced is decreased, the threshold temperature for sweating is increased, and the renal losses seem to be more significant. The renal changes with aging are multiple, but most relevant to this question is the impairment of the maximum concentrating ability of the kidneys (1200 mOsm in the young and < 800 mOsm in the elderly). Furthermore, the elderly are slower to respond to a water deficit. It takes 24 more hours of water deprivation for the older person to reach maximum urine concentrations.

13. How do age-associated changes in body composition affect drug pharmacokinetics?

There is a marked increase in fat mass and corresponding decrease in lean body mass during normal aging. These changes are less dramatic for women, who have significantly more fat mass throughout life. This results in more fat and less muscle (water volume) in which the drug can distribute. Therefore, water-soluble drugs may have higher concentrations due to this decreased volume of distribution, and highly fat-soluble drugs may have lower concentrations at effector sites in the elderly. Furthermore, these drugs are stored in body fat, which then acts as a depot once therapy is discontinued, prolonging the time for drugs to "wash out."

14. How are the three components of hepatic metabolism affected by aging?

1. **Hepatic blood flow** decreases with age in both the arterial and portal systems. This decreased delivery makes an important contribution to increasing the half-life of certain agents and narrowing the oral dose/parenteral dose discrepancies for drugs that are heavily metabolized during the "first pass" through the liver.

2. **Phase I reactions**, oxidations and reductions, decrease with aging.
3. **Phase II reactions**, acetylations and glucuronidations, are generally well-preserved.

15. What is the strongest risk factor for adverse drug reactions?

There are many risk factors, but the strongest is polypharmacy, the number of drugs to which the patient is exposed. Other factors are female gender, small body size, hepatic or renal insufficiency, and previous drug reactions. The presence of multiple diseases, altered compliance, and decreased homeostatic mechanisms may also predispose an older person to such reactions.

16. Are there still more factors to consider when prescribing medications for the elderly?

Albumin levels, renal function, and receptor responsiveness can decrease in otherwise healthy older persons and may change precipitously in the face of acute illness. Therefore, when prescribing anything to the elderly, the specific goals of treatment must be defined. Non-drug alternatives should be considered as a first step if possible, and always "start low and go slow," reviewing all medications and supplements on a regular basis.

17. How large is the age-associated decrease in hemoglobin in healthy men and women?

There is no decrease in hemoglobin in healthy elderly men or women. Anemia is not a normal part of aging.

18. Is there any benefit to smoking cessation for smokers above age 65?

Yes! The most immediate benefit is to the heart and circulation, where the benefits may be seen almost immediately. FEV_1 decreases at a much faster rate in smokers than in nonsmokers. Although the absolute level of FEV_1 does not improve with cessation of smoking, the rate of decline does. The rate of decrease that occurs in smokers (about 75–100 ml/yr) quickly returns to the rate of decrease seen in nonsmokers (about 25–30 ml/yr).

The elderly smoker is difficult to change, and successful cessation rates for those over 65 are not good. Nevertheless, the elderly smoker has much to gain by stopping and should be counseled about the behavioral and pharmaceutical aids available and that nicotine patches should never be used by someone who is likely to continue to smoke.

19. Many old people complain about difficulties sleeping. How many hours of sleep does the average 75-year-old require? Does the requirement change with further aging?

There is considerable controversy in this area, but it is now thought that the number of hours of sleep per 24-hour period changes very little throughout adult life. Older persons seem to increase their daytime sleeping (naps) and decrease their nocturnal sleeping, so the number of hours of sleep at night goes down. There is a large change in the amounts of sleep time spent in the various stages of sleep. Older persons spend more time in stage I (light sleep/sleep-awake transition). There is also an age-associated decrease in stage IV sleep.

20. Sjögren's syndrome is more common than previously thought in older patients. What findings are seen in this syndrome?

Sjögren's syndrome has recently been reported in up to 2% of nursing home residents (predominantly women). This chronic inflammatory disease of unknown etiology primarily involves the lacrimal, salivary, and excretory glands. The symptoms are dry mouth, dry eyes, recurrent salivary pain or swelling, dyspareunia, cough, and dysphagia. In most patients, the ESR is elevated, but because the ESR may be elevated in the healthy elderly, this is non-diagnostic. Antibodies to the Lane SSB antigen are diagnostic. In the elderly population the extraglandular involvement is less frequent than in younger patients with Sjögren's syndrome. Patients with Sjögren's may develop connective tissue disease and may have an increased risk of non-Hodgkin's lymphoma.

21. How much money is spent annually on health care costs for each person over 65? How much of this is their own money?

In 1995, the average spent on health care for an individual over 65 was $7,039 compared with $2,471 for the general population. In 1997, the out-of-pocket expenses for a Medicare recipient ranged from more than $1,700 to nearly $2,500.

22. An older person under your care is unable to live independently at home. What available resources might you consider before concluding that the person needs a nursing home?

Programs such as Meals on Wheels and home health aides may bring food (usually one hot meal daily) or a person to help with personal needs. In addition, nurses, physical therapists, and occupational therapists can often come into the home. If supervision can be provided by the family during the evening and nighttime hours, then adult day centers or psychiatric day hospitals may be valuable. Finally, never underestimate the informal network of friends who can check in on this person and be helpful.

Elon R: Outpatient evaluation for nursing home admission. In Yoshikawa T (ed): Ambulatory Geriatric Care. St. Louis, Mosby, 1993, pp 142–148.

23. What is elder abuse and how significant is it?

The *AMA Diagnostic and Treatment Guideline on Elder Abuse* describes acts of omission or comission that result in harm or threatened harm to the health or welfare of an older adult. This includes not only situations of direct physical and financial abuse but also neglect, abandonment, failure to provide adequate housing and medical care, and even self-neglect. The size of the problem is difficult to gauge since cases are likely underreported and often unrecognized. However, some figures in the United States estimate that at least 3% of community-based elders acknowledge being victimized.

Lachs MS, Pillemer K: Abuse and neglect of elderly persons. N Engl J Med 332:437–443, 1995.

24. What are some of the risk factors for abuse?

Many risk factors identified in the history such as poor health, cognitive deficits, substance abuse by the elder or caregivers, shared living arrangements, external stresses, social isolation, and a history of violence in the home should serve as flags for further questioning or investigation by the clinician. Behavioral withdrawal, agitation or depression, poor hygiene, signs of dehydration or trauma, and missed appointments are just a few signs of possible abuse identifiable on examination.

Lachs MS, Pillemer K: Abuse and neglect of elderly persons. N Engl J Med 332:437–443, 1995.

25. What is the Diogenes syndrome?

The Diogenes syndrome is a syndrome of self-neglect, independent of depression and cognitive impairment, that may represent the evolution of a personality disorder. Individuals are unkempt and may exhibit hoarding behavior. As they retreat socially, their behavior may preclude proper nutrition, so malnutrition is common. The one year mortality rate may be 50%.

Cooney C, Hamid W: Review: Diogenes syndrome. Age Aging 24:451–453, 1995.

26. At what age must a person give up driving?

Driving is without a doubt fundamental to many people's independence, socialization, and sense of self-worth. These factors make driving cessation a very difficult issue for older adults, families, and clinicians. There is no specific age at which one must stop driving, and statutes vary from state to state with regard to driver retesting. Furthermore, published studies have failed to settle the controversy of safety. Some studies suggest that even a diagnosis of early dementia may not preclude safe driving with a copilot present. What is certain is that all older drivers need to be asked about their driving habits and accident history and need to be examined for sensory, cognitive, and neuromuscular function. In some areas, occupational therapists and private agencies can assist in referral for assessment and training.

27. What are some of the risk factors of physical restraints? What are some of the "restraint-free" options for a patient at risk for wandering or falls?

In addition to being dehumanizing, the risk of physical injury with even soft restraints to the wrist, vest, or pelvis is being increasingly recognized. Such measures may only serve to increase agitation and can actually lead to lacerations, fractures, decubiti, thrombosis, and even strangulation. For the individual at risk for delirium, having a family member, sitter, or staff sit with the patient should reduce the risk. For people at risk for falls, physical therapy should be attempted to improve strength and balance. Low beds may be used, and mattresses can be placed on the floor. Even bean bag chairs may minimize the potential for serious injury in some people.

CARDIOVASCULAR DISORDERS

28. What maximum heart rate should be expected for a 75-year-old man wishing to start an exercise program? How about a 75-year-old woman?

Data from men in the Baltimore Longitudinal Study who were vigorously screened for the presence of occult coronary artery disease yielded the following regression equation:

$$\text{Max HR} = 208.2 - 0.95 \times (\text{age in yrs})$$

Thus, in a 75-year-old man, the calculation would be:

$$208.2 - 0.95 \times 75 = 137 \text{ bpm}$$

Women usually only attain 85% of this calculated maximal heart rate. Remember that the target heart rate for training is 50–85% of the calculated increase that occurs with exercise. If a patient's resting heart rate is 75, the target range for training should be 106–128.

29. What percentage of elderly men with congestive heart failure (CHF) have a normal ejection fraction (EF)?

At least 40% of men over age 75 with CHF have normal EFs as determined by echocardiogram or nuclear ventriculography. This result is not different from results found in studies that look at all age groups. In older women, it is likely that the percentage is even higher. This is important because the elderly are most likely to have problems with digoxin. Unless there is a clear indication for this agent (such as atrial fibrillation with rapid ventricular response), elderly patients with CHF and normal EFs should not receive digoxin.

Luchi RJ: Clinical Geriatric Cardiology. Edinburgh, Churchill Livingstone, 1989.

30. How great a decrease in systolic blood pressure (BP) upon standing is considered normal in patients over 75?

One working definition of orthostatic hypotension requires a decrease of systolic BP of > 20 mmHg upon arising. However, decreases of > 20 mmHg have been reported in 20–30% of the community-dwelling elderly. The relative contributions of longstanding hypertension, antihypertensive agents, and age have not yet been clarified. Decreases of > 20 mmHg have little prognostic significance in unselected elders.

Raiha I, et al: Prevalence, predisposing factors and prognostic importance of postural hypotension. Arch Intern Med 155:930–935, 1995.

31. How does Osler's maneuver affect the diagnosis of hypertension?

BP measurement involves the compression of the brachial artery by pressure applied via a cuff. Patients with heavily calcified arteries have rigid, hard-to-compress arteries but may not have high intra-arterial pressures. If the cuff is pumped above the systolic BP and the brachial or radial arteries are still palpable, this is a positive Osler's maneuver. Using cuff measurements of BP in patients with a positive Osler's maneuver results in a gross overestimate of the actual intra-arterial pressures.

32. What is a fourth heart sound (S_4) on the cardiac exam of an older person? Is it of importance?

An S_4 sound likely results from the decreased compliance of the ventricular septum and is very common in older persons. It usually is of limited clinical significance. The presence of an S_3 gallop, however, is never normal in an older person and is characteristic of CHF.

33. How many of those over age 70 will have significant (75% or higher) coronary artery stenoses at autopsy? How many of those over age 90?

The prevalence of coronary artery disease (CAD) increases with age, but for men the prevalence appears to level off after age 70. Over 50% of all persons over age 70 have at least one arterial site with 75% stenosis at autopsy. By age 90, the prevalence increases to about 70%; women account for the increase. By noninvasive testing, the prevalence of CAD is somewhat less prevalent but is still above 50% in the elderly.

34. What clues suggest the presence of renovascular hypertension?

Renovascular hypertension is a common secondary cause of hypertension. It should be considered in the elderly patient with:

1. The sudden development of hypertension (especially systolic and diastolic elevations rather than isolated systolic BP elevation).

2. A history of well-controlled hypertension that suddenly becomes difficult to control.

3. Hypertension in a person who develops acute oliguric renal failure when given an ACE inhibitor.

4. Hypertension in a person who is found to have an abdominal or flank bruit.

5. Known atherosclerotic disease in a person who develops renal insufficiency.
Rosmarin PC: Secondary hypertension. Clin Geriatr Med 5:753–768, 1989.

35. What is the difference between aortic stenosis and aortic sclerosis? Can these be differentiated on physical examination?

Aortic sclerosis is the source of many benign murmurs in patients over 70 years of age. It is due to sclerosis (hardening and fibrosis) of the aortic cusps and is not hemodynamically significant. **Aortic stenosis** is not uncommon in the elderly and is usually due to calcification of a bicuspid valve in the younger elderly patient or degenerative calcification in those older than 75. By definition, there is impedance to flow in aortic stenosis.

Although many physical findings have been reported to distinguish the murmur of aortic stenosis from that of aortic sclerosis, unless the stenosis is severe (producing a thrill or very prolonged ventricular impulse), they are unreliable. It is most prudent to evaluate the patient with echocardiography. For example, the narrowed pulse-pressure characteristic of aortic stenosis in younger people is not often seen in the elderly with the same degree of aortic stenosis. This is probably due to the age-related increase in stiffness of the arterial tree. For the same reason, the "pulsus parvis et tardus" at the carotids also may not be seen in elderly patients with significant aortic stenosis.
Luchi RJ: Clinical Geriatric Cardiology. Edinburgh, Churchill Livingstone, 1989.

36. What is the natural history of an abdominal aortic aneurysm (AAA)? What if it is > 6 cm in diameter?

It appears that all AAAs enlarge progressively, but do so at varying rates. The likelihood of a 6-cm AAA lasting 2 years without rupture is < 50%. It is this threshold (6 cm in diameter) at which elective surgery is most appropriate and probably should be considered. Additionally, not only the size but also the rate of growth may provide prognostic information and dictate timing of surgery. Even small aneurysms that grow rapidly over a 6-month interval may require intervention. The key is frequent evaluation for progression.

37. Are the symptoms of abdominal or low back pain important in patients known to have an abdominal aortic aneurysm?

AAAs tend to rupture, not dissect. Elective aneurysmectomy can be performed with acceptable operative mortality, but emergent surgery is very risky (50% mortality). Hypogastric pain or low back pain in a person known to have an AAA is often due to rapid expansion and may suggest that rupture is occurring or is imminent.

38. How frequently is amyloid protein seen on autopsy in atria of hearts from patients older than 90? What is its significance?

Small amounts of amyloid protein, limited to the atria of the heart, may be seen in 80–90% of autopsy specimens from the very elderly. Isolated atrial amyloid has not been shown to have pathologic importance, and it is considered a benign age-associated marker. Pancardiac amyloid is less common and of clinically greater significance, causing exertional dyspnea, arrhythmias, and congestive heart failure.

39. What is the significance of frequent premature ventricular contractions (PVCs) on routine ECG or continuous ambulatory recordings in asymptomatic, healthy men over 65 with no coronary artery disease (CAD)?

None. In older populations rigorously screened for CAD, 80% have PVCs. At least 20% have frequent PVCs (100 in 24 hours), and 10% may have couplets or other complexity. The presence of these arrhythmias has little impact on prognosis.

Fleg JL, Kennedy HL: Long-term prognostic significance of ambulatory electrocardiographic findings in apparently healthy subjects greater than or equal to 60 years of age. Am J Cardiol 70:748–751, 1992.

40. Why is atrial fibrillation tolerated hemodynamically by young people but produces heart failure in older persons?

In the young, atrial systole provides relatively little of the left ventricular (LV) filling during diastole, and essentially 80% occurs during rapid filling early in diastole. In contrast, left atrial systole provides almost 50% of LV filling in old age. This change in atrial filling fraction occurs in normal elders independent of disease but can result in heart failure when uncompensated.

Kitzman DW, et al: Age-related alterations in Doppler left ventricular filling indices in normal subjects are independent of left ventricular mass, heart rate, contractility, and loading conditions. J Am Coll Cardiol 18:1243–1250, 1991.

NEUROLOGIC/PSYCHIATRIC DISORDERS

41. Why is it important to distinguish patients with cardiovascular syncope from those with syncope from other causes?

Patients with a cardiovascular etiology (anatomic, myocardial, or electrical) for syncopal episodes have a much higher 1-year mortality (20%) than those with a defined noncardiovascular etiology or those whose etiology is uncertain after workup. This is thought to be due to the underlying cardiovascular diseases for which the syncope serves as a marker (especially aortic stenosis).

42. What is the triad of normal pressure hydrocephalus (NPH)? Why is it important?

The three components of NPH are (1) gait abnormalities, (2) urinary incontinence, and (3) dementia. This dementia is often termed a reversible dementia and is treated by ventriculoatrial shunting. A good response among shunted patients is correlated to the presence of all three parts of the triad if treatment is initiated promptly. Incontinence and gait abnormalities are unusual early in the course of other dementias, so their presence should raise a suspicion of NPH.

Black PM: Idiopathic normal-pressure hydrocephalus: Results of shunting in 62 patients. Neurosurgery 52:371–377, 1980.

43. Does jaw pain upon chewing have any significance? How about headache with scalp tenderness?

Both of these unusual complaints may be the symptoms of **temporal arteritis**. Both problems are most common in (but not exclusive to) very elderly white women. Temporal arteritis may rapidly produce monocular or binocular blindness and needs to be addressed urgently when suspected. Corticosteroids can prevent blindness. The ESR is usually 50 mm/hr or greater; however, the definitive diagnosis requires a temporal artery biopsy. This procedure can be performed shortly after the institution of steroid therapy with prednisone at 1 mg/kg per day.

44. How common is dementia? What is its cost?

Rare cases of dementia have occurred early in life, although rarely prior to age 60. For those aged 65 and older, the prevalence of all dementias is 6–8%, while for those over 85, the prevalence soars to 30%. It is estimated that the cost in terms of direct care to the individual and lost wages by caregivers reaches $100 billion annually. The emotional and personal costs cannot be estimated.

45. What percentage of dementia is caused by Alzheimer's disease (AD)?

At least 50–60% of patients with dementia have AD or have a component of AD coexisting with another dementing illness, commonly vascular dementia.

46. What are the two ways to make a definitive diagnosis of Alzheimer's disease?

Autopsy or brain biopsy. The diagnosis of definite AD requires a clinical history consistent with AD and histopathologic confirmation. However, a reasonable approach to exclude other causes of dementia using the history and clinical findings should allow a practitioner to be at least 90% correct when making the diagnosis of AD.

47. What are the currently available treatment options for Alzheimer's disease (AD)?

One of the hallmarks of AD is a decrease in the brain levels of the neurotransmitter acetylcholine. By blocking the enzyme that metabolizes acetylcholine, traditional pharmaceutical agents make more acetylcholine available. The goal is to (at best) improve functional, behavioral, and cognitive performance. The earliest medication approved by the FDA, tacrine, was problematic because of twice daily dosing and the need to routinely monitor for hepatotoxicity. The next drug approved by the FDA, donepezil, is generally better tolerated, is given daily, and needs no special monitoring. The newly approved rivastigmine works in a similar fashion. Numerous trials are underway to test other pharmacologic agents. Vitamin E and seligiline are used by many as neuroprotective agents. Behavioral options, caregiver education, and support remain essential pieces of any therapeutic regimen for the behavioral and cognitive symptoms of AD.

48. Are any neurologic signs present in patients with dementia?

Upon initial evaluation focal neurologic findings may provide a clue that the etiology of the dementia may be vascular and not Alzheimer's disease. Furthermore, cranial nerve findings should suggest the presence of chronic meningitis and prompt further investigation, including lumbar puncture.

There are neurologic findings seen later in progressive dementia, perhaps because of the loss of inhibitory influences. These include the snout reflex, suck reflex, and glabellar blink; however, the sensitivity and specificity of these "soft" neurologic signs in identifying patients with dementia are poor relative to those of a mental status exam.

49. How can you differentiate depression from dementia?

This differential may be very difficult. Apparent dementia by history, examination, or screening tools that actually results from depression is called pseudodementia. On the mental status examination, depressed patients frequently answer questions with "I don't know," whereas demented patients try to answer even though their answer may be wrong. Depressed patients often have complaints about memory impairments that are out of proportion to the severity of findings on exam. The use of a depression questionnaire, such as the Hamilton Depression Scale, is helpful, as is neuropsychological testing. If the uncertainty in the diagnosis persists, then a diagnostic/therapeutic trial of an antidepressant followed by continued surveillance and retesting may be justifiable prior to making any diagnosis of dementia. Remember that in up to one-third of cases, a demented person will have coexistent depression. These people may improve functionally when their depression is treated, even though the underlying dementia is not affected by the treatment.

Reynolds CF, et al: Bedside differentiation of depressive pseudodementia from dementia. Am J Psychiary 145:1099–1103, 1988.

50. Why is depression common after a stroke?

Depression is said to affect up to 60% of stroke victims. The reason is unclear but appears to relate to the physical limitations produced by the stroke as well as the location of the stroke. Patients with left frontal infarctions have the highest risk of depression. This area of the brain may play a key role in maintenance of mood. Commonly used antidepressants are effective and may improve not only affect but also performance in rehabilitation.

51. What neurologic findings are abnormal in a young patient and normal in an older one?

The passage of time has many effects on the normal nervous system. On cranial nerve exam, a marked limitation of upward gaze is seen in most elderly persons as well as relatively constricted pupils. There is a slowing of rapid alternations of movement, which is termed dysdiadochokinesia. In the distal extremity, there may be sensory impairments, and ankle jerks may frequently be absent. Abdominal reflexes may also be absent.

52. How can handwriting help in the differential diagnosis of tremor? What can a glass of wine do in this regard?

Essential tremor worsens with intention and usually improves with ethanol. Parkinsonism patients characteristically have micrographia, a condition in which the handwriting is very small. The administration of ethanol does not significantly alter the tremor of Parkinson's disease.

53. Who gets tardive dyskinesia? How is it treated?

Tardive dyskinesia usually follows prolonged use of neuroleptic agents. Although older patients seem to be more likely to develop tardive dyskinesia, it is not clear that duration of use, the specific agent, or the total dose has any direct relation to the appearance of the involuntary movements. There is little evidence that tardive dyskinesia can be treated with drugs, although in a certain percentage of patients the movements may disappear, even with the continuation of the neuroleptic agent.

54. Does an asymptomatic carotid bruit imply impending stroke?

No. The risk of a cerebrovascular accident (CVA) without warning transient ischemic attacks (TIAs) is only about 1% in the year following the discovery of a bruit. However, the bruit is a marker of widespread atherosclerosis, and the risk of CVA is elevated. The scenario becomes quite different once the bruit becomes symptomatic with ipsilateral TIAs. At this point, therapy is indicated.

DISORDERS OF THE SENSES

55. Other than cataracts, which changes in the eye occur with normal aging?

There are a multitude of changes in the aging eye other than those leading to cataract formation. The periorbital tissues atrophy. The upper lid may droop, and the lower lid can turn inward or outward. The pupil becomes smaller, and adaptation of the eye to changes in lighting is much slower. The lens loses elasticity, leading to an inability to focus on near items (presbyopia), and the ability to distinguish objects from background is impaired, requiring more contrast between objects.

56. Are changes in hearing part of normal aging?

The most common loss of auditory function that occurs with aging is in the high-frequency range, and the minimum sound appreciated by the older ear is increased (louder). This is sensorineural hearing loss, which is usually noted in middle age and becomes problematic in later life.

A parallel finding is the decrease in speech discrimination. When the patient is given words to both ears simultaneously and then asked about information given to one ear, older patients seem to have a large age-related loss in discriminant function. Because this test is performed with sounds above the auditory threshold, it is thought to be due to a central processing deficit independent of the sensorineural problem.

57. How common are macular degeneration and cataracts in those above age 75?

The prevalence of these two eye problems is very high. The Framingham study reported macular degeneration in about 6% of patients aged 65–74 and in 18% of those aged 75 or older. Cataracts were noted in 13% of those aged 65–74 and in approximately 40% of patients aged 75 and older.

58. What are the ophthalmoscopic findings of senile macular degeneration?

There are two types of senile macular degeneration: nonexudative (dry) and exudative (wet). The **nonexudative** type is most common and is characterized by drusen (hyaline excrescences in Bruch's membrane). The underlying changes in the pigmented epithelia can produce geographic atrophy. This disorder produces a slowly progressive central visual loss, although only 10% of patients progress to legal blindness. There is no adequate therapy.

The **exudative** form of senile macular degeneration is accompanied by neovascularization that weeps and bleeds. Laser photocoagulation can be used to slow the progression of visual loss in the exudative type.

59. Are there any types of hearing loss that do not respond to hearing aids?

Though some elderly do not believe that sensorineural hearing loss responds to amplification, it appears that both of the common types of age-associated hearing loss, conductive and sensorineural, respond to amplification provided by hearing aids. The third type of communication defect, a central processing problem in which the words are heard but not properly understood, may be made worse by a hearing aid that also amplifies the background sound. These patients need to have extraneous sound reduced for optimal function.

SKIN DISORDERS

60. Are there any risk factors, aside from immobility, that are associated with developing pressure sores (decubitus ulcer)?

The relative contribution of various factors in producing pressure sores is not clear. Some risk factors, in addition to the pressure itself, include hypoalbuminemia, fecal incontinence, immobility, weight loss, hypotension, and fractures. A depressed sensorium increases the risk of pressure sores, as does any other process that impairs the patient's ability to sense and respond to discomfort.

61. Why do pressure sores heal so much more slowly than similarly sized skin wounds of other types?

Three factors lead to ischemia of the surrounding tissue and slow healing:

1. **Shear forces:** Many pressure sores involve shearing, which occurs because of body position. In addition to producing ischemia by compressing vessels, the shear forces may disrupt the blood supply to the area.

2. **Thrombosis:** At times of low blood flow (or no blood flow), a clot may form in the vascular supply to the area. There is decreased fibrinolytic activity in the area of the ulcer which causes the clot to persist.

3. **Transmission of pressure:** There is a tendency to assume that the skin area that is involved projects cylindrically into the deeper tissues. It appears that the projection is more like a

cone, with a narrow skin site of pressure and a much wider, deeper area of ischemia below the surface.

62. How are pressure sores graded?

All of the popular classification systems to grade pressure sores use maximum depth of penetration to measure the severity of the lesion.

Shea's Decubitus Grading System

Grade 1—Decubiti penetrate into the dermis

Grade 2—Decubiti extend into the subcutaneous fat

Grade 3—Decubiti extend into the fascia

Grade 4—Decubiti extend deeper than fascia and are without apparent boundaries

63. Why is the "head-elevated" bed position so likely to produce pressure sores?

The head-elevated position produces shearing forces at the sacrum. The body is pulled by gravity, while friction holds the skin to the sheet, thus producing the shearing force. The patient should not remain in this position for long periods.

64. What are seborrheic keratoses? What treatments are effective for them?

Seborrheic keratoses are benign epidermal lesions frequently seen in the elderly. These hyperpigmented, hyperkeratotic lesions have distinct borders and an irregular, scaly surface. They are light or dark brown, wart-like papules of varying size, generally described as having a "stuck-on" appearance. They are usually multiple and are most commonly found on the trunk. As they enlarge, they darken and develop a greasy scale.

Although they have no malignant potential, because of their dark color they can sometimes be confused with malignant melanoma. These lesions can be treated with curettage, electrodesiccation, liquid nitrogen, and topical glycolic acid.

Kleinsmith DM, Perricone NV: Common skin problems in the elderly. Clin Geriatr Med 5:189–211, 1989.

INFECTIONS AND IMMUNITY

65. How frequently do elderly persons with active tuberculosis (TB) have a nonreactive skin test?

In as many as 30% of patients with active TB, the initial skin test is negative. Since the frequency of a negative PPD increases with increasing age and a hypersensitivity may exist with a subsequent test, it is generally advisable to give all initial non-responders a second PPD 7–10 days after the first one to help determine if they are truly "negative." In someone who has had a previous mycobacterial infection (tubercular or not), this second test will be more likely to result in a positive test, thus increasing the likelihood of identifying active disease by further investigation.

66. Which age-related changes make the older person more likely to develop pneumonia?

Multiple changes that occur with aging make the older person more likely to develop pneumonia. The most common way for an older person to introduce pathogens into the lungs is aspiration. Older people appear to aspirate more frequently while swallowing and have a poorer cough reflex, thus incompletely clearing the aspirate. Drugs that sedate the patient and allow aspiration to occur are also more frequently administered to the elderly. The organisms that inhabit the oropharynx are usually nonpathogenic in the younger person (with some exceptions), but an increased number of gram-negative organisms appears in the flora in up to 20% of community-dwelling elderly individuals, as well as almost all nursing home residents. Changes in the immune system, especially T-cell changes and antibody affinity changes, may also increase the risk of pneumonia. Finally, the increased frequency of influenza leads to an increased frequency of pneumonia.

67. What are some treatment options for uncomplicated herpes zoster and postherpetic neuralgia?

Antiviral therapy with acyclovir or penciclovir may reduce acute pain and possibly decrease the risk of postherpetic neuralgia (PHN); corticosteroids have not been shown to be effective adjunctive therapy. PHN is more likely to occur in people with advanced age and in those who had extremely painful or sizable rashes. Some commonly used measures to treat PHN include low dose opiates, tricyclic antidepressants (often at low doses), neurontin, and capsaicin. A patch that delivers topical lidocaine has been approved by the FDA for PHN.

68. Are vaccinations useful in preventing illness in the elderly? If so, in which illnesses and in which elderly patients?

Influenza, pneumococcal, and tetanus-diphtheria (Td) vaccinations are all recommended for older patients. The flu vaccine is about 70% effective in elderly patients and should be given annually in the fall to all people over 65, especially those who live in nursing homes.

The pneumococcal vaccine includes antigen from 23 serotypes that cause more than 90% of pneumococcal pneumonia. Antibody levels tend to decline over time, so attention to the latest consensus regarding reimmunization is important.

Tetanus remains a fairly uncommon disease, but the percentage of patients over age 50 has been increasing, and the mortality and morbidity are high. These people often have been immunized in the remote past but not recently. The same is true for diphtheria. Booster immunizations with adult Td vaccine should be done every 10 years throughout adult life.

69. How is the antibody response to an antigen different in an older person compared with a younger one?

The total amount of antibody produced in response to a challenge (perhaps an immunization) is essentially unchanged with increasing age. The quality of the antibody produced is poorer because the affinity of the antibody for its intended antigen may be less than that produced by a young person. The specificity of the antibody is a function of the T cell that is directing the B-cell response. Many of the functions of the T cell, especially those dependent on interleukin-2, are significantly impaired with increasing age.

UROLOGIC DISORDERS

70. What are the indications for and risks of having a chronic indwelling Foley catheter?

There are only a few indications for a chronic indwelling Foley catheter.

- Urinary retention should be treated with chronic catheterization if it produces renal dysfunction, infections, or overflow incontinence, and if it is not treatable with surgery, medications, and intermittent catheterization.
- Decubitus ulcers, or skin irritations, whose healing is complicated by incontinence, may justify a catheter while the wound is healing.
- Severe disability in a patient with a terminal illness or a condition such as severe rheumatoid arthritis in whom any movement is very painful may benefit from a catheter. Rarely, a catheter may be acceptable when used for patient or caregiver convenience.

Risks of long term catheter use include urinary tract infections, pyelonephritis, stones, periurethral abscesses, urosepsis, and colonization with virulent or resistant bacteria and yeast.

71. What can be done to decrease the rate of colonization of indwelling urinary catheters?

Almost all indwelling Foley catheters become colonized with bacteria. Irrigation or antibiotic therapy does not eradicate colonization but does produce changes in the flora. For suspected urinary tract infection, it is important to remove the old catheter and sample urine for cultures from the new catheter. Condom catheters, when twisted, kinked, or clogged have a frequency of infection that is as high as that of the indwelling catheter. Perhaps the most important point is to evaluate the absolute indication for the catheter and be certain that it is not just for nursing convenience.

72. How frequently is urinary incontinence seen in community-dwelling elderly? In those in nursing homes?

The frequency of insignificant loss of urine is quite common in women of all ages. However, the frequency of urine loss of sufficient magnitude to produce social compromise or health problems is found in 10–30% of community-dwelling elderly, with a lower frequency in men. Surveys of elderly nursing home residents have reported urinary incontinence in 50% of inhabitants. The very high frequency in institutionalized populations is primarily due to their underlying diseases, but it is sometimes the product of physical restraints and medications.

73. What are the four different types of urinary incontinence? What are their distinguishing features and causes?

Urinary incontinence is not a part of normal aging, nor is it caused by aging. However, many of the physiologic consequences of aging can contribute to urinary incontinence.

1. **Stress incontinence:** The involuntary loss of small volumes of urine related to events that cause increased intraabdominal pressure (coughing, laughing, and exercise). It is more common in females (present with laughing in 50% of young females) and increases with aging. Its causes include weakness or laxity of pelvic floor muscles, bladder outlet, or urethral sphincter.

2. **Urge incontinence:** The involuntary loss of larger volumes of urine due to the inability to delay voiding when the sensation of bladder fullness (urge) is perceived. Causes include detrusor motor and/or sensory instability, either alone or in combination with one of the following:
   • Local GU conditions such as cystitis, urethritis, tumors, stones, diverticula, and outflow obstruction.
   • CNS disorders such as stroke, dementia, parkinsonism, and suprasacral spinal cord injury or disease.

3. **Overflow incontinence:** Involuntary loss of small amounts of urine resulting from mechanical forces on an overdistended bladder or from other effects of urinary retention on bladder and sphincter function. Causes are anatomic obstruction by the prostate, stricture, or cystocele; acontractile bladder associated with diabetes mellitus or spinal cord injury; and neurogenic (detrusor-sphincter dyssynergy) associated with multiple sclerosis and other suprasacral spinal cord injury.

4. **Functional incontinence:** Leakage of urine associated with inability to toilet because of impairment of cognitive and/or physical functioning, psychologic unwillingness, or environmental barriers. It is seen in severe dementia and other neurologic disorders as well as psychologic factors such as depression, regression, anger, and hostility.

74. How are the four types of urinary incontinence treated?

1. **Stress incontinence:** Pelvic floor (Kegel) exercises, α-adrenergic agonists, estrogen, biofeedback, behavioral training, periurethral injections, surgical bladder neck suspension.

2. **Urge incontinence:** Bladder relaxants, estrogen (if vaginal atrophy is present), training procedures (e.g., biofeedback, behavioral therapy), surgical removal of obstructing or other irritating pathologic lesions.

3. **Overflow incontinence:** Surgical removal of obstruction, intermittent catheterization (if practical), bladder retraining, indwelling catheterization.

4. **Functional incontinence:** Behavioral therapies (e.g., habit training, scheduled toileting), environmental manipulations, incontinence undergarments and pads, external collection devices, bladder relaxants (selected patients), indwelling catheters (selected patients).

75. What are the important causes of acute and reversible urinary incontinence?

Because of the severe physical, psychologic, social, and economic costs of urinary incontinence, it is important to identify reversible cases and render the needed treatment. The causes of acute and reversible forms of urinary incontinence can be remembered by the "DRIP" mnemonic:

D = **D**elirium
R = **R**estricted mobility, retention
I = **I**nfection, **i**nflammation, **i**mpaction (fecal)
P = **P**olyuria, **p**harmaceuticals

Infection and inflammation refer to acute symptomatic urinary tract infection (UTI), atrophic vaginitis, or urethritis. Polyuria may be due to hyperglycemia or volume-expanded states causing excessive nocturia (e.g., CHF, venous insufficiency).

76. What are the complications and adverse effects of urinary incontinence?

Physical health	**Social**
Skin breakdown	Stress on family, friends, and caregivers
Recurrent UTIs	Predisposition to institutionalization
Falls (esp. at nighttime)	**Economic**
Psychologic	Supplies (padding, catheters, etc.) and laundry
Isolation and dependency	Labor (nurses, housekeepers)
Depression	Management of complications

77. Is single-dose therapy for cystitis as successful in older women as it is in younger women? How long should treatment be continued?

No. Even with the lower bacterial load seen in asymptomatic bacteriuria, single-dose therapy was effective in less than two-thirds of elderly women. It is anticipated that symptomatic UTI would be even less responsive to this treatment regimen. Most experts are currently recommending 7–10 days of antibiotic therapy for uncomplicated UTIs.

GASTRIC DISORDERS

78. What are the causes of fecal incontinence?

1. Fecal impaction with overflow diarrhea
2. Laxative overuse or abuse
3. Neurologic disorders (dementia, stroke, spinal cord injury)
4. Colorectal disorders (diarrheal illnesses, rectal sphincter damage, neoplastic or inflammatory processes)

79. Does an enterostomal feeding tube eliminate aspiration in a chronically ill or demented individual?

The risk of aspiration and attendant complications of pneumonia are not eliminated by a feeding tube. Placement of such a tube should only be done after careful consideration of all issues surrounding the patient's functional status, potential for improvement, and previously expressed wishes regarding health care. Such an intervention may only preserve life at the cost of increasing the likelihood of contractures, decubiti, and infection.

80. What are the common causes of lower GI bleeding in an elderly person?

Bleeding from diverticula is the most common cause, followed by bleeding from angiodysplasia. These two conditions make up 75% of lower GI bleeding. Other causes of blood loss in the elderly are colonic polyps, colon carcinoma, ischemic colitis, and inflammatory bowel disease. Older people also can have hemorrhoids as a cause of bleeding. One study has shown that 30% of the elderly known to have diverticula were bleeding because of another reason; therefore, it is unwise to empirically attribute lower GI blood loss to diverticula alone.

CANCER

81. What differences are seen between breast cancers in younger women and older women?

Elderly women are much more likely to have estrogen-receptor-positive breast cancer, implying a malignancy that will be more responsive to hormonal manipulation and possibly slower-growing.

82. What percentage of prostate cancers is confined to the prostate or local pelvis at the time of diagnosis?

Only about 30% of prostate cancers are local at the time of diagnosis. This means that two-thirds are widespread and incurable at diagnosis. Fortunately, the malignancy is usually responsive to hormonal manipulation, which controls the disease and alleviates symptoms.

83. Are patients with shingles very likely to have an underlying malignancy?

No. Although there probably is a small increase in the chance of cancer in patients with herpes zoster recurrence, it is not large enough to merit evaluation for malignancy in every patient who presents with shingles.

Raggazino MW, et al: Risk of cancer after herpes zoster: A population-based study. N Engl J Med 307:393–397, 1982.

84. When an older person is found to a have a monoclonal gammopathy of undetermined significance (MGUS), what are the chances of developing a related malignancy in the next 10 years?

A monoclonal gammopathy is a monoclonal protein noted on serum protein electrophoresis of > 3 g/dl without associated signs or symptoms of hematologic abnormalities. At 10 years of follow-up, 40% of elderly patients with MGUS are stable, 40% have died from other causes, and 10–20% have myeloma, macroglobulinemia, amyloidosis, or non-Hodgkin's lymphoma.

Kyle RA: Monoclonal gammopathy of undetermined significance. Blood Rev 8:135–141, 1994.

85. What treatments are used for early chronic lymphocytic leukemia (CLL)?

Observation is generally chosen for patients in the early stages with alkylating agents and combination chemotherapy being offered to selected other patients.

MUSCULOSKELETAL DISORDERS

86. How is Paget's disease of the bone most often diagnosed in the elderly?

It is frequently recognized via multichannel screening of blood. The elevation of alkaline phosphatase in the absence of liver disease is often found to be a marker of the increased bone turnover that is part of Paget's disease. Confirmation is made radiographically. Paget's disease is present in 10% of those over age 80 and is more common in the northern U.S. than in the southern U.S.

87. What are the clinical manifestations of Paget's disease of bone?

Although most patients are symptomatic at diagnosis, in 90% of cases it has a variety of manifestations:

Bone manifestations (most common):
1. Bone pain in the pelvis, hips, and back
2. Bone deformities due to the remodeling process. Most commonly seen as bowing of the femur and tibia, skull enlargement, and loss of height due to scoliosis and vertebral collapse
3. Pathologic fractures due to bone remodeling
4. Increased warmth over affected areas of bone due to an increase in vascularity

Cardiovascular manifestations (rare):
1. High cardiac output state with or without CHF
2. Hypertension
3. Exacerbation of ischemic heart disease
4. Cardiomegaly
5. Arterial and valvular calcification

Neurologic manifestations (rare):
1. Compression of cranial nerves (most often CN VIII) or blood vessels (causing stroke)
2. Middle ear deafness due to ossification of the stapedius tendon

3. Hydrocephalus due to compression of the foramina of Luschka or Magendie

4. Spinal compression syndromes

Other manifestations:

1. Hypercalcemia and hypercalciuria (with or without renal calculi)

2. Osteogenic sarcoma

88. What are the indications for specific treatment of Paget's disease of bone?

Criteria for Specific Treatment of Paget's Disease

1. Disabling pain not relieved by analgesics or anti-inflammatory medications

2. Progression of skeletal aspects of the disease, as indicated by increasing deformity, head or appendicular bone enlargement, frequent fracture, nonunion of fractures, vertebral compression, or acetabular protrusion

3. Neurologic complications

4. Increasing deafness

5. High-output congestive heart failure

6. Immobilization hypercalcemia, before and after major orthopedic surgery

Lifschitz ML, Harmon CE: Musculoskeletal problems in the elderly. In Schrier RW (ed): Clinical Internal Medicine in the Aged. Philadelphia, W.B. Saunders, 1982, p 193.

89. What treatment modalities are available for Paget's disease of bone?

1. **NSAIDs:** for relief of symptoms

2. **Calcitonin:** Inhibits osteoclast production and activity, which may decrease and improve manifestations of the disease, reverse some of the pathologic changes, and lead to partial normalization of the biochemical markers of the disease. The initial effects are seen in approximately 2 weeks, and therapy reaches maximal effectiveness in 6–12 months. Side effects (which are usually not significant) include nausea, vomiting, facial flushing, and polyuria. Development of resistance due to antibodies against salmon calcitonin may require the use of human calcitonin.

3. **Bisphosphonates:** Cause a slowdown in bone growth and turnover by binding to hydroxyapatite crystals in the bone, blocking their growth and dissolution, and inhibiting osteoclast activity. Bisphosphonates have the advantage of oral administration and are usually given in 6-month courses. Side effects are usually not significant.

4. **Mithramycin:** Although not approved for use in Paget's disease, this cytotoxic antibiotic has been used to suppress the manifestations of the disease in some patients. Remissions of many years' duration have been reported after a single course of therapy. Side effects can be severe and include hepatic, renal, and bone marrow toxicities.

5. **Surgery:** Can be used to increase mobility and joint motion, as well as to relieve nerve compression syndromes. Should be performed after several months of medical therapy to decrease postoperative bleeding and hypercalcemia.

90. What types of falls are most commonly seen in patients with parkinsonism?

Falls are very common in patients with parkinsonism, with the symptoms of bradykinesia, rigidity, gait disturbance, and postural instability contributing to this increased frequency of falls. The typical festinating gait, in which patients appear to be accelerating as if to catch up with their center of gravity, may lead to forward falls. At the time of arising, postural instability may lead to falling backwards. Short steps that do not clear the ground adequately increase the likelihood of tripping over objects.

Johnell O, et al: Fracture risk in patients with parkinsonism: A population-based study of Olmstead County, Minnesota. Age Aging 21:32–38, 1992.

91. List the risk factors for hip fracture.

Since hip fracture is the most severe complication of osteopenia, many of the risk factors are the same for the two conditions.

Risk Factors for Hip Fracture

Female sex	Increasing age
White race	Psychotropic drugs
Thin body habitus	Ethanol use
Hemiplegia	Previous hip fracture
Cigarette smoking	Surgical bilateral oophorectomy
Chronic corticosteroid use	(before natural menopause)
Prior history of falls	

92. How frequently do patients with hip fractures have prior falls?

Hip fractures are very common and one of the most dread sequelae of falling. About 15% of patients with hip fracture report previous falls. Therefore, early intervention in patients who fall may prevent recurrent falls and significantly decrease the number of hip fractures leading to death, disability, or institutionalization.

93. What are premonitory falls? Which diseases are associated with them?

About 5% of falls are premonitory, signaling the presence of a serious systemic illness. These underlying illnesses typically are pneumonia, urinary tract infections, or CHF. However, a fall also can be the presenting complaint in an acute myocardial infarction in elderly patients.

94. Besides menopause, what are the other known risk factors for osteoporosis?

There are two types of osteoporosis, postmenopausal and age-related. Risk factors for osteoporosis include:

Female sex	Hemiplegia
White or Oriental race	Psychotropic drugs
Thin body habitus	Cigarette smoking
Increasing age	Ethanol use
Low calcium intake	Chronic corticosteroid use
Surgical bilateral oophorectomy	Multiple pregnancies
(before natural menopause)	Sedentary lifestyle

95. How effective are supplemental estrogens in preventing hip fractures in postmenopausal women?

Very effective, producing a 50% decrease in the incidence of hip fractures and 80% decrease in the incidence of vertebral fractures. Estrogen replacement retards bone loss and thereby prevents the development of osteoporosis. The most bone mass is conserved if the estrogen replacement is instituted shortly after menopause. However, the evidence that estrogen is not as useful when instituted 5 years after menopause is hypothetical and appears not to be supported by some studies.

96. When might you order a bone mineral density scan?

Bone densitometry, most commonly of the spine and hip, should be considered in anyone with risk factors for osteoporosis, fractures, hyperthyroidism, hyperparathyroidism, Cushing's disease, or hypogonadal men. The results can assess risk and guide therapeutic recommendations.

97. What are the Z and T scores on a bone mineral density (BMD)?

An individual's BMD is calculated in gm/cm^2 and then compared with standard values for the patient's age and standard values for a young adult. The number of standard deviations above or below the standard for the person's age is the Z value and the number of SD above or below the values for the young adult (supposedly replete bone) is called the T value. The World Health Association defines a T of less than 2.5 as **osteoporosis** and a T of 1–2.5 as **osteopenia**. Fracture risk is considered to double for each SD below the mean.

98. What are some considerations for choosing to treat osteoporosis?

The goal of treatment is to stop any further bone loss and to actually increase the BMD to a level that reduces fracture risk. Individual treatment is chosen based on an individual's functional status, other medical conditions, and any possible adverse side effects of therapy. In addition to weight-bearing exercise, calcium, and vitamin D, the most commonly used agents now include hormonal replacement therapy, bisphosphonates, calcitonin, and raloxifene.

99. What are contractures? How do they develop?

Contractures are the result of fibrosis of periarticular structures and shortening of muscles and tendons. The process can occur within just seven days if regular, full motion of the joint is not maintained for whatever reason. Contractures are very difficult to treat once they are present, so preventative measures, such as bedside passive range of motion exercises, should be used in all immobilized patients. If they occur and are addressed early, contractures can be reversed.

100. What is the importance of a positive antinuclear antibody test (ANA) in an older patient?

There is a 15% frequency of a positive ANA in normal older people. These are usually of low titer (1:16 or less) and, in isolation, are of little clinical significance.

BIBLIOGRAPHY

1. Cobbs EL, Duthie EH, Murphy JB: Geriatrics Review Syllabus: A Core Curriculum in Geriatric Medicine. New York, American Geriatrics Society, 1999.
2. Forciea MA, Lavizzo-Mourey RJ: Geriatric Secrets. Philadelphia, Hanley & Belfus, 2000.
3. Gallo JJ, et al (eds): Reichel's Care of the Elderly, 5th ed. Philadelphia, Lippincott-Williams & Wilkins, 1999.
4. Hazzard WR, et al (eds): Principles of Geriatric Medicine and Gerontology, 3rd ed. New York, McGraw-Hill, 1995.
5. Kane RL, et al: Essentials of Clinical Geriatrics, 4th ed. New York, McGraw-Hill, 1999.

INDEX